CAMBRIDGE LIBRARY COLLECTION

Books of enduring scholarly value

History of Medicine

It is sobering to realise that as recently as the year in which *On the Origin of Species* was published, learned opinion was that diseases such as typhus and cholera were spread by a 'miasma', and suggestions that doctors should wash their hands before examining patients were greeted with mockery by the profession. The Cambridge Library Collection reissues milestone publications in the history of Western medicine as well as studies of other medical traditions. Its coverage ranges from Galen on anatomical procedures to Florence Nightingale's common-sense advice to nurses, and includes early research into genetics and mental health, colonial reports on tropical diseases, documents on public health and military medicine, and publications on spa culture and medicinal plants.

The Works of John Hunter, F.R.S.

The surgeon and anatomist John Hunter (1728–93) left a famous legacy in the Hunterian Museum of medical specimens now in the Royal College of Surgeons, and in this collection of his writings, edited by James Palmer, with a biography by Drewry Ottley, published between 1835 and 1837. The first four volumes are of text, and the larger Volume 5 contains plates. Hunter had begun his career as a demonstrator in the anatomy classes of his brother William, before qualifying as a surgeon. He regarded surgery as evidence of failure – the mutilation of a patient who could not be cured by other means – and his studies of anatomy and natural history were driven by his belief that it was necessary to understand the normal physiological processes before attempting to cure the abnormal ones. Volume 3 discusses blood and the vascular system, wounds (especially those suffered in war) and infection

Cambridge University Press has long been a pioneer in the reissuing of out-of-print titles from its own backlist, producing digital reprints of books that are still sought after by scholars and students but could not be reprinted economically using traditional technology. The Cambridge Library Collection extends this activity to a wider range of books which are still of importance to researchers and professionals, either for the source material they contain, or as landmarks in the history of their academic discipline.

Drawing from the world-renowned collections in the Cambridge University Library and other partner libraries, and guided by the advice of experts in each subject area, Cambridge University Press is using state-of-the-art scanning machines in its own Printing House to capture the content of each book selected for inclusion. The files are processed to give a consistently clear, crisp image, and the books finished to the high quality standard for which the Press is recognised around the world. The latest print-on-demand technology ensures that the books will remain available indefinitely, and that orders for single or multiple copies can quickly be supplied.

The Cambridge Library Collection brings back to life books of enduring scholarly value (including out-of-copyright works originally issued by other publishers) across a wide range of disciplines in the humanities and social sciences and in science and technology.

The Works of John Hunter, F.R.S.

Volume 3

Edited by James F. Palmer

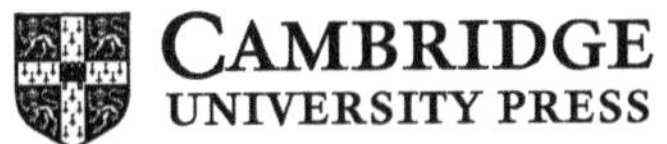

CAMBRIDGE
UNIVERSITY PRESS

University Printing House, Cambridge, CB2 8BS, United Kingdom

Cambridge University Press is part of the University of Cambridge.
It furthers the University's mission by disseminating knowledge in the pursuit of education, learning and research at the highest international levels of excellence.

www.cambridge.org
Information on this title: www.cambridge.org/9781108079594

This edition first published 1837
This digitally printed version 2015

ISBN 978-1-108-07959-4 Paperback

THE

WORKS

OF

JOHN HUNTER, F.R.S.

WITH

NOTES.

EDITED BY

JAMES F. PALMER,

SENIOR SURGEON TO THE ST. GEORGE'S AND ST. JAMES'S DISPENSARY; FELLOW OF THE ROYAL MEDICAL AND CHIRURGICAL SOCIETY OF LONDON, ETC.

IN FOUR VOLUMES.

ILLUSTRATED BY A VOLUME OF PLATES, IN QUARTO.

VOL. III.

LONDON:

PUBLISHED BY

LONGMAN, REES, ORME, BROWN, GREEN, AND LONGMAN,

PATERNOSTER-ROW.

1837.

PRINTED BY RICHARD AND JOHN E. TAYLOR,
RED LION COURT, FLEET STREET.

CONTENTS OF VOL. III.

---

1. Treatise on the Blood, Inflammation, and Gun-shot Wounds.

2. Observations on the Inflammation of the Internal Coats of Veins.

3. On Introsusception.

4. An Account of Mr. Hunter's Method of performing the Operation for the Cure of Popliteal Aneurism, by Sir Everard Home, Bart., from Materials furnished by Mr. Hunter.

5. Additional Cases to illustrate Mr. Hunter's Method of performing the Operation for the Cure of Popliteal Aneurism, by Sir Everard Home, Bart.

6. A Case of Paralysis of the Muscles of Deglutition cured by an Artificial Mode of conveying Food and Medicines into the Stomach.

7. Some Observations on the Loose Cartilages found in Joints, and most commonly met with in that of the Knee, by Sir Everard Home, Bart., from Materials furnished by Mr. Hunter.

8. Observations on certain Horny Excrescences of the Human Body, by Sir Everard Home, Bart., from Materials furnished by Mr. Hunter.

A

TREATISE

ON THE

BLOOD, INFLAMMATION, AND GUN-SHOT WOUNDS.

BY

JOHN HUNTER, F.R.S.

WITH NOTES

BY

JAMES F. PALMER,

SENIOR SURGEON TO THE ST. GEORGE'S AND ST. JAMES'S DISPENSARY; FELLOW OF THE ROYAL MEDICAL AND CHIRURGICAL SOCIETY OF LONDON, ETC.

TO THE KING.

May it please Your Majesty,

In the year 1761 *I had the honour of being appointed by Your Majesty a Surgeon on the Staff in the expedition against Belleisle.*

In the year 1790 *Your Majesty honoured me with one of the most important appointments in the medical department of the army, in fulfilling the duties of which every exertion shall be called forth to render me deserving of the trust reposed in me, and not unworthy of Your Majesty's patronage.*

The first of these appointments gave me extensive opportunities of attending to gun-shot wounds, of seeing the errors and defects in that branch of military surgery, and of studying to remove them. It drew my attention to inflammation in general, and enabled me to make observations which have formed the basis of the present Treatise. That office which I now hold has afforded me the means of extending my pursuits, and of laying this work before the public.

As the object of this book is the improvement of surgery in general, and particularly of that branch of it which is peculiarly directed to the service of the army, I am led by my situation, my duty, and my feelings, to address it, with all humility, to Your Majesty.

That Your Majesty may long live to enjoy the love and esteem of a happy people, is the fervent wish of

Your Majesty's

Most faithful subject,

And most dutiful Servant,

JOHN HUNTER.

Leicester Square,
May 20, 1793.

CONTENTS.

INTRODUCTION.

1. OF Diseased Actions, as being incompatible with each other.—2. Of Parts susceptible of particular Diseases.—3. Of Sympathy.—4. Of Mortification .... *page* 1

PART I.

CHAP. I.

GENERAL PRINCIPLES OF THE BLOOD.

1. Of the Mass of Blood, as composed of different Parts.—2. Of Coagulation and its Effects.—3. Of the Serum.—4. Of the red Globules.—5. Of the Quantity of Blood, and Course of its Circulation. 6. Of the Living Principle of the Blood.—7. Some unconnected Experiments respecting the Blood .... *page* 10

CHAP. II.

OF THE VASCULAR SYSTEM.

1. General Observations on Muscular Contraction and Elasticity.—2. General Observations on the Elongation of Relaxed Muscles.—3. Of the Structure of Arteries.—4. Of the Vasa Arteriarum.—5. Of the Heart.—6. General Observations on Blood-Vessels.—7. Valves of Arteries.—8. Of the Division or Branching of Arteries.—9. Of the Action of the Arteries, and the Velocity of the Blood's Motion.—10. Of Veins .... *page* 145

PART II.

CHAP. I.

UNION BY THE FIRST INTENTION.

1. Of Injuries in which there is no external Communication.—2. Of Injuries where the Wound communicates externally.—3. Practical

Observations respecting Union by the First Intention.—4. Of Scabbing.—5. Accidents attended with Death in a superficial Part. *page* 238

CHAP. II.

FUNDAMENTAL PRINCIPLES OF INFLAMMATION.

1. Of the different Causes which increase and diminish the Susceptibility for Inflammation, either in the whole Body or in Parts.—2. Effects of Strength or Weakness of Constitution and of Parts while under Inflammation.—3. Of Parts of the Body most susceptible of the three different Inflammations to be treated of.—4. Of the two Parts that have the Orders of Inflammation respecting Priority inverted.—5. The Natural Cause of the Adhesive Inflammation being limited.—6. Of Inflammation—its stages.—7. Of the different Degrees and different Kinds of Inflammation . . . . *page* 261

CHAP. III.

THE ADHESIVE INFLAMMATION.

1. Action of the Vessels in Inflammation.—2. Of the Colour, Swelling, and Pain of Inflamed Parts.—3. The Heat of Parts in Inflammation.—4. Of the Production of Cold in Inflammation.—5. Of the Time the Adhesive Inflammation commences after its Cause, and in what Cases and Parts it is imperfect in its Consequences.—6. Of the Uniting Medium in Inflammation.—7. The State of the Blood and of the Pulse in Inflammation.—8. The Effects of Inflammation on the Constitution according to the Structure of the Parts, Situation of similar Structures, and whether Vital or not Vital.—9. General Reflections on the Resolution of Inflammation.—10. Of the Methods of Resolution by constitutional means.—11. The Use of Medicines internally and of local Applications in Inflammation.—12. General Observations on Repulsion, Sympathy, Derivation, Revulsion, and Translation.—13. Of the different Forms in which Medicines are applied, and the Subsiding of Inflammation.—14. Of the Use of the Adhesive Inflammation . . . . *page* 320

CHAP. IV.

OF THE SUPPURATIVE INFLAMMATION.

1. The Symptoms of the Suppurative Inflammation.—2. Of the Treatment necessary in Inflammation when Suppuration must take place.—

3. The Treatment of the Inflammation when Suppuration has taken place.—4. Collections of Matter without Inflammation.—5. Of the Effects such Formations of Matter have on the Constitution.—6. The Effects of the Suppurative Inflammation on the Constitution. *page* 403

CHAP. V.

OF PUS.

1. Of the General Opinion of the Formation of Pus.—2. Of the Properties of Pus.—3. Of the Use of Pus. . . . . *page* 439

CHAP. VI.

THE ULCERATIVE INFLAMMATION.

1. Of the remote Cause of the Absorption of the Animal itself.—2. Of the Disposition of living Parts to absorb and be absorbed.—3. Of Interstitial Absorption.—4. Of the Progressive Absorption.—5. Of Absorption attended with Suppuration, which I have called Ulceration.—6. Of the Relaxing Process.—7. Of the Intention of Absorption of the Body in Disease.—8. The Modes of Promoting Absorption.—9. Illustrations of Ulceration . . . . *page* 459

CHAP. VII.

GRANULATIONS.

1. Of Granulations independent of Suppuration.—2. The Nature and Properties of Granulations.—3. Longevity of Granulations.—4. Of the Contraction of Granulations . . . . *page* 488

CHAP. VIII.

OF SKINNING.

1. The Nature of the new Cutis.—2. Of the new Cuticle.—3. Of the Rete Mucosum . . . . *page* 500

CHAP. IX.

EFFECTS OF INFLAMMATION, AND ITS CONSEQUENCES ON THE CONSTITUTION.

1. Of the Hectic.—2. Treatment of the Hectic.—3. Of Dissolution. . . . . *page* 506

PART III.

THE TREATMENT OF ABSCESSES.

1. The Progress of Abscesses to the Skin.—2. Of the Time when Abscesses should be opened.—3. Of the Methods of opening Abscesses, and treating them afterwards .... *page* 518

PART IV.

CHAP. I.

OF GUN-SHOT WOUNDS.

1. The Difference between Gun-shot Wounds and common Wounds.—2. Of the different Effects arising from the Difference in the Velocity of the Ball.—3. Of the different Kinds of Gun-shot Wounds. .... *page* 541

CHAP. II.

OF THE TREATMENT OF GUN-SHOT WOUNDS.

1. Of the Propriety of dilating Gun-shot Wounds.—2. Of the strange Course of some Balls.—3. Penetrating Wounds of the Abdomen.—4. Of penetrating Wounds in the Chest.—5. Of Concussions and Fractures of the Skull.—6. Of Wounds compounded with Fractured Bones, or containing extraneous Bodies.—7. Of the Time proper for removing Incurable Parts.—8. Of the Treatment of the Constitution. .... *page* 548

PREFACE.

THE philosophic spirit which pervades every part of the ensuing Treatise, and the profound insight which it discovers of the operations of the animal œconomy, both in health and disease, have universally procured for it a high rank among medical writings. We should not perhaps greatly err in stating that its distinctive merit consists in the bold enunciation of the governing laws of life, with reference more especially to the healthy organization, and in the application of those laws to the elucidation of disease. In this respect the Author may justly claim the merit of having originated a new method of investigation, and of having prosecuted this method in a manner and to an extent which was never contemplated by any previous physiologist, either as regards the comprehensive system of illustration which is adopted, or the masterly exposition of the reciprocative influences of the different organic systems on one another. In the introductory discourse to his Lectures on the Principles of Surgery, the Author distinctly declares this to have been his object; for "By an acquaintance with principles," he observes, "we learn the causes of disease, and without this knowledge a man cannot be a surgeon." Those, therefore, who apply the ordinary rules of a petty criticism to the present work will form a very incorrect judgment of its merits, while those who come to its perusal with the expectation of finding a simple exposition of disease, will probably be much disappointed. The reader who would form a just and accurate appreciation of a work of this character, should bring to the task considerable liberality of mind, and at the same time an independency of judgment, which can admit the general propriety of an observation, and yet know how to make those due and necessary abatements which all general propositions require.

The Treatise on the Blood and Inflammation has popularly been considered as Mr. Hunter's chief Work, and that on which his fame as a Physiologist has principally reposed. This opinion in some respects is correct, but in others it does great injustice to the Author; for though undoubtedly the Work in question contains many profound views of the animal œconomy, of unrivalled excellence and value, it never can be regarded as the type and consummation of all his previous researches. In order to evince the absurdity of such an opinion, it is only necessary to glance at the extensive series of preparations contained in his museum, and to reflect on the impossibility of embodying the physiological inferences deducible from such a mass of materials in the limited compass of a volume. From the Author's own allusion to the subject, in his paper on Digestion, as well as from the general nature of the preparations which were made, especially the prolegomena attached to the physiological series of preparations, and the numerous highly finished drawings by which these were illustrated, there can be no question that a general treatise on physiology was designed, which, had the Author been spared to complete his plan, would have exhibited in a more just light the originality and comprehensiveness of his mind. To what purpose would he otherwise have bestowed such extraordinary assiduity in compiling ten folio volumes of notes, but that he might, in the decline of his life, complete from that source the great undertaking to which his whole life was devoted?

In treating of the subject of Inflammation, the Author has commenced the inquiry by an investigation into the general properties of the blood, which he proves, by a new train of argument, to be possessed of life, like the solid parts, so as to constitute the chief bond of union by which recently divided parts are united: he next takes a comprehensive survey of the vascular system, and of its functions in health and in disease; and having discussed the subject of union by the first intention, which he considers to be an act essentially different from inflammation, he at length enters on the main subject of his discourse. This he treats in the order of its terminations, and in reference to the various circumstances which have a tendency more or less to modify the local and constitutional phenomena which it presents; and finally he illustrates the whole subject by a series of cases selected from the different organs and structures of the body, and especially by the subject of gunshot wounds. In the course of these inquiries the author is not unfrequently observed to diverge into collateral disquisitions, especially on physiological topics, which bear only in a remote manner on the main subject of his treatise, but which, from the importance of the principles which they involve, or else perhaps from the habit to which his mind had been accustomed of considering the body as a whole, it fell within his original purpose to consider. I shall not here stay to discuss the propriety of such a course on ordinary occasions, or whether such an example is to be held out to imitation to inferior minds; but such a course I am convinced was admirably calculated to call forth the immense treasures of Mr. Hunter's experience, and to cement more firmly that alliance between Pathology and Physiology which forms the characteristic feature of his doctrines. In one respect such a desultory mode of composition must undoubtedly be considered as a defect, from its tendency no less to embarrass the reader than to divert his attention from the main scope of the discourse. It is, however, a defect which the author would probably have himself corrected, had he lived to superintend his work through the press, and more particularly if his life had been spared to have given to the world a second edition of this great master-piece of his genius.

When I first undertook the office of revising and commenting upon Hunter I was less fully impressed than I now am with the difficulty of the undertaking, and I should probably have entirely abandoned the task but for the reflection that no weight would be attached to the opinions of his commentator beyond what was fairly warranted by the force and justness of his arguments.

The rule which I have chiefly observed in the insertion of notes has been to correct any impressions, arising from the Author's statements, which the progress of science has rendered doubtful. On such occasions, however, I have invariably given my authorities, or assigned the reasons of my dissent, so that, after all, the reader will be left very much to his own judgment. Sometimes I have been able to confirm Mr. Hunter's conjectures by more satisfactory proof, and occasionally I have thought it expedient to collect into one point his scattered statements respecting particular points of doctrine, so that the reader might, in one view, be able to see all that has been said on the subject. I cannot, however, flatter myself that I have attained either of these objects, and still less that I shall escape altogether the imputation of presumption.

Much of the obscurity, so often complained of in the present treatise, is to be ascribed to the peculiar circumstances under which it was given to the world. It was published under circumstances of haste, and at a period of the Author's life when he regarded his state of health as very precarious, and when his faculties, oppressed by repeated illnesses, cannot be considered to have been in their full vigour; in addition to which only a small part of the work was through the press at the time of the Author's death, and therefore it could not receive the full benefit of his corrections, or even of those of his executors, who, in consequence of the numerous professional calls upon their time, were compelled to relinquish the task. Many errors consequently have been allowed to pass unobserved both in the text and punctuation, which often vitiate the sense, and still more frequently render the meaning of the Author extremely difficult of extrication. These have been carefully corrected, and occasionally the correction has been extended still further; but, for the satisfaction of the reader in such cases, the original text has been subjoined at the foot of the page, or the interpolated passages inclosed within brackets.

JAMES F. PALMER.

38, *Golden Square,*
June 1, 1837.

N.B. The Editor's Notes are distinguished from the Author's by being placed below the line, within brackets. They are also further distinguished by initial letters instead of the usual marks of reference.

A TREATISE

ON

THE BLOOD, INFLAMMATION,

AND

GUNSHOT WOUNDS.

INTRODUCTION.

THE following pages, treating of inflammation, were first arranged in the year 1762, at Belleisle, after the complete reduction of that place. They were compiled from notes and memorandums of observations made in the course of twelve years' residence in London. During this space, my time was occupied in my education under the late Dr. Hunter, and partly in assisting him. In the winter season I was principally employed in the dissecting-room, where I taught the practical part of anatomy; in the summer I attended the hospitals. The truth of these observations was during the siege of Belleisle in some degree put to the test, by comparing them with many cases of wounds which were attended with inflammation. From the frequency of gun-shot wounds at that place, I was naturally led to arrange my thoughts upon the subject, and was induced to select them more particularly for the illustration of my opinions on inflammation. About the year 1770, when I began my lectures on the principles of disease, inflammation was the subject of a considerable part of them; and from that time till this, though I have been extending and correcting the materials, my principles remain the same. To distinguish the different species of inflammation*, and to

* In the course of this work I very often make use of the word species or specific, by which I only mean peculiarities or distinctions, and probably the term is much too loose in its application; for, as we are not entirely acquainted with the specific differences in disease, we may call that a species which more properly ranks as a genus, class, &c. Of morbid poisons we can make a correct arrangement; but with regard to disease arising from peculiarities in the constitution, we have no such absolute guides.

express my own ideas the better, I was naturally led to substitute such terms as appeared to me more expressive of what was meant than those usually employed. The best test of the propriety of these terms is, that they have been adopted by many medical writers since that period; and indeed my principles have undergone the same kind of test. In this some medical writers have been very liberal; for, not contented with taking hints, they have even laid hold of large portions of my lectures, screening themselves under the very honourable protection of their not being in print; and, at the same time, quoting authors to show their reading and their *candour*. It would appear that they consider the discoveries and opinions of a lecturer, found probably in a manuscript, as fair game; though their delicate attention to the rights of another would, no doubt, have prevented them from adopting the same doctrines had they been actually in print. Such freedoms have made me anxious to publish; not only because the public interests itself in the origin of every discovery or opinion, but because I wish to preserve my right, and also to give in a more perfect form what was thought worthy of the public even in a mutilated state. My respect for that public, however, has withheld me hitherto from publishing, that I might first be able to complete my subject, as far as time and other circumstances would allow me. I hope this publication will, at least, have equally good effects with those I have before produced, not only enabling persons to write on the same subject who could not otherwise have done it, but even to become critics in matters of which till then they were entirely ignorant.

I have endeavoured, as far as my other pursuits would permit, to form this work into a regular system, one part exactly depending on another. How far I have succeeded, the world must judge. But at the same time it ought to be considered as a new figure composed from rough materials, in which process little or no assistance could be had from any quarter; wherein the author is conscious of many imperfections, more of which he is persuaded he shall himself observe at every successive review.

There are many opinions respecting the animal œconomy peculiar to myself which are introduced, or frequently referred to, in the course of this work. It is therefore necessary to premise a short explanation of some of them, that the ideas and terms which are employed may be better understood. To others of them, however, this method cannot be applied, as they belong essentially to the body of the work, or are so immediately connected with it as to be best understood when treated in connexion with that part.

I shall carry my ideas of life further than has commonly been done. Life I believe to exist in every part of an animal body, and to render it susceptible of impressions which excite action; there is no part which has not more or less of this principle, and consequently no part which does not act according to the nature of the principle itself, and the impressions thence arising, producing thereby infinite variety, both in all natural and diseased acts. How far every part has an equal quantity of life, or of the powers of life, is not easily ascertained; but if we were to estimate them by the powers of action, we should judge tolerably well. Disease would seem to give some intelligence with regard to this matter; but how far resistance to disease, and powers of restoration, depend on the powers of life, or simply on the powers of action[a], I cannot say; but I believe it may be set down as a rule that those parts that are endowed with most action resist disease most strongly, and in disease restore themselves most readily to a healthy state.

§. 1. *Of diseased Actions, as being incompatible with each other.*

As I reckon every operation in the body an action, whether universal or partial, it appears to me beyond a doubt that no two actions can take place in the same constitution, nor in the same part, at one and the same time; the operations of the body are similar in this respect to actions or motions in common matter. It naturally results from this principle that no two different fevers can exist in the same constitution, nor two local

[a] [I believe a distinction should be made between resistance to disease and the powers of restoration. The former would seem to be in proportion to the vital energy residing in a part independently of action, as in a fresh-laid egg subjected to cold, whereas the latter would appear to be in proportion to the vital energy conjointly with the powers of action. Action, in the physiological sense of the word, can neither be supposed to exist in an unorganised body nor in an organised body stiffened by cold, although it is well known that living bodies are capable of resisting the effects of a low temperature under both these conditions; that is, the vital principle resists by a species of simple antagonism, just as gravity resists force, or chemical attraction electricity, although the former powers may be overcome by the latter when the latter are in greater intensity. In disease also, and especially in epidemical and infectious diseases, the weak and debilitated are most liable to catch the infection, and generally fall the first victims; so also in poisons, those parts which are least endowed with life are those which perish most readily. On these occasions, action, it is true, is produced; but then it is a subsequent, or at the most only a concomitant, effect, intended for the reparation of the injury and absolutely necessary for this purpose. However, it is highly probable that the powers of a part or of the system may be temporarily increased by certain species of fevers and inflammations, which may thus indirectly tend to increase the power of resistance. On the same principle, infection is most effectually resisted by those who are actively engaged in the pursuits of life.]

diseases in the same part, at the same time. There are many local diseases which have dispositions totally different, but, having very similar appearances, have been supposed by some to be one sort of disease, by others to be a different kind, and by others again a compound of two diseases. Thus, the venereal disease, when it attacks the skin, is very similar to those diseases which are vulgarly called scorbutic, and *vice versâ.* These, therefore, are often supposed to be mixed, and to exist in the same part. Thus we hear of a pocky-scurvy, a pocky-itch, rheumatic-gout, &c. &c., which names, according to my principle, imply a union that cannot possibly exist.

It has been considered as contradictory to this opinion that a patient might have the scrofula, scurvy, venereal disease, smallpox, &c. at the same time. All of this is indeed possible; but then no two of them can exist in the same part of the body at the same time: but before one of them can occupy the place of another, that other must be first destroyed, or it may be superseded for a time, and may afterwards return.

When a constitution is susceptible of any one disease, this does not hinder it from being also susceptible of others. I can conceive it possible that a man may be very susceptible of every disease incident to the human body, although it is not probable; for I should believe that one susceptibility is in some degree incompatible with another, in a manner similar to the incompatibility between different actions, though not of so strict a kind.

A man may have the lues and the smallpox at the same time; that is, parts of his body may be contaminated by the venereal poison, the smallpox may at the same time take place, and both diseases may appear together, but still not in the same part.

In two eruptive diseases, where both are necessarily the consequence of fever, and where both naturally appear after the fever nearly at the same distance of time, it would be impossible for the two to have their respective eruptions, even in different parts, because it is impossible that the two preceding fevers should be co-existent.

From this principle I think I may fairly put the following queries: Do not the failure of inoculation, and the power of resisting many infections, arise from the existence of some other disease at that time in the body, which is therefore incapable of another action?

Does not the great difference in the time, from the application of the cause to the appearance of the disease, in many cases, depend upon the same principle? For instance, a person is inoculated, and the puncture does not inflame for fourteen days, cases of which I have seen. Is not this deviation from the natural progress of the disease to be attributed to another disease in the constitution at the time of inoculation?

Does not the cure of some diseases depend upon the same principle? —as, *e.g.*, the suspension or cure of a gonorrhœa by a fever.

Let me illustrate this principle still further by one of many cases which have come under my own observation. On Thursday, the 16th May, 1775, I inoculated a gentleman's child, and it was observed that I made pretty large punctures. On the Sunday following, viz. the 19th, he appeared to have received the infection, a small inflammation or redness appearing round each puncture, and a small tumour. On the 20th and 21st, the child was feverish; but I declared that it was not the variolous fever, as the inflammation had not at all advanced since the 19th. On the 22nd, a considerable eruption appeared, which was evidently the measles, and the sores on the arms appeared to go back, becoming less inflamed.

On the 23rd he was very full of the measles; but the punctures on the arms were in the same state as on the preceding day. On the 25th the measles began to disappear. On the 26th and 27th the punctures began again to look a little red. On the 29th the inflammation increased, and there was a little matter formed. On the 30th he was seized with fever. The smallpox appeared at the regular time, went through its usual course, and terminated favourably[a].

[a] [In our ignorance of the essential nature of diseases, the principle which is here laid down may be considered perhaps as too absolutely expressed. The disposition and appearances of specific diseases are unquestionably greatly modified by the existence of peculiar states of the constitution at the time, as of scrofula, gout, rheumatism, &c., and this in so striking a manner as to render the distinction between a *modified* and a *conjoint* disease almost invisible. Thus the affections which result from the abuse of mercury on a constitution affected with syphilis are *sui generis*, and cannot be produced by either of these poisons acting separately. Thus also the phenomena of smallpox and cowpox present many peculiarities which are scarcely reconcileable upon the doctrines laid down by our author. Dr. Willan, for example, found "that when a person was inoculated with vaccine and variolous matter about the same time, (that is, not exceeding a week,) both inoculations proved effective, for the vaccine vesicle proceeded to its acme in its usual number of days, and the maturation of the variolous pustule was attended by a variolous eruption on the skin." (*On Vaccine Inoculation*, p. 1.) Dr. Woodville also has said, "that if the cowpox matter and the smallpox matter be both inserted in the arm of a patient, even within an inch of each other, so that on the ninth day the same efflorescence becomes common to both the local affections, nevertheless inoculating from the cowpox tumour the genuine vaccine disease will be produced," (*Observations on the Cowpox*, p. 12.); but if the inoculation be performed with a mixture of the two matters, then the chance is equal that smallpox or cowpox will be the result, or the varioloid disease, either one of which is capable of conferring an immunity on the patient so affected. Here, therefore, are two diseases acknowledged to be distinct and constitutional, not only coexistent in the system at the same time, but (from the blending of the areolar inflammations) apparently in the same part. These phenomena are probably as uncommon in disease as the hybridous productions of the animal and vegetable world in reference to the usual course of generation. Of the latter there is no question, and I do not perceive any antecedent presumption against the occurrence of the former.]

§. 2. *Of Parts susceptible of particular Diseases.*

There are some parts much more susceptible of specific diseases than others. Poisons take their different seats in the body as if they were allotted to them. Thus, the skin is attacked by what are vulgarly called scorbutic eruptions, as well as many other diseases; it is also the seat of the smallpox and the measles: the throat is the seat of action in the hydrophobia and the hooping-cough. The absorbent system, especially the glands, are more susceptible of scrofula than most other parts of the body. The breasts, testicles, and the conglomerate glands are most commonly the seat of cancer. The skin, throat, and nose are more readily affected by the lues venerea than the bones and periosteum, which however suffer sooner than many other parts, particularly the vital parts, which perhaps are not at all susceptible of this disease. These differences may arise from the nature of the parts themselves, or from some regular circumstances, which must act as a pre-existing cause.

§. 3. *Of Sympathy.*

It is unnecessary to give a definition of sympathy, for it is generally very well understood when applied to the mind, and also by medical men when applied to the body. In the mind its reference is external; it depends upon the state of others, and one of its chief uses is to excite an active interest in favour of the distressed, the mind of the spectators taking on nearly the same action with that of the sufferers, and disposing them to give relief or consolation: it is therefore one of the first of the social feelings, and by many useful operations inclines mankind to union. In the body, sympathy has only a reference internally to the body itself, and is not so evident as the sympathy of the mind, although in some cases we see its effects. It is either natural or diseased; but it is the diseased only that I propose at present to consider. I shall divide the sympathy of the body into two kinds, universal and partial.

By the universal sympathy is meant where the whole constitution sympathises with some sensation or action of a part. By partial sympathy is meant where one or more distinct parts sympathise with some local sensation or action. The universal sympathies are various in different diseases; but those which arise in consequence of local violence are principally three, viz. the symptomatic, the nervous, and the hectic fever. The symptomatic fever is an immediate effect of some local injury, and therefore is a universal sympathy arising from a local cause; the nervous has no determined form nor stages of the disease from the first cause, as delirium, spasm, almost of all kinds and in all parts, locked-jaw, &c. The hectic fever is also a universal sympathy, attended with a local disease which the constitution is not able to overcome. Most of these will be more fully treated of when I have occasion to describe their causes.

I divide partial sympathy into three kinds: the remote, the contiguous, and the continuous.

The remote sympathy is where there appears no visible connexion of parts that can account for such effects. In these cases there is commonly a sensation in the sympathiser which appears to be delusive, and produces a wrong reference of the mind to the seat of the disease, such as the pain of the shoulder in an inflammation of the liver.

The contiguous sympathy is that which appears to have no other connexion than arises from the contact of separate parts. An instance of which we have in contained parts sympathising with the containing; such as the stomach and intestines sympathising with the integuments of the abdomen, the lungs with the chest, the brain with the scalp, and the testicles with the scrotum.

The continuous sympathy is where there is no interruption of parts, and the sympathy runs or is continued along from the irritating point as from a centre, so as to be gradually lost in the surrounding parts in proportion to the distance; and this is the most common of all the sympathies. An example of it we have in the spreading of inflammation, which will be often mentioned in this treatise[a].

§. 4. *Of Mortification.*

Mortification is of two kinds, the one without inflammation, and the other preceded by it. But as the cases of mortification which will be mentioned in this work are all of the second kind, I shall confine my observations to that species.

I consider inflammation as an increased action of that power which a part naturally possesses; and in healthy inflammations, at least, it is probably attended with an increase of power; but in inflammations

---

[a] [See the chapter on Sympathy, Vol. I. p. 317, for a more complete exposition of Mr. Hunter's views on this subject.

It is doubtless in many cases possible to trace the sympathy to a particular distribution of the nerves, as when, for example, the nerves of the affected and sympathising parts derive their origin from the same parts of the nervous centre. Thus, pain in the back is occasioned by irritation of the pelvic viscera, and hemicrania from caries of the teeth. A perfect knowledge of the minute anatomy of the brain, and of the functions of its different parts, would probably unfold the whole mystery of this subject.]

which terminate in mortification there is no increase of power[a], but on the contrary a diminution of it. This, when joined to an increased action, becomes a cause of mortification, by destroying the balance which ought to subsist between the power and action of every part. There are, besides, cases of mortification preceded by inflammation, which do not arise wholly from that as a cause, but rather seem to have something in their nature; of this kind is the carbuncle, and the slough formed in the smallpox pustule.

If this account of mortifications arising from no specific nature be just, we shall find it no difficult matter to establish a rational mode of cure; but before we attempt this, let us take a view of the treatment which has been hitherto recommended, and see how far it agrees with our theory. It is plain, from the common practice, that the weakness has been attended to; but it is plain that the increased action has been overlooked: and therefore the whole aim has been to increase the action in order to remove the weakness. The Peruvian bark, confectio cardiaca, serpentaria, &c. have been given in large quantities, as the case appeared to require, or the constitution could bear, by which means an artificial or temporary appearance of strength has been produced, while it was only an increased action. Cordials and wine, upon the principle on which they have been given, are rationally administered; but there are strong reasons for not recommending them, arising from the general effect which they possess of increasing the action without giving real strength. The powers of the body are by this treatment sunk afterwards in the same proportion as they had been raised, by which nothing can be gained, but a great deal may be lost; for, in all cases, if the powers are allowed to sink below a certain point, they are irrecoverable.

The local treatment has been as absurd as the constitutional. Scarifications have been made down to the living parts, that stimulating and antiseptic medicines might be applied to them, as turpentines, the warmer balsams, and sometimes the essential oils. Warm fomentations have been also applied, as being congenial to life; but warmth always increases action, and therefore should be well adjusted to the case: on the other hand, cold debilitates or lessens powers when carried too far, but at first lessens action. Stimulants likewise are improper where the actions are already too violent.

---

[a] [By "*power*," I apprehend, is here signified the resistance which is offered by a living part to disorganization and death. By the expression, "*the powers of a part*," is generally meant the sum of the vital actions going on in that part, as circulation, growth, secretion, &c. Mr. Hunter employs the expression in a less complex sense, so as simply to express by it the degree and prevalence of the vital principle.]

Upon the principles here laid down, the bark is the principal medicine as yet known that we depend upon, as it increases the powers and lessens the degree of action. Upon many occasions opium will be of singular service by lessening the action, although it does not give real strength. I have seen good effects from it, both when given internally in large doses, and when applied to the part. It is proper also to keep the parts cool, and all the applications should be cold[a].

---

[a] [Notwithstanding the condemnation which is here pronounced on scarifications and warm dressings, yet experience and theory both tend to confirm the utility of this mode of treatment. The former, or scarifications, afford an exit to putrid matters, while the latter by their antiseptic qualities diminish the quantity which is produced, and at the same time modify its virulence. But it is not merely the constitutional effects which are lessened by these means. There cannot be the slightest question that the local effects are equally mitigated, and the pernicious consequences of sloughs and ill-conditioned pus in contact with the living textures materially lessened, by providing a free escape for these matters. This subject will be adverted to more fully when speaking of "diffuse cellular inflammation," in which the bad effects of putrid secretions in contact with the living solids are most conspicuously shown.

In regard to the advantages of bark, I need not here observe that its pretensions in the present day as a medicine in cases of mortification are rated much more moderately than they were formerly. Practitioners no longer think that strength is imparted to the system in proportion to the quantity of bark which the patient is made to swallow.]

PART I.

CHAPTER I.

GENERAL PRINCIPLES OF THE BLOOD.

AS the blood is allowed by all to have a considerable share in inflammation, or at least to be particularly affected by it, becoming, by its appearances, one of the signs or symptoms of its existence, and as the blood is a material object with me in the theory of inflammation, I shall begin my treatise with its natural history, a previous knowledge of which is the more requisite, because the accounts of this fluid hitherto given will hardly explain any of its uses in the machine in health, or of its changes in disease.

The heart and vessels are very active in inflammations; and as their structures and actions have not hitherto been understood, I have subjoined to the natural history of the blood an account of the structure of the heart and vessels, together with their actions in the machine; to which I have added one use of the absorbents not hitherto known.

As every natural action of the body depends, for its perfection, on a number of circumstances, we are led to conclude, that all the various combining actions are established while the body is in health, and well-disposed; but this does not take place in diseased actions, for disease, on the contrary, consists in the want of this very combination; and diseased actions, therefore, vary according to many natural circumstances, of which I propose to point out a few of the most striking instances.

Inflammation must have some exciting cause, and the same cause will produce an effect under one circumstance which it will not under another. I have therefore begun with the supposition of an injury, attended with such circumstances as do not excite inflammation, which will form a strong contrast to those which do, the opposite effects mutually illustrating each other; but as inflammation is a very general action of the vessels in disease, and is of various kinds, I have previously given a short account of several of the most common sorts of inflammation, which will explain the rest.

The whole material world has been very properly divided into solids and fluids, these being the only essentially different states of matter we are able to observe. From one of these states to the other matter appears to be continually passing, but with these restrictions, that no species of matter can assume a solid form without having first been in a fluid state, nor can any change take place in a solid till it be first formed into or suspended in a fluid[a]. The living animal body is obedient to these general laws, for all solid and animal matter has first been fluid, and having passed into this solid form, becomes a recipient for other fluids, out of which the solids may themselves be renovated and increased.

The solids of an animal, although composed of one species of matter, yet admit of great variety in their appearance; and this variety takes place in some animals more than in others. But the fluid part of an animal body, in its natural state, has but one appearance, which is that of blood. There are certain parts of animals which, though hardly solid in their own nature, are yet to be considered as solids, from their being fixed in their situation, and appropriated to local actions; some of them acting on the fluids (which are, to a certain degree, passive in all animals), and disposing of them for particular purposes in the animal œconomy, in the same manner as is done by those which are usually called the solids in animals; of this sort are the gelatinous parts in many of the inferior orders of sea-animals, as the medusa, the vitreous humour of the eye, &c. There appears to be a sympathetic intercourse between the solid and fluid parts of an animal, designed by nature for their mutual support. In disease, when the machine cannot be furnished in the common way, the solids of the body supply the defects, and the person becomes lean ; and the fluids would appear from this to be more an object of attention in the machine than even the solids.

This fluid part of an animal is called the blood, and in the animals with which we are most acquainted it is of a red colour. The nature

---

[a] [See Vol. I. p. 211. Chemistry affords a few exceptions to the universality of this law. Thus chlorate of potash combines with sulphur or charcoal by mere attrition; and the greater number of fulminating powders are examples of the same kind. Crystals of Glauber's salt and nitrate of bismuth are converted into a fluid by being rubbed together in a mortar, and so are the solid amalgams of bismuth and lead. The former part of this sentence is manifestly a pleonasm.]

[b] [Without wishing to question the soundness of this opinion, I would yet venture to suggest that it is contrary to analogy to suppose that the body can subsist on its own materials, unless these have undergone a previous digestion. The fattest people, on this principle, would be the fittest subjects for fevers; repeated losses of blood would produce the greatest degrees of emaciation, and those who have most fat would be the best able to endure privations of food; all which is contradicted by observation. I apprehend

and appearances of the blood have been more attended to in diseases, especially of the inflammatory kind, than in full health, as it is more expressive of disease when removed from the body than any of the solids, and undergoes changes which the solids do not. Some of these changes are produced by the separation of parts from one another; but as the body is seldom in perfect health, we can hardly procure the blood in the same state twice from one person, although it may not be sensibly diseased. In a history of the blood these varieties must be mentioned, although they are often slighter appearances of what we find in disease; for disease certainly throws great light on the natural history of the blood, and the apparent changes which it undergoes must have unavoidably called medical men to consider it with attention.

The only knowledge, however, we have of any difference in the blood, arises from these varieties in its spontaneous changes when extravasated[a]; nor do these differences appear always to affect the real nature of the blood, as the animals often continue in health while they are going on.

---

that fatness and leanness depend on a want of balance between the waste and supply, the waste being principally occasioned by an acceleration of the vascular actions, and the more rapid interchange which thence ensues in the molecular particles of the body. This is seen in caterpillars, in young and growing animals, and in birds, as contrasted with amphibia, adults, and animals of the tardigrade species. The former require a continual supply of food to replace the effete matter, while the latter are enabled to sustain hunger for a long time without injury. Thus hybernating animals retain their fatness during the whole period of their torpidity. Dr. Stevens mentions having seen a rattlesnake as fat after nine months' complete abstinence from food as at the first; and Professor Blumenbach has mentioned similar examples, of a still more remarkable kind. Fevers, on the other hand, rapidly emaciate the body, because in them the supply is cut off at the same time that the waste from excessive action is increased. Thus, also, persons of active minds and bodies are seldom observed to grow fat. Women grow thin during the period of utero-gestation, and animals during the period of the rut.

The uses of fat probably are to preserve symmetry and warmth, consequently in man and the cetaceous tribes it serves as a substitute for external clothing.]

a [The progress of modern chemistry has not only enabled the pathologist to detect many diseased states of the blood which were perfectly unknown in the time of Hunter (see *note*, Vol. I. p. 352), but has enabled the physiologist also to pursue his investigations on entirely a new tack, from which the greatest acquisitions to science may be expected to accrue. In order, however, that the alliance of chemistry with physiology may be really rendered useful, it is important to bear in mind that the object of the chemico-physiologist should be not so much to discover the modes in which the vital principle operates, as the results which those operations give rise to, so as to be able to trace their dependence on one another, or the relation in which they stand, as cause and effect. This can only be done by the most scrupulous and exact analyses of the animal fluids, and particularly of the blood, as the *point de départ* from whence all the others proceed. Hunter did not altogether reject these aids, although, from the state of organic chemistry at the time that this treatise was written, he was little disposed to place reliance on the results which it afforded.]

Blood is most probably as much alike in all animals as the muscle of one animal is like that of another, only with this difference, that some animals have not that part which gives it the red colour; but the other parts, as the lymph and serum, are, as far as I yet know, the same in all[a].

Transfusion of the blood of one animal into the vessels of another proves, to a certain degree, the uniform nature of the blood, for, as far as these experiments have been urged, no alteration has been observed[b].

---

[a] [Berzelius has verified this observation, as far as regards the serum and fibrin in the higher orders of animals, but the globules are found to vary very considerably in size, shape, number, and composition in the different species. The same authority has also stated that there are two thirds less of the muriates in ox-blood than in that from the human subject, but a larger proportion of nitrogen. (*Med.-Chir. Trans.*, vol. iii.) This latter fact would, indeed, be very remarkable if true, considering that man lives for the most part on a highly azotised food, whereas the ox lives on food which contains no nitrogen at all. The recent researches, however, of Macaire and Marcet (*Mém. de la Soc. de Phy. et d'Hist. Nat. de Genève*, v. 389.) have not only shown the error of this particular fact, but, as far as concerns the *ultimate* analysis of the blood, have established the almost entire identity between that of herbivorous and that of carnivorous animals. Certain minor differences in colour, in the relative proportions of crassamentum and serum, in the halitus which exhales from fresh drawn blood, and in the period of coagulation, have been pointed out by Thackrah; but these are not greater than what may occur in the blood of the same individual taken from two different vessels, or at two different periods of life. (*Enquiry into the Nature and Properties of the Blood, by C. T. Thackrah, 2nd Edit.* p. 149.)]

[b] [The honour of this discovery has been sharply contested between the French and English. From certain passages in the classics it seems highly probable that the practice was not unknown to the ancients; at any rate the operation was described by Libavius at least fifty years before the English and French controversy commenced. (*In Def. Synt. Arc. Chy. contra H. Schneumannam, Act. 2. p. 8. Edit. Francof. a.* 1615.)

The operation of transfusion was first performed on the human subject in France, by MM. Denis and Emmerets, on the 15th of June, 1667, and repeated in England by Drs. Lower and King on the 23rd of November of the same year. It speedily grew into great favour; but in consequence of the fatal and dangerous effects which ensued in several cases, it was interdicted by a sentence of the Chastelet, and soon afterwards fell into desuetude. The blood of calves and sheep was generally employed in these operations, and, so far as appears, the blood of the human subject was never thought of.

In 1785 Dr. Harwood revived the inquiry, by making it the subject of his inaugural *thesis*, which he supported by many interesting experiments on dogs, which he performed in public. (*Phil. Trans. Abr.*, vol. i. p. 185, *note.*) MM. Prevost and Dumas, Dr. Leacock, and finally Dr. Blundell followed in the same track.

It was ascertained by Dr. Harwood, that when an animal was bled to complete syncope, it was capable of being resuscitated, by the transfusion of fresh drawn-blood from another animal of the same or a different species; although when the latter was employed, the animal generally perished before the sixth day. MM. Prevost and Dumas ascertained, that although the respiration remained calm, the pulse became remarkably accelerated, the heat of the body was rapidly dissipated, and the dejections and urine became mucous and bloody, and continued so in many instances until death. They found also, that when blood containing spherical globules was injected into a bird, it died, as if poisoned, with violent symptoms of distress of the nervous system, which effects uniformly occurred, whether the precaution of bleeding the animal beforehand

Concerning natural objects, we usually acquire a gross knowledge, from the frequency with which they are observed, and it often requires little more than common attention to have a tolerable conception of their general principles. This is the case with the blood.

Blood is known to be of a red colour in a great number of animals, and to be altogether a fluid while circulating in the living body. It is known to separate into parts when out of the body, and a portion of it to become solid; it is likewise known, that when deprived of a certain proportion of it, an animal dies; it has, therefore, been held in particular veneration, as constituting the life of the animal. Like other things which are discovered to be of great use, the blood has frequently attracted the attention of mankind as an object of curiosity only, from which some have proceeded to a more critical inquiry into its nature and properties, and to a more extensive elucidation of the subject at large. To this practitioners in physic have a great deal contributed, from a conviction that this knowledge would be of much use to them in their profession; and the teachers of the art have been still more industrious

---

had been previously resorted to or not. Sheep's blood restored cats and rabbits for a few days from the exhaustion consequent on excessive hæmorrhage; but it excited rapid and violent convulsions, followed by speedy death, when it was injected into ducks. These experiments, therefore, sufficiently demonstrated the danger attending the transfusion of large quantities of blood from an animal of one species into another animal of a different species. Smaller quantities, indeed, were proved not to be dangerous to life, although unpleasant effects generally followed. Thus Mr. Goodridge, of Barbadoes, has lately injected human blood into the veins of a dog, and the animal afterwards survived.

Dr. Blundell, to whom the profession is indebted for every practical advantage attending this operation, carefully repeated the experiments above mentioned previously to his performing the operation on the human subject. With human blood he nourished a full-grown dog for three weeks by this means alone, and succeeded in reviving another by similar means after it had ceased to respire for full five minutes. In order to prove that the contact of the blood with foreign substances does not deprive it of vitality, or materially deteriorate its qualities, he connected, by means of a syringe, the carotid artery and jugular vein of the same animal, and continued to impel the blood from the artery into the vein for twenty or thirty minutes, until the whole blood of the animal must have passed through the apparatus. (*Med.-Chir. Trans.*, ix. 56. and x. 296.)

In order that the operation may be successfully performed, it is necessary to be exceedingly careful to exclude the ingress of air or clots of blood, and to proceed in so gradual a manner as not to endanger a sudden plethora. With these cautions, transfusion may be regarded as a valuable auxiliary means in the hands of the surgeon, particularly in the treatment of flooding or alarming hæmorrhages from other causes. I may mention that it has succeeded in several cases of this kind where little or no hope could have been entertained from any other resources.

It is unnecessary to add, that the blood should always be taken from a healthy human subject, and be allowed to stagnate in the apparatus as little as possible. (See Vol. I. p. 551, where Hunter appears to have appreciated the value of this means of recovery in the only cases in which it is applicable. The idea of transfusing of human blood does not seem to have occurred to him.)]

in their investigations; but the frequent recourse which is had to the lancet in diseases has afforded the most ample opportunities of observation, almost sufficient to explain every principle in the blood, without the aid of further experiment.

In animals possessed of red blood, two modes of investigation may be adopted. One of these respects the blood while it is circulating, when the colour makes its motion visible, and gives an idea of the circulation in the smaller vessels. Accidents, operations, and anatomical knowledge of the vessels in which the blood is contained, have at the same time assisted us to form more perfect ideas of its motion in the larger vessels. The other mode, which is that of examining the blood when out of the body, enables us to observe whatever relates to its spontaneous changes and separation, together with the apparent properties of each component part. Its chemical properties become known likewise by this second mode, though without throwing much light on the nature of the fluid itself.

The blood is called a fluid because it is always found in a fluid state in the vessels of a living animal while under the influence of the circulation; yet it is not, under all circumstances, naturally so, for of one part of it, when not circulating, solidity is a necessary and essential property, fluidity being only necessary at the time of circulation for its motion, distribution, and the easy separation of its parts.

Without being fluid, it could not be propelled through flexible tubes, and distributed to all parts of the body. It could not be divided into portions, as the vessels branch off; it could not pass through the smaller vessels, nor admit of the various separations of its parts, which are to produce the increase and repairs of the whole body; neither could it be adapted for furnishing the various secretions; nor could it be brought back to the heart*.

The red colour of the blood is produced merely by some red matter diffused through it, but not common to all animals. The blood exhibits a greater variety of changes, and admits of more experiments to determine its nature and properties, than the solids. This, in some degree, arises from its fluidity, in which form it has not yet attained its ultimate state, and is only the substance that furnishes materials out of which the solids are produced or augmented.

* The distribution of water from the sea is similar to the arterial system, and the rivers returning to it have an analogy to the veins; but their effects are different, because the globe works entirely upon its own materials. The waters are continually carrying away the land from one situation, and depositing it in another, taking down continents, and leaving the ocean in their place; whilst at the same time they are raising continents out of the sea. But animals work upon foreign matter, introduced from time to time into the system.

The heat in the animal body, principally in those which are called warm animals, has been commonly considered as depending principally on the blood, or at least as being connected with it as much as with any other portion of the body*. As I shall have occasion to take notice of the increased heat of inflamed parts, it might be expected that I should endeavour to explain this principle in the history of the blood. I profess, however, not thoroughly to understand it, and the theories hitherto brought forward do not in the least satisfy me, as I think that none of them accord perfectly with every circumstance observable in these cases.

§. 1. *Of the Mass of Blood, as composed of different Parts.*

The blood, while circulating in the vessels, appears to the eye to be a homogeneous mass; but when it is passing in vessels so small as almost to separate its visible parts, and is viewed in a microscope, there is no appearance but that of globules moving in the vessels.

In such a situation the other parts, called the coagulable lymph and the serum, are not distinguishable, on account of their being transparent, and the globules do not, strictly speaking, constitute a part of the fluid, but are only diffused through it. These globules being red, give this colour to the blood, and are called the red part, but are not always of the same redness when collected in a mass; this is probably owing to each globule being changed in its tint of colouring. The blood of some animals has no such globules, but is perfectly transparent, indeed more so than the most transparent parts of the red blood, to which it is analogous. A red colour is therefore not essential to constitute true blood; and I believe the slight tinge of colour there is in the blood, independent of the globules, arises from the solution of various substances in the serum. The blood has a peculiar taste, being saltish, but of a peculiar flavour[a]: we can always distinguish by the taste when there is blood in the mouth.

These are the principal observations we can make on the blood when circulating, or in its fluid state; but as one part of it under certain circumstances changes into a solid, or as it is commonly termed, coagu-

* From whence the expression, warm-blooded or cold-blooded animals; but the expression should rather be, the animals of a permanent heat in all atmospheres, and animals of a heat variable with every atmosphere.

---

a [It is also slightly nauseous and alkaline. Turmeric paper is rendered brown, and syrup of violets green, by the very first drops of serum which exude from the clot.]

lates, more of its parts are thus exposed; in this process the blood separates into two distinct substances, a coagulating part, and another which separates from it and remains fluid; but the coagulum entangles the red part, and this alone shows the blood to be formed of these component parts. The parts of the blood so separated have been named according to their apparent properties; the one, the coagulable lymph; the other, the serum; and the red part has been called the red globules; but upon a more intimate knowledge of the different parts of this fluid, we shall find that those terms are not expressive of all their properties.

The term *coagulable* lymph[a] is not expressive of this property, as one which is inherent in the lymph itself, for many substances are capable of being coagulated, though not spontaneously, yet by chemical means. For instance, heat coagulates the farinaceous part of vegetables, and thus forms paste, and also mucus. Spirits of wine coagulates many animal substances; acid coagulates milk, &c.; the term, therefore, to be used respecting this property of the blood should be such as expresses its inherent power of self-coagulation: perhaps *coagulating* might be better applied to what is called *coagulable* lymph, and the epithet coagulable might be reserved for those fluids which require a chemical process to produce that effect. Of this kind is the serum, for I have discovered this fluid to be composed of two parts, which is ascertained by means of the different causes of coagulation. To discover all the various properties and uses of the component parts of the blood in the machine may be impossible; and to determine whether they will act, or are employed conjunctively to produce the effect, is not easy; but there are some properties discoverable which would incline us to believe that particular parts of the blood are employed to compose particular solid parts, which are found to possess properties similar to different parts of the blood[b].

§. 2. *Of Coagulation, and its Effects.*

As coagulation is the first change which the blood undergoes when out of the vessels, and as it even coagulates while in them, under cer-

[a] [*Gluten, fibre of the blood,* and *fibrin* are terms which have also been applied to this principle of the blood. The latter term is now most frequently adopted, from its being in some degree expressive of the fibrous or half-organized texture which this substance exhibits when the serum is expressed from it. The whole coagulum, consisting of the above-named substance, interposed serum, and red globules, has been variously designated by different writers as *cruor, hepar sanguineum, placenta, insula, gluten, clot,* and *crassamentum.*]

[b] [The probability of the opinion expressed in the text will be adverted to in a future part of the work. In the present note I propose briefly to point out the principal

tain circumstances, we shall consider this process first. Though fluidity is necessary to enable the blood to circulate, yet coagulation is no

---

results which have been obtained by modern chemistry, as regards the composition of the blood.

Analysis of healthy serum by M. Le Canu.

	1st Analysis.	2nd Analysis.
Water	906·00	901·00
Albumen	78·00	81·20
Organic matters soluble in water and alcohol	1·69	2·05
Albumen combined with soda	2·10	2·55
Oleaginous matters { Oily matter	1·00	1·30
Oleaginous matters { Crystallizable fatty matter	1·20	2·10
Hydrochlorate of soda and potash	6·00	5·32
Subcarbonate and phosphate of soda, and sulphate of potash	2·10	2·00
Phosphate of lime, magnesia and iron, with subcarbonate of lime and magnesia	0·91	0·87
Loss	1·00	1·61
	1000·00	1000·00

Analysis of serum by Berzelius and Marcet.

	Berzelius.	Marcet.
Water	905·01	900·00
Albumen	80·00	86·80
Hydrochlorate of soda and potash	6·00	6·60
Lactate of soda and extractive matters soluble in alcohol...	4·00	....
Muco-extractive matter	....	4·00
Subcarbonate of soda and phosphate of soda, and animal matter soluble in alcohol	4·10	....
Subcarbonate of soda	....	1·65
Sulphate of potash	....	0·35
Phosphate of lime, iron, and magnesia	....	0·60
	999·10	1000·00

Analysis of healthy venous blood by M. Le Canu.

	1st Analysis.	2nd Analysis.	Average.
Crassamentum deprived of water and salts { Colouring-matter	133·000	119·626	126·313
Crassamentum deprived of water and salts { Fibrin	2·100	3·565	2·833
Serum. Water	780·145	785·590	782·868
Serum. Albumen	65·090	69·415	67·252
Serum. Oleaginous matters { Oily matter	1·310	2·270	1·790
Serum. Oleaginous matters { Crystallizable fatty matter	2·430	4·300	3·365
Serum. Extractive matters soluble in alcohol and water	1·790	1·920	1·855
Serum. Albumen combined with soda	1·265	2·010	1·637
Serum. Chloruret of sodium and potassium, subcarbonate and phosphate of soda, and sulphate of potash	8·370	7·304	7·837
Serum. Phosphate of lime, magnesia and iron, peroxide of iron, and subcarbonate of lime and magnesia	2·100	1·414	1·757
Loss	2·400	2·586	2·493
	1000·000	1000·000	1000·000

(*Journ. de Pharmacie for Sept. and Oct.* 1831. *Med.-Chir. Trans.*, iii. 230.) The great

less necessary when it is to be disposed of out of the circulation, even within the body, and therefore deserves to be considered with no less

---

correspondence of the preceding analyses in all main particulars is a great voucher for their accuracy. I shall only therefore further remark that the muco-extractive matter of Marcet is probably the impure "lactate of soda and extractive matters soluble in alcohol" of Berzelius, the osmazome of Thenard and Denis, and the oleaginous and extractive matters of Le Canu. Likewise also the oleaginous matters of Le Canu, which were first fully investigated by Traill, Christison, and Babington, answer to the "graisse phosphuree rouge et blanche" of Vauquelin and Denis and the "matière cérébrale rouge et blanche" of Chevreul. Berzelius is of opinion that the earthy phosphates, the sulphate of potash, and several other substances, are formed during combustion, or by the process of analysis, and do not exist originally in the blood. (*Op. cit.*, pp. 227, 233.)

We may therefore regard the blood in three lights: 1st, as flowing in the vessels, when we should say that it consists of two substances, the *liquor sanguinis* and red globules; 2nd, as extravasated from the body, when we should say that it is composed of crassamentum and serum; and 3rd, in its chemical relations, when we should say that it is made up of three parts, essentially differing from each other, viz. water, saline or adventitious substances, and nutritive matters; the latter, in consequence of their close chemical correspondence, being now generally regarded as modifications of albumen. According to some chemists, the blood also contains carbon (*Clanny*); carbonic acid (*Vogel, Brande*, &c.); acetic acid (*Hermann*); cruorine, cholesterine, and osmazome (*Denis*); seroline (*Boudet*); a yellow colouring-matter (*Lassaigne, Chevreul*); a peculiar aromatic principle (*Barrueil*); globuline, one of the constituents of the globules, consisting of a modification of albumen and a peculiar colouring-matter (*Le Canu*); a substance analogous to urea (*Raspail, Segalas*); copper (*Meisner, Sarzeau*); soda, either free or in the state of carbonate (*nearly all chemists*); sulphur (*Vogel*); and minute traces of silica, alumina, and manganese (*Turner* and *O'Shaughnessy*). As the presence, however, of these substances in healthy blood has either been disputed or denied by the generality of chemists, it would be improper to include them among the regular constituents of this fluid.

The process employed by Le Canu for obtaining the quantitative results contained in the preceding analyses, I shall transcribe in his own words:

"I evaporated," he says, "a determinate quantity of healthy serum at a gentle heat, and the loss which it sustained gave me the weight of water. Then heating the residue, first with boiling water and afterwards with boiling alcohol, the former dissolved out the soluble salts and extractive matters, and the latter the fatty matters. The aqueous solution being now filtered and evaporated in a sand-bath, and the residue treated with alcohol at 40°, until it ceased to be further coloured, I by this means separated the extractive matters soluble in alcohol. The residue, consisting of salts mixed with extractive matters, insoluble in this menstruum, was calcined, to know the proportion of organic matters, and the new residue treated with boiling alcohol, to separate the hydrochlorates.

"The fatty matters which were taken up by the boiling alcohol were further separated by means of alcohol at 33°, which when cold does not dissolve the crystallizable matter; finally, the albumen, thus deprived of all its soluble contents, was dried, weighed, and afterwards calcined. A very small portion of soluble salts, contained in the residue after incineration, was separated by means of water slightly acidulated, which gave rise to a colourless solution, in which the prussiate of potash clearly indicated traces of iron, undoubtedly in the state of phosphate. Ammonia gave rise to a white precipitate, evidently consisting of phosphate of lime and magnesia; for, upon redissolving it in muriatic acid and precipitating the lime by oxalate of ammonia, the filtered liquor was clouded by solution of potash; and if into the ammoniacal solution thus separated from

attention. There is, I think, more to be learned of the use of blood in the animal œconomy from its coagulation than from its fluidity. The coagulation of the blood, when out of the circulation, would seem to be unconnected with life, yet life could not go on without it; for as all the solid parts of the body are formed from the blood, this could not take place if there did not exist in it the power of coagulating. Many diseases exhibit the blood coagulated in the living body, even in the vessels themselves, but more frequently when extravasated. Coagulation does not belong to the whole mass of circulating blood, but only to the part I have called coagulating lymph, which during this action commonly detaches itself from the other part, called the serum[a].

---

the phosphates, and supposed to contain the muriates of lime and magnesia, I poured oxalate of ammonia, a white granular precipitate was thrown down, consisting of oxalaet of lime, and magnesia remained in the liquor. Thus the ash resulting from the incineration of the albumen yielded carbonate of lime and magnesia, phosphate of lime and magnesia, and traces of iron."

Having established the nature of the immediate principles of the blood, and that they all exist in the serum, with the exception of the fibrin and hæmatosine, M. Le Canu next proceeded to make the complete analysis of this fluid. The process for this purpose, as improved by Dr. O'Shaughnessy, is as follows:

"Divide 1000 parts of the clot into two parts; dry one, and estimate the loss; wash the other, to ascertain the quantity of fibrin. As the water given off from the first exists therein in the state of serum, by subtracting the one proportion of solid matter (which the previous analysis of the serum has shown to be contained in 1000 parts thereof) in the interposed serum, from the weight of the dried clot, the difference affords exactly the weight of the fibrin and colouring-matter together. Subtracting again from this the weight of the fibrin, determined by another experiment, the weight of the colouring-matter is accurately obtained. Incineration, finally, of a given weight of the crassamentum gives the quantity of saline matter."—*Journ. de Pharmacie*, Sept. 1831. *O'Shaughnessy on Cholera*, Appendix, No. IV., p. 67.

The ultimate constitution of the blood, as compared with gelatine, albumen, and fibrin, is exhibited in the following table:

		Carbon.	Hydrogen.	Oxygen.	Nitrogen.
Blood.. Arterial	Macaire and Marcet.	50·2	6·6	26·3	16·3
Blood.. Venous	Macaire and Marcet.	55·7	6·4	21·7	16·2
Gelatine..........	Gay Lussac and Thenard.	47·88	7·92	27·20	16·99
Albumen.........	Gay Lussac and Thenard.	52·88	7·54	23·87	15·70
Fibrin............	Gay Lussac and Thenard.	53·36	7·02	19·68	19·93

The hæmatosine, or colouring-matter, according to Berzelius, has nearly the same composition. Gelatine is not found in the blood, nor in any glandular secretion. It contains from three to four per cent. less carbon than albumen, and is regarded by Dr. Prout as less advanced in the scale of animalization. Besides these elementary bodies may also be mentioned sulphur, phosphorus, calcium, sodium, potassium, chlorine, iron, and perhaps magnesium. Traces also of aluminium, copper, and manganese have been said to have been detected.]

[a] [This has been doubted by some physiologists, who imagine that the clot essentially consists of the central nuclei of the red globules, deprived of their external investment of colouring-matter. (*Prevost and Dumas, Ann. de Chim. et de Phys.*, xxiii. 51. *Young,*

Whether the whole mass of the serum be a distinct part of the blood when circulating is not easily determined, as we have no mode of separating it from the coagulating lymph, while both are fluid. The serum making a part of the whole mass in the fluid state, the first stage in the coagulation is a species of decomposition, forming a separation of the serum. But, on the other hand, there are reasons for considering the coagulating lymph as distinct from the serum, even when both are fluid; since the serum can be separated from the lymph without coagulating, by many actions of the vessels, both natural, preternatural, or diseased. Thus the liquor of the amnios and that of dropsies are formed; and therefore we may conclude that the separation of the serum, when the lymph is coagulated, is not an act necessary to the coagulation, but an effect of it[a].

The circumstances attending the coagulation of the lymph are sub-

---

Med. Liter.) I do not agree, however, in this opinion: first, because there is often a real separation of the coagulable lymph from the red globules previous to these losing their form, and before coagulation; and, secondly, because Professor Blumenbach was able, by the aid of a common microscope, to discover the red globules entangled in the translucent lymph, and retaining their perfect shape after coagulation. If any separation, such as has been supposed, took place of the colouring-matter from the central nuclei, the globules would not be apparent; but the whole would be obscured by a uniform solution of red colouring-matter.

That the coagulation of the blood arises from the concretion or gelatinization of the fibrin alone is rendered evident by the fact that if fresh-drawn blood be briskly stirred by a wisp, so as to remove this principle from it, the residuary liquor will not coagulate. It may perhaps seem surprising that so small a proportion of fibrin as $\frac{28}{10,000}$ should be capable of giving so great a degree of solidity to the whole mass; but in this respect it is nearly equalled by the substance called gelatine, one part of which, dissolved in 100 parts of boiling water, concretes into a solid jelly on cooling.]

[a] [Dr. B. G. Babington, in an admirable paper in the Medico-Chirurgical Transactions, vol. xvi. p. 301, has given unanswerable reasons for believing that the serum and coagulable lymph exist in the circulating blood as a homogeneous compound, and not merely in the form of mixture, as has generally been supposed. "There is no better reason," he says, "for affirming that fibrin exists in a fluid state in *liquor sanguinis* [the term applied by him to this compound] than for affirming that muriatic acid exists in a solid state in muriate of ammonia. The salt indeed is solid of which the muriatic acid forms one ingredient, but the ammonia is essential to the solidity of the compound. In like manner, the compound is fluid of which fibrin forms one ingredient, but the serum is essential to its fluidity." The compound nature of the *liquor sanguinis* is, I think, further shown from the fact that spirits of wine or turpentine does not immediately affect fresh-drawn blood, although they instantly coagulate the albumen of serum which has once separated from the clot.

In answer to the particular objection urged by our author to this view of the subject, it may be replied: 1st, that there is as much reason for believing that the fluids of dropsy, &c. are secreted as there is that they are simply exuded; for, 2nd, these fluids differ in composition from the ordinary serum of the blood; and 3rd, effusions of serum never take place without corresponding effusions of lymph, and *vice versâ*. This latter point has been particularly discussed by Dr. Babington in the paper before cited.]

ject to great varieties. These depend upon or correspond with the state of the body at the time, of which we can best judge by the readiness or difficulty with which the blood coagulates, and by the firmness or looseness of the coagulum. The whole mass of the blood being a compound, of which the parts are in some degree separated, the appearances upon coagulation are attended with still more variety than the lymph alone could exhibit, or than could occur in those animals which are not possessed of red blood, as the red part brings to view many of the changes in the lymph, by the difference of its colour, as well as of its specific gravity.

The three substances, which become visibly distinct when the lymph coagulates, differ as to gravity: the serum is the lightest, and, remaining fluid, swims upon the top; the red globules, which undergo no change, are the heaviest, and sink more or less in the lymph; but being entangled in it, add to its weight, so as to make it sink deeper in the serum[a].

Blood when extravasated coagulates sooner or later, according to the quickness or slowness of its extravasation, and the quantity extravasated: it coagulates late when drawn into a basin rapidly, and in considerable quantity; soon, when allowed to flow slowly, and in small quantities. This will be better understood when I treat of the principles of coagulation.

---

[a] [The specific gravity of the blood has been variously stated by different experimentalists. According to Davy and Scudamore, it is from 1049 to 1051; Ure makes it 1053; Prout, 1030 to 1055; Blumenbach, 1050; Haller, 1053; Fourcroy, 1056; Jurin, 1054; Henry, 1053 to 1126; Whiting, 1055; Denis, 1059; Thackrah, 1041. These differences have no doubt partly arisen from variations in the state of the system at the time the blood was taken. Brande found that the specific gravity of healthy blood occasionally rose to 1071. Blood, whether buffed or not, has generally a greater specific gravity in acute diseases than under ordinary circumstances; but the reverse obtains in diseases of debility. 1050 is the standard which will be assumed in the following notes.

The specific gravity of serum is subject to scarcely less variation than that of the blood; but I shall content myself on the present occasion with merely stating that the medium 1029·5, as mentioned by Dr. Marcet, is now generally admitted. Dr. Davy represents the specific gravity of the red globules as 1087. of the colouring-matter as 1126 to 1130, of the coagulable lymph as 1046 to 1060, and of the whole clot as 1077 to 1084. I conceive, however, in regard to this latter point, that some error must have existed in the experiments; for, as the clot floats in the serum, there cannot, it should seem, be much real difference between them: not to insist on the fact, which will afterwards be adverted to, and which Dr. Babington was the first to point out, viz. that the coagulum which results from the buffy fluid which is skimmed off from inflammatory blood is uniform in density throughout, which could not possibly happen if the fibrin were lighter or heavier than the serum. (See Babington, *Med.-Ch. Trans.*, xvi. 298, *et seq.*) This indeed is one of the arguments which the gentleman above mentioned has ingeniously employed to prove the homogeneity of the *liquor sanguinis*, as stated in the preceding note, and it must be admitted to have considerable force.]

When blood is received into a cup, and is thereby exposed, it certainly coagulates more readily than when extravasated in the cellular membrane or in the vessels; and on the exposed surface it coagulates more readily than anywhere else, except round the edges of the dish in which it is contained. It has been observed that the upper surface of the blood coagulates first, forming a thin pellicle, as milk does when near boiling, while underneath it still remains fluid; but the whole gradually becoming thicker, and losing its transparency, coagulates in about fifteen or twenty minutes into a substance of pretty thick consistence. The time required will vary according to the quantity of blood in one mass and the disposition of the blood at the time[a].

We may observe the following appearances when the blood is coagulated. The coagulum is generally, but not always, swimming in a fluid; for it sometimes happens that the lymph does not squeeze out the serum in the act of coagulation, in which there is an act of contraction. The top of the coagulum is toughest or firmest: and it becomes less and less so towards the bottom, because there is less of the coagulating lymph at the bottom, in proportion as the red globules subside in the lymph before it coagulates. The coagulating lymph has a degree of toughness in proportion as it is free from serum; for while the serum is mixed within it, though there may be no red globules, it is not very tough; but when pressed between the finger and thumb, so as to squeeze out the serum, it becomes nearly as tough and elastic as the

[a] [Coagulation commences in about three or four minutes on an average, and is completed in about ten. In about fifteen or twenty minutes the coagulum assumes a "pretty thick consistence;" but it continues still further to contract and to express the serum for at least three or four hours, and sometimes much longer. The commencement of this process and the degree in which the clot afterwards contracts are subject to be influenced by a great number of disturbing causes: as, for instance, the shape and material of the vessel, the state of the system at the time the blood is drawn, the quantity of blood collected together in one mass, the rapidity with which the effusion has taken place, the temperature of the air, the partial or complete exclusion of the atmosphere, rest, agitation, foreign substances, &c. These will be considered in the subsequent notes.

The period required for the blood of different animals to coagulate has been estimated by Thackrah to be, in general terms, inversely as the size of the animal. Thus, in the horse, coagulation commenced in from 5 to 13 minutes; in the ox, from 2 to 10; in the sheep, hog, and rabbit, from ½ to 2; in the dog, from ½ to 3; in the duck, from 1 to 2; in fowls, from ½ to 1½; in the mouse, in a moment. (*Op. cit.*, p. 154.) There is also a difference in the time required for blood to coagulate from different vessels of the same animal. Arterial blood has generally been conceived to coagulate more rapidly than venous, blood from the vena cava than blood from the jugular vein, and portal blood more readily than either. Thus, while blood from the jugular vein of a dog began to concrete in from 1¼ to 3 minutes, blood from the portal vein concreted immediately on effusion.]

coats of an artery, to appearance becoming fibrous, and even forming laminæ, and indeed appears to be very much the same kind of substance with an artery, which gives us a clear idea how a membrane may be formed, and probably can be varied, according to the impression made on it by the surrounding parts. This is one reason why the lymph, which has the strongest disposition for coagulation, is the toughest, as it parts with more of its serum. The lymph is transparent, but whether tinged as the serum is found to be we can hardly say, as it is seldom possible to catch it in a fluid state free from red globules, and never from serum, which has itself a tinge. When out of the body in a dish, where it is long in coagulating and the red globules sink fast, we find it transparent; but during coagulation it becomes more muddy, till at last it is opake, but with a tinge of colour. On being steeped in water it is often rendered very white, which would not probably be the case if it had a tinge of its own, independent of the serum.

Blood usually requires a considerable time for its complete coagulation, or rather contraction; for if allowed to stand some days, the coagulated part becomes less and less, as more and more of the serum is squeezed out, which cannot arise from the serum being lighter and issuing out spontaneously, for without some expelling force it would be retained mechanically by the capillary attraction, as in a sponge. The blood which is longest in coagulating coagulates most strongly, and produces the most complete separation of its parts. In such instances, as the coagulating lymph continues longer fluid, it allows the red globules more time to subside, and the serum to be more squeezed out from the crassamentum. When the coagulation is slow, and of that kind which will be firm when completed, we may skim off the fluid coagulating lymph, free from the red globules; and the part so taken will coagulate immediately, while that in the cup remains fluid some time longer[a].

Many causes have been assigned for the coagulation of the lymph, which appear to me to be ill founded. It frequently happens that when

---

[a] [This is not merely the coagulating lymph or fibrin, but the fibrin united to the serum, constituting the *liquor sanguinis* of Dr. Babington (See *note*, p. 21.) In itself, and in its mode of coagulation, it does not seem to differ from ordinary blood, except in containing no red globules. When transferred to a globular vessel, it separates into two parts, viz. serum and crassamentum, the coagulation taking place uniformly throughout the mass; that is, every part of the coagulum exhibits the same density, and consequently every part contains the same quantity of fibrin. Hence fibrin cannot exist in a fluid state and be lighter or heavier than the serum; for if lighter, the upper surface of the clot would be more dense than the lower, and *vice versâ* (see *note*, p. 22). Hence also the high probability that the liquor sanguinis constitutes a real homogeneous compound, and not a mere mixture of elements. According to Thackrah, more fibrin was found at the lower third of the crassamentum than at the upper,

changes take place in matter of which the immediate causes are unknown, the mind refers them to some circumstances which accompany these changes, although, perhaps, they may have had no concern whatever in producing them, and may be only attendants. This will always be the case where those changes arise out of the nature of the part itself. A seed put into moist ground grows; but the moist ground is only a necessary attendant, and not the immediate cause. The life of the seed, stimulated to action by the moisture, is the immediate cause of its growth, and it continues to grow because its action is always ex-

---

and least of all in the middle (*op. cit.*, p. 55). I apprehend, however, that the latter part of this statement tends very much to weaken our confidence in these experiments.

In regard to the duration of the contractility of the clot, Mr. Thackrah observes, that "the quantity of serum decidedly increased for three days, was nearly stationary on the fourth day, and on the fifth, sixth, seventh, and eighth progressively diminished." Hence it seems that the contractility of the clot continues for three days, during which time serum is expelled; but after that period relaxation occurs, and a part of the expressed serum is reabsorbed.

As the degree in which the clot contracts is inversely as the rapidity of the coagulation, whatever influences the coagulation of the blood so as to accelerate or retard this process will have a corresponding influence on the contraction of the clot and the relative quantity of serum which is afterwards expressed. About 10 parts serum to 13—14 crassamentum may be assumed as the standard of health; but, like the contraction of muscles after death, it varies infinitely in different cases.

Dr. Babington found the proportion of serum and crassamentum to vary materially in the same blood drawn into differently-shaped vessels. Thus, blood drawn into a pear-shaped vessel and a common basin exhibited the following differences:

	Temperature of blood.	Temperature of serum	Specific gravity of blood.	Specific gravity of serum	Crass. in pear-shaped bottle.	Crass. in basin.	To serum.
Case of Purpura	87°	65°	1050	1027	1495	2230	1000
Vertigo during pregnancy	60	60	1049	1028	945	1716	1000
Phthisis	87	60	1044	1028	960	1090	1000
Diabetes melitus	90	60	1048	1024·6	1292	1717	1000

The nearer the form of the vessel approaches that of a cube or sphere, the greater will be the proportion of serum. "This difference is owing to the greater or less distance of the coagulating particles of fibrin from a common centre, which causes a more or less powerful adhesion or contraction of these particles. Perhaps few facts relating to the phenomena of venesection are of more practical importance than this, since blood is said to be thick or thin, rich or poor, in reference to the quantity of crassamentum it contains, and views of a disease are founded upon these supposed conditions, which, after all, depend not on the blood itself, but on the vessel into which it is received" (*op. cit.*, p. 297). Thackrah found a similar diversity to arise from the composition of the recipient vessel, a circumstance which he attributed to the electric states of the different metals composing it. Thus, while one quantity of the same blood coagulated in a copper vessel in two minutes, and afforded 345·7 serum to 654·3 crass., another equal quantity coagulated in a pewter vessel in 1 min. and 10 sec., and afforded only 54·1 serum to 945·9 crass. (*op. cit.*, p. 66).]

cited. All the water in the world would not make a dead seed grow. The same mode of distinction is applicable to the coagulation of the lymph.

The first observations on the blood were most probably made on that of the more perfect animals, whose heat is commonly greater than the heat of the atmosphere. Such blood when extravasated was found to coagulate on cooling; it was therefore natural to suppose that the coagulation of the lymph arose from its becoming colder, as happens in jelly*; but cold, simply, has certainly no effect upon the coagulating lymph.

If we take a fish out of the sea, the heat of its body perhaps about 60°, and bring it into an atmosphere of 70°, the blood, on being let out of the vessels, will immediately coagulate. This was ascertained on board of a ship lying off Belleisle, in the summer 1761; for immediately upon a fish being caught, I ascertained its heat, and letting out part of its blood, it immediately coagulated, although the blood discharged was become warmer than that remaining in the vessels of the fish; which, however, still continued fluid.

Indeed, common experience and observation show us that cold alone has no power to coagulate the blood. It often happens that particular parts of an animal, such as the fingers, face, nose, ears &c., are cooled nearly to the freezing-point, and frequently are in that state for a considerable time, yet the blood retains its fluidity in those parts, as I have experienced in my own fingers; and indeed in those parts of an animal where the blood has been frozen, and again thawed, the blood appears as fluid as before, and circulates as usual. Heat has the power of exciting action in an animal, and we find that heat even increases the action of coagulation; for if blood be heated to about 120°, it will coagulate five minutes sooner than when kept at its natural heat, and even sooner than the blood of the same animal taken at the same time and cooled to 50°†. Mr. Hewson has laboured this point, endeavouring to show it is not cold that makes the blood coagulate, and he has laboured no less to show the real cause of such a change.

He took fresh blood and froze it quickly; on being thawed, it was again fluid, but soon afterwards coagulated; this he conceived to be a

* This term has been applied to the coagulation of the blood, but I think improperly; for I should only call that jelly which became solid by cold, and fluid again by heat: coagulation is totally different, for it is a new species of combination. The freezing of blood may be called congelation.

† These experiments were made on the jugular veins of dogs, by taking a section of the veins on each side filled with blood, and immersing them in water, either warmer, or colder, or of the natural heat, and observing the comparative difference.

sufficient proof that it was not cold which made the blood coagulate*.

From the above observations and experiments, it must appear that cold, simply, has no influence whatever upon the coagulation of the blood[a].

And in most of the cases in which the blood is observed to coagulate, the air is commonly in contact with it: this was next presumed to be the cause of its coagulation†. But the air has really no more effect than any other extraneous body, in contact with the blood, that is capable of making an impression upon it; for the blood coagulates more readily in a vacuum than in the open air: nor will either of these supposed causes assist in explaining why it is not found coagulated after many kinds of death, nor in the menstrual discharge. Neither will they account for the very speedy coagulation of the blood which usually takes place in all the vessels after death, or when it has been extravasated into cavities, or cellular membranes, where no air has ever been admitted[b].

* Hewson on the Blood, p. 21. † Ibid., p. 23.

---

a [Sir C. Scudamore found that cold retarded coagulation nearly in the same proportion as heat accelerated it. Blood which began to concrete in 4½ minutes in an atmosphere of 53°, underwent a similar change in 2½ minutes at 98°; and blood which coagulated in 4½ minutes at 98°, became solid in 1 minute at 120°: but blood which coagulated firmly in 5 minutes at 60°, preserved its fluidity for 20 minutes at 40°, and required upwards of a full hour for complete coagulation. Hewson had observed that if blood was kept at a temperature of 38° for 24 hours it became thick and viscid, but did not coagulate upon the return of warmth; which fact is capable of generalization, for whatever keeps the blood fluid for a considerable length of time has a tendency to deprive it of the full power of coagulation afterwards. Thackrah asserts, that blood which has once become frozen does not coagulate in any case, but only forms a grumous mass in which there is no separation of parts. (*Op. cit.*, p. 67.) A very high temperature, as 140°—150°, according to Prater, has the same effect, that is, it renders the blood incoagulable; and, what is very remarkable, dilution with water does not restore this property in one case more than in the other (*on the Blood*, p. 13.). It is sufficient at present to notice these facts, which have been considered by some to bear importantly on the question of the vitality of the blood. I may add, however, what is worthy of remark, as bearing on the same question, viz. that low temperatures, (insufficient to prevent coagulation altogether), equally diminish the contractility of the clot and of muscular fibre, while the effect of high temperatures is the very reverse. Thus animals of the order *Batrachia* immediately perish and become rigid by being immersed in water at a temperature of 108° to 120°. The muscular structures of warm-blooded animals likewise become more or less contracted by all temperatures above blood-heat.]

b [Hewson merely contended that air promoted coagulation, not that air was essential to the process. It must be confessed, however, that his expressions are sometimes equivocal, as at p. 123, Vol. I., and in some other parts of his Inquiry.

Scudamore took two portions of blood from a man slightly indisposed, and placed one of them under the receiver of an air-pump and allowed the other to be exposed in the open apartment. The former cooled in five minutes from 84° to 75°; the latter from

Rest is another cause upon which the coagulation of the blood has been said to depend; and although this opinion be not true in the full

---

84° to 82·5° The former, however, was much the most coagulated of the two at the end of this period; although, as we have before shown, cold retards the coagulatory process. But if blood be received into a close vessel, so as completely to fill it, and care at the same time be taken to exclude it from the contact of the atmosphere, the process will be considerably retarded.

To account for this apparent anomaly, Scudamore not only attempted to prove that carbonic acid is extricated from the blood during coagulation, and that the time required for the concretory process in great measure depends on the quick or slow extrication of this gas, but that its evolution is "an essential circumstance" in this process. (*Op. cit.*, p. 103.)

With respect to the fact on which this explanation turns, viz. the extrication of carbonic acid gas, nothing can be more discordant than the results of experimentalists. One party, as Vogel, Scudamore, Brande, &c. (*Ann. de Chimie*, tom. xciii. *Essay on the Blood*, p. 28. *Phil. Trans.* 1818, p. 181.), affirming its existence in arterial and venous blood alike in considerable quantities. Another, as Clanny, Prout, and Stevens, (*Edin. Med. and Surg. Journ.*, xxxii. 40. *Bridgewater Treatise*, p. 524. *Observations on the Blood*, p. 21.) that it exists in venous blood only; and a third, as Davy, Thackrah, and a number of others, (*Edin. Med. and Surg. Journ.*, xxix. 254. *Enquiry into the Blood*, p. 63.) that it has no existence in either. But this question has lately been investigated and set at rest by Mr. Squire of Oxford-street; who, by a series of accurate and ingenious experiments, has succeeded in obtaining notable quantities of carbonic acid from *venous* blood, when, from the nature of the apparatus which was employed, it was impossible that any portion of the gas so obtained could have been derived from the atmosphere. It has been urged, indeed, that the alkalinity of the blood is inconsistent with the admission of this fact; but Dr. Davy has shown that the admixture of a fourth part of an inch of carbonic acid to an ounce of fresh blood did not destroy its alkaline properties. (*Edin. Med. and Surg. Journ.*, xxix. 254.)

Admitting, therefore, the fact of the presence of carbonic acid in the blood, the question arises how far the escape of this gas affords a reasonable explanation of the cause of coagulation. Now it must be apparent that the coagulation and non-coagulation of the blood under circumstances not at all connected with the escape of carbonic acid is a sufficient answer to this question; for if coagulation can take place in the interior of the body, where no gas can escape, or be prevented from taking place when effused from the body by the mere circumstance of cold, it is evident that the extrication of carbonic acid is not necessary for this process. Still the experiments which have been referred to render it extremely probable that coagulation *in vacuo* is accelerated by the free escape of carbonic acid, and that atmospheric air, in addition to its action as a foreign body, promotes coagulation by promoting the escape of carbonic acid.

Majendie has observed (*Phys.*, 4eme edit., Brux., p. 306.) that enormous quantities of atmospheric air may slowly be injected into the veins of an animal without producing any inconvenience, or without imparting to the blood any tendency to coagulation; but Hewson found that blood confined within a living vessel by two ligatures remained two thirds fluid for 3¼ hours, although it coagulated in fifteen minutes when air was blown into the vessel. Hence there would appear to be a difference in regard to the effects of atmospheric air, according as the blood happens to be at rest or in motion in the vessels.

As to the effect of gases generally on coagulation, Sir H. Davy has informed us that he could discover no difference in the time required for coagulation when blood was exposed to nitrogen, oxygen, nitrous oxide, carbonic acid, hydro-carbon, or atmospheric air. (*Researches on Nitrous Oxide*, p. 380.) Nitrous oxide injected into the veins con-

extent in which it has been taken, I think that rest has greater influence in the change than any other circumstance whatever. But though rest seems greatly to dispose the blood to coagulation, it is the operation of rest alone, without exposure, which we are to consider; as otherwise we shall be apt to confound it with the two foregoing causes, viz. cold, and the contact of air[a].

---

verts the blood to a chocolate brown colour, and destroys its coagulating power. Sulphuretted hydrogen has the same effect, and renders it viscid and greenish. Carbonic oxide gives it a brownish tint. (*Christison on Poisons*, p. 691 *et seq.*) When the experiment of breathing pure oxygen is kept up for some time, or until the animal dies, the blood in the veins is found to present the same florid hue as that in the arteries, and to coagulate with remarkable rapidity. (*Broughton in Lond. Quart. Journ. of Sc.* 1830.) For the effect of other gases on the blood the reader is referred to the able work of Dr. Christison above cited, to the *Recherches Chim.-Phys.* of Nysten, and to Thenard's *Sys. de Chim.*, iii. 513.]

[a] [The question which will here be considered is rest or stagnation of the blood within the vessels or living textures of the body.

In the preceding note I have adverted to the experiments of Hewson as to the effect of rest combined with the insufflation of air into the living vessels. Mr. Thackrah (*op. cit.*, p. 76.) repeated and varied these experiments in the following manner. By means of double ligatures he secured the jugular veins of two rabbits and two dogs, and examined the state of the blood at different intervals. In the veins of the two rabbits the blood was perfectly fluid after 45 minutes; and in the veins of the two dogs it was perfectly fluid after 60 minutes in one case and 20 minutes in the other. Sir Astley Cooper performed similar experiments on dogs, and found the blood perfectly fluid after three hours; although by varying the form of the experiment and allowing the blood to flow into a portion of vessel unequivocally dead, the blood was found to be perfectly coagulated in 15 minutes. The blood in the heart and vessels of struck cattle is commonly fluid for half an hour or upwards after the apparent death of the animal; although if it be effused from the vessels during any part of this interval, it speedily coagulates. In the same manner extensive extravasations of blood into the cellular membrane or into the tunica vaginalis testis remain fluid for weeks or even months, notwithstanding that the same blood when let out readily coagulates. Thus also Mr. Hunter found the blood in the stomach and intestines of a leech still fluid ten weeks after it had been sucked.

It must be evident, therefore, that some other principle is concerned in keeping the blood fluid in these cases besides motion, which principle must previously be ascertained before we can determine anything concerning the effects which are due to mere rest. This principle I believe to be the vitality of the vessels, which maintains the blood in a fluid state, and counteracts its coagulating tendency in exact proportion to the energy of the system at the time, or the tonic powers of the vessels. In proof of this I shall offer the following arguments in corroboration of those which have preceded. 1st, It is well known that struck cattle retain a residual vitality in their muscles for some hours after apparent death; consequently it is not surprising, upon the hypothesis, that the blood should preserve a fluid state in virtue of a like residual vitality in the vessels. 2nd, If a leech die soon after it has fallen off, the blood in its body will be found coagulated. 3rd, In asphyxia, syncope, and other cases in which the system is depressed, the blood coagulates rapidly as contrasted with those cases in which the energies of the system are in full vigour, as in inflammatory fever. 5th, Upon the same principle, the

Since, therefore, the blood may coagulate in the vessels either of a living or a dead body, and since it coagulates when extravasated into different parts of a living body, rest, like cold or air, might be supposed to be the sole cause of the coagulation of the blood: yet it is not rest considered simply, but rest under certain circumstances, which appears to possess such a power; for motion given to the blood, out of the vessels, will not of itself prevent its coagulation; nor will it even in the vessels themselves, if all the purposes of motion are not answered by it. Motion seems to retard coagulation*[a]; yet we know for certain that

* This is motion given to it in a vessel, without any empty space, and having beads put into it, which are shaken.

---

second and third cups of blood in a common venesection coagulate more rapidly than the first; but if the blood be taken in the commencement of an inflammatory attack, while the system still labours under oppression, the first cup will coagulate more rapidly than the second. In the same manner, blood from the extreme parts of the body coagulates more rapidly than that which is near the source of circulation. 6th, Fontana found that although the poison of a viper had no effect on extravasated blood, it immediately promoted coagulation when it was injected into the veins. 7th, The blood coagulates in mortified limbs, and in the capillaries of inflamed parts.

The following, however, are supposed to be proofs that rest, even in the living vessels, promotes the coagulation of the blood. Kellie remarked that blood which had been mechanically impeded by the tourniquet speedily coagulated. The formation of coagula in the cavities of the heart and great veins during life is by no means of unfrequent occurrence, and is generally found to be preceded by some obstruction in the circulation, accompanied with a depressed state of the vital powers. (*Bright's Medical Reports*, ii. 63. *Andral's Précis de Pathologie*, ii. 340.) Fibrinous vegetations about the valves of the heart in diseases of that organ, the formation of coagula in aneurismal sacs, the concretion of fibrinous clots in vessels which have been secured by ligature, and the coagulation of blood which has been effused into the interstices of the cellular membrane, are all evidences of the same nature. It must not be forgotten, however, that in all these cases the blood is placed under very different conditions to those which exist in a normal state, in as much as either the system or the parts which contain the blood are diseased, and consequently not possessed of a full power of life. Hence the great difficulty of assigning the real share which rest has in producing coagulation in these cases; for the effects which seem to arise from mere rest may in fact arise from the diminished vitality of the vessels. "It is not rest considered simply, but rest under certain circumstances, which appears to possess such a power;" but when we reflect further that rest out of body has a contrary effect (see next note) we may, I think, "conclude," with Hunter, "that rest does not of itself in the least assist the coagulation of the blood." It is difficult to conceive that rest can have opposite effects on the blood in and out of the vessels.]

[a] [When blood is briskly stirred or shaken immediately on its effusion, it retains a homogeneous character, and apparently loses its coagulating properties: but this appear ance is fallacious; for if blood thus treated be placed on a filter, the fibrin will become apparent. It has, in fact, assumed the solid form; but being in a state of minute division, it is diffused through the turbid liquor, and thus escapes observation. (*Davy in Edin. Med. and Surg. Journ.*, xxix. 244.) Indeed it is very probable that coagulation is really accelerated in such cases, just as it is by a more moderate agitation. To prove the latter point, three portions of blood being taken; the first and third were moderately

blood will in time coagulate even in the vessels themselves, and under certain circumstances sooner, perhaps, than anywhere else: as, for instance, when there is a disposition to mortification. In this case we find the blood coagulated even in the larger vessels. I have seen a mortification come on the foot and leg, and when it had advanced only to a certain degree, the patient died. On examining the parts above the mortified part, I found the crural and iliac arteries filled completely with strong coagulated blood: we may thence infer that the tendency to mortification in the vessels produced this disposition in the blood. If the coagulation should be supposed to have arisen from the blood being stopped in the large vessels at the mortified part, let us reflect that this cannot account for it: the same thing ought then to happen in an amputation, or in any case where the larger vessels are tied up.

In a priapism the blood does not coagulate, except it threatens mortification.

The separation of the blood, either from itself, that is when divided into small portions, or separated from the living body, becomes one of the immediate causes of the coagulation of the lymph; therefore the contact of blood with blood, or with living vessels, in some degree retards coagulation: this is the reason why blood which comes from the vessels slowly, or falls from some height, or runs some way on the surface of a dish, coagulates sooner than when the contrary circumstances happen; and upon this principle it is, that blood when shaken in a phial will coagulate the sooner, even if shaken in a vacuum. A deep mass of blood is also, from the same cause, longer in coagulating than a shallow one.

From the above observations it must appear evident that neither cold, nor air, nor rest, alone, has any influence on the coagulating power of the blood; there must, therefore, be some other principle on which this process depends; and, as it retains its fluid state while circulating, and even for a long time when at rest in the living vessels, and coagulates when the vessels or the body dies, it might naturally be supposed that

---

stirred with a stick for two minutes, while the second was allowed to rest. The two former concreted in 3½ to 4 minutes, the latter or second portion did not concrete till 6 minutes, and at the end of eight minutes the coagulum was much less firm than that of the other two. (*Thackrah*, p. 68.) Scudamore observed a difference of one minute. (*Op. cit.*, p. 40.) Prater observed a difference, but it was not so considerable. (*Op. cit.*, p. 18.) It should be noticed, however, that these experiments were made in open vessels, while those which were made in close vessels were much less decisive. Agitation promotes coagulation by bringing the interior particles of the mass into contact with the sides of the inert vessel, which will necessarily have the effect of rapidly dissipating its residual vitality. It is on the same principle, that a small portion of crassamentum dropped into fresh-drawn blood accelerates coagulation.]

it was the life of the body or vessels which kept it fluid; we know, however, that life in the body or vessels does not hinder the blood from coagulating under certain circumstances, but often rather excites coagulation. Nor does death, in the body or vessels, in all cases become a cause of coagulation; for we find that in many who die suddenly from a strong impression of the mind, the blood does not coagulate; there is, therefore, something more than the mere situation of the blood, surrounded with dead parts, that allows of coagulation; and that must be a something in the blood itself.

From these observations it must be evident that the fluid state of the blood is connected with the living vessels, which is its natural situation, and with motion; and that where there is a full power of life, the vessels are capable of keeping the blood in a fluid state. I believe, however, very little motion is required to keep up this fluidity when the other is present. A total stagnation of the blood while the body is alive, as in a trance, or where the circulation has been stopped for several hours, as in the case of persons apparently drowned[a], does not make it coagulate; yet where there are no actions going on in a part, if the blood stagnates for a much shorter time than in a trance, it will be found coagulated, as in mortifications; but then this coagulation is to answer a good purpose, and arises from necessity*, which appears to act as a stimulus in disposing the blood to coagulate.

As a proof that blood will not coagulate in living vessels, in a perfect and natural state, and ready to act when powers were restored to it, I found that the blood of a fish, which had the actions of life stopped for three days, and was supposed to be dead, did not coagulate in the vessels; but, upon being exposed or extravasated, soon coagulated.

The blood of a lamprey-eel, which had been dead to appearance some days, was found fluid in the vessels, because the animal was not really dead; there had, however, been no motion in the blood, as the heart

* By action taking place from necessity, effects are meant which arise in consequence of some unusual or unnatural change going on in the parts, which becomes a stimulus to action. The stimuli, from this cause, may vary exceedingly among themselves; but as we are unable to investigate them, I have included them under this general term, stimulus of necessity. (See note, Vol. I. p. 236, and Index, art. *Stimulus*.)

---

[a] [It is difficult to reconcile the results of physiological experiment with the accounts which have been given of recoveries from protracted asphyxia. It is extremely doubtful, under the most favourable circumstances, whether in drowning the heart ever continues to pulsate for so long a period as five minutes after the cessation of respiration, or whether, having stopped its actions, it can ever be renewed. In trances also and the ordinary forms of syncope it is questionable whether the functions of respiration and circulation are ever wholly arrested. The statements which have been made on these subjects are certainly without foundation, and no better than extravagant fables.]

had ceased acting; but upon its being exposed, and extravasated into water, it soon coagulated*: yet, under certain circumstances in life, it has been observed that the blood will in a small degree coagulate: this is in the state of torpor. It is asserted by some author, whom I now do not recollect, that the blood of a bat coagulates when in that state; and Mr. Cornish, (surgeon, at Totnes, in Devonshire,) to whom I applied for some bats in the torpid state, sent me them, but in the carriage they always died: however, he took opportunities of examining them, and he found that the blood was in a certain degree coagulated; but it soon recovered its fluidity on motion and heat[a].

From these remarks, I should conclude that rest does not of itself in the least assist the coagulation of the blood, but that this effect arises from the blood being separated from the living vessels, and being deprived of motion; and that it happens sooner or later, according to other circumstances. It might be supposed that these are rather negative causes of coagulation than positive ones; but it is to be considered, that in a living body the cessation of a natural action, the absence of an usual impression becomes a cause of action, of which innumerable instances may be given.

I have now considered the circumstances under which the blood coagulates, and shown that none of them alone, nor all them combined, induce the blood to coagulate. My opinion is, that it coagulates from an impression; that is, its fluidity under such circumstances being improper, or no longer necessary, it coagulates to answer now the necessary purpose of solidity. This power seems to be influenced in a way in some degree similar to muscular action, though probably not entirely

* There are some circumstances which hinder the coagulation of blood in living bodies, although extravasated. Two leeches had been applied, and had sucked till full. These were preserved for ten weeks, and then contained considerable quantity of blood, which appeared like that recently drawn from a vein, and coagulated when exposed. I have known, in tapping a hydrocele, that a small vessel has been wounded, and the blood, as it extravasated, got into the sac, and when tapped sixty-five days after, the blood has come out thickish; but when extracted it coagulated, and separated into different parts[b].

---

[a] [I am informed by Dr. Marshall Hall, that in his experiments on hybernating animals, he found the blood quite as fluid as under ordinary circumstances. This is not different from what might have been expected; for notwithstanding that the respiration is almost wholly, if not entirely, suspended during the state of hybernation, the heart still continues to beat, and to circulate black blood, at the rate of twenty-eight strokes in a minute. (*Hall* in *Phil. Trans.* 1834.)]

[b] [A sanguineous tumour of the leg, which had existed upwards of eight months, and was supposed to be a chronic abscess, was punctured by Mr. Cæsar Hawkins, at St. George's Hospital, in the course of the last year (1834), and about five ounces of fluid blood discharged, which immediately coagulated.]

of that kind; for I have reason to believe that blood has the power of action within itself, according to the stimulus of necessity, which necessity arises out of its situation.

I shall now consider the simple act of coagulation, abstracted from causes.

Coagulation I conceive to be an operation of life; and I imagine it to proceed exactly upon the same principle as the union by the first intention; it is particle uniting with particle, by the attraction of cohesion, which, in the blood, forms a solid; and it is this coagulum, uniting with the surrounding parts, which forms the union by the first intention; for union by the first intention is no more than the living parts when separated, whether naturally or by art, forming a reciprocal attraction of cohesion with the intermediate coagulum, which immediately admits of mutual intercourse, and, as it were, one interest.

To produce coagulation of the blood, however, something more is required than merely the reverse of the causes above mentioned, as having the power to keep it fluid; for the blood becomes in many cases instantaneously incapable of coagulation, either in or out of the vessels, even when nothing has been added or taken away, and must be therefore under the influence of some other cause. This, I believe, must be sought in some property inherent in the blood itself: besides, some natural operations destroy this principle in the blood when extravasated.

In many modes of destroying life the blood is deprived of its power of coagulation, as happens in sudden death produced by many kinds of fits, by anger, electricity, or lightning[a]; or by a blow on the stomach, &c. In these cases we find the blood, after death, not only in as fluid a state as in the living vessels, but it does not even coagulate when taken out of them. As in the bodies of such persons no action of life takes place, the muscles do not contract. There are partial influences likewise which destroy the power of coagulation, as a blow on a part producing a considerable extravasation. This forms an ecchymosis, in which we shall often find the blood not in the least coagulated. In healthy menstruation the blood which is discharged does not coagulate;

---

[a] [Although this statement has been impugned by Sir C. Scudamore (*op. cit.*, p. 54.), yet general testimony has evinced the accuracy of Mr. Hunter's observation. Scudamore found that the blood coagulated as usual in animals which had been killed by the discharge of an electric battery. It is worthy of remark, that electricity and galvanism rather accelerate coagulation out of the body, and also occasion a sensible elevation of temperature.

Mayo has observed, that when any accidental extravasation happens in a person that has been hanged, the blood speedily coagulates (*Physiology*, 3rd edit. p. 26); but Thackrah has carried the observation still further, and affirmed that such is generally the case in all instances of violent death. (*Op. cit.*, p. 168.)]

in the irregular or unhealthy it does. The healthy menses, therefore, show a peculiar action of the constitution; and it is most probably in this action that their salubrious purposes consist; for if twice the usual quantity is evacuated, with the power of coagulation, even from the same vessels, the same benefit is not produced, much less when taken away from another part by art[a].

Many substances, when mixed with the blood, prevent coagulation; bile has this effect out of the body; but we cannot suppose that in a living body it can be taken into the blood in such quantity as to produce this effect; for we find in a very severe jaundice that the blood is still capable of coagulating strongly.

That probably every inanimate fluid in nature, which is capable of being rendered solid, produces heat during that change, and in the contrary change cold, is commonly known. It is on this principle that Dr. Black has established his very ingenious theory of latent heat. Thus, in the freezing of water heat is produced.

To see how far the coagulation of the blood was similar in this respect to the same change in other substances, I first coagulated the white of an egg, by applying to it rectified spirits of wine: the heat of both was the same before their union; but I found, upon uniting them, that the white of the egg was immediately coagulated, and that the heat of the mixture was increased four, sometimes five degrees, according as it coagulated slowly or quickly[b].

As the blood in the animals upon which we most commonly make our experiments is warm, it becomes a difficult matter to ascertain whether it produces heat upon coagulation. In holding the ball of the thermometer in the stream of blood coming from the arm, I found the heat raised to 92°: I then took a cup of human blood, allowed it to coagulate, and put it up to the brim in water warmed to 92°, till the whole mass was heated to this point. I bled afterwards another person to the same quantity, in a similar cup, which was put into the same water. Having two well-regulated thermometers, one in each cup of blood, I observed which cooled first, for I did not expect so much heat to be produced in the second as to make it warmer, but conceived, if any heat

[a] [The healthy menstrual discharge, which is probably a true secretion, does not coagulate, because it contains no globules or fibrin. Brande found that "it had the properties of a very concentrated solution of the colouring matter of the blood in a diluted serum." (*Phil. Trans.* 1812, p. 113.) Unhealthy menstruation is attended with actual hæmorrhage.]

[b] [The disengagement of caloric in this case is to be ascribed to the union of the water contained in the albumen with the spirits of wine, and the consequent condensation which takes place. Albumen coagulated by dilute nitric acid does not evolve any heat.]

was formed, it would retard the cooling of the fresh blood; but it rather cooled faster, which I imputed to the coagulated blood parting with its heat slower than the fluid blood. These experiments I have repeated several times, with nearly the same effect. I then conceived the experiment would be more conclusive if I could get blood in a fluid state which was naturally of the heat of the atmosphere, for which purpose I took the blood of turtles.

A healthy turtle was kept in a room all night, the floor of which was about 64° and the atmosphere 65° In the morning the heat was nearly the same. The thermometer was introduced into the anus, and the heat of that part was 64°. The animal being suspended by the hind legs, the head was cut off at once, and the blood caught in a bason; the blood while flowing was 65°, and when collected was 66°, but fell to 65° while coagulating, which it did very slowly: it remained at 65°, and when coagulated was still 65°. These experiments had been made several times, but not with that nice accuracy which was obtained by causing all the heats to correspond exactly; yet, as they were all known and marked down, if any heat had been produced upon coagulation its exact quantity would have been ascertained in each; and, indeed, in some it seemed to cool, but in none it became warmer. From these experiments, I should say that in the coagulation of the blood no heat is formed[a].

Coagulated blood is an inorganized animal substance. When the blood is thinly spread before coagulation, or oozes out on surfaces, (in which act it immediately coagulates,) and coagulates in that form, it may then be said to form an inorganized membrane, of which there are many; and organization is seemingly so simple in many (which we

---

[a] [The change in the capacity of bodies for heat depends on the change of their densities; but no change takes place in the sum of the densities of the constituents of the blood during, or as the effect of, coagulation, for what the fibrin gains in specific weight is exactly balanced by what is lost by the serum; and were this otherwise, we should still not expect any appreciable degree of heat to be evolved, when we reflect on the extremely small proportion which the fibrin bears to the whole mass of the blood, and that it is this principle alone which undergoes coagulation. The opinion in the text has, nevertheless, been controverted by several experimentalists. Fourcroy, in one instance, observed the heat to rise during coagulation from 20° to 25° Cent., or nearly 11° Fahr. (*Ann. de Chimie*, vii. 147.) Dr. Gordon also, in some experiments, estimated the rise to be as much as from 6° to 12°. (*Ann. of Phil.*, iv. 139.) And Dr. Scudamore was led to a similar conclusion, viz. "that a slight evolution of heat takes place during the coagulation of the blood." (*Op. cit.*, p. 75.) I am of opinion, however, that the experiments of Davy on the blood of sharks and turtles, and those of Thackrah on warm-blooded animals, are more to be depended on, and these fully confirm the accuracy of Mr. Hunter's observations. (*Thackrah*, p. 60.) Raspail has even gone into the opposite opinion, and imagined that the temperature of the blood is actually reduced by the act of coagulation. (*Syst. Chim. Org.*, p. 361.)]

know to be constituent parts of the body), that these coagula, more especially the thin ones, cannot easily by their appearances be distinguished from them.

The coagulating lymph of the blood being common probably to all animals, while the red particles are not, we must suppose it from this alone to be the most essential part; and as we find it capable of undergoing, in certain circumstances, spontaneous changes, which are necessary to the growth, continuance, and preservation of the animal, while to the other parts we cannot assign any such uses, we have still more reason to suppose it the most essential part of the blood in every animal[a].

---

[a] [There seems good reason for this opinion, and yet Fourcroy was unable to detect any fibrin in the blood of the fœtus; an observation which has since been repeated by different experimentalists, and confirmed by the statement of Bichat, that fœtal blood does not coagulate.

Dr. Grant has stated that the proportion of fibrin in the blood of the less perfect animals is considerably smaller than that which exists in the higher classes.

Davy, Thackrah, and Scudamore found that the proportion of fibrin was relatively increased during inflammation. Scudamore even found that it varied during the same venesection. "In one instance," he says, "I found the proportion in the first cup for 1000 grains of clot twelve grains, and in the last cup not quite six grains: the highest proportion that I have found in healthy blood has been, for 1000 grains of clot, 4·43 of fibrin. It is in the inflammation of the fibrous textures of the body that the greatest quantity of fibrin is found in the blood; for example, in inflammation of the heart, when the blood is drawn we meet with the strongest example of the buffy coat; and next, probably, in pleurisy and acute rheumatism." (*Op. cit.*, p. 119.) Mr. Thackrah found that this variation in the relative proportions of the constituents of the blood during the same venesection was not confined to the fibrin, but was equally applicable to the serum and hæmatosine. (*Op. cit.*, pp. 146, 209.) It is remarkable, however, that the increase of fibrin, which is observable both in inflammation and in breeding animals, is uniformly found to take place at the expense of the albumen of the serum, from which it may be inferred that the former is formed out of the latter, or is in fact in a higher and more perfect state of animalization, a view of the case which is still further corroborated from the fact of its containing more nitrogen.

The generality of modern chemists have been disposed to regard the fibrin, albumen, and hæmatosine of the blood as modifications of the same animal principle. In its coagulated state, the chemical relations of albumen are undoubtedly closely allied to those of fibrin, so as with difficulty to be distinguished from them: still there are certain well-marked differences which distinguish these substances; as, for instance, albumen contains less nitrogen than fibrin; it is soluble in water at common temperatures; it undergoes coagulation at a temperature of 160°, and it is also coagulated by all the mineral acids. Whether these points of dissimilarity are sufficient to characterize it as a distinct and separate organic principle, I shall not pretend to decide. I will only observe, that in deciding this question it would be right to reflect that the doctrine of definite proportionals does not obtain, in regard to organic principles, in the same manner or to the same extent as it does with respect to inorganic compounds, so that the former class of bodies are far less distinctly characterized in general than the latter, and pass, by a series of easy transitions, from one into the other, so as often to be convertible. It signifies, however, very little in fact whether we regard the fibrin, albumen,

Besides a disposition for coagulation under certain circumstances, as before described, the blood has also a disposition for the separation of the red globules, and probably of all its parts; for I think I have reason to believe that a disposition for coagulation, and a disposition for a separation of the red part, are not the same thing, but arise from two different principles. Indeed, a disposition to coagulation would counteract the effect, and hinder the separation of the red particles from taking place. Thus we see that rest, or slow motion of the blood in the vessels, gives a disposition towards the separation of the red part, as well as when it is extravasated; since the blood in the veins of an animal acquires a disposition to separate its red parts more than in the arteries, especially if it be retarded in the veins; the nearer, therefore, to the heart in the veins the greater will the disposition for separation be; though it does not seem to retard coagulation. This is always observable in bleeding; for if we tie up an arm, and do not bleed immediately, the first blood that flows from the orifice, or that which has stagnated for some time in the veins, will soonest separate into its three constituent parts: this circumstance exposes more of the coagulating lymph at the top, which is supposed by the ignorant to indicate more inflammation, while the next quantity taken suspends its red parts in the lymph, and gives the idea that the first small quantity had been of such service at the time of its flowing as to have altered for the better the whole mass of blood. Rest, therefore, may be regarded as one of the immediate causes of the separation[a].

---

and hæmatosine as distinct and separate principles or merely as modifications of the same principle. There can be little doubt that the offices which they fulfil in the œconomy are perfectly distinct, and therefore it is probable that the substances themselves are so.

In order to explain the variations above mentioned in the constitution of the blood during one and the same venesection, we have only to remember the extraordinary rapidity of the circulatory, secretory and absorbent functions. A solution of prussiate of potash introduced into the jugular vein of a horse was detected by the appropriate test in the opposite jugular vein in from twenty to thirty seconds, and in the serous cavities of the pericardium and pleura in from two to six minutes; and if we may be allowed to judge from the effects of poisons, or from the rapid manner in which enormous ascitic collections are sometimes suddenly dispersed, the rapidity of the action of the absorbents would appear to exceed even that of the secretories. (*Hering* in *Med. Gazette*, xiv. 745.) From these sources it is not difficult to account for the change in quality which the blood undergoes during venesection, which ordinarily occupies from two to five minutes. The first portions of blood which pass are abstracted under natural circumstances; but the new impression which is thus produced on the constitution by the first loss of blood, may easily affect the residual mass; 1st, through the medium of the absorbents; 2nd, through the secretory vessels, which rapidly take up the fluid parts of the body, and convey them into the circulation.]

[a] [*Buffy Blood.*—The reason why more buff appears in the first than in the second quantity of blood (a fact which is by no means universal,) will be intelligible from what

§.3. *Of the Serum.*

The serum is the second part of which the whole mass of blood appears to be composed, or is one of those substances into which the

---

has been said in the preceding note respecting the superabundance of fibrin in inflammatory blood, as well as from the circumstance that the first portions of blood are generally slowest in coagulating, by which a greater time is allowed for the red globules to subside. It is not difficult, however, to prove that an increased disposition to separate must also exist in the red globules, and aid in producing the buffy crust. Take, for example, blood from a patient labouring under acute rheumatism, and set it aside; in less than thirty seconds the surface will be covered with a bluish transparent lymph, although no traces of coagulation will be apparent for several minutes afterwards. Thus Hewson found that of two portions of the same blood, one afforded a buffy crust, and the other none, although the latter remained fluid full ten minutes after the buffy coat had begun to be formed on the former (*Exp. Enq.*, p. 90). I think, therefore, it must be apparent that the buffy coat of blood undoubtedly depends on thesé three circumstances acting conjointly, viz. the increased quantity of fibrin, the slowness of the coagulation, and the increased tendency to separation.

Dr. Davy (*Edinb. Med. Surg. Journ.*, xxix.) and Dr. Stoker (*Pathol. Observ.*, p. 37.) have irrefragably proved that mere slowness of coagulation is not alone a sufficient cause to account for this phenomenon. The latter has furnished twenty-seven experiments, in fifteen of which buff was formed, and in the other twelve it was not. In the former coagulation was never delayed beyond fourteen minutes, and in all but three it took place in less than five minutes. Out of the latter there were four instances in which coagulation was delayed eight, and three in which it did not take place in less than from twenty to forty minutes; the real cause, therefore, of the buffiness in the former instances was certainly not the slowness of coagulation: yet slowness of coagulation has a very marked effect in increasing the quantity of buff; for if blood be drawn from a small orifice into a shallow vessel, the quantity of buff will be infinitely less than if it is drawn from a large orifice into a deep vessel; the difference in these cases depending in great measure on the more rapid manner in which the blood coagulates in one case than it does in the other. For the same reason Dr. Babington (*Med.-Chir. Tr.*, xvi. 298.) found that when blood was drawn into two vessels, one empty and the other half-filled with olive oil, the buffy crust which formed under the oil was twice or thrice as thick as that which formed in the empty jar. Nay, the same author has even gone so far as to affirm that healthy blood placed under these conditions will sometimes exhibit a buffy surface.

I may also advert to one other circumstance, which is, that the quantity of buff will be greatly influenced by the shape of the vessel into which the blood is received, for it must be evident that the space left by the gravitation of the red particles will bear a proportion to the whole perpendicular depth of the blood, and consequently be much greater in one case than in another, although the same blood be employed. This circumstance is frequently overlooked in judging of the degree of inflammation from the appearance of the blood previously abstracted.

To account for the buffy coat, it has been imagined that the fibrin of the blood becomes specifically lighter, or the red globules specifically heavier than usual; but nothing has been offered in the shape of proof for either of these statements. Hey attributed the sizy crust to a more intimate admixture of the constituent parts of the blood; and

blood spontaneously separates itself. So far it appears as a simple fluid, in which light I shall first consider it; though we shall find

Hewson to the greater tenuity of this fluid; but both of these opinions are directly contradicted by experience, for nothing can be more clear than that there exists in the blood a greater disposition to separate into its component parts in inflammation than in a healthy state, while nothing has been more clearly proved than that the specific gravity of the whole blood is increased under the same circumstances, at the same time that the fibrin and albumen are separately and collectively in greater relative proportions than in a state of health. (*Thackrah*, pp. 206–212.) Rapidity of circulation is another cause which has been adduced in explanation of this phenomenon; but rapidity of circulation does not necessarily precede a sizy state of the blood, nor would it, if it did, throw any light on the proximate cause of this appearance.

The question now naturally occurs, Does the buffy crust consist of the original fibrin of the blood, or of the fibrin of the blood modified by disease, or of altogether a new substance? I think there can be no doubt that it consists of the fibrin of the blood deprived of the red globules, that is, of a net-work of fibrin containing a more or less considerable portion of serum. It is difficult to imagine that this substance has not undergone some modification from disease; for although the fibrin thus obtained does not chemically differ from ordinary fibrin, yet it is firmer, denser, more contractile, and more like an ordinary membrane than the fibrin of healthy blood; physiologically speaking, therefore, it has undergone some modification. It would also appear from the researches of Trail, Gendrin, and Dowler, that the serum which is interposed in its meshes is more charged with albumen than the rest of the serum, although this statement has been denied by Thackrah. The ratio of solid and liquid elements in the buffy crust varies considerably in different cases, but in general there is more fibrin and less serum than in the ordinary crassamentum of healthy blood. The cases in which the buffy coat is most strikingly exhibited are those of rheumatic inflammation, and inflammation of serous and fibrous structures. The quantity of buff present may generally be considered as an index to the strength of the constitution and the acuteness of the disease conjointly; but this is not universally the case, for the blood is very often found to be buffed in scurvy and diabetes as well as in the latter stages of phthisis and acute diseases, so that this circumstance taken singly is an extremely unsafe guide to act on. On the other hand, it is found deficient in children, and has rarely been observed to form in arterial blood, or blood abstracted by cupping. It is also very often found to be wanting in plethoric people; in cases of smallpox previous to the appearance of the eruption; in violent and extensive inflammation, involving several textures of the body at the same time, and running into rapid suppuration; in diffuse inflammation of the cellular membrane; in inflammation of mucous membranes; in the first attack of the endemic and common remittent fevers of hot climates: "Imo in morbis maxime inflammatoriis, in nullo sanguine, quotiescunque misso, aliquoties crusta ulla est." (*De Haen, Rat. Med.*, iii. c. 2.) Under these circumstances it must be apparent that the mere absence or presence of buff is no sure indication in practice, but must be judged of, like other symptoms, from concurrent circumstances.

Mr. Vines (*Lancet*, xi. 294.) has stated a very extraordinary fact relating to this subject. Asses, he says, that feed on hay and live in the open air at a temperature of 45°–55° exhibit a buffy crust, which disappears as soon as the temperature is raised to 60° or depressed to 35°. Also that if an animal in health, his blood being buffy, be made to undergo moderate exercise, it will become wholly red, and will continue so for some hours afterwards. But when the circulation becomes tranquil, it will again put on the buffy appearance. If the exertion, however, be continued to an immoderate degree, the blood becomes again buffy. The fact of excessive exercise rendering the blood buffy,

hereafter that it is composed of two substances, which in many of our experiments separate. Serum, I believe, is common to the

---

although it has been disputed by some, is now generally admitted. Horses, after a full gallop, have often been observed to have buffy blood.

Dr. Todd and Dr. Stoker of Dublin conceive that the colour and figure of the buff may point out the seat of the inflammation; but this is very questionable: others, again, have affirmed that they could distinguish buffy blood from the mere colour of the stream as it flowed from the vein.

I intimated in the preceding note that the origin of the buffy crust is probably to be sought for in the conversion of the albumen into fibrin. The final intention of this provision obviously is, to answer the increased demand which is made for this substance in inflammation, as without some additional supply it is probable that the work of reparation could not go on in cases of extensive injury, nor the adhesions consequent on inflammation be duly formed. Thus in diffuse cellular inflammation, no adhesions are formed, and no buff is observed on the blood, but the reverse of these circumstances is observable when the seat of the inflammation is in fibrous or serous structures.

The Coagulation of the Blood has generally been referred to a physiological or a chemical cause. The first of these opinions was maintained by Hunter, the latter is most prevalent in the present day. In reference to the author's ideas on this subject, it will be necessary to premise a distinction between his statements as to the cause of fluidity and the cause of coagulation of the blood. The former I think are borne out by every fact (*note*, p. 29.), the latter are open to considerable differences of opinion.

Having considered the effects of exterior causes on coagulation, viz. heat, cold, motion, and rest, and "shown that none of these alone, nor all of them combined, induce the blood to coagulate," he comes to the conclusion "that it coagulates from an impression;—that the blood has the power of action within itself;—that to produce coagulation something more is required than merely the reverse of the causes above mentioned to keep it fluid, for the blood becomes in many cases instantaneously incapable of coagulation, either in or out of the vessels, even when nothing has been added or taken away.—There is therefore something more than the mere situation of the blood surrounded with dead parts that *allows* of coagulation; and that must be a something in the blood itself.—Coagulation I conceive to be an operation of life."

Now as these opinions are greatly dependent on another, namely, the vitality of the blood, which opinion has not yet been considered, it might seem expedient that I should in the first place examine the truth of this *datum*. I believe, however, that this will not be necessary, but that it will be extremely possible to assign a reasonable cause of coagulation without adverting to this subject.

In regard to the cause of the blood's fluidity, Mr. Hunter is perfectly clear. "It must be evident," he says, "that the fluid state of the blood is connected with the living vessels, which is its natural situation, and with motion; and that where there is a full power of life, the vessels are capable of keeping the blood in a fluid state," &c. &c. Now if the fluidity of the blood depends, under ordinary circumstances, on motion and contact with the living vessels, (which opinion can scarcely I think be doubted,) then the conditions under which this fluid is placed when removed from the living vessels and set at rest are essentially changed, and the difficulty of accounting for the act of coagulation on simply chemical principles is entirely removed.

For let it be assumed, in the first place, that the whole mass of blood consists of liquor sanguinis and red globules (*notes*, pp. 22, 24.); secondly, that the liquor sanguinis is

blood of all animals; but there is more of it, I think, in those animals which have red blood: perhaps it may bear some proportion

---

really and *bonâ fide* a compound body, and no mere mixture of elements (*id.*); thirdly, that the existence and integrity of this compound depends on, or is preserved by, the living vessels or other containing parts (*note*, p. 29.); and fourthly, that the natural or inherent condition of fibrin is that of a solid (and as yet it has never been known to exist as an uncombined fluid); admit, I say, these *data* and the difficulty of accounting for the coagulation of the blood at once disappears, for the cause being removed which kept the elements of the liquor sanguinis in a state of combination, the effect also ceases; in other words, the conditions ceasing under which this compound can alone exist, the principles of which it is constituted necessarily revert to those states which are most natural to them, which state, as regards the fibrin, is that of a solid.

This opinion was first maintained by Schultz (*Journ. des Prog. des Sc. Méd.*, vi. 85.), and has since found an able supporter in Dr. Babington, who has given additional reasons for believing in its truth. It is not, as might at first appear, opposed to Mr. Hunter's peculiar doctrines concerning the vitality of the blood, but presupposes and confirms them; for without admitting the vitality of the blood, it would be impossible to explain many circumstances connected with coagulation, and particularly why the blood does not immediately solidify on extravasation whenever it is removed from the influence of those causes which kept it fluid. But this does not happen, and therefore it is plain that coagulation, instead of being an act of life (as Hunter supposed), is in fact an act which can only take place on the cessation of life, or, in the language of our author, an act of death. A residuum of vitality certainly adheres to the blood for some considerable time after it is extravasated from the body, and it is not until this is partially or wholly dissipated that coagulation takes place; hence, as I have observed before, the disposition to coagulation is always inversely as the powers of the animal, and is promoted by all those circumstances which are calculated to exhaust or carry off the living principle.

But this explanation does not account for every circumstance, nor remove the specific objections which the author himself has urged against all such hypotheses. It does not, for example, account for the coagulation of the blood in the vessels of mortifying limbs, or for the incoagulability of this fluid in cases of sudden death.

With regard to the first of these objections, I think we may be allowed to suppose that the effects of sympathy extend to a considerable distance beyond the mortified parts, so that these parts, and particularly the great vascular trunks, are weakened and deprived of those full powers of life which are necessary to preserve the blood in a fluid state. Many analogous cases might be adduced to show that any one part of a system of organs being injured, the effect is participated in by the whole; and I think we must refer to this principle, viz. to the sympathy which exists between the heart and its various prolongations, the great disposition which is manifested by the blood to coagulate during the existence of syncope.

With respect to the second objection which has been mentioned, I confess my inability to propose any hypothesis capable of explaining the variety of circumstances under which the blood remains fluid after death. That it depends, as Hunter supposed, on the sudden and entire abstraction of life, or as Mayo has imagined, on a greater residual vitality in the solids of the body, are explanations diametrically opposed; and totally irreconcileable, as it appears to me, with the diversity of circumstances under which this phenomenon is exhibited. The blood has been found uncoagulated in every variety of common and epidemic fever, and in almost every variety of local phlegmasia,

to the quantity of red particles in the blood, and may be of use to dilute it[a].

The serum is lighter than the other parts of the blood, and therefore swims above them when separated. It is commonly separated from the coagulating lymph when that fluid coagulates, and is therefore almost

---

in hanging, drowning, hydrophobia, coup-de-soleil, lightning, blows on the stomach, overwhelming affections of the mind, intoxication, apoplexy, severe and mortal injuries of vital parts, and in most cases of poisoning; and, as opposed to these, in almost every respect in overdriven animals, typhoid and low fevers, cholera, scurvy, death from putrid food or putrid inoculations, &c. The former for the most part are examples of the sudden extinction of life attended with all the signs of previous health, the latter of the gradual decay of life attended with all the evidences of previous debility. There requires, therefore, evidently some more general principle than has yet been discovered to explain these diversities. The chemical and physiological explanations are in this respect both on a par; they both equally fail, as theories, in explaining all the circumstances of the case.

Mr. Hunter compared the coagulation of blood to union by the first intention, and in a larger sense to the act of nutrition and organical formations; but this opinion, as I shall have occasion hereafter to show, does not seem to be supported by any sufficient data. At present I shall content myself with remarking one striking difference, which is, that organized structures when once formed continue to live and to manifest an interior activity, whereas the blood when once coagulated undergoes the common changes of dead matter.

The act of coagulation has also been compared to muscular contractility; but it differs from this in two essential respects: first, in not being followed by any relaxation; and secondly, in not being stimulated to action by any of those agents which are apt to excite muscular contraction. It is further remarkable that prussic acid and extract of belladonna, one of which is so fatal to life, and the other so destructive of muscular action, do not in the least prevent a strong contraction of the coagulum; but according to my judgment, no other argument is required to subvert the physiological hypothesis, than the fact that blood which has been kept fluid for an indefinite period of time by common salt, may yet be made to coagulate by the addition of water. It is remarkable that blood may be kept fluid and of a bright arterial colour for many months, or even years, by this means, and yet retain its coagulating property.]

[a] [I shall take the liberty of extending the inquiry which is suggested in the text, to the following points:

First, As to the relative proportion of nutritive to non-nutritive matters in the blood under different circumstances of age, sex, constitution, &c.;

Secondly, As to the relative proportion which the red globules bear to the serum;

Thirdly, As to the variations which may occur in the quantity of albumen in common serum; and

Fourthly, As to the relative quantity of salts.

The *data* on which my observations on these points will be founded may be seen at large in M. Le Canu's second memoir on the blood, contained in the *Journal de Pharmacie* for October 1831.

I. *As to the relative proportion of nutritive to non-nutritive matters in the blood under different circumstances of age, sex, constitution, &c.*

1000 parts of healthy blood being taken, the proportion of water and salts to the nutritive matters (fibrin, globules, and albumen) varied—

always found when the blood is taken out of the blood-vessels, and kept together in a considerable mass. When the lymph coagulates strongly,

---

			Water.	Salts.	Nutr. matt.
1st, In individuals of different ages and sexes.		Max.	853·135	9·760	137·105
		Min.	778·625	11·541	209·834
		Average of twenty analyses.	796·846	10·316	192·838
2nd, In individuals of the same sex but of different ages.	Female.	Max. Æt. 22	853·135	9·760	137·105
		Min. Æt. 58	790·394	11·220	198·386
		Average of ten analyses	804·371	9·944	185·685
	Male.	Max. Æt. 50	805·263	12·120	182·617
		Min. Æt. 26	778·625	11·541	209·834
		Average of ten analyses	789·320	10·689	199·991

It appears, therefore, from the above table, that a variation of 72·729 in 1000, or nearly 7½ per cent., in the nutritive parts of the blood is consistent with a state of health, and that the blood of males is richer in this respect by 14·306 in 1000, or nearly 1½ per cent., than females. Age (within the period of twenty to sixty years) does not seem to make much difference. The proportion of nutritive matters in the sanguine is about 1 per cent. more in the female, and 1½ per cent., more in the male, than in those who are lymphatic. Venesection and considerable hæmorrhages have a marked effect in impoverishing the blood of its nutritive parts. Thus the blood of a patient who had been subject to copious uterine hæmorrhages (*pertes uterines*) yielded only 137·120 parts, or nearly 5 per cent. less than the usual average, while the blood of another patient was impoverished as much as 4 per cent. after a single venesection. These facts accord with experience, and afford a rational account of the advantages of depletion in cases of over-excitement. The principal change in the blood in cholera consists in the great relative increase of the solid parts and deficiency in the carbonated alkalies, the fibrin, albumen, and colouring matter not undergoing any changes which can be detected by chemical analysis. Thus the average of the following analyses shows an extraordinary increase of the solid contents in choleric blood:

$$\text{Water....}\begin{Bmatrix} 66{\cdot}0 \\ 74{\cdot}9 \\ 48{\cdot}1 \end{Bmatrix} \text{ solid contents } \begin{Bmatrix} 34 \\ 25 \\ 52 \end{Bmatrix}$$

$$\text{Average } 63{\cdot}0 \quad + \quad 37 = 100.$$

Amounting to little less than double the ordinary quantity. From other observations it would appear that acute diseases generally tend to increase, and chronic ones to diminish, the nutritive parts of the blood. Thackrah has related a case of pleurisy in which the proportion of serum to crassamentum was as 10· to 54·9 (*op. cit.*, p. 197.); and according to Langrish the relative quantities of serum to crassamentum in acute fevers, tertians, and quartans, were respectively as 10 to 33, 10 to 25, and 10 to 16. Of sixteen cases of acute disease taken indiscriminately from ordinary practice, only one fell below the ordinary standard, while the average of solid contents for 12 out of the 16 was 207·9 in 1000, the healthy standard being estimated at 160. (*Thackrah*, p. 208.) The blood is proportionally more rich in those who have long fasted than in those who have recently eaten; in wild and predatory animals, in persons who subsist on rich animal diet, and in females during the period of utero-gestation. Sickness, syncope, salivation, insufficient nutriment, and, above all, hæmorrhage, impoverish the blood. The blood of a calf which was killed 16 hours after a copious venesection and subsequent

we commonly find more serum, because it is then squeezed out more forcibly than when the coagulation is formed loosely; it is not, however,

---

refusal of food, afforded only 3·4 crass. to 10 serum, instead of the usual proportion of 8 to 10.

II. *As to the relative proportion which the globules (inclusive of fibrin) bear to the serum.*

			Red globules	Serum.
1st, In individuals of different ages and sexes.		Max.	148·450	851·550
		Min.	68·349	931·651
		Average of twenty analyses	124·227	875·773
2nd, In individuals of the same sex but of different ages.	Female.	Max. Æt. 53.	129·999	870·010
		Min. Æt. 22.	68·349	931·651
		Average of ten analyses.	115·963	884·037
	Male.	Max. Æt. 40.	148·458	851·550
		Min. Æt. 34.	115·850	884·150
		Average of ten anlayses.	132·491	867·509

It appears, therefore, that the superior richness of the blood of men depends principally upon the superabundance of the red globules, in the proportion 16·528, or upwards of 1½ per cent. The proportions of this element of the blood are not influenced so much by age (within the limits of twenty to sixty years) as by the temperament of the individual. In the sanguine it exceeds by nearly 2 per cent. in the male, and 1 per cent. in the female, the proportion in the leucophlegmatic, a conclusion which strikingly corroborates the opinion of Hunter that the red globules are in some manner connected with the strength or vital energies of the individual, while it points out also the importance which this element probably has on the full development of animal heat. Dr. Christison found that the changes which were wrought on the air by respiration were always in proportion to the quantity of red globules present in the blood; while MM. Prevost and Dumas ascertained the fact that birds (which are the most active of all animals, and possess the highest range of animal temperature,) have the greatest number of red globules, next to them carnivorous quadrupeds, and least of all cold-blooded animals. The constitution does not easily repair considerable losses of the red globules. A single venesection reduced their amount nearly one third, and a severe uterine hæmorrhage upwards of 34 per cent. In a case of purpura hæmorrhagica, Dr. Whiting found that the red particles did not exceed 40 in 1000 parts of blood, although the common proportion was estimated at not less than 100 to 130. (*De Sang. Ægrorum.*) Mr. Andrews found that the red globules were diminished upwards of 50 per cent. in calves after the fourth venesection to syncope. (*Dubl. Journ.*, No. 19.) Their quantity is also much diminished by improper or insufficient nutriment, obesity, chronic diseases, and the absence of solar light.

III. *As to the variations which may occur in the quantity of albumen in common serum.*—The serum essentially consists of water and albumen, the proportions of which preserve a remarkable uniformity both in health and disease. The difference in the quantity of albumen seldom exceeds 2 per cent. even after considerable losses of blood. It is sometimes deficient in milky serum, and in the serum of patients suffering from dropsy, attended with albuminous urine. In the former cases the albumen is apparently converted into an oleàginous principle, and in the latter into fibrin. The specific gravity of the serum in such cases is generally exceedingly low. Dr. Babington found that milky serum varied from 1019 to 1024, and that in a case of albuminous urine it did not ex-

necessary for the lymph to coagulate, in order to separate the serum, for we find that it separates in disease, as in the dropsy. It is separated

---

ceed 1020 at 60°, nor the solid contents amount to more than 1·61 per cent., the usual averages being 1029·5 spec. grav. and 10·00 per cent. solid contents. (*Med.-Chir. Trans.*, xvi. 57, 315.) M. Denis is of opinion that albumen predominates in the young and aged, and suggests that it may probably depend on a transference of this substance from the crassamentum to the serum, the former being most abundant in adult life. (*Sur le Sang*, pp. 288, 290; *see note*, p. 37.)

IV. *As to the relative quantity of salts.*—The uses of the salts of the blood can only be conjectured, for we have very little knowledge on the subject. Dr. Stevens indeed has spoken on this matter with much confidence, and assigned to the salts of the blood an importance inversely proportionate to their quantitative amount, appropriating to them the office of preserving the blood in a fluid state (*On the Blood*, p. 6.), of rendering it stimulating to the heart (pp. 14, 43.), of giving to it its scarlet colour (p. 8.), and of influencing in some unknown and indefinite manner the nutritive and respiratory functions (pp. 43, 51. *et passim*). The ground on which these statements rest is, that "in every part of the world where healthy blood has been analysed, it has invariably been found to contain a *given proportion* of certain salts." Now there certainly appears to be some mistake here respecting the fact, for if by given proportion is meant a fixed proportion, this is contrary to experience. It is not indeed to be doubted that the salts of the blood are sometimes deficient in cholera and other malignant fevers, but in order to constitute this any argument to prove that fevers and cholera depend on this cause, it will be necessary in the first place to prove that the salts are never deficient in a healthy state, and secondly, that this variation in regard to the salts is greater than what occurs in regard to the other elements of the blood.

With respect to the first of these points, I may observe that the extreme plus and minus quantities of salts present in healthy blood, according to Le Canu, were 11·11 and 5·10 in 1000 parts,—allowing, therefore, of a difference of just one half. But, according to Dr. Thompson, the diminution of the quantity of salts in cholera blood was very inconsiderable (*Phil. Mag.*, May 1832); while, even in the two cases which are reported by Dr. O'Shaughnessy, the proportions were 5·60 and 2·92 in 1000 parts of serum (*Report on Malignant Cholera*), the average standard being, according to Le Canu, 9·01. The utmost diminution, therefore, of the salts in cholera did not amount to more than 2·18 below the minimum, or 6·09 below the average standard of health. Now, as a cause of disease, this is surely not to be compared with the extraordinary increase already mentioned of solid contents, or the extraordinary disorganization of the blood in other respects. The truth is, that neither the increase of solid contents, nor the diminution of the saline, are to be looked upon as *causes*, but rather as *effects* of the disease. The serous, and therefore the saline, parts of the blood pass off by the stools, but the cause of these stools must necessarily be antecedent.

The second condition is equally incapable of proof, for beyond all question, every other element of the blood is subject to as great a variation as the salts, and much greater. Thackrah has referred to two cases of cholera in which there was an increase of solid contents to 400 and 500 in 1000 parts of blood, which is considerably more than double the common average, and exceeds the maximum quantity of healthy blood much more than the deficiency of salts in disease falls short of the minimum quantity of this element in a healthy state of the system. The fibrin, according to Le Canu, varies from 1·360 to 7·235 consistently with a state of health, and according to Dr. Whiting, it sometimes rises from 2·8 to 6· or even 9·7 in acute rheumatism and pleurisy. An equal variation is observable in regard to the hæmatosine and red globules. Shall we, also from the mass of blood in uterine-gestation, being the fluid in which the fœtus is immersed or swims[a].

I have seen it separate from the remaining mass before the coagulation of the lymph. I observed once in the blood of a lady, that a separation between the two fluids almost immediately took place, the serous part swimming on the top, while the lymph remained still fluid. From this appearance I had pronounced that there would be a great deal of buff, supposing that the transparent fluid at the top was coagulating lymph; but I was mistaken, for when the lymph was coagulated, there was no buff, and the transparent fluid remaining at top, proved to be the serum.

In this there could be no deception, as there was no buff, or size; for if there had been size at the top of the coagulum, it might have been supposed that this fluid, which appeared so soon after bleeding, had

---

then, make no account of these alterations in the primary constituents of the blood, because the salts happen to be affected at the same time, especially when we reflect on the known and paramount importance of these substances? With all respect for the abilities of Dr. Stevens, and for the contributions which he has undoubtedly made to our knowledge of the blood, I cannot but regard his reasoning on this subject as liable to the greatest objection.

Dr. Prout has indeed brought forward some happy illustrations concerning the effect of infinitessimal quantities of foreign matter in modifying the composition of organic bodies, from which it may fairly be inferred that the salts in the blood perform an important, although to us as yet unknown, office in the animal œconomy. This distinguished chemist has even gone yet further, and endeavoured to assign a particular use of one of the individual salts; for having remarked that chlorine or muriatic acid is sometimes evolved during the process of digestion, he thinks it probable that the muriate of soda undergoes decomposition in the stomach; the chlorine or muriatic acid being secreted into this organ to aid in the act of digestion, while the soda is retained in the blood to confer on this fluid its alkaline properties. (*Bridgewater Treatise*, p. 499.)

[a] [The average specific gravity of serum being taken, at a temperature of 60°, as 1029·5, that of hydrocephalic fluid varies from 1000·5 to 1019, a middle term being most frequent. The fluid of hydatids is about 1004, sometimes not containing a trace of albumen. Effusions into the chest 1019 to 1024, and ascitic effusions 1014 to 1026.

The ratio of serum to crassamentum is extremely variable, depending on many circumstances. Whatever accelerates the coagulation diminishes the contractility of the clot; to which head belongs the shape of the receiving vessel. "If this be shallow, the crassamentum will be abundant; if approaching the form of the cube or sphere, it will be scanty. This difference is owing to the greater or less distance of the coagulating particles from a common centre, which causes a more or less powerful adhesion and contraction of these particles." (*Babington, loc. cit.*) There is also another circumstance to be considered; for in proportion as the form of the vessel departs from that of a sphere, the blood is subjected to a more extensive contact with dead matter, which accelerates the coagulating process. Hence the quantity of clot is inversely as the mass of the blood; because when the mass is small, the surface of contact is usually great. The actual quantity of fibrin in these cases is the same; but the quantity of serum involved in the interstices of the clot is greater in one case than it is in the other.]

been the coagulating lymph, and that the serum had been separated in the act of coagulation as usual. The serum is commonly of a yellowish colour, sometimes more so than at others; and this I should conceive arises from the substances dissolved in it*, by means of the water it contains; for it probably suspends every salt soluble in water, many of which are dissolved in it. If serum be not coagulable in itself, though it contains a large quantity of coagulable matter, yet I conceive it to be in a more fluid state when circulating. As it is separated from a compound mass, it appears in this respect to be somewhat similar to the whey of milk, though not exactly. This fluid undergoes no spontaneous changes, but what may arise from its separation from the coagulating lymph, except putrefaction. Though not coagulable in itself, yet one of its properties out of the body is to coagulate upon the application of certain substances. This is the principal change it undergoes; and during this process, it more or less separates into two parts, one of which is not coagulable by such means.

The coagulable part, which I now mean to describe, seems to be in some degree the same with that in the white of an egg, synovia, &c., and many other secretions, but not exactly; for those secretions contain, as I conceive, a quantity of the coagulating lymph united to them, which makes them in part coagulate after secretion; and the further coagulation of those secretions afterwards, by mixture with other substances, is owing to this part of the serum. Though the serum is coagulable under certain circumstances, and with certain mixtures, yet this power or effect may be prevented by other mixtures. Heat, to a certain degree, coagulates this part; and probably this is the only test necessary to know whether a fluid found anywhere in the body, not coagulable in itself, is this part of the serum; but as many substances do also coagulate it, I shall mention a few of them, although to me their effects do not seem to throw any light on the subject. Heat coagulates the serum at 160° or 165°; it stood at 150° for some time perfectly fluid. There is a great deal of air contained in the serum, which is let loose by heat; but not when it is coagulated by other means. The serum which was a little whitish coagulated in that degree of heat necessary for separating its air, which was extricated in very large quantities. This coagulum becomes first like the synovia, and then thicker. Many substances which do not coagulate this part of the serum do not, however, hinder its coagulation by heat; such as vinegar, acid of lemon, salt of wormwood, nitre, sea-salt[a].

* The red globules are suspended without being dissolved in the serum, in which they are commonly examined.

[a] [According to the best analyses, synovia and the white of egg do not contain any

Serum coagulates with spirits of wine, in about equal quantities, into a sort of curd and whey, which upon heating becomes something like a jelly, but the spirit seems to evaporate. It coagulates with volatile spirits into a milky fluid, which becomes like a jelly upon heating; it requires a greater proportion of the spirit than the serum, and the spirit seems chiefly to evaporate. When mixed with salt of hartshorn it does not coagulate with heat, but makes a large effervescence till the whole is formed into froth. This again becomes a fluid by the froth subsiding, but at last it forms a sort of coagulum which is not tough. Being mixed with water, and let to stand for twelve hours, it coagulates like pure serum upon heating. If this be mixed with sal. cornu cervi, as above, it rather becomes more fluid, and continues so for a long time,

---

fibrin, consequently these substances have no resemblance to the coagulable lymph of the blood. Undiluted albumen coagulates at a temperature of 160°, and is rendered opake at 212°, even when diluted with 1000 parts of water, unless excess of free or carbonated alkali be present, in which case it will not be coagulated by heat. (See Burrows in *Med. Gazette*, xiv. 555.) It is a singular fact that serum when diluted with 20 parts of water is not precipitable by a temperature of 165°. Galvanism and the mineral acids are very excellent tests of the presence of albumen, and so are the solutions of the ferrocyanate of potash and corrosive sublimate. Albumen diluted with 2000 parts of water may easily be detected by the two latter.

The mode in which heat, galvanism, alcohol, acids, and a variety of other agents produce coagulation of the albumen has long been the subject of debate. The most general, and, as it appears to me, the most rational, explanation of the matter is as follows, viz. that the albumen of serous fluids is held in solution by means of a free alkali; but by heat the free soda of the serum is transferred to the water or united to the carbonic acid of the atmosphere; by acids it is neutralised, and by galvanism it is attracted to the negative pole of the trough. However, this explanation is not quite satisfactory. Dr. Bostock has shown not only that excess of acetic acid does not coagulate albumen, but that the quantity of free alkali present is too inconsiderable to produce the effect ascribed to it. Others have supposed that alcohol and acids coagulate albumen by abstracting the water; but it is possible to desiccate albumen by slow evaporation without necessarily destroying its distinctive property, which is that of being again soluble upon the addition of water. The mineral salts do not merely precipitate albumen from its solution, but chemically combine with it, so as to produce specific compounds. Dr. Turner has suggested "that albumen combines directly with water at the moment of being secreted, at a time that its particles are in a state of minute division; but as its affinity for that liquid is very feeble, the compound is decomposed by slight causes, and the albumen thereby rendered quite insoluble. Silica affords an instance of a similar phenomenon," (*Elem. of Chem.*, 4th edit., p. 868.). But the cases are not analogous. Albumen admits of being dried at a temperature below 150°, and even of being heated to 212°, without losing its solubility; whereas silica remains perfectly insoluble after it has once been precipitated.

The truth seems to be that albumen is one of those compounds which allow of a new arrangement of their molecular particles with exceeding facility, similar to muscular fibre, which is rendered permanently rigid by a temperature at least 20° below that which is required to coagulate albumen. It is scarcely therefore correct to say that albumen before and after coagulation are identical substances.]

with a strong effervescence; but it forms at length into a jelly or paste, although not a solid one. Here I suspect that the salt is evaporated, and likewise the water in the paste, so that it is not a true coagulation. When mixed with common water it is coagulated by heat; but the water separates with the other substance, and does not unite with the coagulum.

Upon the coagulation of the serum by heat I have observed that it separates a fluid which is not coagulable by heat, and I have reason to believe by none of the other means, viz. spirits of wine, &c., though this is not so easily ascertained; for the other coagulating substances, as spirits of wine, &c., are applied in a fluid form, and therefore a fluid may remain after the coagulation of the serum, which might be supposed to be the fluid separated; but from other experiments it is proved that those substances coagulate the coagulating part and unite with the other. It is also observable in meat, either roasted or boiled, that when cut there flows from it a fluid more or less tinged with the red part, commonly called gravy. I conceived that this must be different from the coagulating part of the serum, believing that the heat had been sufficient to coagulate it; but I chose to try it further, and therefore gave it such heat as would have produced the effect if it had been coagulable by heat; but I found it did not coagulate. The fluid separated from the coagulable part of the serum, I conceived to be the same with this. Thus then I saw there was in the serum a matter coagulable by heat, and a fluid which was not so.

Pursuing the above observations on dressed meat, I observed that the older the animal had been, the more of this fluid was contained in the meat. In lamb we have hardly any of it. in young mutton of a year old but little; but in mutton of three, four, five, or six years old it is in large quantity: in veal also we have but little, while we have it in great quantity in beef. But perhaps we know less in general of the age of our beef than of our mutton*.[a]

Poultry is commonly killed young in this country, therefore we have not the comparative trials; but in wild fowl, and what is commonly

* It may be observed here that this is very different from the jelly formed in boiling or roasting meat; that which forms the jelly is part of the meat itself, dissolved down in this very fluid, and the water in which it is boiled; and we find that this effect is just the reverse of the above, for in young meat there is most of this jelly.

---

[a] [This fluid, which is termed the serosity, may be obtained from the coagulum by gentle expression. It contains a little muriate of soda, a little free alkali, and about one fiftieth of its weight of animal matter, principally albumen, which is immediately coagulated by galvanism or the mineral acids. Brande supposes that the albumen is held in solution in this case, as in the serum, by virtue of the free alkali which is present; but Dr. Bostock has objected to this view of the case, for reasons which have

called game, we find the above observations hold good. I likewise observe that animals which have not had exercise, such as house-lamb, veal, &c., have less of this fluid than those of the same class which have been allowed to go at large. Nothing can be drier than the English veal, though kept to a greater age than anywhere else; while it is juicy in every other country, though killed much younger.

In many of the trials respecting the coagulation of the serum, I observed that it had in some cases much more coagulum than in others; and of course a less proportion of the fluid part that separated, and *vice versâ*; from the above observations too I conceived that a deficiency of this fluid part bespoke a greater quantity of coagulating matter in the serum; and to ascertain this I took the serum of persons of different ages. This fluid, like the serum itself when united with the coagulating lymph, appears only to be mixed with the serum; for it is separated in the living body for many purposes of the œconomy; it is not therefore serum in another form, but a distinct fluid, which before coagulation is mingled with the serum, and seems to make a part of it.

The following experiments are, perhaps, not perfectly conclusive, for many were obliged to be made on blood taken from those who were not perfectly in health; peculiar dispositions in the body may make a material difference in the serum. It is probable, however, that disease may not have any great effect upon the serum; for I found, from experiment, that the serum of blood taken from a person labouring under an inflammatory complaint, and the serum of blood in a case not at all inflammatory, were nearly the same respecting coagulation and the quantity of matter not coagulable by heat.

The serum of a man fifty-six years of age, who had met with a slight accident, and was of a healthy constitution, coagulated by heat almost wholly into a pretty firm coagulum, separating only a small portion of that fluid which is not coagulable by such means. The serum of the blood of a man seventy-two years of age, of a healthy constitution, hardly coagulated by heat, became only a little thicker, and formed a small coagulum, adhering to the bottom of the vessel. With spirits it formed but a very small quantity of coagulable matter. On putting about three fourths of water to the blood of the person aged fifty-six, and heating it as above, it coagulated much in the same way with the

been adverted to in a previous note. The serosity does not appear to merit any particular attention.

The basis of muscular fibre, or meat properly so called, is fibrin, which is insoluble, except in very minute quantities, by the continued action of boiling water. Jelly is a solution of gelatine, which is a distinct animal principle, with which young animals abound, but which, according to Prout, is a less animalized product than either albumen or fibrin.]

serum of seventy-two. The serum of a boy fifteen years of age coagulated wholly; there was hardly any of the fluid part that could be squeezed out: at the same time I coagulated the serum of a man sixty-three years of age, in which there was but a small quantity of the fluid part.

Conceiving that the whey of milk, made with rennet, was the serum of the blood, I made experiments on it analogous to the above. I heated some of the whey, and found it formed a coagulable matter, which floated in flakes in a fluid, which did not coagulate by this means.

As this less coagulable fluid is a substance hitherto not taken notice of, and makes perhaps as interesting a part as any of the whole mass of blood, it will be necessary to be more descriptive in giving an account of it than of the other parts. Urine does not coagulate by heat; but as I found that it coagulated with the extract of Goulard*, and as I also knew that this extract coagulated the whole mass of the serum, I conceived that the fluid in question might be similar to urine, and that the coagulation of the serum might be owing to the coagulation of this part: I therefore put the fluid to this test, and found that it was coagulated by the extract, which led to a series of experiments.

As several fluids, apparently different from each other, appear to be thrown out from the blood on many occasions, I wished to see how far they consisted of the common serum, viz. of a pretty equal quantity of matter coagulable by heat, or principally of that coagulable by Goulard's extract; I therefore collected the several kinds; not only those which may be called natural, but also those proceeding from disease, which appear more like serum than the others. Of the natural, I took the aqueous humour of the eye, and first heated it in a spoon, to see what quantity of coagulable matter by heat was in it, and I found it became gently wheyish: therefore it had a small portion of matter coagulable by heat; but upon adding the extract to it, it coagulated immediately. The same exactly happened with the water in the ventricles of the brain; and also with the tears.

Water was taken from the leg of a dropsical boy, who was extremely reduced by a compound fracture of the opposite thigh-bone, which water was much clearer than any serum. Upon heating it in a spoon over a candle, it became a little wheyish, and had a few flakes of coagulum

* What led me to the above knowledge was mixing this extract of Goulard with solutions of gum arabic in water for injections, when I found that the whole always became a solid mass; while injections with saccharum saturni had not that effect. I then tried it upon many other vegetable juices, and found it coagulated every one of them. In some of these experiments I put some of the compounds into a vessel where there was some urine, and I found that, when the extract had been in too large a quantity the urine was also coagulated.

floating in it. The water from the abdomen of a lady, which was a little wheyish, coagulated before it gave out its air; but the coagulum was not one half of its quantity. In another case of ascites, the water coagulated wholly, although not to a firm coagulum. Water drawn from the abdomen of a gentleman, which was pretty clear, when held over a lamp to coagulate, became at first wheyish. The liquor amnii has but very little coagulable matter in it. In coagulating all the above kinds of serum by heat, and taking the incoagulable parts and putting extract of Goulard to them, they coagulated immediately[a].

Whether this fluid is of the same specific gravity with the other I do not know; for though when part of it is coagulated by the extract of lead it is the heaviest, yet as it is united with the lead, it may acquire its additional weight from this union.

The use of the serum is probably to keep suspended and undissolved the red globules; for we find it in largest quantity when these globules are most abundant. It is also intended to suspend and dissolve any foreign substances in the blood, whether they are of use to the body or otherwise, acting upon them as a common solvent. Thus we see in a jaundiced person the serum is yellower than common. When a person has taken rhubarb the same thing happens. It is probably the solvent of all our secretions.

I conceive it to be unnecessary to say how much water enters into the composition of the blood. In order to constitute a perfect body or compound it is necessary that all its parts should be in due proportion. But as the blood in many animals is made up of four distinct parts, viz. the coagulating lymph, serum, which we find is composed of two parts, and the red globules, each must have its due quantity of water when in a perfect state; and I think it is probable that the lymph and red part cannot have more water than a certain quantity, but that the serum may be diluted with any proportion of it. Yet, as serum, it can have a certain proportion only; and indeed this was in some degree proved by the experiment of mixing some water with serum, and then coagulating the whole with heat: the water separated and did not make a part of the coagulum.

Some of the juices of a living animal, whether circulating or out of circulation, as those which lubricate surfaces, are in a volatile state while the animal is alive; for when the scarf-skin is taken off, the part soon dries; and if the skin is removed from a new-killed animal, it immediately dries; or if a cavity is opened, the surface of the cavity

---

[a] [These are merely examples of the precipitation of albumen or mucus by means of Goulard's extract in variable proportions.]

dries quickly; this shows that some part of the juices must have evaporated from the surface: but let the animal cool before it is skinned or the cavity is opened, and then give it the same degree of heat that it had when alive, you will find, on taking off the skin, no immediate sensible evaporation, but the parts so exposed will remain moist. This volatility I conceive therefore to be connected with life, and not with the circulation; for that is stopped in both cases before the experiment. Whether it is this volatile part that gives the smell that most recently-killed animals have upon being skinned or opened I do not know; but it may be observed that it follows the same rules, for if the animal is allowed to cool it loses this smell, although warmed to the same degree of heat as when alive[a].

The serum of the blood is sometimes wheyish, and then upon settling it often throws up a white scum like cream. This was most probably first observed in the human blood, but is not peculiar to it. Although these appearances pretty often happen, yet few instances fall under the observation of one man in the common course of bleeding. When they have occurred to myself I have made inquiry after the state of health of

---

[a] [The halitus, or vapour, which is emitted from fresh-drawn blood, is of this kind, and consists almost exclusively of water holding in solution minute quantities of animal matter and salts, together with a peculiar aromatic principle. It occasionally happens that this effluvium is exalted to a very intense degree, so as to occasion headache, sickness, fainting, dysentery, and even death. In suppression of urine it acquires a strong urinous character. Orfila and more recently Barrueil (*Ann. d'Hygiène*, i. 274, 550. *Revue Méd.*, Sept. 1829,) have attempted to establish the possibility of distinguishing the different tribes of animals by the peculiarity of smell disengaged from blood-spots or stains upon the addition of strong sulphuric acid. The odour which exhales is said to resemble strongly the perspiration or respiration of the animal from which the blood is derived, which in men having dark hair and complexions and in carnivorous animals is said to be peculiarly characteristic. M. Leuret, in order to test the accuracy of M. Barrueil's assertions, sent four specimens in phials containing ox blood, horse blood, and blood from the human subject both male and female. M. Barrueil detected the two former, but in regard to the two latter he mistook the male's for the female's; a mistake, however, which, under the circumstances, strongly confirmed his own views of the case, for it so happened that the man from whom the blood was taken was fair, whereas the woman had dark hair and was remarkably strong. These statements have been supported by Leuret and Chevallier, and as stoutly denied by Raspail, Villermé, and Soubeyan, so that considerable doubt at present hangs over the subject; and evidence founded on these data would not, I apprehend, be admissible in a court of justice on any medico-legal question. (Raspail, *Chim. Organ.*, p. 383. *Ann. des Sc. d'Obser.* 1829, ii. 183. 465.)

Blood-spots on linen clothes or steel instruments may be distinguished from any other marks: 1st, by the evolution of ammonia on dry distillation; 2nd, by the effects of acids and neutral salts on solutions of the colouring matters; 3rd, by the usual tests for albumen; and 4th, by blood scaling off from steel instruments on being heated, and leaving them tolerably clean and free from rust.]

the patient, as well as examined the nature of this change and whether there was any variety in it. So far as I have been able to observe, it can hardly be said to have any leading cause: having found it, however, more frequently in the blood of breeding women, I conceived it might have some connexion with that state; but I have seen it in others, and sometimes in men. Yet it is possible that the state of pregnancy may adapt the constitution for forming such appearances, as well as for producing other symptoms in the blood like those of inflammation; for we often find the same effect or disease arising from various causes which have no immediate connexion with each other.

There have been many opinions formed about the nature and cause of this appearance of the serum. It has been supposed to be occasioned by chyle not yet assimilated; but it does not occur frequently enough to be attributed to this fluid. Mr. Hewson supposed it to be absorbed fat or oil; which certainly is not the case, for it is not the same in all cases[a].

---

[a] [Opaline or milky serum would appear to depend on certain principles (stearine and oleine) naturally present in the blood (see *Analysis*, p. 18), but which under certain circumstances superabound in the system. In a very well marked case of this kind, Dr. Babington estimated the proportion of oleaginous matters at three per cent. of the whole serum. (*Med.-Chir. Trans.*, xvi. p. 46.) Dr. Traill, in two other cases, estimated it at 2·44 and 4·50 per cent. (*Edin. Med. and Surg. Journ.*, xvii. 235. 637. *April* 1823.), and Dr. Christison at five per cent. (*Ib., October* 1829.) The proportion in healthy serum does not exceed ·257, or about one quarter per cent.

Milky serum varies in specific gravity from 1019 to 1024, that of healthy serum being 1029·5. This loss of specific gravity in milky serum is apparently dependent on a corresponding deficiency of albumen, and affords an example of the easy convertibility of one animal principle into another under peculiar conditions of the system, somewhat analogous to the conversion of dried fibrin, and perhaps also of albumen, into adipocere, by digestion with ether and alcohol (see *note*, p. 46.). Dr. Babington did not observe that the degree of milkiness bore any proportion to the quantity of oily matters present. By agitating serum and ether together, and decanting and evaporating the latter, the oily matter may easily be obtained. Collected on bibulous paper or amianthus, it may be burned like any other oil.

When the quantity of oily matter is very considerable the blood is observed to have a chocolate or milky colour even while flowing from the vessel; which is a clear proof that the oil primarily exists in the blood, or in other words that it is an educt and not a product of the processes for obtaining it. (*Le Canu* in *Journ. de Chim. Med., June* 1835.)

The circumstances under which milky serum has been observed to exist are so unlike as to render it impossible to assign any probable state of the constitution as leading to its production. (*Journal de Pharmacie,* No. X.) Marcet, Berzelius, and Thackrah have partaken of the opinion that this appearance is derived from a mixture of unassimilated chyle with the blood; a conjecture which derives some support from the fact that chyle taken from an animal which has recently fed on fat animal diet presents precisely similar appearances. Mr. Thackrah has affirmed "that when the lacteals are fully distended (in dogs), this cream-like appearance is almost always presented in the blood Indeed, we may generally produce it at will by taking blood a certain time after a full

The globules forming this wheyish appearance are not of the same specific gravity in every case; for though they always, I believe, swim on the serum, and often on water, yet they sometimes sink in water. The white cream that swims on the top of the serum I believe to be formed after the serum is separated from the mass, for if it existed as such prior to this, it would be retained in the coagulum, as the red globules are, which is not the fact, and therefore it does not exist in the blood while circulating.

I bled a little woman who seemed half an idiot, and was big with child: this happened in the afternoon, about three or four hours after she had eaten some veal cutlets. The day following I went to see the blood, and found the serum of a milky white, with a white pellicle swimming at the top like cream. I bled a lady in the arm, who was six months gone with child. It was about two o'clock in the forenoon: she had only eaten a dry toast and drank a cup of chocolate for breakfast, about ten o'clock, which was four hours before she was bled. On seeing the blood the next day, I found it inflamed rather more than is common in women who are pregnant, and I also found a thin white scum on the top of the serum: this scum I examined in the microscope, and found it to be globular. I diluted it with water, and found the globules did not dissolve as the red globules do. I put some of them into water, and found that they rose to the top, but not so fast as in the serum. About six days after I bled the same lady again, after she had eaten the same kind of breakfast, and about the same interval of time from it. The blood was still sizy, but the serum had no white appearance at the top.

I examined the wheyish serum taken from the blood of a man at St. George's Hospital, who had received a severe blow on the head, which had stunned him, but had produced no bad symptoms. In this serum,

---

meal." (*Op. cit.*, p. 120.) The same appearance had also frequently been observed in the serum of animals that are very fat. Dr. Prout regards the fatty matter of chyle as incipient albumen.

From some cause therefore, such as the absorption of a peculiarly rich chyle after a full meal, or the sudden and temporary increase in the action of the absorbents, an undue proportion of fat is absorbed and carried into the blood, where, being suspended in the serum in the form of an emulsion, it becomes visible. M. Raspail endeavours to account for this appearance upon the supposition that an acid is generated in the blood which saturates the free alkali of the serum and precipitates the albumen.

The irregularity of the action of the absorbents is well exemplified by several cases recorded in the 4th volume of the Dublin *Journal of Medical and Chemical Science*, in which extraordinary quantities of fatty matters were discharged by the bowels. In the *Annali Universali* a case is related in which thirty pounds weight of fat were discharged from the bowels in twenty-four hours. "The patient nearly sunk, and his skin hung in folds as though all his fat had been absorbed."]

when viewed in the microscope, I could not observe anything like globules or flakes, although the magnifier was a deep one. The red globules when mixed with it were the same as in common serum. It dried uniformly like size.

Blood was taken away from the arm, being of no particular quality, except in having a wheyish serum, and was allowed to stand quiet in order to see the spontaneous changes of this serum. The white part came to the top like cream, being therefore lighter than the serum, and was very white when collected. When viewed in a microscope it was plainly globular, but the globules were smaller than those of red blood. They did not seem to be dissolved when mixed with water, as red globules are.

Thomas Skelton, a publican, forty-seven years of age, being rather lusty, and subject to frequent colds, attended with coughs, hoarseness, and a discharge of matter from the lungs or throat, but otherwise enjoying a good state of health, was attacked with a violent cold, together with a difficulty of breathing, for which he applied to Mr. Wilson, apothecary, who took twelve ounces of blood from his arm, which relieved him greatly. He had taken some bread and butter, with some tea without milk, about four hours before he was bled. The blood coagulated firmly, and the serum which separated was of a white colour with a yellowish tinge, appearing like the colour of cream; upon the top of this floated a whiter scum, like another cream. On viewing this cream in a microscope it had a flaky appearance; it did not coagulate sooner than common serum. In spirits of wine a white mixture was produced, which, on standing, fell to the bottom of the glass: this most probably arose from the serum, with which it was mixed, coagulating.

The globules of white serum differ from the red globules in colour, specific gravity, size, and in not dissolving in water.

To see how far this is chyle, it would be proper to try the chyle in the same way in serum, &c.

After dipping a bit of blotting-paper into the cream, and absorbing all of it, and also dipping a piece of the same paper into the serum, and drying them, I burnt them both, to see if one burnt more briskly than the other; but there appeared to be no difference.

The white part of the white serum sunk in water.

§. 4. *Of the Red Globules.*

The red part of the blood I choose to consider last, although it has been more the object of attention than the other two, because I believe it to be the least important; for it is not a universal ingredient in the blood of animals, like the coagulating lymph and serum, neither is it to be found in every part of those animals which have it in the general mass of their blood*.

The blood, as I have already observed, in those animals we are most acquainted with appears to the naked eye to be a red mass of fluid, having a part which coagulates upon being extravasated. The red part, however, may be washed out of this coagulum, so as to leave it white; and this shows that the blood is not wholly red, but only has a red matter diffused through its other component parts[b].

* The blood of the insect tribe of every kind is free from any red parts, as is probably that of most animals below them; yet it has been asserted and supposed that their blood contains globules, although not red. I have examined the blood of the silk-worm, lobster, &c., and with considerable magnifying powers, but never could discover anything but a uniform transparent mass[a]

[See Professor Grant's Lectures on Comparative Anatomy, as reported in the *Lancet*, 1833-4, vol. ii. p. 868 *et seq.*, where the existence of globules in the blood of insects is assumed as an indisputable fact. See also Bowerbank in *Entom. Mag.*, i. 239, who not only admits their existence, but affirms that they lose their peculiar elliptical form, and acquire the form of those of Mammalia when they are deprived of their external envelopes.]

[b] [The red colouring matter, or hæmatosine, of the blood in the higher animals is not diffused through the whole mass, as in the class *Annelides*, but belongs exclusively to its globular particles, constituting the external or investing tunic of their fibrinous nuclei. This matter, when separated from the other parts of the blood and dried, is a tasteless inodorous substance, red by transmitted and dark garnet-coloured by reflected light, very soluble in water, and capable of being preserved a great length of time without undergoing any change from the putrefactive process. Dissolved in 50 parts of water it begins to coagulate at a temperature of 149°, and is precipitated in the form of insoluble brown flocculi. Prevost and Dumas have attempted to show that the colouring matter is not really dissolved in the water, but exists in a state of extremely minute division; so that though the fragments are sufficiently small to pass through a filter, they are yet plainly discernible through the microscope. I have already observed that hæmatosine is now generally regarded as a modification of the albuminous principle. According to Berzelius it contains about ·625 per cent. of iron, in some peculiar state of combination, which may be rendered manifest by the appropriate reagents for this metal, after decolorating the mixture by chlorine gas. The same authority states that 400 grains of colouring matter yielded on incineration five grains of ashes, which on accurate analysis were found to contain

Oxide of iron	50·0
Subphosphate of iron	7·5
Phosphate of lime with a small quantity of magnesia	6·0
Pure lime	20·0
Carbonic acid and loss	16·5
	100·0

(*Med.-Chir. Trans.*, iii. 216; Engelhart in *Edin. Med. and Surg. Journ.*, *Jan.* 1827; and Rose *in the Ann. de Chim. et de Phys.*, xxxiv. 268.)

The exclusive presence of iron in this element of the blood, joined to the known tendency of the peroxide of this metal to form salts of a red colour, has generally induced

Any further information we receive concerning the red part of the blood is by means of magnifying glasses, which appear to give a good deal of information. They show us that the red part is composed of bodies of a globular form, swimming in the lymph and serum of the blood. This circumstance of the red part having form probably led anatomists to pay more attention to it than it deserves; as if they could thence explain any essential principle in the blood or animal œconomy.

This knowledge is of late date; for such examinations of minute bodies could only have taken place since the invention and application of magnifying-glasses. Malpighi was probably the first who employed the microscope for this purpose; and he, in 1668, wrote a description of the appearance of the globules in the blood-vessels of the omentum, which he mistook, however, for globules of fat. Microscopical observations were pursued with great ardour by Antonius Van Leewenhoeck, who saw the red globules, August the 15th, 1673. These early observers probably imagined more than they saw.

When an old opinion is partly exploded and a new one brought forward, it becomes only necessary to see how far the new one is just; because if it be not proved, we must revert to the old opinion again, or to some other.

Mr. Hewson has been at great pains to examine the blood in the microscope, and has given us figures of the different shapes of those

---

chemists to suppose that the colour of the blood is due to this cause. Those who wish to consider the arguments on this subject are referred to Berzelius (*ubi ut supra*) and Dr. Bostock (*Physiology*, i. 460.). I shall here only observe, 1st, that the tints produced by reagents on the blood and on the compounds of iron are wholly dissimilar; and 2ndly, that the intensity of colour is too great to allow us to refer it to the minute quantity of iron present in the blood. Dr. Ure has ingeniously suggested that the colour of the blood may possibly depend on the sulphocyanate of potash, this substance having been discovered in the saliva, at the same time that it strikes with the peroxide of iron a very deep and abundant tint much resembling that of the blood. Dr. Williams, on the authority of Dr. Maton, mentions "the case of a lady whose perspiration, when profuse, dyed the clothes on some parts of her person, particularly the wrists and neck, of a bright crimson colour, which was supposed by Dr. Prout to be caused by the sulpho-cyanate of iron." (*Med. Gazette*, xvi. 724.) But the explanation of this subject by Mr. Brande is by far the most plausible. He supposes that the tint of hæmatosine is owing to a peculiar colouring principle, capable, like cochineal or madder, of acting as a dye and of combining with metallic oxides. Pieces of calico impregnated with solutions of corrosive sublimate or nitrate of mercury, and afterwards immersed in an aqueous solution of hæmatosine, acquired a permanent dye of a fine lake red, unchangeable by washing; and solutions of oak bark gave a colour very nearly equal to that of madder and tolerably permanent. The Armenian dyers have for a long while been in the habit of employing it in combination with madder, in order to insure the permanency of that colour. (*Phil. Trans.* 1812.)]

globules [*Phil. Trans.* 1773, p. 303.]; but there is reason to think he may have been deceived in the manner I have just mentioned.

The red globules are always nearly of the same size in the same animal, and when in the serum do not run into one another as the oil does when divided into small globules in water. This form, therefore, does not arise simply from their not uniting with the serum, but they have really a determined shape and size. This is similar to what is observed of the globules in milk; for milk being oily, its globules are not soluble in water; neither do they consist of such pure oil as to run into each other; nor will they dissolve in oil. I suspect, therefore, that they are regular bodies, so that two of them could not unite and form one.

What this property in the red part is I do not know, for it has something like the nature of a solid body; yet the particles seem not to have the properties of a solid, for to the touch they yield no feeling of solidity. When circulating in the vessels they may be seen to assume elliptical forms, adapting themselves to the size of the vessels; they must therefore be a fluid, with an attraction to themselves while in the serum which forms them into round globules, yet without the power of uniting with one another, which may arise from their central attraction extending no further than their own circumference. If they are found, however, of an oval figure in some animals, as authors have described, that circumstance would rather oppose the idea of their being a fluid having a central attraction; but this is probably an optical deception. Whatever their shape is, I should suppose it to be always the same in the same animals, and indeed in all animals, as it must depend upon a fixed principle in the globule itself. Hence the less credit is to be given to those who have described the globules as being of an oval figure in some animals; for they have also described them as being of different and strange shapes even in the same animal*.

* I am led to believe that we may be deceived by the appearances viewed through a magnifying glass; for although objects large enough to be seen by the naked eye are the same when viewed through a magnifying glass which can only magnify in a small degree, yet as the naked eye, when viewing an object rather too small for it, is not to be trusted, it is much less to be depended upon when viewing an object infinitely smaller brought to the same magnitude by a glass. In such a situation, respecting our eye, all the relative objects by which the eye, from habit, judges with more nicety of the object itself, are cut off. The eye has likewise a power of varying its forms, adapting it to the different distances of the parts of an object within its compass, making the object always a whole; but a magnifying glass has no such power. For instance, in viewing a spherical body, a magnifying glass must be made to vary its position, and bring in succession the different parts of the hemisphere into so many focal points, every part separate not having the same relative effect on our organ of vision as when they are all seen at the same time; and the eye, under such circumstances, being unable to vary itself sufficiently to alter the focal distance of the glass, is the reason why rounded

The globules of the blood are endowed with a number of properties. They are the only part of the blood which has form or colour; two

bodies appear of different shapes, giving the shape only of the part that is within the focus of the glass, placed upon an undefined plane; and if it should have more focal points than one then there is an increase of parts; and this will vary according to the opacity or transparency of the body. It may also be remarked that from habit our minds are informed by the necessary actions of our body; therefore the eye, taking on the necessary actions (as it were instinctively), adapting itself at once to the circumstances of the object, gives an intelligence to the mind, independent of the real impression of the object; so that both the impression and the consequent action give information. But this cannot be effected by glasses; for the different focal distances of the hemisphere do not accord with those to which we vary our eyes in adapting them to the distances of the different parts of a rounded body. We are, therefore, left to the impression alone, which is new and consequently imperfect, the centre being too near for the circumference to be seen at one distance, and the circumference, when seen, bringing the centre within the focus, so as to obscure it: for an eye with a given focus which can vary it in a certain degree when viewing objects alone, yet when looking through a magnifying glass of any power must now vary the distance of the object according to the magnifying power in the glass, the eye not being able to vary the focal distance of both; and this, probably, in an inverse degree to the magnifying power of the glass. This may be observed to take place in very short-sighted people, for in them the eye has the least variation respecting distance. A rounded body may be just of such a size as shall have either of its parts out of the focal distance of the eye, and must be moved to and fro alternately before the centre and circumference can be seen; and indeed it is only having a spherical body, of a size proportional to the length of focus, to produce the same effect in every eye.

The appearances in a transparent body when viewed through a magnifying glass are still more fallacious than of an opake one: for an opake body gives only the reflected light, which however will vary according as the rays come on the object. The moon, an opake body, gives us various shapes, and therefore shows only the light and shade arising from the irregularity of the surface; but a semitransparent body, like a red globule, gives both the reflection of the light from the surface and also the refraction of other rays of lights, which vary according to the direction of the light thrown upon the object respecting our eye.

In some transparent bodies we have still a greater variety, for we have both the reflex and refracted light, and these vary according to the distance of the object from the eye or the distance of the light.

If the transparent body is not perfectly round, or is by any circumstance broken in the uniformity of structure on which transparency depends, which I conceive happens to the red globules when diluted in the serum, then the different reflections and refractions will give to the eye the impression of so many shapes*.

---

* [The improvements which have been effected in the construction of microscopes by the adoption of achromatic object glasses has only partially removed the scepticism which still justly attaches to observations made with this instrument. There still exists the greatest imaginable disagreement between the statements of different microscopical observers. "An historical detail," Dr. Bostock observes, "of the errors into which this instrument has led even those who have been the most skilful in its application, would have the effect of inducing us to place little confidence in hypotheses and speculations which are derived from objects which can only be detected by the use of high

properties which are ready to catch the eye and render the mass more visible. In the living body, by making it an object of sight, they give

---

magnifiers." No one I imagine that has examined the conflicting accounts which have been given respecting the globules of the blood will be disposed to doubt the justness of this observation.

Hewson, Home, Meckel, Bauer, Prevost, and the greater number of authorities describe the globules of the blood as consisting of a central nucleus surrounded by a transparent vesicle; Hodgkin affirms that they are flattened cakes, and rejects the notion of a vesicle; others that they are elliptical, spherical, or ovoid; and others again that they are mere rings with central depressions, or mere discs with central elevations.

The same discrepancy is observable in the accounts which have been given of the size of these bodies. Twine estimated their diameter at $\frac{1}{1524}$ to $\frac{1}{1940}$ of an inch, Bauer $\frac{1}{2000}$, Hodgkin $\frac{1}{3000}$, Cavallo $\frac{1}{3333}$, Rudolphi $\frac{1}{3000}$ to $\frac{1}{3500}$, Wollaston $\frac{1}{4000}$, Prevost and Dumas $\frac{1}{4076}$, Raspail $\frac{1}{2,500}$ to $\frac{1}{5000}$, Haller, Home and Kater $\frac{1}{5000}$, and Young $\frac{1}{6060}$. Amidst these discordant statements it would be absurd in any one to pretend to accuracy. The following account, therefore, of these bodies by Professor Mayo can only be regarded as an approximation to the truth; and I take the liberty of inserting it in this place, first, because it accords most accurately with my own observations, and, secondly, because it approaches as nearly as possible to the mean of all the preceding observations.

" The form of the globules (in man) may be compared to a silk-worm's egg. They are circular and extremely thin, with rounded edges and a central depression on either flat surface. Their diameter is very exactly $\frac{1}{3000}$ part of an inch. They are flexible, and, when, rolling upon their edges, are often bent in such a manner that they appear to consist of a central nucleus projecting from a thin disc. Plate XX. fig. 5—10 [which see] represents six squares of a glass micrometer, each side of a square being $\frac{1}{500}$ part of an inch. In the squares 5. 6. 7. different appearances of the particles of the human blood are delineated, their central depression, and various positions in which they may be seen when rolling down an inclined surface—fig. 8. 9. 10 represent the particles of the blood of a skate: they appear to differ from the particles of human blood principally in being of a much larger size, in their oval outline, and in the oval figure of their central depression." (*Outlines of Human Physiology*, 3rd edit., p. 23.)

The size and shape of the globules differ very remarkably in different animals. In the skate, for example, they are elliptical and about twice as large as in human blood. In fishes they are about $\frac{1}{2000}$ to $\frac{1}{2500}$, and in the frog, about $\frac{1}{1000}$ of an inch in diameter; in the water-sow they are about ten times as large, and in the land salamander, nearly thirteen times as large as those of the human blood. These last are the largest which have yet been discovered. It may be observed that the globules are larger in all cold-blooded animals, and represent the oval or ellipse more decidedly than those of mammalia.

Sir Everard Home has stated that the blood-globules, when they have discharged their external envelope of colouring matter, are disposed to coalesce like beads in a row, so as to form fibrils; from which he was led to believe that the ultimate muscular fibre was composed of these corpuscles lineally arranged, an opinion which has been participated in by MM. Prevost and Dumas, Dutrochet, and many other eminent physiologists. Dr. Hodgkin agrees as to the fact of the disposition of the globules to form piles or rouleaux, but affirms that this disposition only exists when they are in their entire state.

Sir Everard Home has also stated, upon the authority of Bauer, that a different and

some idea of the motion of the blood in the smaller vessels, where it is much divided: being there viewed with microscopes, the red globules

---

smaller series of globules (lymph-globules) are generated during coagulation, being in diameter about $\frac{1}{2800}$ of an inch. These are said to be generated in greatest abundance immediately after coagulation; but Professor Faraday has observed them to form so late as the eighth or tenth day; and Dr. Stevens, who examined them by the solar microscope, found that they were equally numerous at all periods, and as abundant as the red globules. He says they varied in size amongst themselves, the largest being at least six times larger than the smallest; but then the latter resembled the globules in rain-water, which are generally believed to consist of air in a state of very minute division.

The prevalence of globules in several of the animal secretions, and in chyle, has led some physiologists to suspect that these particles are identical with the blood globules; those which are found in the secretions, as the milk, the semen, &c., being deprived of their external tunics of colouring matter, while those which are found in the chyle are destined to receive these tunics during the blood's passage through the lungs; nay, the globular structure of the ultimate textures of the body has even induced some to suppose that these particles of the blood form the pabulum of nutrition, not merely of the muscular fibre, but of every other part: but these are mere conjectures, too vague and indefinite to support any physiological argument, which not only do not advance science, but tend rather to retard it, by seducing the mind from the substantial evidence of facts into the ideal regions of imagination. The diversified magnitudes of the globules, according to micrometrical measurement, not only in the blood of different species, but in the textures of the same animal, are circumstances clearly against the notion that these constitute the ultimate molecules of organic structures; not to add that the structure of many parts is such as not easily to admit the red globules at any period of their growth.

In reference to the objection urged by our author to the solidity of the globules, viz., that they show no disposition to coalesce, I may observe, first, that when the capillary circulation is viewed under a good microscope, the globules are often observed to meet and repel one another, from which it has been supposed that the principle of life may confer (like electricity) a new power of repulsion on these bodies, or at least control the aggregative tendency; and secondly, that the nature of the circulation must be admirably adapted to diffuse the globules through the whole mass of the blood, as well as to prevent their coalescence in any particular part. It is not, however, necessary to answer specifically this or any other objection in order to prove the solidity of the globules, for if they were not solid, it must be evident they would always assume the form of spherules, and those spherules would always be of the same size; whereas the fact is, the shape and size of the globules are different in almost every different species of animal, but uniformly the same in the same species; not to mention that the colouring matter of the globules forms a leading constituent of the blood, and may be collected and examined like any other solid body.

The spontaneous volvular and rotary movements which have been observed in the globules of the blood and semen by G. L. Treviranus, Schultz, Dutrochet, Tiedemann, and other microscopical observers, must (if true) materially tend, with the circumstances before mentioned, to promote their diffusion through the whole mass of blood. (*Revue Méd.* i. 136—8.) These movements are conceived by the German physiologists to be as much spontaneous and a property of life as the movements of the infusorial animalculæ. But Brongniart has shown that the granules which issue from the pollen of plants, when it explodes in water, are equally endowed with an automatic motion; and Brown, that all impalpable molecules, whether organic or inorganic, are endowed with the same kind

are seen moving with different velocities in different parts, and taking retrograde or lateral motions, according as mechanical obstructions or those arising from contractions in the vessels may happen to retard or change their motion.

They are heavier than the coagulating lymph, and of course heavier than the serum; which is known by their falling to the bottom of the cup when blood is taken out of a blood-vessel. This allows the coagulating lymph to be seen more or less at the top, and produces on the surface various hues, according as the red globules subside. When they subside much, the buff is then of a yellowish colour; when the buff is thin at the top, then we have the red globules shining through it, of various colours, such as blue, purple*,&c., according to the reflection or refraction, which is according to the depths.

* The blood in the veins, when near the skin, gives the same hues.

---

of inherent or self motion, by virtue of which they exhibit a variety of gyratory evolutions when placed on the surface of liquids. If, therefore, these observations of Brown are correct, the idea of an intestine vital motion in the globules of the blood must be abandoned; but as the Germans have attributed a variety of effects to this cause, it will be necessary to revert to this subject when speaking of the circulation of the blood.

Majendie says that a uumber of globules are developed in the serum of the blood by the action of galvanism very similar to those of the blood (*Phys.*, p. 234.); and a similar result was experienced by Prevost and Dumas on applying galvanism to the white of an egg. (*Ann. de Chim.*, xxiii. 53, and *Bib. Univ.*, *Juillet* 1821.) Raspail regards the globules not as organized particles, but as particles of albumen undissolved in, or precipitated from, the serum, and has attempted to show that albumen, dissolved in an excess of hydrochloric acid, forms minute spherical and equal globules, scarcely distinguishable from the globules of the blood. "If a portion of the albumen of a pullet's egg," he says, "be placed in an excess of hydrochloric acid, it will at first form a white coagulum, but presently it will be dissolved by the acid acquiring at the same time a violet colour, which passes into blue. If the hydrochloric acid be then poured off, and left to evaporate spontaneously, it will deposit a white powder, which, when observed by the microscope, will be seen to consist of spherical globules, of uniform size, and which the most practised eye might well mistake for the globules of the blood." The same phenomenon is also noticed when lactic acid is saturated by barytes; "the precipitation in this case is composed of beautiful globules, some of which even show a nucleus in their centre." (*Org. Chem.*, *transl. by Dr. Townsend*, p. 406.) Dr. Elliotson observes, that "one takes breath while reading M. Raspail, after the strange and varying statements of so many experimenters, especially of those who use microscopes" (*Physiology*, p. 148.); but the justness of this eulogium may I think be questioned. M. Raspail has entirely failed to account, 1st, for the colouring matter of the red globules; 2nd, for their precipitation; 3rd, for the difficulty with which they are regenerated, although the regeneration of the albumen is easily effected; 4th, for their importance in relation to the function of respiration, and the production of animal heat: 5th, for their various forms and sizes in different animals, and their uniformity in these respects in the same animal; and 6th, for the presence of iron in one and not in the other.]

In healthy blood, however, the coagulum is commonly formed before the red part has time to subside; but we may always observe that the lower part of the mass contains more red globules than the top, and will sink more quickly in water. The red globules do not retain their globular form in every fluid, but are dissolved and diffused through the whole; and this probably happens sooner in water than in any other fluid. The red globules are not soluble in the serum of the blood, yet it is not the only fluid in which they are insoluble; the urine does not dissolve them; but urine might be supposed to be principally serum. Water itself, however, ceases to dissolve them when saturated with many of the neutral salts, or with some of the acids. The red globules are not soluble in water mixed with common sea-salt, sal ammoniac, Epsom-salt, nitre (potassæ nitras), Glauber's-salt (sodæ sulphas), soluble tartar (potassa tartras), Lymington-tartar; nor in the fixed vegetable alkalies when saturated with fixed air. As they do not dissolve in the serum or urine, it might be imagined to arise from the neutral salts which they contain; but I should believe that neither of these fluids has a quantity sufficient for that purpose.

The vitriolic acid does not dissolve the red globules when diluted so low as to have less pungency of taste than common vinegar.

The red globules are soluble in common vinegar, but take a longer time to dissolve than in water; and they also dissolve much sooner when the vinegar is diluted with water.

In muriatic acid, diluted so as to be more pungent to the tongue, and three times stronger than the vinegar, the red globules are not dissolved, but lose their red colour: by adding more water to the red globules, they dissolve; lemon juice dissolves the red globules: all this, however, throws but little light on this part of the blood.

When the globules are put into water they dissolve, which destroys their globular form; it is therefore the serum, and probably the coagulating lymph also, when circulating, which confines them to this form; but when the serum is diluted with water they dissolve in it; and this appears to take place at once, as quick as water unites with water[a]. I could not observe that it was like the solution of a solid body, as a salt, for instance: a drop of blood requires about two drops of water added to it to dissolve its globules: if urine also be diluted with water, the

[a] [According to Dr. Young, the outer coat only, or colouring matter, is dissolved by water, in consequence of which the central (fibrinous) nucleus becomes spherical, and specifically lighter than water. Sir Everard Home states that the globule loses $\frac{1}{3}$rd in diameter, and $\frac{2}{3}$rds in substance, whenever it is deprived of its colouring matter by solution.]

globules dissolve in it. However, after standing some days the globules dissolve both in serum and urine; but I think later in the last. When the globules are not dissolved in any fluid the whole looks muddy, not transparent; but when dissolved in water the whole is a fine clear red. What are the properties of the serum, and those other substances that preserve the red part of the blood in a regular form, I do not know[a].

The red globules, when dried in the serum, and moistened in the same, do not again resume their regular form; nor do they dissolve in it, as they do in water, but form rather a sort of flakes. As the serum and solutions of many kind of salts do not dissolve the red globules, I conceived that it might be possible for them to resume their globular figure (after having been dissolved in water,) by adding such a quantity of serum as to make the proportion of water very little; but I could not produce this effect, although the menstruum was such as not to dissolve fresh globules.

The red globules not dissolving in the serum, nor in the coagulating lymph, become separable from those parts when circulating, and therefore may be prevented from going where the coagulating lymph passes in a natural state, which they certainly do not*, and which also is the reason why they are so perfectly retained in the coagulum when extravasated. The globules, besides being heavier than the serum, and the coagulating lymph, appear to have more substance; for they do not lose so much upon drying, and when dried with serum they give a kind of roughness to the surface, which serum has not by itself. They appear not to be a natural part of the blood, but, as it were, composed out of it, or composed in it, and not with it; for they seem to be formed later in life than either of the other two; thus we see, while the chick is in the egg, and the heart beating, it then contains a transparent fluid before any red globules are formed, which we may suppose to be the serum, and the lymph. The globules do not appear to be formed in those parts of the blood already produced, but rather to rise up in the sur-

* This will be more fully explained when on the colour of parts from the blood.

---

[a] [Many circumstances induce the belief, that the cohesion of the colouring matter of the globules to their central fibrinous nuclei is a manifestation of vitality. In adynamic fevers, in cases of death from poisoning, and under many other circumstances, this cohesion is destroyed, in consequence of which the colouring matter of the blood transudes through the coats of the veins, or else exudes into the serous cavities. Under such circumstances also, the blood, when abstracted from the body, instead of coagulating, is apt to let fall a pulverulent deposit, and to pass rapidly into a state of putrefaction. I have already observed that the catamenial fluid is devoid of red globules, and consists merely of a solution of colouring matter.]

rounding parts*. It would also seem to be formed with more difficulty than either of the other two parts. When an animal has lost a consi-

* Thus, on some of the first appearances of the chick we find a zone surrounding it, composed of dots, which contain red globules, but not in vessels, and which zone becomes vascular afterwards. Vide Plate XVI.

* [This account has been amply confirmed by Dœllinger and Wolff, who noticed the formation of blood-globules in the chick previously to the existence of either heart or vessels. Similar phenomena have also been related by Gruithuisen and Kaltenbrunner, who observed sanguineous puncta to arise in inflamed and regenerating parts, which at first were placed in regular order, but afterwards united, so as to represent, and actually to constitute, new vessels, which in the further process of development formed interconnexions with each other, and with those which previously existed. (*Tiedemann's Phys., trans. by Lane and Gully*, p. 150.)

Having already adverted to M. Raspail's account of the origin of the red globules, I would here further observe that these bodies are probably formed much earlier in the process of sanguification (*note*, p. 64). MM. Prevost and Dumas detected globules in the chyle of rabbits, hedgehogs, and dogs, which they conceived might form the rudiments of the future blood globules; for although the chyliferous globules have not all the same diameter, yet the largest among them are smaller than those of the blood, and consequently may admit of a further enlargement by the addition of their coloured envelopes. (*Journ. des Prog. des Sci. Med.*) Leuret and Lassaigne affirm that they have discovered fibrinous globule seven in the chyme, in the stomach, and still more numerously in the duodenum, which globules they say exactly resembled those of the chyle, and ran together so as to form fibrils, precisely in the same manner as the globules of the blood. (*Op. ut supra.*)

The striking analogy which exists between the chyle and the blood unquestionably must be allowed to be in favour of this opinion. If an animal be killed three or four hours after a full meal, and the chyle be collected, it will be found to exhibit an opake milk-white colour if the food has consisted of fat animal food, opaline if the diet has consisted of animal food without fat, and transparent if it has merely consisted of vegetables; after it has coagulated, the serum exhibits the same general properties as the serum of the blood, and the coagulum consists of pure fibrin, of a slightly roseate hue. Still the composition of chyle and blood is not exactly the same; for, like the globules, the albumen and fibrin of chyle differ in some unimportant respects from those of blood, and appear, in short, to be in an incipient state, requiring some further elaboration (which is probably effected in the lungs,) to render their conversion into blood complete. (*Prout, Bridgewater Treatise*, p. 520, *and Ann. of Phil.*, xiii. 12.)

The coagulum which forms from lymph collected from the thoracic duct of an animal which has fasted for several days, exhibits so deep a roseate hue as nearly to approach that of the blood; and, like it, it is converted to scarlet by oxygen, and to purple by carbonic acid gas. (*Majendie, Physiologie, 4eme edit.: Brux.*, p. 220.) I am not aware, however, that this fact has ever been observed of chyle collected in a pure state from the lacteals. Tiedemann and Gmelin have asserted that pure chyle has very little disposition to coagulate, and that it contains no globular or reddish particles previously to its having passed the mesenteric glands: but as these particles instantly appear after the chyle has passed this point, and particularly after it has become mixed with the lymphatic fluid proceeding from the spleen, they conceive it not improbable that the globules are formed in one or other of these organs. (*Recherches sur la Digestion.*)

The opinion that the red globules are elaborated in the spleen is of very old date. It does not, however, appear to be well founded, for after the most accurate microsco-

derable quantity of its blood, the other parts seem to be sooner made up than the red globules; the animal looks long pale; but this is only conjecture, for we have no method of knowing the quantity of the other parts.

From the above account it appears that whatever may be their utility in the machine, the red globules certainly are not of such universal use as the coagulating lymph, since they are not to be found in all animals, nor so early in those that have them; nor are they pushed into the extreme arteries, where we must suppose the coagulating lymph reaches; neither do they appear to be so readily formed. This being the case, we must conclude them not to be the important part of the blood in contributing to growth, repair, etc. Their use would seem to be connected with strength, for the stronger the animal the more it has of the red globules; and the strength acquired by exercise increases their proportion, not only in the whole body, but, as we shall find, occasions them to be carried into parts where, in either a quiet or debilitated state of the animal, they were not allowed to go; the use, therefore, of a part, and the quantity of red globules passing through it, are probably pretty well proportioned to each other. This effect is so well known to feeders of young animals for the table of the epicure, that bleeding, to lessen the quantity, is immediately practised; as also debarring the creature from exercise, in order to prevent their increasing, and being carried so far from the heart as they otherwise would be.

These three substances are of different specific gravities: the serum, or fluid part, is the lightest; the solid part, or lymph, is the next in order; and the red globules are the heaviest. This is seen in such blood

---

pical observations of the blood of a dog whose spleen had been removed several months previously, Dr. Babington was unable to discover any deficiency of red particles, as compared with the blood of another dog in perfect health whose blood was examined at the same time. (*Med.-Chir. Trans.*, xvi. 318.) The idea that they are formed in the mesenteric glands is rebutted, first, by the testimony of Leuret and Lassaigne, before mentioned; and, secondly, by the fact that many of the lacteals enter the thoracic duct without passing through the glands, and yet contain as many globular particles as those that do. Upon the whole, therefore, I am induced to believe that rudimentary globules are formed during the earlier periods of digestion, and that these are afterwards perfected in the system by means with which at present we are wholly unacquainted. This appears to me to accord better with the general law of progressive development which characterizes the whole organic world, than to suppose that they are perfectly formed at once by any individual organ. We see a gradually ascending scale of animated beings, a progressive formation of the different parts of each individual organism during the different periods of its growth, and a successive elaboration of its various proximate principles before they are applied to their final purposes in the œconomy. It seems, therefore, reasonable to suppose that the formation of the globules is governed by the same law.]

as separates readily into its constituent parts. The serum swims upon the top, and the red globules fall to the bottom, while the lymph would be suspended between the two if the red part were not retained in the lymph, from its coagulation: but this constant effect is no absolute proof of the difference in the specific gravities of the serum and coagulating lymph; for we still do not know but that the red globules, which are evidently the heaviest, make the coagulating lymph to sink in the serum. To ascertain this circumstance I made the following experiment: I took some blood, which separated easily into its constituent parts; I then suspended in a portion of serum a piece of coagulating lymph, which was free from red globules, and it sunk to the bottom, but not very quickly: this proves that the lymph, when coagulated, is somewhat heavier than the serum.

I then took as much of the bottom of the coagulum containing the red globules, and put it into the serum along with the lymph, to see which of them sunk the fastest, and found that the piece with the red globules sunk much more quickly than the other; I should think three times as fast. The serum itself is much heavier than common water, for when the parts before mentioned were put into common water, in the same manner as into the serum, they both sunk much faster, and there was not that disproportion between the times of their falling as in the serum. But if the blood has a strong disposition to coagulate, and is not in large quantity, it will coagulate soon, and involve the red globules; yet there will then be fewest at top, and they will be more and more crowded towards the bottom; though there would appear in such blood to be no coagulating lymph at top free from the red globules, yet in most of it a thin pellicle may be found, which can be pulled off.

I have already observed that the whole mass of blood, taken together, in a great variety of classes of animals, appears of a red colour; and I shall now further remark, that it is of a much deeper colour in some classes of animals than in others, which I believe arises from a greater number of red globules being contained in a given quantity of lymph and serum. This, I think, evidently appears to be the case when we examine a portion of the blood itself belonging to different classes of animals. In the class called quadruped I believe it has the deepest body of colour; I am not, however, certain that it is not nearly as deep in some birds; and even in the same class of animals it appears to have a much greater body of colour in some species than in others. Thus, it appears to be deeper in the hare than in the rabbit.

It is the red part itself which makes the difference in depth of colour in different parts of the animal; and the common mode of judging is by the colour of the parts in different classes of animals that have red blood;

on these we generally form our opinion; for though in some animals which have white muscles the liver, kidney, and heart may be nearly as red as in others whose muscles are universally as red, yet, as the muscles are white, there must be a deficiency in the red globules on the whole; for if these parts which are red in animals having white muscles, as the heart, liver, etc., have no more than their due proportion with other animals that are universally red, there must be in such animals a deficiency of red globules on the whole. This idea may be gradually carried on, from the animal which has fewest red muscles, to those whose muscles are universally red and of a high colour; even in the same species the colour of all the muscles is not equally high. What are called different temperaments have their muscles redder or paler; the darker the colour of the skin, hair, etc. of any one species, I believe the blood is in proportion redder. When a part, of whatever kind, is red, it takes place in consequence of its vessels being large enough to carry red blood; and therefore, when we find a muscle red we know it arises from the same cause. When a part, on the contrary, is white, as a tendon, it is because its vessels are small, and have little or none of the red blood passing along them, although it may probably be as vascular as the muscle to which it belongs*; and those animals that have no red blood have white flesh universally†, and this, probably, no less vascular than the flesh which receives red blood.

The blood in the same animals is not equally deep-coloured in every part; that is, every part of the body has not its blood equally loaded with red globules, or, at least, it is not equally red, even in parts of the same construction and use, such as muscles; this arises from the red globules not being carried into those parts in equal proportion: these are the white parts of animals; such muscles, in animals used for food, are called white meat. In animals which have these muscles there is commonly not so much red blood as in others where these parts are more universally red; and perhaps the red part of the blood is not pushed so far in them as in those which have it in a larger proportion. There are some animals, however, which have a larger quantity of red globules in the blood, yet have some of their muscles of a lighter colour than others:

* Conceiving that the amnion of a calf might have but few vessels, I injected a piece of it with quicksilver, first drying its edges all round on the edge of a dish, while the middle of it lay in the dish, in water; but the whole became one mass of vessels. The intention of this experiment was to see, if possible, the communication between the arteries and the veins; but the mass of vessels prevented every view of this kind.

† The redness of the blood is of great use towards the knowledge of diseases; many inflammations are known by it when on the skin, and even the kind of inflammation is distinguished by the kind of redness: also putrid diseases are distinguished when the blood is extravasated. The quantity in the face is a sign of health or disease.

even in the human subject all the muscles are not equally red; the muscular part of the intestines, for instance, is not equal in redness to the heart, and many other muscles. To what is this owing? Does it arise from mechanical causes? Do the vessels become suddenly so small beyond a certain limit as not to allow the red blood to pass? or are the other parts of the blood less tenacious? Is the red part in such not allowed to go so far? or is it a separating principle in the vessels themselves? Many circumstances in life either increase the quantity of the red globules, or make them more universal in the muscles of the same animal; thus, exercise increases the quantity of the red globules and the red colour of muscles, while there is the same quantity on the whole; or perhaps we should rather say that indolence decreases the quantity: this is particularly remarkable in woman; and probably the whiteness of the muscles of young animals may arise from the same cause; I suspect, however, something more; I conceive it arises from the principle of life, influenced by accidental or mechanical causes, for the muscles of young animals are increasing in colour till they arrive at the age of maturity, and not afterwards, although they continue to use exercise. Diseases lessen the quantity of the red globules, and often render their distribution unequal.

From the above account we may reason, upon the whole, that the animals which are reddest, or have the greatest number of red parts, have their blood furnished with the greatest proportion of red globules[a].

One would naturally suppose that the red globules were of the same colour everywhere in the same animal; this last is perhaps the case; but now we find that these globules are of different hues in the different systems of vessels in the same animal. In the more perfect animals, where there are two systems of vessels carrying the blood, viz. arteries and veins, the blood is not of the same species of red in both of them in the same animal; one red is the scarlet, which takes place in the arteries of the body, the other is the modena, which takes place in the veins; and as every part of the body possesses such systems of vessels,

---

[a] [This mode of reasoning is extremely questionable. It may be doubted, for example, whether any degree of exercise would ever occasion the wing muscles of certain birds to assume the dark tint which characterizes the muscles of the legs, and *e converso*. According to Prevost and Dumas, birds are more vascular than mammiferous quadrupeds, and possess a greater number of red globules; and yet there can be no doubt that the colour of their flesh is generally paler. The same observation is equally applicable to the young of all animals. Bichat has endeavoured to show that the colour of muscles depends on some foreign substance combined with their fibres; but this colour is certainly not essential to their perfect structure, for the lightest-coloured muscles are often those which are most contractile. (*Bichat, Anat. Gen.*, ii. 327.)]

the parts which are visited by red blood must have a mixture of both. As there are two circulations in every animal above the insect, one in the lungs in those that breathe air, or in the gills, as in fish, in those that breathe water, and the other the general circulation to the body in both, we find the two colours of the globules not corresponding to the same system of vessels in each. The scarlet is the venal blood in the lungs, which afterwards becomes the arterial in the body, where it is commonly seen, and hence it is called the arterial blood: the modena is the venal blood of the body, and is the blood also of the pulmonary artery; but as it is commonly seen in the veins only of the body, it is called the venal blood; the scarlet colour, therefore, is acquired in the lungs, and the modena in the body. There are so many proofs of this that it hardly requires any illustration; yet many circumstances and experiments may be brought in direct proof of it. I bled a man in the temporal artery and in the vein of the arm at the same time, each into a phial. The blood of the artery was of a florid red, and the venal was dark. The arterial kept its colour, and did not separate its serum; but this was singular, for in others it does separate its serum and coagulum: the venal separated into its constituent parts as usual.

Although this, however, is a general rule, yet there are many exceptions; for we find in many cases the scarlet colour of the blood in the arteries not changed in the veins, and under some circumstances the modena taking place in the arteries, as well as where blood is extravasated in the body*.

* [In ordinary bleeding it is not uncommon to find the blood which issues from the vein of a bright arterial tint; or sometimes the stream appears to be composed of dark- and light-coloured blood in nearly equal proportions, as if the artery and vein had both been punctured. This is particularly observable in excited states of the circulation, when at the same time the function of respiration is carried on without impediment. Baglivi noticed this appearance of the blood in bleeding patients who were labouring under hectic fever; but it is certainly much more frequent in rheumatic attacks and after brisk exercise. Sometimes this appearance is produced by the warm bath (*Thackrah*, p. 181), and in a less degree by warm climates; sometimes by fits, paroxysms of palpitation and syncope, and not unfrequently by common inflammation and fever. Broughton found the blood in the veins of animals which had been made to respire oxygen gas as florid as in the arteries. Thackrah remarked that a similar effect was generally produced by a full dose of prussic acid. It would seem, therefore, either that the blood is unduly oxygenized in the lungs, or else that it is hurried through the circulation with too great rapidity to allow it to undergo the usual changes in the periphery of the body. The peripheral and pulmonary circulations being antagonized to each other, either of these causes may produce the effect by destroying the balance which necessarily subsists between them in a normal state: besides which, it is extremely probable that this balance may sometimes be disturbed through the mere influence of the nervous system, independently of any alteration in the physical conditions under which the vital functions are performed. Thus, Dupuytren found that the blood was only imper-

It becomes a question how the change is produced in each.

More attention has been paid to the mode in which it gets the scarlet colour than the modena (though both probably are of equal importance), because it was believed that life in some degree depended on this colour.

---

fectly arterialized in the lungs when the eighth pair of nerves was divided; and, as the counterpart of this fact, it is notorious that the blood is not venalised in inflamed parts. There is no improbability, therefore, in supposing that the whole function of nutrition may be more or less partially suspended for a time, in consequence of which the blood may pass through the capillaries of the body without undergoing any change, or at least any change commensurate with the effect produced in the lungs.

It more frequently happens, however, that the blood is black in the arteries than red in the veins; this appearance depending on the reverse of those causes which have been above mentioned. Thus, during the congestive stage of fevers the blood exhibits a black appearance arising from the remora of the circulation. The same thing also happens in cholera, apoplexy, epilepsy, asphyxia, poisoning from opium, and under a variety of other circumstances where the respiration is impeded or the circulation materially retarded.

The principal points of difference which distinguish arterial from venous blood are comprehended in the following table:

		Arterial.	Venous.
Specific gravity	(*Davy, Phil. Trans.* 1814.)	1051	1049
Capacity for heat	(*Ib.*)	913	903
Temperature	(*Ib.*)	1° more.	1° less.
Carbon	(*Macaire and Marcet, op. cit.*, p. 400.)	50·2	55·7
Oxygen		26·3	21·7
Nitrogen		16·3	16·2
Hydrogen		6·6	6·4
Electricity	(*Bellingeri, Exper. in Elect. Sang.*)	less.	more.
Colour		bright scarlet.	brownish or modena red.
Odour	(*Magendie, Physiologie.*)	strong.	faint.
Coagulation	(*Thackrah.*)	quicker.	slower.
Clot to serum	(*Ib.*)	more.	less.
Fibrin	(*Alison, Physiology.*)	more.	less.
Carbonic acid	(*Stevens, op. cit.*)	none.	appreciable quantities.
Functions	(*Kay on the Physiology of Asphyxia.*)	great supporter of life.	weak supporter of life.

Besides these differences, there are probably some others, arising from the different degrees of vitality possessed by the two bloods; but these can only be investigated in their effects upon the solids.

In connexion with this subject it may not be improper to advert to the diversities of the blood in different vessels of the same body. Thackrah found that the portal blood of dogs differed from blood from the jugular veins in containing much less albumen and hæmatosine, in coagulating more rapidly, in having a muddy brownish colour, as if it had been defectively elaborated, and in some other minor particulars. (*Op. cit.*, p. 70.) Stoker made similar observations. (*Op. cit.*, part ii. p. 31.) Now it must be manifest that these remarks are only applicable to blood from different parts of the venous system. In the arteries it must be the same everywhere; but in the veins it must be continually liable to variation, in consequence of the abstractions which are

Many substances change the colour of the blood from the modena to the scarlet: respirable air has this effect, and many of the neutral salts, more especially nitre, which occasions the florid colour in meat that has been salted also with sea-salt. But as the air produces this effect in the living body, and as we find that without air the animal dies, great stress has been laid on this change of colour, whereas it should only be considered as a sign that the blood has been in contact with the air, but not that it must be fit for the purpose of circulation. This effect takes place readily under many circumstances: it takes place out of the circulation as readily as when in it; as readily when blood is coagulated as before; it takes place in blood whose coagulating principle has been destroyed, as by lightning, sudden death, &c.: it does not, therefore, depend upon life. It is the cause only of this change in the colour by respirable air which becomes an object of consideration; for if we suppose the change of colour in the red globules to be all that respiration is to perform, we shall make the red globules the most essential part of the blood, whereas they are the least so. Most probably the effect of air upon the blood is greatest on the coagulating lymph; and

---

made by the different secretory organs. (See M. Le Gallois' Essay, entitled "*Le Sang est-il identique dans tous les vaisseaux qu'il parcourt?*" Par. An. xi.)

Allied also to this subject is the alteration which the blood undergoes in regard to its chemical constitution during one and the same venesection. This point has been already adverted to in reference to the diminution of fibrin (see *note*, p. 37); but it remains to be noticed that the quantity of serum is proportionally increased under the same circumstances, probably because the absorbent system is roused to increased action by whatever depresses the vital powers (*Pharmacologia, by J. A. Paris, M.D.*, 5*th edit.* p. 174.), or else because the first evacuation of blood causes the return into the larger vessels of much of the thinner parts of this fluid previously divergent in the invisible capillaries. Such at least are the opinions of Davy (*De Sang.*, 1814) and Schrœder Van der Kolk (*Com. de Sang. Coag.*, 1820, l. c.), and the same views have more recently been adopted by Dr. Alison (*Physiology*, p. 58.). The attenuation of the blood in these cases has been assigned as the cause why it coagulates more rapidly the nearer an animal approaches to the state of syncope. Prater found that blood which was diluted with equal parts of water coagulated only one minute sooner than a similar quantity not diluted, but that dilution with one half, one third, one sixth, or even one tenth of serum accelerated concretion at least six minutes; from which facts he argued "that dilution takes place by a provision of nature, and that such dilution is the principal if not the sole cause why the blood flowing from a dying animal coagulates so quickly." (*Op. cit.* pp. 109, 111, 114.) Now it is not to be disputed that repeated venesections, at considerable intervals of time, will have the effect of increasing the tenuity of the blood (see *note*, p. 44.); but it is extremely doubtful whether this effect is uniformly or even generally produced during a single venesection, however copious. Thackrah did not find this to be the case, but, on the contrary, that the fluid parts of the blood were often diminished in the last cup. The same thing also occurred to Prater, whose experiments, however, are open to many sources of fallacy; and, even though we should admit the fact, yet it would not explain all the circumstances of the case, for timidity and alarm not unfrequently occasion the first portions of blood to coagulate more rapidly than the last,

this conjecture is rendered more likely when we consider that in animals which have no red globules of any kind respiration is as essential to their existence as in any other, and we find that the blood may lose this effect and yet retain its salutary effects in the constitution. Thus, when any large artery is tied, the parts beyond must be supplied with blood that shall have lost its florid colour; and in the chick in the egg the blood in the arterial system is dark, while in the veins of the temporary lungs it is florid. We are led by daily experience to observe that the dark blood taken from a vein becomes red on that surface which is exposed to the common atmosphere, and that if it be shaken in a phial with air the whole becomes red*. If blood also be allowed to stand exposed to the air and to coagulate, its upper surface will become of the scarlet red, while the bottom remains dark, or even of a darker colour than common venal blood, because it contains a greater quantity of red globules. If the coagulated blood be inverted, and the bottom

* This does not arise from motion, for fill the phial with blood without air, and put into it glass-beads, and shake them, so as to give it motion, the colour will not be altered.

---

while of three portions of blood taken from a slaughtered animal, the third is often observed to be slower in coagulating than the second: besides, "Pithing, poisoning by prussic acid, and the injection of air into the veins, show as strongly as death from hæmorrhage the last-drawn blood to concrete with greatest rapidity." (*Thackrah*, p. 139.) I conceive, therefore, that these differences in the coagulating power of the blood may best be referred to the varying conditions of the vital powers.

The following Table exhibits the differences of time in regard to the blood's concretion:

	1st Cup.		2nd Cup.		3rd Cup.	
	′	″	′	″	′	″
From a dog bled to death......	1	10	0	40	—	—
From a slaughtered sheep	1	30	1	00	0	30
Ditto	1	10	0	50	—	—
Ditto	2	10	1	45	0	55
From a slaughtered ox	3	40	6	45	0	55
Ditto	2	29	8	30	0	30
Ditto	2	50	1	10	2	15
Ditto	2	30	1	35	1	10
Ditto	1	30	0	50	0	20
From a stuck horse	11	10	9	55	3	20

Accordingly, Thackrah found that in venesection syncope reduced the time required for concretion from 5′ to 2′, or from 90″ to 40″. (*Op. cit.*, p. 132.) Blood taken during the actual state of syncope rarely separates its serum, and in proportion as an animal approaches to this state, the separative change is less and less; thus, from a stuck calf the first portion of blood (which was taken on the infliction of the wound,) yielded 412·3 serum to 587·7 crassamentum, while in the second portion (which was taken when the hæmorrhage had nearly ceased,) the proportions were as 361·7 to 630·3.]

exposed to the air, this part will also assume the scarlet red, and become even redder than that exposed before, because it contains a greater number of red globules, which undergo this change. The red colour will even penetrate to some depth, which shows that the effect can be produced through a thick substance. We often find the vessels of the lungs full of blood, and the whole substance of the lungs of a dark colour; but if we inflate the lungs the cells will become of a florid red, the small vessels on those cells, both arteries and veins, having the colour of their blood changed by the air in the cells affecting it through their coats. We find the same thing on the surface of flesh or muscles, liver, &c. We may observe in the gills of fish that they retain their florid colour as long as the fish is fresh, from being exposed to the air, for they naturally have the air applied externally in the act of breathing. It is from these facts we reason respecting the scarlet colour which the blood acquires in the lungs but loses in the body, and why therefore it is found of the modena colour in the veins, and of course in the right side of the heart and larger trunks of the pulmonary artery. As the blood is florid in the pulmonary veins as far as we can trace them, we reasonably suppose that it acquires this appearance in the small vessels of the lungs, and as the lungs constantly take in fresh air, we conceive that by exposure to the air (perhaps both in arteries and veins) it acquired the scarlet colour; for we shall see that the air, or the influence of the air, is capable of passing through animal substance.

In the living body, when the breathing is imperfect, we can plainly see the change taking place in the colour of the blood in proportion as the breathing becomes more perfect, of which the following experiments are proofs. They were made with a view to observe the motion of the heart, by producing an artificial breathing, and exhibited a vast variety of satisfactory phenomena, of which the change in the colour of the blood in the lungs was one.

I invented a pair of double bellows, each of which had two openings, but their actions were reversed: two of the openings were inclosed in one pipe or nozzle, and the other two were on the sides. The lower chamber had its valve placed exactly similar to that of the common bellows; but it had also a valve at the nozzle, which did not allow any air to enter there. The upper half had a valve placed at the nozzle, which allowed the air to enter but not to escape, and the opening on the upper side allowed the air to escape but not to enter; so that, on dilating the bellows, the upper side or chamber drew in the air by the nozzle only, and at the same time the under chamber drew in its air by the side only. On closing the bellows, or expelling this air, the air drawn in by the nozzle passed out at the opening on the upper side, and the air that was drawn in by the under side passed out by the nozzle. By this means I could, by fixing the nozzle into the trachea, draw the air out of the lungs into the upper chamber of the bellows, and at the same time draw fresh air into the lower chamber: on emptying these cavities of their air, the pure air in the lower chamber passed into the lungs, and that which had been just taken from the lungs into the upper chamber passed into the open air alternately. The action of these bellows, though double, is exactly as simple as breathing itself; and they appear to me to be superior to any invention made since for the same purpose[a] I fixed the nozzle of these bellows into the trachea of a dog, and immediately began the artificial breathing. I then removed the sternum and cartilages, and opened the pericardium. While I continued the artificial breathing, I observed that the blood in the pulmonary veins, coming from the lungs, the left auricle, the aorta, &c., was florid or dark just as I threw air or not into the lungs.

I cut off a piece of the lungs, and found that the colour of the blood which came from the wound corresponded with the above effects. When I threw air into the lungs, so as to render the blood florid in the pulmonary veins, two kinds of blood issued from the wound; and when I left off blowing, the whole blood which passed out by the wound was of the dark colour. If the air is confined in the lungs of a quadruped, it soon loses its power over the blood, which remains dark, or has the appearance of becoming dark, because dark-coloured blood is thrown in and it undergoes no change; but if the same experiment is made on an amphibious animal it is a considerable time before the whole blood becomes dark, because in such animals the lungs are a reservoir of air, which of course continues its influence over the blood for a longer time.

---

[a] [The principal inconvenience of this bellows consists in the extreme difficulty of regulating the artificial respiration. The researches of Magendie and Leroy have fully established the fact of the great liability of the air-cells to become ruptured when the quantity of air impelled is either too great or too rapidly effected, in consequence of which the pulmonary tissue is rendered emphysematous, and the chances of recovery much diminished; and to so great a degree are the lungs exposed to this danger, that it has even been doubted whether the proportion of recoveries from asphyxia has not been considerably reduced since the introduction of this means of resuscitation.

To obviate this inconvenience, M. Leroy has recommended the adaptation of an arc of degrees to the handles of Hunter's bellows, graduated in such a manner as at once to show the proportions requisite for the different ages of life, to which are added moveable pipes to correspond, so as only to allow of the escape of the air in such quantities and in such periods of time as shall closely represent natural respiration. There can be no doubt that this is a very great improvement upon the old bellows, and ought universally to be adopted in all institutions for the recovery of drowned persons. (*Magendie's Journ. de Phys.*, vii. viii. xi.)]

This experiment I have repeated upon several animals, and commonly for half an hour at a time, which was sufficient to allow me to make my observations with coolness and accuracy. In this part of the experiment it was curious to see the coronary arteries turn darker and darker, becoming like the veins which run on each side of them, and on blowing again resume gradually a brighter colour, till they became of a florid red. As respiration was generally prevented in the first part of the experiment, the blood was found at first wholly of a dark colour, and the heart large and hardly acting; but on throwing into the lungs fresh air, the heart began to act, upon which both auricles and ventricles became gradually smaller; then by stopping the respiration they again became larger and larger.

The diminution of the heart's motion upon stopping respiration does not depend upon the immediate impression of improper blood on the left auricle and ventricle as a sedative, but upon the sympathetic connexion which exists between the heart and lungs (one action ceasing the other also ceases); which sympathy is established, because if the heart were to continue acting it would send improper blood into the body, by which it can be supported only a little while. The right auricle and ventricle also cease acting, although not so early, and for the same reason; because on the cessation of the function of the lungs the blood cannot receive any benefit in passing through them.

These actions and cessations are all dependent on life and the connexion of one action with another. It is upon the same principle that the first effect of recovery is the act of breathing[a].

---

[a] [The cessation of the heart's action, in cases of asphyxia, would appear to depend,

1st, On the circulation of black blood through its substance, by which its irritability is more or less impaired;

2nd, On the effect of black blood on the brain producing universal depression,—lowering still further the tone of the heart, and paralysing the muscles of respiration, as well as the pulmonary capillaries;

3rd, On the insufficient supply of blood which is sent to the left side of the heart in consequence of the paralysis of the pulmonary capillaries.

We may therefore trace a sort of reaction in a circle among the vital organs, each concurring towards the same effect. What is the exact order of their cessation, or the precise share which each of them has in producing the ultimate effect, is not easily assigned. In syncope the series of phenomena would appear to commence with an impression on the brain, which is thence propagated to the heart, and thence to the lungs; but in asphyxia the first effect is probably felt by the heart, the second by the brain, and the third by the lungs.

Goodwyn conceived that the heart ceased to act because the left side, being only arterio-contractile, was incapable of being stimulated by venous blood; but this idea was fully disproved by the experiments of Bichat, which render it certain that the blood stimulates the ventricles not by its quality, but by its bulk. (*Goodwyn on the Connex. of Life with Resp.* pp. 82, 83; and *Bichat, Sur la Vie et la Mort.*) On the other hand, Bichat's

The following cases illustrate this still further.

I bled a gentleman in the temporal artery, while in a fit of apoplexy; he breathed seemingly with great difficulty; the blood flowed very freely, and he continued to bleed longer than we commonly find from the same wound, which made me suspect that the artery had lost some of its contracting power. The blood was as dark as venal blood; he became somewhat relieved, and his breathing more free. About two hours afterwards we opened the same orifice, which still bled freely, but now the blood was become florid as usual.

Mrs. ——, in Norris-street, Haymarket, fell into an apoplectic fit, in which she was insensible respecting ideas: her breathing was very imperfect, attended with a rattling in her throat, and a snort; the pulse was very steady, but rather slow. I opened the temporal artery, which bled very freely. But I observed that when she breathed freely the blood from the artery became red; and when her breathing was difficult, or when she hardly breathed at all, the blood became dark, and this alternated several times in the course of bleeding; yet all this made but little alteration in the pulse.

In many diseases of the heart, as well as of the lungs, we may often observe the same appearance. In many diseases of the heart, producing what is called angina pectoris, (the symptoms of which arise from a vast variety of causes, palpitations being commonly one,) we shall see that upon any exertion the heart acts with great violence, and the breathing is very laborious, or rather imperfect, not corresponding with the violence of the motion of the blood; the face will become of a dark

---

theory that the heart is poisoned by its own blood, is disproved, first, by the experiments of Kay and Edwards, which tend to prove that venous blood contributes, although feebly, to support muscular irritability; secondly, by the post mortem appearances, which exhibit the right side of the heart and the whole venous system gorged with blood, while the left side is almost wholly empty, contrary to what might be expected, considering that the left ventricle ceases to act first in ordinary death; and thirdly, by the difficulty of accounting for the renewal of the contractions of the heart on the reestablishment of respiration. Resuscitation from asphyxia would, if Bichat's doctrine were true, be impossible, because the very power by which it must owe the restoration of its irritability would be destroyed; whereas by admitting that the heart retains a certain portion of irritability, it is not difficult to account for the renewal of its contraction as soon as the stagnation in the pulmonary capillaries is removed. It would obviously be inconsistent with the object of these notes to enter on this subject more fully; at the same time it appeared necessary to guard the reader against the notion, that "these actions, or cessations of actions, are all dependent on life" abstractedly considered. The fact is, all the phenomena of asphyxia primarily arise out of the interruptions to those chemical changes which atmospheric air produces on the blood, in consequence of which venous blood is circulated through the system, and produces a series of effects which are plainly capable of being analytically examined. (*See Cyclop. of Pract. Med., art.* ASPHYXIA, *by Dr. Roget.*)]

purple colour, the patients will be nearly expiring, and nothing but rest relieves them. Of this the following case is a strong instance.

A. B. when a boy could never use the same exercise that other boys did; he could not run up stairs nor ascend a hill without being out of breath, and had almost through his whole life an irregular pulse, more especially when he used more exercise than he could well bear. Upon the least increase of motion he had a palpitation at the heart, which was often so strong as to be heard by those that were near to him; and his becoming soon fatigued was by his acquaintance supposed to be owing to a want of spirit or courage. With all this he grew to be a well-formed and common-sized man; but still he retained those defects, which indeed rather increased as he extended his views, and with them extended his actions. About the age of thirty he took to violent exercise, such as hunting, and often in the chase would be seized so ill with palpitations and almost a total suffocation that he was obliged to stop his horse and be held upon the saddle. At such times he became black in the face, and continued so as long as the fit lasted. It was often several days before he perfectly recovered his usual health, and frequently he could not lie down in his bed, but was obliged to sit up for breath. All these symptoms gradually increased upon him, and at times, without any violence of exercise or action, he would feel as if dying, and used so to express himself; but as the cause of these feelings did not appear to his friends, they rather treated them slightly. At last mere anxiety of mind would bring on these feelings, palpitations, and suffocations in some degree.

In the winter 1780 and 1781 he hunted very violently and also caught cold, which together brought on the above-mentioned complaints with greater violence than ever. He consulted two gentlemen of the profession: the palpitation, the difficulty of breathing, the great oppression, with the blackness in the face (I suppose) they thought either arose from spasms, or was nervous, for they ordered cordials, such as spirit of lavender, wine, &c.

I was sent for, to give a name to the disease. Upon inquiring into all the symptoms, my opinion was that there was something very wrong about the construction of the heart, viz. about the source of the circulation; that the blood did not flow at any time freely through the lungs, so as to have the proper influence of the air, but much less so when he was hurried; that a stagnation of the blood in any one part about the heart would produce in some degree suffocation, and want of due influence of the air upon the blood (being the same thing), which was the cause of the darkness of the face at those times; that the means to be practised were in some degree contrary to what had been advised, viz.

rest, gentle bleeding, care to eat moderately, to keep the body open and the mind easy: and as he had got the better of former attacks (although those were not so violent), I saw no absolute reason why he should not get the better of the present. Eight ounces of blood were taken from him that day, which relieved him. The symptoms still continuing, though not so violently, I saw him once more; he lost about four or five ounces more blood, which also relieved him, but still he did not get materially better. At last, as an addition to the above symptoms, he became yellow, his legs began to swell with water, and all his other complaints gradually increased, which made me suspect that a deposit of water was begun in the chest. He was now attended by a physician; was blistered on his legs, which threatened a mortification, and a caustic was applied to the pit of his stomach (I suppose for a pain there): nature was at last worn out, and he died. I solicited to open him, and was allowed.

On opening the belly there was found in the abdomen a very small quantity of bloody yellowish serum. Every viscus appeared to be sound; the gall-bladder was pretty full of bile, which was thick, but not ropy, as if the thinner parts had been strained off; the ducts were clear, both to and from the gall-bladder. Upon opening the chest the lungs did not collapse, being a good deal œdematous, but otherwise appearing sound; there was also a little bloody serum in both sides of the chest: these I conceive were the consequences of the last attack. The heart was very large, and very full of blood. Upon opening the right side of the heart, I found nothing uncommon either in the heart or the pulmonary artery. Upon opening the left side, I found the valves of the aorta thicker and harder than usual, having at the same time the appearance of being very much shrivelled. This diseased structure of the valves accounts for every one of what may be called his original symptoms, and was such as to render them of very little use; the blood, therefore, must have fallen back into the cavity of the ventricle again at every systole of the artery.

Whether this shrivelled state of the valves of the aorta was a natural formation, or a disease, is not easily ascertained; but if it was a disease, it must have begun much earlier in life than such diseases commonly do, as the symptoms appeared when he was young*. From this construction of valve we must see that it required the greatest quiet to allow the motions of the blood from the left side of the heart to go on sufficiently, and that whatever interrupted this produced a stagnation, or an accumulation of the blood almost in every part of the body; first, in the left ventricle, then the left auricle; pulmonary veins, pulmonary

* I have seen it at a very early period.

arteries; right ventricle, right auricle, and all the veins in the body: however, a smaller quantity than usual could get to the veins of the body through the arteries, so that a kind of circulation went on.

If we consider the effect arising from this construction of valves simply on mechanical principles, we cannot account for the darkness of the arterial blood, which must have passed through the lungs when there was no mechanical obstruction to respiration; but since it happens that when the heart either ceases to act, or cannot get rid of its blood (which must have been the case in the present instance), respiration ceases, or is performed so imperfectly as to have nearly the same effect*, the person is in reality in a state of suffocation. Suffocation is no more than imperfect respiration, which is the cause of imperfect blood passing to and from the left side of the heart; and it is therefore immaterial, as to consequences, whether a stoppage to respiration is the first cause, or is an effect, for in either way it is the cause of imperfect blood being introduced into the arterial system.

It may be difficult to account for the increased size of the heart; whether it was a mechanical effect, as the blood would be thrown back into it at every systole of the aorta and diastole of the heart, or whether it arose from a particular affection of that viscus. The first idea is the more natural; but it is not necessary that the cause should be of this kind, for we see every day enlarged hearts, where the symptoms have been somewhat similar, and yet no visible mechanical cause existed; and indeed it is a common effect where there is an impeded circulation.

It is easy to be conceived, first, that the circulation could not, in the case of this patient, be carried on regularly and perfectly; secondly, that a stoppage to the blood's motion in either arteries or veins, but much more a retrograde motion of the blood in any part, must produce a stagnation, which will be more or less extensive, according to the quantity of blood passing that way; thirdly, that if it was only in a branch of an artery, or vein, the stagnation would probably be only partial; but when in an artery, or the veins of the whole body, as the aorta or vena cava, it must then be pretty universal; and as the retrograde motion in the blood began in the aorta, we can easily trace its effects. We also find, in imperfect constructions of the heart, etc., where there is a communication between the right and left side, kept up after birth, that the same circumstances and appearances take place; cases of this kind frequently occur, of which the following is a strong instance.

I was several times consulted about the state of a young gentleman's health, and though it could not be said anatomically, with precision,

* In such inspirations I conceive that so little air is taken in as hardly to reach the cells of the lungs, so as to be able to influence the blood circulating on those cells.

what the real conformation of the heart was, yet it was imagined that the symptoms arose from some imperfection in that organ. From his infancy, every considerable exertion produced a seeming tendency to suffocation; and as suffocation always arises from a want of the due effect of air on the blood, while the circulation is going on, the whole body must change from the scarlet tinge to the modena or purple; and in those parts where the blood gives its colour most, there will this effect be greatest, which is commonly in the face, and particular parts of the face, at the finger-ends, etc. While very young nothing but crying brought on those fits, but when he was grown so as to take bodily exercise, as running, etc., then they became more frequent and more violent; and it is to be observed, that the older he grew the worse he was likely to be; for, with years approaching to maturity, his actions were likely to increase: great care, however, was taken to suppress such actions as were found from experience to bring on the fits. No medical advice could be of the least service, further than to inform him what experience had already taught, unless to recommend occasionally, when his friends found that the fits of suffocation were more easily excited than usual, that he should lose a little blood, so as to lessen the necessary action of breathing; putting, in this way, the quantity and motion of the blood more upon a par, and at the same time not to indulge too much his appetite; but all these precautions hardly kept him tolerably well. The heart, in proportion to the difficulty, acted with more violence; and one could rather have wished the contrary to have taken place. As he could hardly use any exercise of his own, motion was given him, such as riding slowly on horseback, in carriages, etc. He lived to the age of between thirteen and fourteen; and though the disorder did not destroy him, yet it is most probable that he could not have lived long, as he was every day arriving more and more at an age of action, but not in the same proportion acquiring prudence. When he died he was opened by Dr. Poultney, who transmitted an account of the appearance of the parts to the College of Physicians of London, which is published in the third volume of their Medical Transactions: such parts as are immediately connected with my subject I shall transcribe.

"Both lobes of the lungs were remarkably small, and some parts of them flaccid to such a degree as to suggest an idea of their having been incapable of performing their functions*. The liquor pericardii was in due quantity, and the heart was firm in texture, and of the natural size†. On examining the ventricles and the beginning of the aorta, a canal, or

* Although I have transcribed this, yet I do not lay much stress upon it.

† This shows there was no disease.

passage, was found communicating with both ventricles, situated in an oblique direction near the basis of the heart, so large as to admit the end of the finger from the aorta with equal facility into either ventricle, the septum of the ventricle appearing to terminate with this canal. On examining the entrance of the pulmonary artery within the ventricle, it was judged that this entrance was much smaller, and more firm than common." It is difficult here to say what would be the exact effect of this communication on the motion of the two bloods; that is, whether the blood of the right side was received into the left, or *vice versâ*; if the oblique direction of this passage had been further described, it might have explained this doubt; for if the passage was direct, the blood would most probably pass from the left to the right, as the left ventricle acquires the greatest strength: the word oblique, however, and the expression, that the finger, from the aorta, passed with equal facility into either ventricle, would make us suppose that the obliquity led out of the right ventricle into the aorta; but, even with this obliquity, I should not think it probable that the blood would pass from the right to the left, because the left acts with so much more force: the description leaves us to account for the defect in respiration another way. If the blood passed from the right to the left, then it would have had the same effect as the canalis arteriosus, and probably was the only one in the fœtus. In this case too little blood would pass through the lungs; but I do not conceive that this circumstance would affect respiration, because no stagnation would take place in the lungs; but if the blood got from the left to the right, then too much blood would be sent to the lungs, as it would be found to take its course twice. On the other hand, if the lungs be not capable of allowing a full distension equal to the actions of the heart, though naturally framed, the same thing takes place. In natural deaths the pulsation of the heart commonly stops before breathing ceases; but in deaths arising from a stoppage of breath, such as hanging or drowning, the reverse must take place; and in such we shall always find dark blood in the left side, which plainly took place in the experiment above mentioned.

It may be supposed that in the lungs the blood cannot come in contact with the air; but the circumstances above related, that the florid colour will extend some depths into the blood, shows that the effect of air can and does pervade animal matter. Not attending to this fact at first, I covered the mouths of vessels filled with venal blood with gold-beaters' skin, touching the surface of the blood, and the blood constantly became of a florid red on the surface, and even for some depth.

I put some dark venal blood into a phial, till it was about half full, and shook the blood, which mixed with the air in this motion, and it became immediately of a florid red*.

As the globules are the coarsest part of the blood, and they appear to be fully affected by the air in the lungs, we may suppose that the vessels of that viscus do not run into extreme minuteness, by which, apparently, no other purpose would be answered.

The blood of the menses, when it comes down to the mouth of the vagina, is as dark as venal blood; and as it does not coagulate, it has exactly the appearance of the blood in those where the blood continues fluid. Whether this arises from its being venal blood, or from its acquiring that colour after extravasation, by its slow motion, it is not easily determined; but upon being exposed it becomes florid: it is naturally of a dark colour, but rather muddy, not having that transparency which pure blood has. Whether this arises from its mixing with the mucus of the vagina, or from the cessation of life in it, I will not pretend to say. The red globules, however, are not dissolved; they retain their figure.

Does air in the cellular membrane of an emphysematous person produce or continue the floridness of the blood or not†?

The surface of the blood becoming of a scarlet red, whether exposed immediately to the air, or when only covered by membranes, through which we may suppose its influence to pass, is a circumstance which leads us to suppose that it is the pure air which has this effect, and not simply an exposed surface‡. To ascertain this, I made the following experiment:

I took a phial, and fixed a stop-cock to its mouth, and then applying an air-pump to the cock, exhausted the whole air: in this state, keeping it stopped, I immersed its mouth in fresh blood flowing from a vein, and then turning the cock, allowed the blood to be pressed up into the phial. When it was about half full I turned the cock back, and now shook the phial with the blood, but its colour did not alter as in the former experiments; and when I allowed the blood to stand in this vacuum, its exposed surface was not in the least changed[a].

* These experiments I made in the summer 1755, when I was house-surgeon at St. George's Hospital, and Dr. Hunter taught them ever after at his lectures.

† Vide Chester on Cases. Case first, the venal florid. St. George's, a man emphysematous; blood very dark.

‡ I may here observe, that fixed air [carbonic acid gas], as also inflammable airs, have contrary effects.

---

a [I have much pleasure in referring the reader to Faust and Mitchell's papers on Endosmose and Exosmose, and on the Penetrativeness of Fluids, in the American Journal of the Medical Sciences, vol. vii. pp. 22, 36. See also *note*, p. 35, respecting the menses.]

The vast number of cells into which the lungs are divided, the whole arterial and venal system ramifying on the surface of those cells, and of course the whole of the blood passing through them in every circulation, together with the loss of life upon the missing three or four breathings in the most perfect animals, show the great nicety that is required in preserving the due properties of the blood for the purposes of animal life: the time that we can live without air, or breathing, is shorter than that in which we die from a defect in any other natural operation; breathing, therefore, seems to render life to the blood, and the blood continues it in every part of the body. This nicety is not nearly so great in many of the more imperfect animals.

The amphibia have not this division of lungs, nor does the whole of the blood pass through the lungs in them, and they can live a considerable time without breathing. This, at present, I only mention as a fact, not meaning to give my opinion of the mode of preserving life, either in the blood or body, by the application of air to it; though I will say that mere life in both is supported by the air, and probably few of the other properties connected with the blood depend so much upon air as its life. But we may observe, that it was not necessary for the blood to undergo this change to render it fit for every purpose in the animal œconomy, for we find that venal blood answers some purposes: thus, the blood from the intestines, spleen, etc., going to the liver, as we suppose for the secretion of the bile, shows that venal blood will do for some secretions, though probably not absolutely necessary[a]. This application of venal blood is a saving of blood; and it is not necessary for the formation of bile that the venous blood should proceed from the parts above mentioned, for in birds, amphibia, etc., other veins, besides those, enter the liver.

I have shown that several substances mixed with dark-coloured blood have the property of rendering it of a florid red; and it must have appeared that by circulating through its body its dark colour is restored. As it is capable of being rendered florid by several substances, so it may be rendered dark by several when florid: vital air [oxygen gas] has the power of rendering it florid; but the other vapours, or gases, which

---

[a] [This question was for a long while agitated, many physiologists contending that the blood acquired in its passage through the spleen, omentum, intestines, &c., peculiar qualities which fitted it for the secretion of the bile. However this may be, it certainly is not indispensable. The trunk of the vena portæ has been found in several instances to terminate in the inferior cava, instead of branching out into the liver. Mr. Abernethy found this in a child about ten months old (*Phil. Trans.*, 1793, p. 59.), and Mr. Wilson in a young female (*Med. Gaz.*, viii. 443.), the gall-bladder in both cases being perfectly full; and in the last case the hepatic artery increased to a great size. Saunders, Huber, and Lawrence have referred to similar cases.]

have the name of airs, such as fixed air, inflammable air, etc., render it dark. This change is peculiar to the living body, for if arterial blood is taken away, it retains its florid colour, although not in the least exposed to the air[a]. As it is found dark in the veins, and as it performs some offices in the course of the circulation which perhaps render it unfit for the purposes of life, we may conceive that the loss of colour and this unfitness are effects of the same cause; but, upon further observations on this fluid, it will be found that it may be rendered unfit for the purposes of life without losing its colour, and may lose its colour without being rendered unfit for life[b]: slowness of motion in the blood of the veins is one circumstance that causes the alteration; but this alone will not produce the effect, for I have observed above, that arterial blood put into a phial, and allowed to stand quiet, does not become dark; but rest, or slowness of motion in living parts, would appear, from many observations, to be a cause of this change in its colour. We know that the blood begins to move more and more slowly in the arteries; we know that its motion in the veins is slow in comparison to what it is in the arteries; we should therefore naturally suppose (considering this alone,) that it was the slowness of the motion that was the immediate cause. Rest or slowness of motion, in living and probably healthy parts, certainly allows the blood to change its colour; thus, we never see extravasations of blood but they are always dark. I never saw a person die of an apoplexy, from extravasation in the brain, but the extravasated blood was dark; even in aneurism it becomes dark in the aneurismal sac; also when the blood escapes out of the artery, and coagulates in the cellular membrane, we find the same appearance.

These observations respecting apoplexy struck me much. I conceived

---

[a] [Arterial blood is rendered dark by being placed in the vacuum of an air pump. There appears, therefore, no good reason for believing that any of the effects, relating to change of colour, which take place in the lungs, are peculiar to the living body.]

[b] [Bichat's opinion respecting the deleterious effects of venous blood, has been already briefly adverted to. Dr. Kay, however, found that when venous blood was injected in small quantities into the arteries it did not destroy life, or manifest any directly poisonous effects. Hybernating animals continue to circulate black blood during the period of their torpidity, with the effect of rather increasing their muscular irritability. (*Hall* in *Phil. Trans.* 1832.) Mr. Owen found that in the kangaroo the ovum did not connect itself with the mother, or the chorion put forth any villi until the period of gestation had two thirds elapsed, although the fœtus continued to grow during this time without respiration, or any office vicarious of it. (*Phil. Trans.* 1834.) In cholera, the blood in the arteries is perfectly black, and yet the functions of the brain remain perfect to the last, although undoubtedly the animal and vital functions are much enfeebled. Besides which, many other facts are mentioned in the present treatise which clearly require some modification of Bichat's doctrine, in order to explain all the phenomena which relate to this subject.]

at first that the extravasations there must consist of venal blood; but, from reasoning, I could hardly allow myself to think so; for whatever might be the beginning of the disease, it was impossible it could continue afterwards wholly venal, especially when the blood was found in a considerable quantity; because, in many cases, great mischief was done to both systems of vessels, and the arteries once ruptured would give the greatest quantity of blood: but to ascertain this with more certainty, I made the following experiment.

I wounded the femoral artery of a puppy obliquely; the opening in the skin was made at some distance from the artery, by a couching needle; the blood that came from the small orifice in the skin was florid. The cellular membrane swelled up very much; about five minutes afterwards I punctured the tumour, and the blood was fluid. In ten minutes I punctured it again; the blood was thinner, and more serous, but still florid. In fifteen minutes I punctured it again: at first only serum issued; upon squeezing, a little blood came, but still florid: the mass now seemed to be principally coagulated, which prevented further trials. Some days after, when I cut into the swelled part, I found the blood as dark as common venal blood; so that here the change had taken place after coagulation.

When I had plaster of Paris applied to my face to make a mould, in the taking it off it produced a kind of suction on the fore part of the nose, which I felt; and when the plaster was removed, on observing the part it was red, as if the cells of the skin were loaded with extravasated blood; this was then of a florid red, but it soon became of a dark purple, which showed that it was arterial blood, and that by stagnating in the cells of the body it became of the colour of venal blood.

Blood may even be rendered dark in the larger arteries by a short stagnation. I laid bare the carotid artery of a dog for about two inches in length; I then tied a thread round it at each end, leaving a space of two inches in length between each ligature, filled with blood; the external wound was stitched loosely up: several hours afterwards I opened the stitches, and observed in this vessel that the blood was coagulated, and of a dark colour, the same as in the vein. Thus, I have also seen, when a tourniquet has been applied round the thigh, and the artery divided, that when it was slackened, the first blood came out of a dark colour, but what followed was florid. This I have seen in amputations, when a tourniquet had been applied for a considerable time; and it is commonly observed in performing the operation for aneurism.

July, 1779, Mr. Bromfield had a patient in St. George's Hospital with an aneurism of the crural artery, about the middle of the thigh: the artery had been dilated about three inches in length. The operation was performed, in which the artery was tied up above the dilatation, three or more inches, for security. When this was done, the tourniquet was slackened, and a pretty considerable bleeding was observed, seemingly at the lower orifice, leading from the dilated part, which, at first, was supposed, from its colour, to be the venous blood that had stagnated in the veins by means of the tourniquet; but this it could not be; and it was found to flow from the lower orifice of the artery, which was immediately tied: we must suppose that the motion of the blood; in making this retrograde course, was very slow, for it had first to pass off into small collateral branches above where it was tied, then to anastomose with similar small ones from the trunk below, and then to enter that trunk, all of which must very much retard its motion; and, indeed, the manner of its oozing out of the vessels showed such a retardation. This motion of the blood, though in the arterial system, was in some respects similar to the motion of the blood in both systems of vessels.

This last circumstance plainly indicates a communication of the arteries above the aneurism with those below, by means of the anastamozing branches.

The blood from the lower orifice flowed without any pulsation, which must have been owing to its coming into the large artery below by a vast number of smaller ones at different distances, and of course at different times; but probably the chief cause of this want of pulsation in the great artery was, that the power of the heart was lost in the two systems of smaller arteries above and below; for the second system, or those from below, became in a considerable degree similar to veins, and the great artery in the leg below the aneurism was like a considerable vein.

A young man, servant to Henry Drummond, Esq., having had a knife run into his thigh, which wounded the crural artery, a considerable tumour came on the part, consisting chiefly of blood extravasated, and lodged in the cellular membrane. This in some degree stopped the flowing of the blood from the cut artery, and on dilating the wound, so as to get to the artery, I observed that the extravasated blood in the cellular membrane was of the venal colour. On exposing the artery, which was first secured from bleeding by a tourniquet above, and then slightly slackening that instrument, the first blood which flowed from above was dark, and even was taken for venous blood by the operator; but he was soon convinced that it was arterial by the florid colour of that which almost immediately ensued. I observed that the colour of the blood was as dark as that of any venous blood I ever saw.

From these experiments and observations, we must conclude that the colour of the blood is altered, either by rest or slow motion, in living parts, and even in the arteries; this circumstance takes place in the vessels as the motion of the blood decreases[a].

Another observation occurs, viz., that the whole of the limb below the ligature, where the crural artery had been taken up, must have been entirely supplied with such altered blood; and as it kept its life, its warmth, and the action of its muscles, it is evident that the colour of the blood is of little service to any of those properties. It is probably from this cause that granulations on the lower part of the lower extremity look dark when the person stands erect, as well as in very indolent sores, however situated.

Another observation strongly in favour of the supposition that rest is a cause of the change of blood from the scarlet colour to the dark, or modena, is taken from the common operation of bleeding; for we generally find the blood of a dark colour at its first coming out, but it becomes lighter and lighter towards the last. Some reasons may be given for this: first, it has stagnated in the veins while the vein was filling, and the orifice making, which occupy some time, and may render it darker than it otherwise might have been in the same vein: secondly,

---

[a] [Arterial blood is also blackened in vacuo, and when placed in media which exert no apparent chemical action upon it, such as hydrogen and nitrogen (*Priestley on Air*, iii. 363–4.); nay, arterial blood gradually blackens when confined in pure oxygen, and cannot be again brightened by this agent (*Thompson, Sys. of Chem.*, iv. 474.), although, by the addition of any neutral salt having an alkaline or earthy base, the colour is instantly restored. These facts are clearly against the notion, to be adverted to presently, of free carbon being the cause of the black colour of the blood, because as much of this substance must exist in the blood at the commencement of the experiment as at the termination. Neither is it easy to reconcile these phenomena with Dr. Stevens's theory of arterialization; for if carbonic acid is the cause of the dark colour, how is it that arterial blood (which, according to this author, contains no carbonic acid,) is rendered black, and venous blood still blacker, by being placed in vacuo; since the salts remain the same, while the effect of a vacuum whould evidently be rather to extract a part of the carbonic acid than to increase its amount? It is possible that these phenomena may depend on some alteration in the constitution of the clot, arising from a mutual play of affinities between its proximate elements, thus the blood is also observed to become venalized in the living body from the mere fact of stagnation. Sir Astley Cooper found that those changes which constitute the venalization of the blood in the body were not effected under extreme cold, so that the blood remained florid throughout the whole system of those animals which perished from cold (*Dr. Hodgkin's Notes to Edwards*); whereas, under the influence of moderate warmth, such as that of the body, these changes take place, slowly on extravasated or stagnating blood, but instantly in the extreme capillaries.

It will be sufficient to have noticed in this place the analogy which subsists between the venalization of the blood under these different circumstances, without pretending to decide whether these phenomena depend on the gradual union of carbon and oxygen with each other, or on any other cause. The subject will be resumed in a future note.]

when there is a free orifice the blood may pass more readily into the veins from the arteries, and therefore may be somewhat in the state of arterial blood, which may occasion the last blood to be rather lighter. What amounts almost to a proof of this is, that although a ligature is tied so as to stop the passage of the blood to the heart, and therefore it might be supposed not to have so free a passage from the arteries as in common, yet, from the following observations, it appears that it certainly has a much freer; for if the orifice be large in a full-sized vein, the arm beyond the orifice will be much paler than the natural colour, and the blood will become more florid; but if, on the contrary, the vein be small, and little blood passes, it will retain its dark colour; this, however, would appear not always to be the case.

I bled a lady, whose blood at first was of a dark colour; but she fainted, and while she continued in the fit the colour of the blood that came from the vein was a fine scarlet. The circulation was then very languid.

We may observe that venal blood in the most healthy is commonly, if not always, the darkest; and that whenever the body is the least out of order, it is then not so much changed from the florid to the very dark purple. This I have often observed, and particularly recollect a striking instance of it in a gentleman who had a slight fever; his venal blood was quite florid, like arterial blood. This could not have arisen from the increase of the blood's motion, or from being kept up in the veins by the fever, for it was slight*.

The blood will change its colour from the scarlet to the modena in different situations, according to the mode of circulation. In animals which have lungs and a complete double circulation, the darkest blood will be where it comes (if I may be allowed the expression) to get anew its bright colour; for instance, in the arteries of the lungs, and of course the brightest in the veins of the same part, which will be continued more or less into the arteries of the other circulation, where again it will begin to change, except in one stage of life of some animals which do not use their lungs, such as fœtuses; but in such fœtuses as convert animal matter into nourishment, (and therefore, most probably, must have it influenced by the air, although not by means of the lungs of the chick, such as the chick in the egg,) we find the blood in the veins of

* I believe the blood does not become dark by standing in an inflamed part. I have seen cases of apoplexy where the person died some days after the attack. I have found the pia mater inflamed in several places, even to the length of inflammatory transfusion, forming dots, all of which were of a florid red colour, while the other parts of the same membrane, the blood in the larger vessels, and also the extravasated blood, were of the usual dark colour.

their temporary lungs of a florid colour, while it is dark in the arteries; so that it has become of a dark colour, in its passage to and from the heart; but in the more perfect animals the blood, I believe, becomes darker and darker as it proceeds from the heart, till it returns to the heart again; but this change is very little in the arterial system, more especially in vessels near the heart, as the coronary arteries. The change of colour is more rapid in the veins, but it is not equally made through the whole venous system; for it will be produced more quickly in the lower parts of the lower extremities than in the veins near the heart: it begins, most probably, where the motion first has a tendency to become languid; and this usually takes place in the very small arteries; for in bleeding in the foot, or on the back of the hand, I have observed, in general, that the blood is of a more florid red than in the bend of the arm[a].

---

[a] [In order to complete the general view of the changes which the blood undergoes during the course of its circulation, I propose very briefly to advert to the subject of respiration, relying upon my reader's indulgence for the imperfection of a sketch which is not capable of being well comprised within the limits of a note.

Mr. Hunter, although no chemist, had sufficient sagacity to perceive the insufficiency of all existing theories of respiration, and therefore confined himself to the bare statement of facts, leaving it to future observation to discover the clue by which these might be explained. He admits that the arterialization of the blood, so far at least as change of colour is concerned, is wholly irrespective of vital causes; but he seems to have regarded the renewal of the vitality of the blood as dependent on some inexplicable effect of the vital air, from which the idea of any chemical changes is wholly excluded. Undoubtedly we shall not err in regarding change of colour as merely expressive of some other more important changes effected by respiration; but then these changes are essentially chemical, and it is on these alone that the vitalizing properties of the blood depend. I shall also premise that the principal seat of these changes is in the pulmonary and systemic capillaries; for although, under certain circumstances, a similar change may undoubtedly occur, as well in the great vessels as in extravasated blood, yet the change is generally instantaneous in the natural course of the circulation; that is, the blood enters the capillaries of the lungs black, and is immediately converted to red; and on the other hand, it is scarlet in the smallest arterioles of the body, but black in the minutest radicles of the veins. These systems antagonize each other, so that whatever the blood acquires in one it loses in the other, and *vice versâ.*

If venous blood be exposed to atmospheric air, its colour is soon converted from black into scarlet; a portion of oxygen is absorbed, and an equal proportion of carbonic acid is disengaged. If, instead of atmospheric air, pure oxygen is employed, these effects are more quickly and more characteristically developed; but they are not produced by any gases (with the exception perhaps of carburetted hydrogen,) which have not oxygen as an element. Such are the simple phenomena of arterialization, which equally take place in and out of the body, although not with equal rapidity.

Thus, Allen and Pepys found that a man of average size breathed about nineteen times in a minute, and took in about 16½ cubic inches of air at each inspiration. About 26·6 cubic inches, at 50°, of oxygen were calculated to be withdrawn from the atmosphere per minute, and the same quantity of carbonic acid to be emitted from the lungs,

§. 5. *Of the Quantity of Blood, and course of its Circulation.*

It appears to me impossible to ascertain the quantity of blood in the body, and the knowledge of it would probably give very little assistance

---

making of the latter about 38,232 cubic inches per day, or nearly 10¾ oz. troy of solid carbon. (*Phil. Trans.* 1808, p. 256.)

Atmospheric air consists of 79 parts of nitrogen and 21 of oxygen; but, according to Allen and Pepys, the nitrogen remained unaffected by the process of respiration, which consisted solely in the abstraction of a quantity of oxygen exactly sufficient to convert the carbon of the blood into carbonic acid, bulk for bulk, equal with that of the oxygen abstracted. It was therefore natural to suppose that the black colour of venous blood depended on the presence of free carbon, or carbon in some peculiar state of combination, which was given out from the lungs in the act of respiration. The blood, in short, was supposed to be carbonized in the extreme capillaries of the body, and to be decarbonized in the lungs.

It has been ascertained, however, by more correct experiment, first, that the quantity of oxygen lost does not always correspond with the quantity of carbonic acid emitted from the lungs; 2nd, that nitrogen is absorbed or given out under certain circumstances; and 3rd, that carbonic acid exists ready formed in venous blood (see *note*, p. 28.). Dr. Edwards found that the quantity of oxygen consumed above the quantity of carbon produced, varied in the lower tribes of animals from nothing to one third of the whole (*De l'Influence des Agens physiques sur la Vie*); while, on the other hand, it has been remarked by Dr. Prout that the amount of carbonic acid produced also varied according to the age of the animal, the diet, the time of the day, the season of the year, the state of the atmosphere, the quantity of exercise, and many other physical circumstances. (*Ann. of Phil.*, ii. 330., and iv. 331–4.) Edwards found similar variations in the quantity of nitrogen (*op. cit.*, p. 420.). When pigeons were confined in oxygen gas containing from one to two per cent. of nitrogen, the volume of gas remained undiminished, and only so much oxygen was found to have been abstracted as would have happened if the pigeons had been made to respire common air; but then a much smaller quantity of carbonic acid was formed, the deficiency being made up by an evolution of nitrogen.

By varying the experiment, and mixing oxygen and hydrogen with a small proportion of nitrogen (the oxygen being in the same proportion as in common air), no loss of oxygen was sustained, but a quantity of hydrogen disappeared, which was exactly replaced by an equal proportion of nitrogen. (*Allen and Pepys, Phil. Trans.* 1829, p. 279.) During the month of March Dr. Edwards confined frogs in pure hydrogen, from which he found that volumes of carbonic acid, nearly equalling the whole bulk of the animals employed, were evolved, although the lungs had previously been exhausted by pressure. A young kitten also, confined for nineteen minutes in the same manner in hydrogen, evolved twelve times more carbonic acid than could be accounted for by the residual air in the lungs when the experiment began. (*Op. cit.*, pp. 437–465.)

It may be distinctly concluded, therefore, from these facts, that the lungs are capable of absorbing and giving out gaseous matters, particularly oxygen and carbonic acid. In man the quantity of oxygen abstracted from the atmosphere pretty exactly equals the quantity of carbonic acid produced; but whether the whole oxygen is absorbed, and the whole carbonic acid evolved from the blood, or whether the lungs are merely the seat in which the carbon of the blood combines with the oxygen of the air to form carbonic acid, remains at present a question. From the system of antagonism which is

towards better understanding the œconomy of the animal. The quantity of blood is probably as permanent a circumstance as any, and

---

evinced in many of the functions of the animal œconomy, Dr. Edwards is disposed to regard the former of these opinions as most probable (*op. cit.*, p. 437.); and certainly, when we reflect on the importance of the respiratory functions, it is reasonable to suppose that this is actually the case. What the exact changes are which are wrought on venous blood, so as to restore to it its vivifying properties, are unknown, but it seems to fall infinitely short of our notion of the importance of this function to suppose that it merely rids the blood of a little carbon. This would be merely to ascribe to respiration a negative effect, whereas it is scarcely possible to refrain from the conclusion that this important function confers on the blood new and positive qualities, by more completely animalizing its various elements.

Such, then, are the phenomena of respiration; but what are the immediate causes of the change of colour in the blood? The scarlet colour is instantly restored to venous blood by the contact of oxygen, and hence it was universally supposed that the arterialization of the blood depended on the absorption of this gas. But this has been denied by Dr. Stevens (*On the Blood*, p. 8. *et passim*), whose views are: 1st, That the colouring matter of the blood is naturally black, but that "scarlet is the natural colour of the vital current; and this it owes to another cause." 2nd, "That carbonic acid is the cause of the dark colour in the venous circulation," having "ascertained by numerous experiments that all the acids blacken the blood." 3rd, "That oxygen brightens its colour, not by *addition*, but by *attracting* or removing the carbonic acid." And 4th, "That the scarlet colour is produced by the action of the saline ingredients on the colouring matter." He affirms that "the scarlet colour exists in the blood independent of oxygen, or, at all events, oxygen of itself cannot produce either the red or the arterial appearance, for when we cover the crassamentum, when it first coagulates, with a layer of distilled water, or any other fluid which does not contain saline matter, the acid may be removed by the oxygen, or absorbed by the water, but the colour becomes darker than it had been before. On the other hand, when we immerse the black and saltless crassamentum in any clear saline fluid, the colour instantly changes from dark venous to bright arterial; and when the fluid which we use is sufficiently impregnated with saline matter, this change is produced *when we make the experiment, as I have frequently done, even in an atmosphere of carbonic acid.* Oxygen, however, is essential to life, for without this the heavy deleterious gas, which is the cause of the impurity of the venous circulation, would not be removed in the pulmonary organs; the blood in the extreme circulation is converted from arterial to venous, partly by the loss, or rather by the change of form in the oxygen which it contains, and partly by the addition of carbonic acid; but when this dark or acidified blood is exposed to the air in the lungs, the oxygen instantly removes the acid from the circulation." Such is a brief outline of Dr. Stevens's views, according to which oxygen plays the following part in respiration, namely, at first it lifts out or carries off the carbonic acid of the blood by virtue of a "latent power of attraction"; and secondly, having performed this office, it is absorbed into the circulating fluids, where it gradually attracts carbon, from the proximate principles of the blood working important changes on these substances, and giving rise to the production of carbonic acid. This union of carbon and oxygen may slowly take place, as we have seen in the preceding note, even out of the body, and still more rapidly in the great vessels of the living animal; but undoubtedly the principal seat of these changes is in the extreme capillaries of the periphery, where the change from arterial to venous is instantaneous, and where, it must be evident, the affinity of oxygen for carbon must be exercised under the most favourable circumstances, in consequence of the minute

not depending on immediate action: we have not one hour less and another hour more; nothing but accident or disease can lessen the quan-

---

state of division in which the combining elements are presented to each other, not to mention the controling influences of the nervous power over this system of vessels, as evinced in the functions of secretion and nutrition, which are merely parallel examples of the exercise of complicated chemical affinities.

Whatever may be thought of several parts of these views, it seems to be an incontestible fact that oxygen *alone* is incapable of restoring the arterial tint to blood which has been rendered black by immersion in water. Dr. Turner, with the assistance of his friend and colleague Mr. Quain, records the following experiment, which I shall recite in his own words. "I collected," he says, "some perfectly florid blood from the femoral artery of a dog; and, on the following morning, when a firm coagulum had formed, several thin slices were cut from the clot with a sharp penknife, and the serum was removed from them by distilled water, which had just before been briskly boiled and allowed to cool in a well-corked bottle. The water was gently poured on these slices, so that while the serum was dissolved, as little as possible of the colouring matter should be lost. After the water had been poured off and renewed four or five times, occupying in all about an hour, the moist slices were placed in a saucer at the side of the original clot, and both portions shown to several medical friends. They all, without hesitation, pronounced the unwashed clot to have the perfect appearance of arterial blood, and the washed slices to be as perfectly venous; the colour of the latter in fact was quite dark. On restoring one of the slices to the serum of the same blood, it shortly recovered its florid colour; and another slice, placed in a solution of bicarbonate of soda, instantly acquired a similar tint. In thus brightening a dark clot by a solution of salt or a bicarbonate, the colour is often still more florid than that of arterial blood; but the colours are exactly alike when the salt is duly diluted.

"I am at a loss to draw any other inference from the foregoing experiment than the following;—that the florid colour of arterial blood is *not* due to oxygen, but, as Dr. Stevens affirms, to the saline matter of the serum. The arterial blood which had been used had been duly *oxygenised*, as it is called, within the body of the animal, and should not in that state have lost its tint by mere removal of its serum. The change from venous to arterial blood appears, contrary to the received doctrine, to consist of two parts essentially distinct: one is a chemical change essential to life, accompanied with the absorption of oxygen and evolution of carbonic acid; the other depends on the saline matter of the blood, whch gives a florid tint to the colouring matter after it has been modified by the action of oxygen. (*Elem. of Chemistry*, 4th edit. 1833, p. 903.)

As it would lengthen too much the discussion of the present subject to examine fully all the objections which may be urged to this theory, I shall content myself with making two or three observations which strike me as being most important.

1st. Oxygen is said to have no *positive* concern in producing the red colour of the blood; but a stream of oxygen passed through a solution of colouring matter, previously rendered florid by a neutral salt, unquestionably exalted the vividness of the tint. Consequently oxygen is not entirely a passive agent.

2nd. Oxygen is said to possess a "latent power of attraction" for carbonic acid, by which it lifts this gas out, and, as it were, carries it off from the blood; but the ascription of such a property to oxygen is unphilosophical, as the phenomenon in question may be referred with more propriety to the general law of endosmose and exosmose, according to which, gases, by virtue of their elasticity, mutually penetrate and displace one another, such penetration and displacement being always reciprocal. (See *Amer. Journ. of Med. Sci.*, vii. pp. 23, 36.) Besides, as the rate of penetration for carbonic

tity; the first probably immediately, the other slowly; but even then, although under par, it is so slowly made up as not to constitute sudden

---

acid and oxygen is respectively as 5½ and 113 minutes, while that for nitrogen is too inconsiderable to be assigned, it would not be possible, even admitting an attraction between gases to exist, to explain this property of oxygen; for whatever may be the rate of penetration, the attraction between gases must be equal; consequently, as the proportion of nitrogen to oxygen is as 79 to 21, the *attractive* power of the former will be nearly four times greater than that of the latter, and be moreover constantly present (in consequence of the low rate of penetrativeness of this gas) to aid in "lifting out the carbonic acid." From these considerations, therefore, I conclude that the ascription of a latent power of attraction to oxygen is both an unfounded and an inadequate supposition.

3. The presence of oxygen and the absence of carbonic acid in arterial blood have never been satisfactorily ascertained by accurate experiment; for, notwithstanding the assertion of Dr. Stevens that arterial blood contains no carbonic acid, a different result has been obtained by MM. Tiedemann and Gmelin (*Poggendorf's Annal.*, xxxii.), so that this point must certainly be regarded at present as undecided.

4. It has also been objected, 1st, that venous blood coagulated in vacuo parts with a portion of its carbonic acid, and yet remains black, nay blacker than before, although if oxygen be admitted in this state the red colour is restored; and 2nd, that arterial blood (as has been remarked in the preceding note) grows black when coagulated in vacuo, or even when confined in pure oxygen. In answer to the first of these objections, it has been replied that the attraction between carbonic acid and blood is greater than can be overcome by one atmosphere, so that the air-pump is an insufficient means of ridding the blood of this gas, but only draws it to the surface, by which it blackens it still more. But this explanation is not satisfactory; because although the air-pump cannot draw out the whole, it yet draws out a part; besides which, hydrogen and nitrogen, which draw out the whole, strongly blacken the blood, although they have no chemical action upon it. (*Dublin Journ.*, ii. 72; *Lancet*, 1831-32, ii. 659; *Med. Gazette*, xi. 881.) In respect to the gradual blackening of arterial blood in pure oxygen, it has been replied that the blood acts on itself when out of the body in a way somewhat analogous to what happens to it in the capillaries of the living animal (see preceding *note*), that is, various complex affinities are brought into exercise from the union and gradual action of the oxygen on some of the component parts of the blood, in consequence of which the whole composition of this fluid is altered, and probably carbonic acid produced. But this explanation is not more satisfactory than the preceding, because, in the first place, a number of things are here assumed which are not proveable, and in the second place it is reasonable to suppose that the blackening effect on the blood is always due to the same cause; which cause cannot be the one here assumed; because, if it were, the oxygen which is present would invariably carry off the carbonic acid as fast as it is generated, and restore the red colour. (See Williams in *Med. Gazette*, xvi. 813.) With respect to the readmission of oxygen restoring the red colour to arterial blood which has been blackened in vacuo, I believe no explanation has yet been attempted, although the fact itself has been partly denied. Upon the whole, therefore, these are real objections, which must be allowed their due weight in considering this subject.

5. The objection that carbonic acid does not blacken the blood (*Lancet ut supra*) has been completely removed by Mr. Hoffman, who found that a stream of carbonic acid passed through oxygenized blood gradually converted it to a black colour. (*Med. Gazette*, xi. 881.) The same author has also confirmed the statement of Dr. Stevens that a

variations: yet, when we come to consider the varieties in the pulse, we should imagine there would be great varieties in the quantity of blood. The quantity I think must be considerable when we reflect on the use of this fluid; the quantity of supply or food necessary to keep it up; that it supports the body and life everywhere; and that it forms the pabulum of many secretions. All these cannot depend on a very small quantity of this fluid without conceiving at the same time an extremely quick change. There seem to be two modes of judging, both of which are evidently liable to objections in point of accuracy, and they differ so much as to show that neither can be right. One is, to calculate how much may be in an animal from the quantity it will lose in a short time. I have seen several quarts thrown up from the stomach in a few hours, even by a very thin puny person; and, on the other hand, if we had not this proof we should suppose there could be but very little, when a few ounces will make a person faint. I have an idea, however, that people can bear to lose more by the stomach than in any other way. Besides,

---

stream of carbonic acid gas passed through blood which has been previously reddened by a neutral salt renders it irrecoverably black.

6. A dark clot is equally arterialized when covered with milk or white of egg (*Priestley on Air*, iii.; *Wells in Phil. Trans.*, 1797.) as when covered with its own serum. The effect indeed is more slowly produced, but it is accompanied with the same loss of oxygen and the same evolution of carbonic acid, consequently the salts of the serum cannot be the cause of the red colour. But this objection is of little weight, 1st, because a minute portion of salts is contained in milk and white of egg; and 2nd, because the further contraction of the clot may extrude a still further portion of serum, which coming in contact with the surface of the clot may arterialize it.

7. Upon the supposition that free carbonic acid is the sole cause of the dark colour of the blood, by suspending the reddening tendency of the salts, the addition of a minute quantity of any pure alkali, sufficient to neutralize the acid, ought immediately not only to restore this property to the salts, but to increase it, by adding to the previously existing salts a carbonated alkali; but the addition of any quantity of a pure alkali is found rather to increase the blackness of the blood. (*Williams in Med. Gaz., ut supra.*)

Considerable weight is undoubtedly due to several of these objections, although they do not appear to me to be of that nature that they may not possibly be removed by further inquiries.

The following inferences seem at least fairly deducible from the preceding considerations: 1st, that air or oxygen without salt has no power of reddening the blood; 2nd, that salt without air has this effect; 3rd, that carbonic acid is *probably* the cause of the black colour of venous blood, by overpowering the natural reddening tendency of the serum; and 4th, that the removal of the carbonic acid is the cause of the red colour, by allowing the serum to exercise this tendency unobstructed. Independently of any theory these are novel and interesting facts, for which we are mainly indebted to Dr. Stevens. It cannot, however, be concealed that the theory of respiration, calorification and arterialization which he has built upon them is defective in many main points, although I consider it on the whole as open to fewer objections than any other, and as fully deserving of being followed up with further and more accurate experiments.]

it becomes a matter almost of surprise how little is commonly found in the dead body: but I believe in disease it in some degree diminishes with the body; for more is to be found in those who die suddenly, or of acute diseases; and even in some who die of lingering diseases, as of dropsy, we have a considerable quantity of blood. The only way of accounting for this is, that in a common lingering illness there is less blood, and in a dropsy it coagulates less; for the strong coagulation squeezes out the serum, which, I imagine, transudes after death, and is not observable.

It would appear upon the whole, that the quantity of blood in an animal is proportioned to the uses of that blood in the machine, which, probably, may be reckoned three in number: the first is simply the support of the whole, which includes the growth or increase of parts, the keeping the parts already formed to their necessary standard, and also the supply of waste in the parts. The second is the support of action, such as the action of the brain and muscles, in which is produced uncommon waste; and thirdly, secretion; all of which will fluctuate except the simple support, but more particularly the support of action. I have already observed that the anastomosing of vessels gives greater space for blood. Probably a paralytic limb would give the necessary quantity for simple support[a].

There is nothing particular in the veins, so as to give an idea that they were intended to increase the quantity of blood: they hold, however, more than the arteries, which certainly adds to the quantity; but the increase of size lessens the velocity. They form plexuses, and what are called certain bodies; as the plexus reteformis in the female, and corpora cavernosa and spongiosa in the male. We see how little blood supports a part in an aneurism; and, probably, slowness of motion is suitable to little blood.

It must have appeared in the account of the different colours of the different parts of the body, arising from the proportion of red blood,

---

[a] [On bleeding a young ass to death, of the weight of 79lbs., Percival obtained 5½lbs. of blood, that is, it perished from a loss of about $\frac{1}{15}$th of its weight: Sir Astley Cooper estimated the proportion which an animal might lose before death at about $\frac{1}{16}$th. Probably Haller's estimate of the actual quantity of blood in the body approaches as nearly to the truth as any, viz. $\frac{1}{5}$th its weight; of which $\frac{3}{4}$ths or more were supposed to be in the veins, and $\frac{1}{4}$th or less in the arteries. (*El. Phys.*, v. i. 3.) As the proportional quantity of blood varies very considerably in different animals, it is probable that age, temperament, food, exercise, and other external circumstances have also a considerable influence in this respect in man. Thackrah found that the quantity of evaporable fluid in a dog was 621·6, the solid being 378·4 (*op. cit.*, p. 232.): but this gives no idea of the actual quantity of blood in the body, for all the animal textures contain abundance of water, which would necessarily come into the account.]

that some parts must have much more blood than others; and we have now to mention that some parts have much larger vessels going to them than others. This idea is confirmed, by the blood being the moving material of life, and taking a part in every action of it: its quantity is to be found in proportion to those actions; and since the body is a compound of parts, or rather of actions, whose uses are known to vary considerably, we find blood directed to those parts in proportion to their actions; and this we judge of by the size of the vessels and redness of the part in those animals which have red blood, and we may suppose the same in those which have not this part of the blood. The brain has considerable vessels, &c. going to it, yet its substance is white, which is in some degree owing to its opacity; the tongue is vascular; the thyroid gland is vascular; the lungs allow of the passage of the whole blood in most animals, and therefore have always a current of blood through them equal to the whole; the liver is extremely vascular, which is known from its proportion of vessels, as well as its colour; and as there is in this viscus a peculiar circulation, the very great quantity of blood passing through it adds to the quantity in the whole body. The spleen is extremely vascular, as are likewise the kidneys; the stomach and intestines have considerable vessels going to them, and the muscles in general, more especially those of labouring people; for labour increases the quantity of blood in the whole, beyond simple nourishment in the full-grown, or beyond the mere growth in the young.

In tracing the course of this nourishment in animals (which consists ultimately of the blood), from the most simple to the most complicated there is a pretty regular series; although this regularity is interrupted whenever there is a variety in the circumstances, which are to be taken into the account; but the whole of this forms too extensive a subject for our present consideration.

If I were to begin at the formation of the blood, I should first treat of digestion in those animals which have stomachs; but this is a distinct subject. We may, however, begin with its immediate consequences, as digestion produces the first and most essential change, viz. the conversion of the food into a fluid called chyle. The chyle is the immediate effect or product of digestion, and is the seed which, as it were, grows into blood, or may be said to be the blood not yet made perfect. The chyle, to appearance, varies in different animals. In the quadruped and in the crocodile it is white; but in most other animals it is transparent: where it is white its parts are more conspicuous than where it is transparent. In this respect it is similar to the red blood, and is found to consist of a coagulating matter, a serum, and white globules, which render it of a white colour, so as in some degree to resemble milk. These globules are smaller than the red globules of the blood, and about the size of those in the pancreatic juice; they retain their figure in water, and therefore are not similar to the red globules; they retain their round form in the serum; they are also specifically heavier than their own lymph and serum.

One would naturally suppose from observing the chyle to have globular particles in certain animals that they formed the red globules in the blood; but when we consider that the chyle in fowls has no globules, and yet that they have red blood, we must conclude that they do not answer this purpose[a].

The first motion of the nourishment in most animals consists in the absorption of the chyle from the appendages of the stomach; and in many this alone appears to constitute the whole, as they have no such organ or viscus as a heart, to which it may be carried; and in such it may be supposed to be, in its mode of distribution, somewhat similar to the mesenteric veins and vena portæ: the parts therefore assimilate, and dispose of it themselves; but this structure belongs only to the most simple, or the first class of animals. In those which are more perfect, where parts are formed for each particular purpose, the chyle is brought to one organ, called the heart, having first joined the venous blood, which now requires a similar process, and both are sent to the lungs, where most probably the chyle receives its finishing process; and from thence it comes back to the heart again, to be sent to every part of the body*.

In those animals that have hearts we are to take into the account a number of particulars. First, the blood's motion in consequence of that organ; secondly, the principal intention of that motion, viz. that it may be prepared in the lungs, which introduces breathing; thirdly, the variety in the kinds of lungs; fourthly, the different kinds of media in which animals are obliged to breathe for the purpose of extracting matter employed in the preparation of this fluid.

In this investigation we shall find there is not an exact or regular correspondence in all the parts so employed. This irregularity arises from animals breathing different substances: such as some breathing the common atmosphere, in which is included the respirable air; others water, in which air is included, as fish. Some breathe both air and water; while there are others which breathe air in their perfect state, but water in their first periods or imperfect state of life†. If we were

* The circulation in fish is an exception to this.

† In this account I do not include animals in embryo, and some others, which do not breathe at all.

[a] [See *note*, p. 67.]

to take a view of all these systems, each should be considered apart, with all its peculiarities or connexions, together with the different systems, as they gradually creep into one another, some being perfectly distinct, while others partake more or less of both. The complete system is always to be considered as the most perfect, although it may belong in other respects to a more imperfect order of animals.

It has been supposed by physiologists that as the blood is found to consist of different parts, or rather properties, that certain parts or properties were determined to certain parts of the body, for particular purposes; but from the frequent anastomosis of arteries, the great variety in their number and origin, and the different courses which they take in different bodies, it is very evident that there can be no particular blood sent to any part of the body, where the whole blood can circulate. Many unnatural situations of parts show this. For instance, the kidneys sometimes have one artery only on one side, and two, three, or four on the other: on one side they may arise from the aórta as high nearly as the superior mesenteric, and on the other as low almost as the division into the two iliacs; and in some cases a kidney has been formed in the pelvis, and the artery has arisen from the iliac. The spermatic arteries too, sometimes, arise on one side from the aorta, and on the other from the emulgents or the arteria capsulæ renalis. If there was a particular blood sent to every gland, we should expect to find urine secreted in the testicle, when its artery arose from the emulgent; but as the blood visibly consists of different parts in those animals we are most acquainted with, and whose physiology is probably best known to us, and as one part of the blood can be traced in the vessels, we can determine with sufficient accuracy the proportions of blood sent, as well as the different kinds. Thus, the red part of the blood informs us how far it is carried; and we find that our coloured injections nearly correspond with this information.

I may here first remind the reader that the red globules are the grosser part of the blood, and therefore wherever these exist we have the blood with all its parts in due proportion and unseparated; but the construction in many parts of an animal is such that the red blood is excluded, and this also excludes every coloured powder we can inject; the vascularity, therefore, of such parts is not known, as has been mentioned already. Through them the coagulating lymph only can pass, and probably the serum, for the simple nourishment of the parts. Of this nature are tendons or tendinous parts, ligaments, elastic ligaments, cartilages, especially those of joints, the corneæ of the eye, &c. Even the brain and nerves have not the red blood pushed so far into their substance as many other parts have: we see therefore that the whole blood is not conveyed to all parts alike, and this we must suppose to answer some good purpose; yet, upon a more particular view of this subject, we may find it difficult to assign causes for this selection of the blood; for in many animals we find parts similar in construction and use, such as muscles, which are furnished, some with the whole blood, others with the coagulating lymph only, with all the gradations; some animals having both red and white muscles, others having them wholly red, and others wholly white, as will be more fully explained. Even venous blood can be rendered useful when it is not to answer the purpose of nourishment; for we find the blood of the intestines and spleen going to the liver, we may presume, for the secretion of the bile, as has been already observed (p. 86.).

The idea of particular kinds of blood being sent to parts having particular uses, more especially where the part is employed solely in disposing of this fluid, such as glands, is now, I believe, pretty well exploded; and it is supposed therefore that the whole mass of blood is such as to be fitted for all the purposes of the machine. This idea gives to the parts themselves full power over the blood so composed, and makes us consider the circulation or motion of the blood simply[a].

As the blood is composed of different parts, it might be supposed that if any particular part had been expended in any process, the remainder, as returned by the veins, would show this by its different appearance or qualities. The only visible difference that I could conceive to take place was in the appearance or quantity of coagulating lymph. To ascertain this, however, I made the following experiments.

Exp. 1. I opened the right side of the thorax in a living dog, and tied a ligature round the vena-cava inferior, above the diaphragm. I then applied my hand upon the opening, which allowed him to breathe, that the circulation might go on and fill the larger veins. When the inferior vena-

[a] [It seems extraordinary that the question, whether the blood sent to any one part of the body differs from that sent to any other part, should ever have been agitated. (See *note*, p. 73.) But to assign distinct and appropriate offices to the several elements of the blood in the functions of secretion, nutrition, &c., is altogether another question, which may plausibly enough be entertained. The observations of Bauer, Prevost and Dumas, and, lastly, of Milne Edwards, on the globules of the blood and several of the animal secretions, agreeing in this respect with the apparent globular constitution of the animal tissues, seemed for a time to establish a simple system of homogenesis of structure for the whole body, consisting, on the one hand, of an infinity of elementary molecules diffused through the nutritive fluids of plants and animals, and on the other hand, of these same molecules arranged in definite but diversified manners, so as to constitute the various tissues of the body. Unfortunately, however, for the beauty of this hypothesis, the very fact of the globular constitution of the animal tissues has been recently denied by Hodgkin and Lister. (*Phil. Mag. and Annals*, Aug. 1827, and also *App. to Tr. of Edwards's Influence of External Agents on Life*, &c.) Tiedemann also affirms the same thing, and says that even where organic particles do exist they present various forms and sizes, and are unlike those of the blood (*Phys., tr. by Gully and Lane*, p. 397.). So far, therefore, as relates to the use of the globular particles we are just as much in the

cava became turgid, I killed him. On the day following I examined the blood in the different veins, and found a coagulum in the emulgent, mesenteric, vena-cava inferior, splenic, and in the venæ-cavæ hepaticæ, of sizes proportionable to the sizes of the vessels; nor was there any difference in any other way.

Exp. 2. Some blood was taken from the mesenteric vein of a living dog, and similar quantities from the splenic vein, the emulgent vein, and the vena-cava inferior, below the openings of the emulgents. These four quantities were taken in four separate cups. They all soon coagulated; and if there was any one later of coagulating than another, it was that from the mesenteric veins. On standing twenty-four hours, the coagula were all of the same firmness.

§. 6. *Of the Living Principle of the Blood.*

So far I have considered the blood, and in the common way; but all this will explain nothing in the animal œconomy, unless we can refer it to some principle which may show the nature of its connexion with the living solids in which it moves, and which it both forms and supports. If we should find this principle to be similar to life in the solids, then we shall see the harmony that is supported between the two, and we shall call it the living principle of the blood. Without some such principle, all we have been examining is like dissecting a dead body without having any reference to the living, or even knowing it ever had been alive. But, from the account I have given of the blood, it must have appeared that I have still in reserve a property not hitherto explained; for in treating of the coagulation of the coagulating lymph I have not

---

dark as ever; for though Hunter has pointed out their connexion with the strength and vigour of the animal (p. 68.), Prevost and Dumas the relation which they bear to animal heat (*Ann. de Chim.*, xxiii.), and Dr. Christison the correspondence which exists between them and the consumption of oxygen in respiration (*Edin. Med. and Surg. Journ.*, xxxv. 94.), yet the exact relation which either of these phenomena bears to the cause from which it is supposed to spring is altogether a secret.

It has also, with equal confidence, been asserted that the fibrin of the blood constitutes the basis of muscular fibre, and that it is the great intermedium by which recently divided parts are united; the albumen also has been said to afford the basis of the dermoidal, ligamentous, and membranous tissues of the body. These, however, at present must be regarded as mere conjectures, in favour of which no definite or satisfactory kind of proof has as yet been offered. If, as very probably is the case, the act of assimilation carried on in the parenchymatous structure of parts is to be regarded as of the same nature with secretion, then there seems no greater reason for supposing the preexistence of muscle, or brain, or ligament, ready formed in the blood, than for imagining that bile, or milk, or semen, previously exist in this fluid; and yet no one has yet been hardy enough to affirm that either of these secretions is discoverable in healthy blood.]

been so full in my account as I might have been. As many phenomena respecting the coagulation or non-coagulation of the blood develop this principle, I have chosen in part to reserve it for this place; nor shall I be so full upon the present occasion as I should otherwise be were I writing on this subject expressly; my intention being rather to explain many appearances in the animal œconomy, and particularly the diseases I am to treat of, than to discuss this single principle. I reserve the illustration of my doctrine for such parts of the treatise as shall be employed on these subjects; the explanations and illustrations, therefore, will be interspersed through the work, by which means they will come more forcibly on the mind. From many circumstances attending this fluid, it would seem to be the most simple body we know of endowed with the principle of life. That the blood has life is an opinion I have started for above thirty years, and have taught it for near twenty of that time, in my lectures; it does not, therefore, come out at present as a new doctrine, but has had time to meet with considerable opposition, and also acquire its advocates[a]. To conceive that blood is endowed with life, while circulating, is perhaps carrying the imagination as far as it well can go; but the difficulty arises merely from its being fluid, the mind not being accustomed to the idea of a living fluid*. It may

* It is just as difficult for a man born in the West Indies to conceive water becoming a solid. I recollect a gentleman from Barbadoes walking out with me one frosty morning when there was ice on the gutters, and I, without having anything else in my mind than just common observation, said, "It has been a frost in the night." He immediately caught at the word frost, and asked me, "How I knew that?" Without thinking particularly of the cause of his question, I said, "Because I see the ice on the gutters." He immediately said, "Where?" and I answered, "There." Having been told that ice was a solid, he put his fingers down upon it; but with such caution as bespoke a mind that did not know what it was to meet; and upon feeling the resistance it gave, he gently pulled his hand back, and looked at the ice, and then became more bold, broke it, and examined it.

---

[a] [Although the doctrine of the life of the blood did not originate with Hunter, we are unquestionably indebted to him for its erection on a solid basis. His comprehensive mind enabled him to see more clearly than any preceding physiologist the real bearings of the question, and to devise experiments by which the specific difficulties which lay in the way might be removed. It is not alleged that the doctrine in question is demonstrable; but only that the evidence before us warrants and requires this inference,—the falsity of which has never yet been demonstrated by any of its opponents.

I am not afraid of diminishing Hunter's just fame by citing the following passages from Harvey, which fully prove that the life of the blood was maintained by that celebrated man, and maintained too by the same kind of arguments. But Hunter, in the spirit of the true English maxim, acquired his right to the property by blending his own labours with the soil; the originality of his mind improved the least thing that he borrowed, and stamped it with the *imprimatur* of his own genius.

" Vita igitur in sanguine consistit (uti etiam in sacris nostris legimus,) quippe in ipso

therefore be obscure at first, and it will be the more necessary that I should be pretty full in my account of it; yet the illustration of it in my account of inflammation will perhaps do more to produce conviction than any other attempt, although strongly supported by facts. It is to me somewhat astonishing that this idea did not early strike the medical inquirers, considering the stress which they have laid on the appearances of this fluid in diseases; since it (i. e. the blood) is probably more expressive of disease than any other part of the animal œconomy: and yet all this, according to them, must have arisen from, what shall I call it? a dead animal fluid, on which a disease in the solids must have had such an effect. This, I think, is giving too much to the solids, and too little to the fluids. When all the circumstances attending this fluid are fully considered, the idea that it has life within itself may not appear so difficult to comprehend; and indeed, when once conceived, I do not see how it is possible we should think it to be otherwise, when we consider that every part is formed from the blood, that we grow out of it, and if it has not life previous to this operation, it must then acquire it in the act of forming; for we all give our assent to the existence of life in the parts when once formed. Our ideas of life have been so much connected with organic bodies, and principally those endowed with visible action, that it requires a new bend to the mind to make it conceive that these

---

vita atque anima primum elucet, ultimoque deficit....... Sanguis denique totum corpus adeo circumfluit et penetrat, omnibus ejus partibus calorem et vitam jugiter impertit; ut anima primo et principaliter in ipso residens, illius gratia, *tota in toto et tota in qualibet parte* (ut vulgo dicitur) inesse, merito censeatur...... Clare constat sanguinem esse partem genitalem, fontem vitæ, primum vivens et ultimo moriens, sedemque animæ primariam; in quo, tanquam in fonte, calor primo et precipue abundat, vigetque; et a quo reliquæ omnes totius corporis partes, calore influente foventur et vitam obtinent...... Ideoque concludimus, sanguinem per se vivere et nutriri; nulloque modo ab alia aliqua corporis parte, vel priore vel præstantiore dependere....Utrumque autem, *sensum* scilicet, et *motum*, sanguine inesse, plurimis indiciis fit conspicuum....Id nunc solum dicam: licet concedamus, sanguinem non sentire; inde tamen non sequitur, eum non esse corporis sensitivi partem, eamque præcipuam....Habet profecto in se animam, primo ac principaliter, non vegetativam modo, sed sensitivam etiam et motivam; permeat quoquoversum, et ubique presens est, eodemque ablato, anima quoque ipsa statim tollitur: adeo ut sanguis ab anima nihil discrepare videatur; vel saltem substantia, cujus actus sit animus estimare debeat....Hic, ne à proposito longius aberrem, sanguinem (cum *Aristotele*) accipiendum censeo, non ut simpliciter intelligitur et cruor dicitur, sed ut corporis animalis pars vivens est." (*De Generatione, Exer.* li. lii.)

The following extracts from Aristotle's first and third books, on the history of animals, are probably those which are alluded to in the last paragraph:—"Sanguis nempe, instar laris familiaris, est anima ipsa in corpore...... et semper quamdiu vita servatur, sanguis unus animatur et fervet...... In sanguine reperitur divinum quid, respondens elemento stellarum." With more or less explicitness, the same doctrine was advanced by Willis (*De Motu Muscul.*, p. 71.), Hoffman (*Opera*, i. 33.), Huxham (*Essay on Fever*), and several other authors.

circumstances are not inseparable. It is within these fifty years only that the callus of bones has been allowed to be alive*; but I shall endeavour to show, that organization and life do not depend in the least on each other; that organization may arise out of living parts, and produce action; but that life never can arise out of, or depend on, organization. An organ is a peculiar conformation of matter (let that matter be what it may), to answer some purpose, the operation of which is mechanical: but mere organization can do nothing even in mechanics; it must still have something corresponding to a living principle, namely, some power. I had long suspected that the principle of life was not wholly confined to animals, or animal substances endowed with visible organization and spontaneous motion: I conceived that the same principle existed in animal substances devoid of apparent organization and motion, where there existed simply the power of preservation.

I was led to this notion about the year 1755 or 1756, when I was making drawings of the growth of the chick in the process of incubation. I then observed, that whenever an egg was hatched, the yolk (which is not diminished in the time of incubation,) was always perfectly sweet to the very last; and that part of the albumen, which is not expended on the growth of the animal, some days before hatching, was also sweet, although both were kept in a heat of 103° in the hen's egg for three weeks, and in the duck's for four. I observed, however, that if an egg did not hatch, it became putrid in nearly the same time with any other dead animal matter; an egg, therefore, must have the power of self-preservation, or in other words, the simple principle of life. To determine how far eggs would stand other tests, to prove a living principle, I made the following experiments†.

Having put a new-laid egg into a cold about 0, which froze it, I then allowed it to thaw; from this process I imagined that the preserving powers of the egg might be destroyed‡.

I next put this egg into the cold mixture, and with it one newly laid; the difference in freezing was 7½ minutes, the fresh egg taking so much longer time in freezing.

A new laid egg was put into a cold atmosphere, fluctuating between 17° and 15°; it took above half an hour to freeze; but when thawed, and put into an atmosphere at 25°, viz. nine degrees warmer, it froze in half the

* Dr. Hunter was the first who showed callus to be endowed with the principle of life, as much as bone.

† Phil. Trans. xlviii. pp. 28, 29; also Obs. on certain Parts of the Animal Œconomy, 1st edit., p. 106; and vol. iv. of the present edition.

‡ However this was at first not so certain; but the result of the experiment proved it was so. To be more certain of killing a part by freezing it, I believe it should be frozen very slowly, for simple freezing does not kill.

time: this experiment was repeated several times, with nearly the same result.

To determine the comparative heat between a living and a dead egg, and also to determine whether a living egg be subject to the same laws with the more imperfect animals, I made the following experiments. A fresh egg, and one which had been frozen and thawed, were put into the cold mixture at 15°; the thawed one soon came down to 32°, and began to swell and congeal; the fresh one sunk first to $29\frac{1}{2}$°, and in twenty-five minutes after the dead one it rose to 32°, and began to swell and freeze. The result of this experiment upon the fresh egg was similar to what was observed in the like experiments upon frogs, eels, snails, &c., where life allowed the heat to be diminished 2° or 3° below the freezing point, and then resisted all further decrease; but in both the powers of life were expended by this exertion, and then the parts froze like any other dead animal matter.

This is not a principle peculiar to life, but is common in many other cases: it has been observed that water could be so circumstanced as to be brought below the freezing point without freezing; but just as it began to freeze it rose to 32°. In my experiments on the heat of vegetables, I observed that the sap of a tree would freeze at 32°, when taken out of the vessels; but I found the trees themselves often so low as 15°, and the sap not frozen.

From these experiments, it appears that a fresh egg has the power of resisting heat, cold, and putrefaction in a degree equal to many of the more imperfect animals, which exhibit exactly the same phenomena under the same experiments; and it is more than probable that this power arises from the same principle in both. Similar experiments have been made on the blood: after a portion of blood had been frozen, and then thawed, it has again been frozen with a similar quantity of fresh blood, drawn from the same person, and that which had undergone this process froze again much faster than the fresh blood*.

As all the experiments I had made upon the freezing of animals, with a view to see whether it was possible to restore the actions of life when they were again thawed, were made upon whole animals, and as I never saw life return by thawing[a], I wished to ascertain how far parts were, in this respect, similar to the whole, especially since it was asserted, and with some authority, that parts of a man may be frozen, and may afterwards recover; for this purpose I made the following experiments upon an animal of the same order with ourselves.

* Vide Corrie on the Vitality of the Blood, p. 45.

---

[a] [Leeches have been frozen, and yet recovered. See *note*, vol. i. p. 284.]

In January 1777 I mixed salt and ice till the cold was about 0; and on the side of the vessel containing them was a hole, through which I introduced the ear of a rabbit. To carry off the heat as fast as possible, the ear was held between two flat pieces of iron, that sunk further into the mixture than the ear; the ear remained in the mixture nearly an hour, in which time the part projecting into the vessel became stiff; when taken out, and cut into, it did not bleed; and a part being cut off by a pair of scissors, flew from between the blades like a hard chip. It soon after thawed, and began to bleed, and became very flaccid, so as to double upon itself, having lost its natural elasticity. When it had been out of the mixture nearly an hour, it became warm, and this warmth increased to a considerable degree; it also began to thicken, in consequence of inflammation; while the other ear continued of its usual temperature. On the following day the frozen ear was still warm; and it retained its heat and thickness for many days after. About a week after this, the mixture in the vessel being the same as in the former experiment, I introduced both ears of the same rabbit through the hole, and froze them both; the sound one however froze first, probably from its being considerably colder at the beginning, and probably, too, from its powers not being so easily excited as those of the other: when withdrawn, they both soon thawed and became warm, and the fresh ear thickened, as the other had done before. These changes in the parts do not always so quickly take place; for on repeating these experiments on the ear of another rabbit, till it became as hard as a board, it was longer in thawing than in the former experiment, and much longer before it became warm; in about two hours, however, it became a little warm, and the following day it was very warm, and thickened.

In the spring, 1776, I observed that the cocks I had in the country had their combs smooth, with an even edge, and not so broad as formerly, appearing as if nearly one half of them had been cut off. Having inquired into the cause of this, my servant told me that it had been common in that winter, during the hard frost. He observed that the combs had become in part dead, and, at last, had dropt off; and that the comb of one cock had dropped off entirely; this I did not see, as the cock by accident had burnt himself to death. I naturally imputed this effect to the combs having been frozen in the time of the severe frost, and having, consequently, lost their life from this cause. I endeavoured to try the solidity of this reasoning by experiment. I attempted to freeze the comb of a very large young cock (being of a considerable breadth), but could only freeze the serrated edges (which processes were fully half an inch long); for the comb itself being very thick and warm, resisted the cold. The frozen parts became white and hard, and when I cut off a little bit it did not bleed; neither did the animal show any signs of pain. I next introduced into the cold mixture one of the cock's wattles, which was very broad and thin; it froze very readily, and, upon thawing both the frozen parts of the comb and wattle, they became warm, but were of a purple colour, having lost the transparency which remained in the other parts of the comb and in the other wattle: the wound in the comb now bled freely; both comb and wattle recovered perfectly in about a month: the natural colour returned first, next to the sound parts, and increased gradually till the whole had acquired a healthy appearance. Finding that freezing both the solids and the blood did not destroy the life in either, nor the future actions depending on organization, and that it also did not prevent the blood from recovering its fluidity, I conceived the life of every part of the body to be similar: what will affect, therefore, the life of any one part, will affect also that of another, though probably not in an equal degree; for in these experiments the blood was under the same circumstances with the solids, and it retained its life; that is to say, when the solids and blood were frozen, and afterwards thawed, they were both capable of carrying on their functions.

The following experiments were made in the same manner, on living muscles, to see how far the contractions of living muscles, after having been frozen, correspond with the coagulation of the blood.

A muscle removed from a frog's leg, with a portion of its tendon, was immediately placed between two pieces of lead, and exposed to a cold about ten degrees below 0. In five minutes it was taken out, when it was quite hard and white; on being gradually thawed it became shorter and thicker than while frozen; but on being irritated, did not contract; yet if at all elongated by force it contracted again, and the tendinous expansion covering the muscle was thrown into wrinkles: when the stimulus of death took place it became still shorter.

From a straight muscle in a bullock's neck, a portion, three inches in length, was taken out immediately after the animal had been knocked down, and was exposed between two pieces of lead, to a cold below 0, for fourteen minutes; at the end of this time it was found to be frozen exceedingly hard, was become white, and was now only two inches long: it was thawed gradually, and in about six hours after thawing it contracted so as only to measure one inch in length; but irritation did not produce any sensible motion in the fibres. Here, then, were the juices of muscles frozen, so as to prevent all power of contraction in their fibres, without destroying their life; for when thawed, they showed the same life which they had before: this is exactly similar to the freezing of blood too fast for its coagulation, which, when thawed, does afterwards coagulate, as it depends in each on the life of the part not being destroyed. I took notice in the history of the coagulation of the lymph, that heat of 120° excited this action in that fluid: to see how far muscular contraction was similar in this respect, I made the following experiment*.

As soon as the skin could be removed from a sheep that was newly killed, a square piece of muscle was cut off, which was afterwards divided into three pieces, in the direction of the fibres; each piece was put into a bason of water, the water in each bason being of different temperatures, viz. one 125°, about 27° warmer than the animal; another 98°, the heat of the animal; and the third 55°, about 43° colder than the animal. The muscle in the water heated to 125°, contracted directly, so as to be half an inch shorter than the other two, and was hard and stiff. The muscle in the water heated to 98°; after six minutes, began to contract and grow stiff; at the end of twenty minutes it was nearly, though not quite, as short and hard as the above. The muscle in the water heated to 55°; after fifteen minutes, began to shorten and grow hard; after twenty minutes it was nearly as short and as hard as that in the water heated to 98°. At the end of twenty-four hours they were all found to be of the same length and stiffness.

Here, then, is also a similarity in the excitements of coagulation in the blood, and of contraction in muscles, both apparently depending on the same principle, namely, life†.

If it should still be difficult to conceive how a body in a fluid state, whose parts are in constant motion upon one another, always shifting their situation with respect to themselves and the body, and which may lose a portion without affecting itself or the body, can possibly be alive, let us see if it is also difficult to conceive that a body may be so compounded as to make a perfect whole of itself, having no parts dissimilar, and having the same properties in a small quantity as in a great. Under those circumstances, the removing a portion is not taking away a constituent part, upon which the whole depends, or by which it is made a whole, but is only taking away a portion of the whole, the remaining portion being equal in quality to the whole, and in this respect is similar to the reducing a whole of anything. This might be perfectly illustrated, without straining the imagination, by considering the operation of union by the first intention. Union by the first intention is an immediate sympathetic harmony between divided parts when brought simply into contact, which I call contiguous sympathy. In this case it

* Vide Phil. Trans. lxvi. p. 412, Paper on Drowning; also, Obs. on certain Parts of the Animal Œconomy, vol. iv. of this edition.

† The application of this principle in disease I shall not at present take notice of.

is not necessary that the very same parts should oppose each other, else harmony, and consequently union, could never take place; it is simply necessary that the two parts be alive, and they might be shifted from one sort of a living creature to another for ever, without any injury to either, or without exciting irritation, and the whole would still be as perfect as ever. Neither can the motion of one living part upon another affect the body, because all its parts are similar, and in harmony with each other. It is exactly the same with the blood, for neither its motion on itself, nor its motion on the body, can either affect it or the body, since all the parts are similar among themselves. This is the case with all matter, where the property does not depend upon structure, or configuration, but upon the compound; for water is still water, whether its parts are moving on each other, or at rest; and a small portion has the same property with the whole, and is in fact a smaller whole. One of the great proofs that the blood possesses life depends on the circumstances affecting its coagulation; and, at present, we are only to explain the principles upon which these are founded, which it will be in some degree necessary to recapitulate: but perhaps the strongest conviction on the mind will arise from the application of this principle to diseases, especially inflammation. While the blood is circulating it is subject to certain laws to which it is not subject when not circulating. It has the power of preserving its fluidity, which was taken notice of when treating of its coagulation; or, in other words, the living principle in the body has the power of preserving it in this state. This is not produced by motion alone, for in the colder animals, when almost in a state of death during the winter, when their blood is moving with extreme slowness, and would appear to preserve simply animal life through the whole body, and keep up that dependence which exists between the blood and the body already formed, the blood does not coagulate to accomplish these purposes. If the blood had not the living principle, it would be, in respect of the body, as an extraneous substance. Blood is not only alive itself, but is the support of life in every part of the body; for mortification immediately follows when the circulation is cut off from any part, which is no more than death taking place in the part, from the want of the successive changes of fresh blood. This shows that no part of the body is to be considered as a complete living substance, producing and continuing mere life, without the blood; so that blood makes one part of the compound, without which life would neither begin nor be continued[a]. This circumstance, on its first ap-

[a] [The form of the argument is here changed from mere passive life to life such as it exists in completely organized bodies, where it always is active, and where, consequently, as it is quaintly enough expressed in the text, its continuance seems to be the

pearance, would seem a little extraordinary, when we consider that a part, or the whole, are completely formed in themselves, and have their nerves going to them, which are supposed to give animal life; yet that perfect living part, or whole, shall die in a little time, by simply preventing the blood from moving through the vessels: under this idea, it is not clear to me whether the blood dies sooner without the body, or the body without the blood. Life, then, is preserved by the compound of the two, and an animal is not perfect without the blood: but this alone is not sufficient, for the blood itself must be kept alive; because while it is supporting life in the solids, it is either losing its own, or is rendered incapable of supporting that of the body. To accomplish all this it must have motion, and that in a circle, as it is a continuance of the same blood which circulates, in which circle it is in one view supersaturated, as it were, with living powers, and in another is deficient, having parted with them while it visited the different parts of the body. Life is in some degree, in proportion to this motion, either stronger or weaker, so that the motion of the blood may be reckoned, in some degree, a first moving power; and not only is the blood alive in itself, but seems to carry life everywhere; however, it is not simply the motion, but it is that which arises out of, or in consequence of the motion. Here, then, would appear to be three parts, viz. body, blood, and motion, which latter preserves the living union between the other two, or the life in both. These three make up a complete body, out of which arises a principle of self-motion, a motion totally spent upon the machine, or which may be said to move in a circle, for the support of the whole; for the body dies without the motion of the blood upon it, and the blood dies without the motion of the body upon it; perhaps pretty nearly in equal times.

So far, I have considered the blood when compounded with the body and motion, in which we find it preserves its fluidity, and continues life in the body; but fluidity is only necessary for its motion to convey life, and the continuance of life is probably owing to its being coagulated, and becoming a solid; or at least the support of the body is owing to this cause. For this, however, it requires rest, either by extravasation, or by being retained in the vessels till the utility of circulating is lost;

---

result of "body, blood, and motion." I apprehend, however, the real line of argument to be, to prove that the blood and the solids possess life independently of each other,—not to make it the result of a compound of the two. It might be, and has been, with full as much propriety argued that the life of the blood is derived from the vessels, as that the life of the body is derived from the blood, for neither can continue without the other. The life of the blood is soon lost out of the body, and the body soon dies without the blood; nevertheless, a residual and independent vitality seems to reside in both for a limited space after they are separated from each other.]

or till it can answer some good purpose by its coagulation, as in mortification. Under any of these circumstances it becomes a solid body; for the moment it is at rest it begins to form itself into a solid, and changes into this or that particular kind of substance, according to the stimulus of the surrounding parts which excites this coagulum into action, and makes it form within itself, blood, vessels, nerves, etc.

The coagulation is the first step towards its utility in the constitution, and this arises from its living principle; for if that principle be destroyed, it does not coagulate at all, that is, naturally, for I do not here speak of any chemical coagulation.

I shall now endeavour to prove that the coagulation of the coagulating lymph bears some analogy to the actions of muscles, which we know to depend upon life, and which affords one of the strongest proofs of the existence of this principle; and though the action of coagulation itself be not similar to the actions of muscles, yet, if we can show that they are governed by the same laws, we may reasonably conclude that the first principle is the same in both. When I was treating of the coagulation of the lymph, I took notice that cold did not cause it, and supported the opinion by several experiments; at the same time I mentioned an experiment of Mr. Hewson, to prove the same thing, and which he conceived to be conclusive, but which does not appear to me in any way to affect his hypothesis (p. 26.). This experiment I had often made, but with another view, viz. to illustrate the living principle of the blood, which to me it in some measure does, more especially when compared with similar experiments on living muscles.

As the coagulation of the blood is a natural process, and as all natural processes have their time of action, unless influenced by some exciting causes, and since cold is not a cause of the blood's coagulation, even when removed out of the circulation, the blood may be frozen much more quickly than it can coagulate, by which change its coagulating power is suspended. To prove this by experiment, I took a thin leaden vessel with a flat bottom, of some width, and put it into a cold mixture below 0, and allowed as much blood to run from a vein into it as covered its bottom. The blood froze immediately; and when thawed became fluid, and coagulated, I believe, as soon as it would have done had it not been frozen.

As the coagulation of the blood appears to be that process which may be compared with the action of life in the solids, we shall examine this property a little further, and see if this power of coagulation can be destroyed: if it can, we shall next inquire if, by the same means, life is destroyed in the solids, and if the phenomena are nearly the same in both. The prevention of coagulation may be effected by electricity, and often is by lightning: it takes places in some deaths, and is produced in some of the natural operations of the body; all of which I shall now consider.

Animals killed by lightning, and also by electricity, have not their muscles contracted: this arises from death being instantaneously produced in the muscles, which therefore cannot be affected by any stimulus, nor consequently by the stimulus of death[a]. In such cases the blood does not coagulate. Animals that are run very hard, and killed in that state, or, what produces a still greater effect, are run to death, have neither their muscles contracted nor their blood coagulated; and in both respects the effect is in proportion to the cause *.

I had two deer run till they dropped down and died: in neither did I find the muscles contracted nor the blood coagulated[b].

In many kinds of death we find that the muscles neither contract nor the blood coagulate. In some cases the muscles will contract while the blood continues fluid, in some the contrary happens, and in others the blood will only coagulate to the consistence of cream.

Blows on the stomach kill immediately, and the muscles do not contract, nor does the blood coagulate. Such deaths as prevent the contraction of the muscles or the coagulation of the blood are, I believe, always sudden. Death from sudden gusts of passion is of this kind; and in all these cases the body soon putrefies after death. In many diseases, if accurately attended to, we find this correspondence between muscles and blood; for where there is strong action going on, the muscles contract strongly after death, and the blood coagulates strongly.

It is unnecessary, I imagine, to relate particular instances of the effects of each of these causes; I need only mention that I have seen them all. In a natural evacuation of blood, viz. menstruation, it is

* This is the reason why hunted animals are commonly more tender than those that are shot.

---

[a] [These sort of expressions are evidently vague and unsatisfactory. It is a fact that muscles contract at death; but to say that this is caused by the "stimulus of death" adds nothing to our knowledge of the fact. It is the ascription of a negative cause, and serves but to cover our ignorance of the real cause with the cloak of a name, and that name a bad one. See p. 32, *note* *; and vol. i., p. 236, *note*.]

[b] [Brisk exercise rather tends to accelerate coagulation (*Mayo's Physiology*, p. 38; *Prater on the Blood*, p. 94.), although, if carried to the point of exhaustion, this effect is altogether prevented; that is, according to the physiological hypothesis, the stimulus of exercise, by being in excess, becomes a sedative. It is to be observed, however, that the clot, although it forms more rapidly, contracts less, both in extent and duration, than under ordinary circumstances, and runs more rapidly into putrefaction. But muscular contraction is obedient to precisely the same laws, and hence the argument for the analogy of these phenomena, and that coagulation must consequently be a vital process.]

neither similar to blood taken from a vein of the same person, nor to that which is extravasated by an accident in any other part of the body, but is a species of blood changed, separated, or thrown off from the common mass by an action of the vessels of the uterus, similar to that of secretion; by which action the blood loses the principle of coagulation, and I suppose life (p. 35.).

The natural deduction from all these facts and observations I think is perfectly easy; it is impossible to miss it.

This living principle in the blood, which I have endeavoured to show to be similar in its effects to the living principle in the solids, owes its existence to the same matter which belongs to the other, and is the materia vitæ diffusa, of which every part of an animal has its portion*: it is, as it were, diffused through the whole solids and fluids, making a necessary constituent part of them, and forming with them a perfect whole; giving to both the power of preservation, and the susceptibility of impression, and, from their construction, giving them consequent reciprocal action. This is the matter which principally composes the brain; and where there is a brain, there must necessarily be parts to connect it with the rest of the body, which are the nerves; and as the use of the nerves is to continue, and therefore convey, the impression or action of the one to the other, these parts of communication must necessarily be of the same matter; for any other matter could not continue the same action.

From this it may be understood that nothing material is conveyed from the brain by the nerves, nor, *vice versâ*, from the body to the brain; for if that was exactly the case, it would not be necessary for the nerves to be of the same materials with the brain: but as we find the nerves of the same materials, it is a presumptive proof that they only continue the same action which they receive at either end.

The blood has as much the materia vitæ as the solids, which keeps up that harmony between them; and as every part endued with this principle has a sympathetic affection upon simple contact, so as to affect each other, (which I have called contiguous sympathy,) so the blood and the body are capable of affecting and being affected by each other; which accounts for that reciprocal influence which each has on the other. The blood being evidently composed of the same materials with the body, being endued with the same living powers, but from its unsettled state

* I consider that something similar to the materials of the brain is diffused through the body, and even contained in the blood; between this and the brain a communication is kept up by the nerves. I have, therefore, adopted terms explanatory of this theory; calling the brain the materia vitæ coacervata; the nerves, the chordæ internunciæ; and that diffused through the body, the materia vitæ diffusa.

having no communication with the brain, is one of the strongest proofs of the materia vitæ making part of the composition of the body, independently of the nerves, and is similar in this respect to those inferior orders of animals that have no nerves, where every other principle of the animal is diffused through the whole[a]. This opinion cannot be proved by experiment; but I think daily experience shows us that the living principle in the body acts exactly upon the same principle with the brain. Every part of the body is susceptible of impression, and the materia vitæ of every part is thrown into action, which, if continued to the brain, produces sensation; but it [the materia vitæ] may only be such as to throw the part impressed into such actions as it is capable of, according to the kind of impression; so does the brain or mind. The body loses impression by habit, so does the brain; it continues action from habit, so does the brain. The body, or parts of the body, have a recollection of former impressions when impressed anew; so has the brain: but they have not spontaneous memory as the brain has, because the brain is a complete whole of itself, and therefore its actions are complete in themselves. The materia vitæ of the body being diffused, makes

---

[a] [Thus no muscular fibres have yet been detected in the homogeneous parenchyma of the freshwater Polype, the Medusa, and several other species of zoophytes, although a species of contractility plainly resides in every part of these animals. In the Acrita there are no distinct nervous filaments; the digestive organ is excavated in the parenchyma of the body, and is devoid of distinct parietes; the vascular system consists merely of reticulate canals, in the substance of the body, devoid of proper tunics, in which a cyclosis of the nutrient fluids is observed, analogous to that of plants, but not a true circulation; and generation is accomplished by spontaneous fission, or gemmation. All the different systems, in short, are blended together in these polymorphous animals, analogous to what occurs in the ova or germs of the higher classes; and where even a distinct organ happens to be eliminated, it is often repeated indefinitely in the same individual, as in polypi, where the nutritious tubes of one individual are generally supplied by numerous mouths, which give it the semblance of a composite animal. The Polygastrica derive their name from an analogous multiplication of their digestive organ; and in the Tæniæ, each joint of the animal is the seat of a separate ovary. In these, which may be considered as the first steps of animal organization, we may observe a close resemblance to vegetables. There is no attempt or approach to centralization, but all the properties or functions of the animal (for which in the higher orders distinct organs are appropriated) are enjoyed by and reside in equally every part, and confer on every part an individuality of existence which enables it, when separated from the whole, to exist, to grow, and to reproduce as a complete animal.

The knowledge of these facts by Hunter may serve to show the extent of his information on comparative anatomy, and the powers which he possessed of generalization; but I look upon it as a still higher proof of the activity of his genius, to have applied so unexpected a truth to the illustration of the life of the blood. In the ensuing note I shall have occasion to notice the error into which many physiologists have fallen in expounding this part of Mr. Hunter's doctrines. See *note*, vol. i. p. 260; and *Cyclop. of Anat. and Phys.*, art. ACRITA.]

part of the body in which it exists, and acts for this part, and probably for this part alone. The whole, taken together, hardly makes a whole, so as to constitute what might be called an organ, the action of which is always for some other purpose than itself: but this is not the case with the brain. The brain is a mass of this matter, not diffused through anything for the purpose of that thing, but constituting an organ in itself, the actions of which are for other purposes, viz. receiving, by means of the nerves, the vast variety of actions in the diffused materia vitæ which arise from impression and habit, combining these, and distinguishing from what part they come. The whole of these actions form the mind, and, according to the result, react so as to impress more or less of the materia vitæ of the body in return, producing in such parts consequent actions. The brain, then, depends upon the body for its impression, which is sensation, and the consequent action is that of the mind; and the body depends upon the consequence of this intelligence, or effect of this mind, called the will, to impress it to action; but such [sensation and action] are not spent upon itself, but are for other purposes, and are called voluntary.

But mere composition of matter does not give life; for the dead body has all the composition it ever had. Life is a property we do not understand; we can only see the necessary leading steps towards it.

If nerves, either of themselves or from their connexion with the brain, gave vitality to our solids, how should a solid continue life after a nerve is destroyed? or, still more, when paralytic? for the part continues to be nourished, although not to the same full health as where voluntary action exists: and this nourishment is the blood; for deprive it of the blood, and it mortifies.

The uterùs, in the time of pregnancy, increases in substance and size, probably fifty times beyond what it naturally is; and this increase is made up of living animal matter, which is capable of action within itself. I think we may suppose its action more than double; for the action of every individual part of this viscus, at this period, is much increased, even beyond its increase of size, and yet we find that the nerves of this part are not in the smallest degree increased. This shows that the nerves and brain have nothing to do with the actions of a part, while the vessels whose uses are evident increase in proportion to the increased size: if the same had taken place with the nerves, we should have reasoned from analogy. It is probably impossible to say where the living principle first begins in the blood; whether in the chyle itself, or not till that fluid mixes with the other blood, and receives its influence from the lungs. I am, however, rather inclined to think that the chyle is itself alive; for we find it coagulates when extravasated; it has the same powers of separation with the blood; and it acquires its power of action in the lungs as the venal blood does [p. 67, *note*.]. I conceive this [viz. the action of the air on the chyle] to be similar to the influence of the male and female on an egg, which requires air and a due warmth to produce the principle of action in it, and somewhat similar to the venal blood coming to the lungs to receive new powers, which it communicates to the body. To endeavour to prove whether the chyle had the power of action in itself, similar to the blood, I made the following experiment.

I opened the abdomen of a dog, and punctured one of the largest lacteals at the root of the mesentery, out of which flowed a good deal of chyle, I then allowed this part to come in contact with another part of the mesentery, to see if they would unite, as extravasated blood does; but they did not. However, this experiment, though performed twice, is not conclusive; for similar experiments with blood might not have succeeded.

From what has been said with regard to the blood, that it becomes a solid when extravasated in the body, we must suppose that some material purpose is answered by it; for if the blood could only have been of use in a fluid state, its solidity would not have been so much an object with nature. It appears to me to be evident that its fluidity is only intended for its motion, and its motion is only to convey life and living materials to every part of the body. These materials, when carried, become solid; so that solidity is the ultimate end of the blood, as blood.

The blood, when it naturally increases the body or repairs a part, may be said to be extravasated, although it is not commonly so considered: what is usually understood by extravasation is when blood is effused from some accident, or from disease in the vessels, when of course it becomes obvious to the sight; but even this extravasation is of use, by the blood coagulating, although too often it is in too large a quantity. Accident does not calculate the size of the vessel ruptured to be just equal to the effect wanted by the rupture; but nature has made a wise provision for this overplus.

As extravasation arises from a rupture of a vessel, it is of service in the reunion of that vessel: if there are more solids ruptured than a vessel, as in a fracture of a bone, it becomes a bond of union to those parts; and this may be called union by the first intention: but the union is not that of the two parts to each other, but the union of the broken parts to the intermediate extravasated blood; so that it is the blood and parts uniting which constitutes the union by the first intention.

This blood, so extravasated, either forms vessels in itself, or vessels shoot out from the original surface of contact into it, forming an elongation of themselves, as we have reason to suppose they do in granulations. I have reason, however, to believe that the coagulum has the power, under necessary circumstances, to form vessels in and of itself; for I have already observed, that coagulation, although not organic, is still of a peculiar form, structure, or arrangement, so as to take on necessary action, which I should suppose is somewhat similar to muscular action. I think I have been able to inject what I suspected to be the beginning of a vascular formation in a coagulum, when it could not derive any vessels from the surrounding parts. By injecting the crural artery of a stump, above the knee, where there was a small pyramidal coagulum, I have filled this coagulum with my injection, as if it had been cellular; but there was no regular structure of vessels. When I compare this appearance with that of many violent inflammations on surfaces where the red blood is extravasated, forming, as it were, specks of extravasation like stars, and which, when injected, produce the same appearance with what I have described in the injection of the coagulum; when I compare these again with the progress of vascularity in the membranes of the chick; where one can perceive a zone of specks beyond the surface of regular vessels close to the chick, similar to the above extravasation, and which in a few hours become vascular, I conceive that these parts have a power of forming vessels within themselves, all of them acting upon the same principle. But where this coagulum can form an immediate union with the surrounding parts, it either receives vessels at this surface, or forms vessels first at this union, which communicate with those of the surrounding surface; and they either shoot deeper and deeper, or form vessels deeper and deeper, in the coagulum, till they all meet in its centre. If it is by the first mode, viz. the shooting of vessels from the surrounding surfaces into the coagulum, then it may be the ruptured vessels, in cases of accident, which shoot into the coagulum; and where a coagulum, or extravasation of coagulable lymph, is thrown in between two [sound] surfaces only contiguous, there it may be the exhaling vessels of those surfaces which now become the vessels of the part. In whatever way they meet in the centre, they instantly embrace, unite, or inosculate. Now this is all perfectly and easily conceived among living parts, but not otherwise.

As the coagulum, whether wholly blood or coagulating lymph alone, has the materia vitæ in its composition, which is the cause of all the above actions, it soon opens a communication with the mind, forming within itself nerves. Nerves have not the power of forming themselves into longer chords, as we conceive vessels to have; for we know that in the union of a cut nerve, where a piece has been taken out, it is by means of the blood forming a union of coagulum, and that the coagulum gradually becomes more and more of the texture, and has, of course, more and more the use, of a nerve, somewhat similar to the gradual change of blood into a bone in fractures.

It would appear, then, that the blood is subservient to two purposes in an animal: the one is the support of the matter of the body when formed, the other is the support of the different actions of the body [a].

---

[a] [ON LIFE.—Although it would be foreign to the object of these notes to enter into a lengthened discussion on the nature of *life in general*, I shall, I trust, need no apology for presenting the reader with a condensed view of Mr. Hunter's opinions on the subject, since by so doing I shall furnish him with the means of more clearly comprehending the nature, and more exactly estimating the value, of the arguments adduced by the author in support of his peculiar views respecting the *life of the blood.*

Mr. Hunter had a great dislike to definitions, for, said he, a definition allows one "to bring together a thousand things that have not the least connexion with it;" and for this reason probably he has abstained from setting forth, in the shape of a formal definition, his notions of life in the abstract. As it is necessary, however, when speaking of life, to fix on at least some of its essential properties by which to recognise its presence or absence, I shall take as a definition the short statement Mr. Hunter has made in his lectures, Vol. i. p. 223, of what he calls the most simple ideas of life. 1. "The first and most simple idea of life," says he, "is its being the principle of self-preservation." 2. "The second is its being the principle of action," or, as he has elsewhere stated it, "the susceptibility to impression, with a consequent power of action." "These are two very different properties, though arising from the same principle," and will require separate consideration.

I. *Of the principle of self-preservation.*—"By the living principle," says Mr. Hunter, "I mean to express that principle which prevents matter from falling into dissolution,—resisting heat, cold, and putrefaction......I have asserted that life simply is the principle of preservation, preserving it from putrefaction." Bodies belonging to the animal and vegetable kingdoms, considered as mere chemical compounds, must, from the energetic affinities of their component elements, be exceedingly prone to spontaneous decomposition; nevertheless, we find them, when in a living state, existing unchanged, often for a great length of time, although placed under external influences the most favourable for the operation of these affinities. Thus, seeds retain their vitality for years, if not for centuries, when buried deep in the soil; during the process of incubation, the yolk, and also a part of the albumen, of the egg, remain perfectly sweet to the last, though subjected from three to four weeks to a temperature of 103°; or, on the other hand, a fresh egg will resist the influence of a freezing mixture considerably longer than an egg the vitality of which has been destroyed by previous freezing, and, as in the case of some of the inferior animals, it will not allow its temperature to be reduced more than two or three degrees below the freezing-point, until the powers of life are exhausted, when it congeals, and assumes the temperature of the surrounding medium. Again, animals will exist and grow in the stomach, resisting the powers of digestion as long as they live; but where, as their vitality ceases, they are immediately digested. What, then, is it that confers on animal and vegetable substances this power of resistance to the influence of external agents tending to their destruction?

The theory which Mr. Hunter maintains is, that life is a *simple principle*, superadded to the common properties of matter in these bodies. "Animal and vegetable sub-

§. 7. *Some unconnected Experiments respecting the Blood.*

The following experiments have rather been imagined than fully executed, and the subject is rather broached and touched upon than pro-

---

stances," says he, "differ from common matter, in having a power superadded totally different from any other known property of matter, out of which arise various new properties: it cannot arise out of any peculiar modification of matter, but appears to be something superadded......Mere composition of matter does not give life, for the dead body has all the composition it ever had......This principle exists in animal substances devoid of apparent organization and motion......Organization and life do not depend the least on each other;" or rather, are not necessarily connected. "Organization may arise out of living parts, and produce action; but life can never arise out of, or depend on, organization......Organization and life are two different things."

This opinion respecting life in its most simple form seems, from the frequency and explicitness with which it is announced, and from its being that which he adopted in his work on Inflammation, to be the opinion which Mr. Hunter considered as most probably true. We do, however, find him here and there propounding views somewhat at variance with the above; but this arose probably from the habit of always keeping his mind open to conviction; or from an unwillingness to bind himself to any opinions which did not rest on the most unequivocal proofs, rather than from his considering these as affording more satisfactory explanations of the phenomena of life than the former.

First, he seems to have had some doubts whether life might not be regarded as an effect of the arrangement of the ultimate molecules of matter, as distinguished from organization of a more apparent kind. "Life, then, appears to be something superadded to this peculiar modification of matter; *or* this modification of matter is so arranged, that the principle of life arises out of the arrangement; and this peculiar disposition of parts may be destroyed, and still the modification from which it is called animal matter remain the same. If the latter be the true explanation, this arrangement of parts on which life should depend would not be that position of parts necessary to the formation of a whole part, or an organ, for that is probably a mechanical, or at least an organical arrangement; but just a peculiar arrangement of the most simple particles, giving rise to a principle of preservation.....the arrangement for preservation, which is life, becomes the principle of action, not the power of action......We have hitherto traced animal matter from its change from common matter to animal matter, the particles of which have possessed such an arrangement as to produce life."

It must, I think, be conceded, that such an arrangement of the ultimate molecules as is above alluded to, may exist even in those forms of animal and vegetable matter which, to our limited powers of observation, appear to possess no traces of organization, as the albumen and yolk of an egg; and further, that those phenomena of life which are perceptible to our senses, may be necessarily connected with, nay, dependent on, such an arrangement. But even this admission only carries us back one step further, namely, to inquire what is the agent or cause, under the influence of which this arrangement of molecules is effected and preserved? Is it one of those agents under the control of which the arrangements and changes in unorganized matter are effected, as attraction, galvanism, &c.; or is it a principle distinct from these? Now it is evident that here our reason is at fault, and will not enable us to reply conclusively to this question, since neither the cause itself, nor the first links in the chain of effects, supposing the above

secuted; but as I have not time at present to go through with the experiments, so as to arrive at some general result, I thought it better to

---

notion of a peculiar arrangement of ultimate particles be correct, are within the reach of our observation. We want data, and therefore we must be content to limit our inquiries to the more obvious phenomena of life; to examine its laws and modes of action, and to ascertain how far these coincide with those of the other agents above mentioned. If we adopt this course,—and it is the only one by which we can hope to arrive at a solution of the problem,—we shall, I think, be obliged to admit the existence of some principle or agent distinct from those which govern unorganized bodies. In these we find nothing analogous to the vital phenomena of irritability, contractility, the nervous influence, &c., not to mention that a broad line of distinction seems also to exist in regard to the chemical composition, intimate structure, mode of growth, form, duration, &c. of these two classes of bodies. These marks of distinction are broad and obvious, and should make us careful in admitting the identity of the causes by which they are produced with others of which the effects are so very dissimilar, merely on the ground of some hastily admitted analogy. We are by no means to abstain from inquiring how far the ordinary laws of matter are employed in producing effects in organized bodies; but we should at the same time be prepared, when these laws will not account for the phenomena observed, to admit the influence of another agent, the vital principle, the laws of which are to be patiently sought out and understood before we undertake to decide on its identity with other and apparently dissimilar agents.

In reference to this subject, Mr. Hunter was accustomed to employ the illustration of magnetism, which may be generated by holding a bar of iron at a particular angle with the horizon. "A bar of iron without magnetism may be considered like animal matter without life; set it upright, and it acquires a new property of attraction and repulsion at its different ends. Now is this any substance added? or is it a certain change which takes place in the arrangement of the particles of iron giving it this property?" I apprehend that no one will be disposed to object to this illustration as a simple help to apprehension, however unphilosophical it may be to extend the parallelism to its utmost limits, as Mr. Abernethy has done with respect to electricity. I have met with nothing in Mr. Hunter's published or posthumous writings which warrants, or in the least degree countenances, the opinion that these principles are identifiable; the analogy is wholly fallacious; nor is there, so far as I am aware, any single instance in which the principle of electricity has ever produced the proper and genuine effects of the principle of life.

It has I know been asserted by Dr. Wilson Philip (*Exper. Enquiry*, 2nd edit. p. 246), that galvanism performs all the functions of the nervous influence; that it excites the muscles; that it effects the secretions of the stomach; and that it occasions the evolution of caloric: but it may be replied, 1st, that many other stimuli affect the muscles besides gaivanism; 2nd, that digestion is not materially affected when the eighth pair of nerves is divided on the œsophagus; and 3rd, that the phenomena of animal heat are more easily explicable on chemical principles. Dr. Alison (*Physiology*, 2nd edit. p. 116 *et seq.*) has fully and in my opinion most satisfactorily refuted this doctrine, to the support of which the name and authority of Hunter have been most unwarrantably adduced.

Secondly, the existence of the living principle is ascribed to the *materia vitæ diffusa*, "of which every part of an animal has its portion; *i. e.* something similar to the brain diffused through the whole solids and fluids, making a necessary constituent part of them, and forming with them a perfect whole, giving to both the power of preservation, &c."; but this, I apprehend, is not to be taken literally, for "as the brain and nerves are composed of animal matter, and as that animal matter has life, or the first principle

bring forward what, in my opinion, should be done, than to omit the subject altogether*.

* Many of these experiments were repeated, by my desire, by Dr. Physic, now of Philadelphia, when he acted as house-surgeon at St. George's Hospital, whose accuracy I could depend upon.

---

of action in common with all the other matter composing the whole body," it must be evident that the author did not mean to identify the living principle with a tangible material substance; I presume his meaning to be simply that something corresponding to cerebral matter is diffused through all living substances, and serves as the intermedium by which the sympathy of living parts is maintained. This is rendered probable by what has been said in the previous note; but to suppose that he considered this cerebral matter as identical with life, is totally irreconcileable with the supposition formerly made, of a superadded principle.

Every part, then, whether organized or unorganized, solid or fluid, "where there exists simply the power of preservation," is supposed to possess this simple principle of life. It is on this principle that the horticulturist performs the operation of grafting; that the testicles of a cock may be made to grow in the belly of a hen, and a man's tooth in the comb of a cock. It must be evident that the detached parts would, if not alive, act as foreign substances in these cases, and stimulate the living parts to throw them off. Perhaps the most striking proof that life is not a mere emanation from the brain, or any other individual centre, but inheres in every part, is to be found in the irritability of muscles when separated from the body after death. In warm-blooded animals this does not last many minutes, but it endures for a long time in cold-blooded animals. Thus, according to Sir B. Brodie, "the head of a turtle was still alive, and bit at objects which were presented to it, many hours after it had been separated from the trunk"; and "the heart of a sturgeon, inflated from the mouth and hung up to dry, pulsated regularly for ten hours, the auricles continuing their action even when so dry as actually to create a rustling noise.....Oxygen, hydrogen, carbonic acid, and nitrogen produced the same effect on the heart of a snapper." (*Mitchell in Amer. Journ.*, vii. 58.) "The living principle [therefore] is essential to every part, and is as much the property of it as gravity is of every particle of matter composing a whole......Every individual particle of the living body, then, is possessed of life, and the least imaginable part which we can separate is as much alive as the whole."

But it by no means follows, because every particular part of the body possesses a principle of life independent of the effect which arises from their union as one system, that therefore this principle is independent of matter. We can with difficulty conceive of any of the powers of matter apart from, and independent of, the substances in which they reside; although, from the manner in which heat, electricity, magnetism, &c. are capable of being transferred from one substance to another, we conventionally agree to speak of these agencies as independent substances, or at least as superadded principles.

Blumenbach supposes every living particle to be endowed with a formative principle (*nisus formativus*), as contradistinguished from the peculiar mode of life (*vita propria*) enjoyed by each organ or structure. The former is the same in all parts, and in that energy by which, under different modifications, nutrition, reparation, and generation are accomplished; the latter is peculiar to each part, and is that by virtue of which, concurring with other parts, the complex phenomenon of systemic life is preserved (*über den Bildungstrieb*, &c.). This appears to me to be only another mode of expressing what was meant by Hunter, who says, that "although life may appear very compounded

I wished to see if blood that coagulated with an inflammatory crust putrefied later than that which coagulated without it; for I conceived that the strength of coagulation was something similar to the strength

---

in its effects in a complicated animal like man, it is as simple in him as in the most simple animal, and is reducible to one single property in every animal."

The resistance to putrefaction which arises from the possession of the principle of life, and which, in fact, is the only genuine indication of its presence in many cases, is not, as Richerand supposes, a "secondary effect, depending on the exercise of the functions," because function presupposes organization, but proceeds from a simple principle of antagonism, just as gravity resists force, or one chemical affinity is balanced by another. I am speaking here only of the most simple substances; for in completely organized bodies the resistance which is opposed to external agencies is undoubtedly to be regarded as a phenomenon of a mixed kind.

Life then, according to this first and most simple idea of it, consists in a property of matter superadded to and different from all other known agencies, whereby substances otherwise extremely prone to be acted upon by external causes are enabled to preserve themselves from dissolution. It exists independently of visible organization and spontaneous motion, and it inheres more or less in every living part, although not perhaps always in every part in equal intensity. Of its nature or immediate proximate cause we are entirely ignorant, except that a peculiar chemical and perhaps organical constitution of bodies always accompanies it, which may be either its cause or its effect, or a collateral effect of the same cause; but at present we are compelled to regard it as an ultimate fact.

II. *The principle of action*, or *susceptibility to impression and consequent power of action.*—"It was not sufficient that animal matter should be endowed with this first principle of self-preservation; it was necessary that it should have action or motion within itself. This does not necessarily arise out of the arrangement for preservation. On the other hand, the arrangement for preservation, which is life, becomes the *principle* of action, not the power of action; for the power of action is a step further. The power of action must arise from a particular formation of those living parts; for before action can take place, the matter must be arranged with this view. This is generally effected by the union of two or more living parts, so united as to allow of motion on each other, which motion the principle of action is capable of effecting when so disposed." The impressions and actions thence ensuing will vary infinitely amongst themselves, according to the complexity of the organization, "producing thereby infinite variety, both in all natural and diseased acts."

Now incitability and the power of acting under stimuli are the common fundamental properties of all organized beings, and of all the parts of those beings; but these qualities are differently designated, according to the different tissues in which they are manifested: irritability in muscles, sensibility in nerves, contractility in membranes, and so forth. This state of receptivity and action are carefully however to be distinguished from that power on which these qualities depend, viz. the vital principle, of which we know nothing except from its effects. "Life is a property we do not understand: we only see the necessary steps leading to it."

But although "life is not action," yet "it is continued and supported by it when it takes place. Action creates a necessity of support, and furnishes it. It is not necessary that action should continue in all parts; in some it is necessary that the principle or power of action should be continued, but in others it is necessary that action should take place even for the preservation of the power of action."

Such are the leading outlines, as they appear to me, of Mr. Hunter's doctrines of life;

of contraction in a muscle, resisting putrefaction. For this purpose I ordered the following experiments to be made.

Four ounces of blood were taken from the arm, which, after coagula-

---

according to which it would appear that the principle of life may exist both in a *passive* and in an *active* state; in a passive state generally only where there is no apparent organization, but in an active state wherever organization is developed. It has been considered by several modern physiologists, that as we are entirely ignorant of the nature of life, we ought to reject all such expressions as *principle of life, vital principle,* &c. as vague and indeterminate abstractions; but surely the same grounds exist for banishing the term principle altogether from our vocabularies. In the analysis of complex phenomena we ascend to ultimate facts, for which we assign some unknown causes, differently denominated *forces, principles,* or *powers* of matter, which have been likened to the unknown algebraical quantities x and y; and the determination of the laws by which these operate, constitutes the sole business of the philosopher. I do not, therefore, agree in the following observation of Majendie: "De toutes les illusions dans lesquelles sont tombés quelques physiologistes modernes, l'une des plus deplorables est d'avoir crus, en forgeant un mot *principe vital,* ou *force vitale,* avoir fait quelque chose d'analogue à la découverte de la pesanteur universelle;" (*Physiologie,* p. 14.) but rather in the remark of Prout, "that it is absolutely necessary to assume the existence of some agency different from and superior to that which operates among inorganic matters," (*Bridgewater Treatise,* p. 442.) whether this agency be called *life,* the *principle of life,* or merely *organic agencies.*

The circumstances under which this principle is usually manifested are infinitely complicated, arising partly from the reaction of the different parts on each other, and partly from the introduction into the living organism of most of those powers which operate on inorganic bodies, which the principle of life has the power more or less of modifying and counteracting, in subserviency to its own purposes. The animal body may be regarded as an intricate piece of machinery, arranged in perfect accordancy with the pre-existing properties of matter, so as to admit of the agency of those properties for the accomplishment of its own ends: thus we see various apparatuses, as the eye, the ear, the heart, the joints, &c., contrived in perfect conformity with the laws of light, of sound, of fluids, and of force. Gravity is still gravity in organized as well as in unorganized bodies; and the phenomena of endosmose and exosmose, of evaporation, elasticity, imbibition, and chemical affinity, plainly evince that these properties exist as well in living as in dead bodies, and even enter as essential elements into all the vital and most important functions of the body. Physiology, in short, is a complex science, presenting phenomena which proceed from the combined operation of chemical, physical, and vital agencies, harmoniously intermixed, but in which the vital principle holds a sort of supremacy, directing and modifying all the subordinate agencies to its own definite ends, besides producing effects which are not referrible to any other power. It seems, however, as Sir E. Home observes, "to be a rule of the animal œconomy, that the laws o life should not be employed when the mechanical or chemical laws of matter will answer the purpose." (*Lect. on Comp. Anat.,* v. 477.)

Having admitted the possibility of the self-organization of blood and coagulable lymph, it appears to me that Hunter has not been quite consistent in limiting his notion of action so strictly as he has done. He speaks as if action could only take place in parts visibly organized, as, for instance, in the muscles; but we know that action does and must commence in the egg, where no previous organization of parts has existed, and therefore necessarily precedes organization; somewhat, perhaps, as crystals are seen to gather in a fluid evaporating under the microscope. It may perhaps be replied, that the

tion, had the inflammatory crust upon its surface, and was also cupped. On the same day, four ounces of blood were taken from another per-

---

albumen and yolk of the egg are imperfectly organized, in as much as they exhibit evident traces of stratification and a granular arrangement after they are boiled, just in the same manner as the crystalline lens of the eye: this latter body, which appears of a perfectly homogeneous and gelatinous consistence in its natural state, is found, on more minute inquiry, to be composed of upwards of five millions of fibres, which curiously interlock one another by an elaborate mechanism. I do not see, however, how this removes the difficulty; for as the albumen is unquestionably secreted, in the first place, into the oviduct as a fluid, it must on this supposition organize itself; which is all that is pretended to be said. To argue, as some have done, that because life proceeds only from life, by an uninterrupted succession from the creation, therefore life is the result of organization, appears to me an instance of false logic, unless it can previously be proved, either that the albumen is not alive, or that, being alive, it is secreted already organized into the oviduct; neither of which propositions appears to me tenable.

I shall now briefly advert to the opinions of other physiologists, especially of those who have rejected the idea of a vital principle. These have been compelled to give some definition of life, and the following are examples. "L'ensemble des fonctions qui resistent à la mort." (*Bichat.*) "Une collection des phénomènes qui se succedent, pendant un temps limité." (*Richerand.*) "Life is the assemblage of all the functions, and the general result of their exercise," or, in other words, "the result of the mutual actions and reactions of all parts." (*Lawrence.*) "Life, then, consists of a continued series of actions and reactions, ever varying, yet constantly tending to definite ends." (*Roget.*) The term life "is applied to a certain assemblage and succession of phenomena." (*Alison.*) "Life is constituted by the conjoined operation of many actions." (*Bostock.*) "Life is simply an effect, the efficient cause of which is beyond the limits of human investigation. It is not a principle or source of action." (*Grainger.*) "L'idée de la vie est une de ces idées générales et obscures produites en nous par certaines suites de phénomènes, que nous voyons se succéder dans un ordre constant, et se tenir par des rapports mutuels. Quoique nous ignorions la nature du lien qui les unit, nous sentons que ce lien doit exister, et cela nous suffit pour nous les faire designer par un nom que bientôt le vulgaire regarde comme le signe d'un principe particulier, quoiqu'en effet ce nom ne puisse jamais indiquer que l'ensemble des phénomènes qui ont donné lien à sa formation......Ce mouvement général et commun de toutes les parties est tellement ce que fait l'essence de la vie." (*Cuvier.*)

Now the objection to all these definitions is, that they deal merely with the effects arising from the presence of life, or of the vital principle, and do not touch the question at issue, viz. of the nature of the principle itself. Let us apply these sort of definitions to some analogous subject of inquiry, and we shall more readily understand this. Suppose, for instance, that a person wanted to ascertain the cause of motion in any complicated piece of machinery, as a watch or a steam-engine, and he were to be informed that "it was the combination of motions which resisted rest," or that it was a "collection of phenomena which succeeded one another for a limited time," or "that it was the result of the united actions and reactions of all the parts," &c., he would at once perceive that his informant either did not understand his question, or could not answer it.

If by the term life we are to understand the complex assemblage of phenomena exhibited in a perfect animal, let it be so; in the same way as by the term movement we may understand the complicated actions and reactions in a piece of machinery: but let us not mistake such a definition for expositions of the original cause of the phenomena of life, or of the motions of machinery. Such a cause does exist, however, in the one

son's arm, which, on coagulating, showed no inflammatory crust on its surface. Both these quantities of blood were kept, in order to see which

---

case as in the other, and that quite independently of the particular form or structure of the animal or the machine, and perhaps independently of form or structure of any kind. Such definitions of life, therefore, as the preceding are plainly liable to the objection of making life dependent on organization and action, which appears to me to be nothing less than a complete reversal of the actual relations of cause and effect: for in regard to the cause, we cannot say that there is invariable antecedence or connexion; while in regard to the effect, it is not found invariably to follow the existence of the cause. We recognise the presence of life antecedently to all visible organization and action; and we also recognise its presence posteriorly to all action, as when an animal is frozen or asphyxiated. On the other hand, life is sometimes suddenly and completely extinguished, without any apparent change having taken place in the organization of the body.

On the Life of the Blood.—The difficulty of conceiving that the blood is endowed with life "arises merely," as Mr. Hunter observes, "from its being a fluid;" but we have not the smallest reason for assuming *à priori* that in the nature of things there is a more intimate connexion between life and a solid than between life and a fluid. Let us, therefore, dismiss this prejudice entirely from our minds, and examine the real grounds on which the doctrine of the life of the blood rests.

"From many circumstances attending this fluid, it would seem to be the most simple body we know of endowed with the principle of life;" consequently we should expect that the proofs of its vitality would be deducible chiefly from the resistance which it offers to external agencies.

1st. If a dead frog or eel be exposed to a freezing mixture, it sinks to 32°, freezes, and continues to fall to the temperature of the mixture. If the animal be alive it will sink to a few degrees below 32°, and remain at that point for a certain time, until the power of resistance be exhausted: it then dies, congeals, and sinks to the temperature of the mixture. If two eggs be similarly treated, one of which has had its powers of resistance destroyed by previous freezing, and the other is fresh, a like result is obtained: the former sinks uninterruptedly to the temperature of the mixture, the latter resists for a time at a few degrees below 32°, then congeals, and becomes cold as the former. If two portions of blood, one of which has been previously frozen and the other not, be exposed in a similar way to a freezing mixture, precisely the same thing occurs. Now are we not justified in concluding that the resistance to cold arises in each instance from the same cause? If it is the possession of life which enables the eel and frog to maintain their temperature for a time, it is the possession of life which also enables the fresh egg and the fresh blood in like manner to maintain their temperature. The objection that the resistance in the blood may be merely from a remainder of vital influence imparted to it by the solids, rests on the notion that there is in the nature of things a greater connexion between a solid and life than between a fluid and life: but this is a mere assumption, the contrary of which may be the fact; for in a perfect animal, as the eel or frog, it is not until the fluids, viz. the blood, &c., have become frozen that the animal is congealed. A solid deprived of blood is as little able to bear cold as blood separated from the solids.

2nd. Parts of animals, such, for example, as the ears of rabbits, and even whole animals, such as several insects in their chrysalis state, admit of being completely frozen without the necessary extinction of life. The blood, in the same manner, admits of being frozen without destroying its coagulating property. As, however, the ears of a rabbit become flaccid, so the coagulum of blood which forms after it has been frozen is

would resist putrefaction longest. By the fourth day, that without buff was putrefied; but the blood with the inflammatory crust did not putrefy

---

exceedingly loose. Cold acts as a sedative to the whole system, and if its action is sufficiently prolonged extinguishes life; but its action on the coagulation of the blood is precisely analogous, retarding or altogether preventing this act, in proportion to its intensity and continuance.

3rd. In all vegetables and animals, particularly those which are high in the zoological scale, there is a disposition to maintain a uniform temperature. Thus "blood taken from the arm in the most intense cold that the human body can bear, raises the thermometer to the same [or nearly the same] height as blood taken in the most sultry heat." Thus also fresh blood is slower in parting with its heat than other fluids of a similar consistency and specific gravity, even before coagulation.

4th. The analogy of heat is not so well marked as that of cold, yet the blood resists any considerable increase of temperature, which is seldom found to exceed by more than 3° or 4° that of the standard. Again, "Heat has the power of exciting action in an animal; and we find that heat even increases the action of coagulation." Thus also the muscles of cold-blooded animals are rendered perfectly rigid by being immersed in a fluid at a temperature not exceeding that of the human blood, while a similar effect is produced on the muscles of warm-blooded animals when immersed in a fluid at 125°, or if a fluid of this temperature be injected into the vessels; but as the effects of heat on the blood are precisely similar, it is reasonable to presume that they are analogous phenomena, and depend on the same cause.

5th. Notwithstanding that the blood is constantly in a temperature the most favourable possible to putrefaction, yet, like the egg in the process of incubation, it resists every approach to this state; and even out of the body it undergoes no decomposition for several days, but, like the muscles of the body, continues still further to contract. In proportion as the body is strong, so is the period during which the blood continues to contract and remain sweet prolonged; but in diseases characterized with great debility, it speedily runs into the putrefactive state. Thus blood from old and infirm persons uniformly began to putrefy two or three days sooner than that from young and strong persons. Blood which had been violently agitated putrefied three days sooner than blood from the same person allowed to remain in perfect repose; which may be compared to the effect of hard running on the solids. So also blood which was first frozen at a temperature of zero, and then heated to 126°, putrefied three days sooner than another portion which was not meddled with. But as muscles exhibit exactly the same phenomena under the same circumstances, it is reasonable to suppose that they both depend on the same cause.

6th. Sir Charles Scudamore found that when animals were killed by the discharge of an electric battery, the temperature of the whole body was exalted precisely in the same manner as has been observed in regard to the blood. Caldwell also found that the blood, subjected to very powerful shocks of electricity, was five times longer in coagulating than blood allowed to coagulate in the natural way; and after all it only coagulated imperfectly: effects which exactly correspond with those produced by electrical shocks on the muscular tissue.

7th. The effects of stimulants and sedatives on the blood and muscular fibre exhibit another train of analogies. Thus heat, electricity, exposure to air, motion, and very small proportions of salt and other extraneous substances, all hasten coagulation, and excite muscular contraction. "The blood," Mr. Hunter says, "coagulates from exposure as certainly as the cavity of the thorax or abdomen inflames from the same cause." Many observers have professed to have remarked a manifest contraction of the clot on the application of salt (*Stevens*, p. 132.) or galvanism (*Reil's Archiv für die Phys.*, x. 417; and

till the seventh day. In these two experiments it would appear that the inflammatory blood preserved its sweetness longest; but, from a repe-

Biologie, iv. 654.); but whatever effect is produced by the latter agent is probably due to the coagulation of the albuminous part of the serum interspersed in the meshes of the clot; the solidification of which may easily be supposed to occasion a sudden contraction of the whole mass. Tourdes, in his translation of Spallanzani, saw, or supposed he saw, a mass of blood agitated by an undulatory motion, analogous to the feeble oscillatory movements of a muscle; while Rosa has affirmed that the blood possesses an expansile and contractile property, by which it experiences alternate movements of dilatation and contraction, corresponding to the rhythm of the pulse, wherever it is removed from the living vessels of the body (*Lettere Philos.*). These observations, however, have not been confirmed. Mr. Hunter says that the more the blood is alive, the more readily it obeys stimulants, in consequence of which it coagulates more rapidly in health than in inflammation, and in the arteries than in the veins: but there are numerous facts of a contrary nature. (See *notes*, pp. 39, 42.)

8th. On the other hand, the opposite effects of sedatives have been adduced to prove the same point. Thus, it has been argued, that as opium, belladonna, and other narcotic extracts retard or prevent coagulation, or diminish the subsequent contractility of the clot, in the same manner and degree as these substances are known to affect the contractility of muscles, so it is probable that they both depend on the same cause. But the value of this argument is entirely destroyed, in my opinion, by the fact that the extracts of cinchona, gentian, and sarsaparilla, and many other substances of an equally inert kind, affect the coagulation of the blood much more strongly than the narcotic extracts, while many of the most powerful sedatives, as the hydrocyanic acid, have no appreciable effect on this process. The premiss, in short, is incorrect which assumes that any such actual relation exists between the effects produced by different agents on the blood and muscular fibre as to justify one in concluding from one to the other in any case. The most obvious and characteristic example of this sort is probably that of common salt, which equally and powerfully prevents the contraction of the crassamentum, the coagulation of the blood, and the contraction of muscular fibre; but as this agent has a similar effect in preventing the contraction of the coagulum of milk, even after the acescent fermentation has commenced, it must be evident that such an effect can only proceed from a chemical operation. It is impossible, as it appears to me, to account *physiologically* for the fact that the extracts of belladonna and opium have less effect in preventing the coagulation of the blood than the extracts of sarsaparilla and gentian, and the infusions of tobacco and hydrocyanic acid than the infusions of tea or coffee.

9th. The coagulation of the blood has been already several times referred to, so that it will here only be necessary to advert to it again as a specific point of analogy. However we may account for this phenomenon, it is impossible to overlook the strict parallelism which exists between it and the tonicity of muscles. In nineteen cases out of twenty, or ninety-nine out of the hundred, the same physiological causes which accelerate, retard, or entirely destroy the coagulability of the blood, increase, diminish, or entirely destroy the irritability of muscles. Coagulation has been compared to the last act of life, corresponding to the convulsion of the muscles which takes places at the moment of death, and also to union by the first intention. "Coagulation," Mr. Hunter says, "I conceive to be an operation of life; and I imagine it to proceed on exactly the same principle as the union by the first intention;" that is, particle unites to particle, because they are endued with the same living principle, and consequently have a sympathetic affection upon simple contact, so as to affect each other.

The circumstances connected with coagulation formed the chief of Mr. Hunter's

tition of these experiments, it did not appear upon the whole that there was much difference.

---

arguments for the vitality of the blood, and have also been considered by Majendie as affording "une preuve démonstrative que le sang est doué de la vie." In a previous note, however, (p. 41.) I have offered a different explanation of this process, and therefore think it right to mention here that I consider the present argument as a real objection to that explanation, although not a sufficient one to overturn it. The subsequent and uninterrupted contraction of the clot for several days after coagulation, exactly corresponds with the gradual stiffening of the muscles after death, and therefore the presumption is that both depend on a physiological cause. I apprehend, however, that the same chemical affinity which first produced coagulation may still continue to act and to increase the effect; for acescency and even putrefaction in the coagulum of milk do not prevent a still further contraction of the clot, although it cannot be pretended that the coagulation of milk is a vital process, (since freezing and boiling have no effect in preventing it,) and still less that the contraction which subsequently occurs is due to such a cause. The analogy between the coagulum of blood and the coagulum of milk is at least fully as much to the point as the analogy between the contraction of muscles and the contraction of the coagulum of blood: so that the argument from this subject, in respect of the theories before mentioned, is ambidexter, and will receive its quality from other circumstances.

10. Another argument is derived from the fluidity of the blood, which manifestly depends on its vitality, whether this quality be conceived to proceed merely as an emanation from the surrounding living solids, or to be inherent in the blood itself (see *note*, p. 29.). The former opinion is certainly favoured by what is mentioned in the next paragraph respecting the effect of poisons on the blood; but the latter appears to me the most probable; first, because it makes the body one consistent whole; and secondly, because it assigns a sufficient reason why the blood does not instantly solidify when it is extravasated from the body, and when, therefore, it must necessarily be placed beyond the reach of that influence which previously kept it fluid. A certain time is required before the blood concretes, and this time is generally found to bear a direct relation to the extent of contact which it has with foreign substances, which appear to conduct away the living principle somewhat in the same manner as heat, electricity, and some other imponderable substances are conducted away under the same circumstances.

11. The celerity with which impressions made on one part of the blood are propagated by sympathy throughout the mass. Fontana found that almost infinitesimal quantities of certain poisons instantly rendered the whole mass of the blood incoagulable; while, on the other hand, other substances having a styptic quality had a contrary effect. (*Op. cit.*, ii. 135.) Now as the poisons above mentioned had no influence whatever on the blood when extravasated from the body, it necessarily follows that the effect which they produced on the blood, while in the body, was physiological, and not chemical, either directly on the blood itself, or, as is most probable, intermediately through the containing vessels; a reciprocative sympathy, that is, must have existed, to have allowed of this action and reaction on each other, although it is impossible to conceive of any sympathy in a dead part. This harmony between the containing and the contained parts is preserved under all circumstances, and can only be ascribed to the sympathy which exists between vital parts. If the body is strong, the contraction of the clot is strong, and the period at which it begins to putrefy protracted; but the reverse of these circumstances universally obtains in proportion as the powers of the whole system are debilitated. But the blood is not only believed to sympathize with the body, but with

To see whether the blood in a young person or an old one become soonest putrid, I desired that the following trials should be made:

---

itself: that is, blood sympathizes with blood in the same manner as the solid parts of the body sympathize with one another.

12. As I have already adverted (*note*, p. 63.) to the volvular or rotary motion of the globules of the blood, I shall here only add further, that were this property clearly proved to belong exclusively to the products of organization, it would constitute in itself a sufficient and convincing proof of the vitality of the blood. The researches of Schultz, Dollinger, and more recently those of Dr. Alison (*Supplement to Physiology*, p. 18.), are full on this point, and seem at least to render it extremely probable that the globules of the blood are endowed with vital attractions and repulsions, distinct from any motion impressed on them by the living solids; that, in fact, the blood possesses all the properties of self-motion enjoyed by the solids. To the same head may be referred the adherence of the coloured external tunics of the globules to their central nuclei, which is uniformly found to be strong in proportion as the strength and health of the animal is perfect. The repulsion also which exists among the globules themselves, by which their individuality is preserved, and their diffusion through the whole mass effected, can only be explained on the same principle.

13. The blood is the first part which is formed in the embryo, being, in fact, the primordial rudiment to which the principle of life is attached, and from which, by successive elaborations, the various solids of the body are formed. This is one of Harvey's chief arguments, who denominates it the "particula genitalis prima," the "pars primigenia corporis," the "primum vivens et ultimo moriens" of animals.

14. Allied to the last argument is that of Hunter: "The blood preserves life in the different parts of the body. When the nerves going to a part are tied or cut, the part becomes paralytic, and loses all power of action; but it does not mortify. If the artery be cut, the part dies, and mortification ensues......No part of the body is to be considered as a complete living substance, producing and continuing life, without the blood. .....It is not clear to me whether the blood dies sooner without the body, or the body without the blood......Every part is formed from the blood, and if it has not life previously to this operation, it must acquire it in the act of forming." Thus, the vascularity of a part is the measure of its vitality, and the extraordinary exercise of any function necessitates an extraordinary supply of blood. But it may be argued that the blood is no otherwise necessary to life than food is necessary: both are essential; but both may equally be regarded as simple aliments, on which the organization of the body operates so as to convert them into living structures.

In continuation of the same argument, Mr. Hunter further says, "The blood has motion in a circle, in which circle it is in one view supersaturated, as it were, with living powers, and in another is deficient, having parted with them while it visited the different parts of the body." Dr. Davy consequently asks, whether we are to regard the circulation as "a perpetual miracle, in which material particles are, without cessation, dying and reviving"? But how does Dr. Davy know that the venous blood is dead? It is plain also that the same question might with equal force be asked respecting the whole body, which cannot subsist without a continual supply of fresh blood; the solids require fresh blood as much as the blood requires fresh air, in order to continue life, so that a something is acquired in both cases, and that something is essential to life, or at least to its continuance.

15. "If the blood had not the living principle, it would be in respect of the body as an extraneous substance"; wounds would not unite as they do, by the first intention, because the coagulated blood would have first to be thrown off as a foreign body, by suppura-

June 24th. Some blood was taken from a woman twenty years of age, and its surface, after coagulation, was covered with an inflammatory crust. On the same day some blood was taken from a woman aged

---

tion, and all ecchymoses would form abscesses: but the contrary of all this happens, for we see the blood everywhere adhere to fresh-cut surfaces without irritating them, on exactly the same principle that cut surfaces themselves adhere to one another. The case of certain fluids, such as bile, urine, &c., not irritating their respective receptacles, is no argumemt against this view of the subject; since there is not one of the secretions of the animal body which would not irritate a cut surface, and prevent union by the first intention. The scorpion can destroy itself by its own poison, although that substance is perfectly innocuous in its proper vessels.

16. "A body may be so compounded as to make a perfect whole of itself, having no parts dissimilar, and having the same properties in a small quantity as in a great." If, then, the blood be of this kind, motion or division cannot affect it, for all the parts are similar, and independent of the rest. "The blood has as much the materia vitæ as the solids, which keeps up that harmony between them." The value of this argument may be estimated by referring to note, p. 116.

17. Blood, when it coagulates, has an unquestionable disposition to assume a peculiar arrangement, corresponding to the organization of the most simple membranes; the globules of the blood, that is, arrange themselves into piles or rouleux, so as to constitute fibrils, which variously intersect one another, unlike any other thing in nature, except the chyle, which Hunter supposed to be endowed with life equally with the blood. Sir E. Home imagined that the blood, on coagulating, formed a sort of tubular structure, in consequence of the escape of carbonic acid gas; but this notion has been completely exploded by more correct observation. The incipient organization of the clot seems entirely to depend on the polarizing forces of the ultimate globules. I apprehend also that it would be difficult to deny that the globules themselves may possess an incipient organization, in as much as they evidently consist of separate parts, have a determinate shape, and are larger than the ova of many animalcules, or even than the animalcules themselves, of whose organization there can be no doubt. Some have regarded these particles as distinct monads, possessing an independent vitality.

18. The last argument for the coagulation of the blood is derived from the phenomenon of union by the first intention, and the power which the blood has of originating and carrying on organization and action within itself. "Animals and vegetables have a power of action within themselves," by which they are capable "of working themselves into a form and a higher state of existence. Now the blood seems to possess this characteristic property of life as well as the solids, for extravasated blood "forms either vessels in itself, or vessels shoot out from the original surface of contact into it....I have reason to believe that the coagulum has the power, under necessary circumstances, to form vessels in and of itself.....I think I have been able to inject what I suspected to be the beginning of a vascular formation in a coagulum, when it could not derive any vessels from the surrounding parts." But it may be asked how could these vessels be injected if there was no connexion? The decision of this point would afford a true "crucial instance" decisive of the vitality of the blood; but unfortunately the present state of science does not enable us to come to any satisfactory conclusion in this matter. I have already intimated (*note*, p. 43.) that Hunter's notions on the subject of union by the first intention do not seem supported by sufficient data; but I must beg leave to refer the reader to part ii. chap. i. for the evidence which at present exists on this subject. There can be little doubt, I think, that effused lymph has a power of self-organization; but I apprehend it is taking too much for granted to suppose that

sixty, the crassamentum of which was also covered with an inflammatory crust. These quantities of blood were set by. The blood from the old woman putrefied in two days. That from the young woman kept quite sweet till the fifth day, when it began to smell disagreeably; in this state it continued two days more, and then emitted the common odour of putrid blood.

Several experiments were made in the course of the summer, of a similar nature with the last, in all which it appeared that the blood from young people kept longer sweet than that which was taken from the old.

In October 1790, when the weather was cold, some blood was taken from two men, one of whom was seventy-five years of age, and the other eighty-three, about six ounces from each. The blood from each kept sweet till the fifth day; but on the sixth both quantities smelt equally putrid, which uniformity accords with the preceding experiment.

To see if recent blood or coagulated blood lost its heat soonest, four ounces of blood, after coagulation, were heated till the mercury of a thermometer, placed in the middle of the coagulum, was raised to the 98th degree. The thermometer was then put into a similar quantity of blood, immediately after it was taken from the vein, in which the mercury stood at 90°. These were placed by each other, and the thermometer put alternately into each, to observe how they parted with their heat.

	Coagulated Blood.	Recent Blood.
At the beginning of the experiment	98°	90°
After two minutes	97	89
After four minutes more	93	88
After two minutes more............................	92	87
After two minutes more............................	91	86

This experiment was not accurately made, for the two bloods should

lymph effused from a cut or inflamed surface is identically the same as lymph as it exists in the circulating blood.

I shall only further observe, that the argument for the vitality of the blood is strictly a cumulative one, and must be viewed in its totality in order to estimate its real force. Taken altogether, the preceding facts raise at least a strong presumption in its favour, not to say a high probability. It may seem inconsistent, after having rejected two of the most material arguments (viz. those founded on coagulation and union by the first intention), that I should introduce them into the present argument; but it should be remembered that these are the arguments employed by Hunter. The explanation of these facts by Mr. Hunter is not demonstrated to be false, but only another explanation is offered, which appears to me to account more easily for the phenomena in question. It is a balance of probabilities, and therefore I conceive it perfectly legitimate to introduce the minor probability into the question, which will carry weight in proportion as it is corroborated by other circumstances.]

have been of the same temperature, because the warmer any body is, the faster it will lose its heat to any neighbouring colder body; yet I believe that the coagulated blood lost its heat faster than the fluid blood.

To see whether a stimulus can be applied to the blood, so as to make it coagulate faster than it does naturally, I desired the following experiment to be made:

Three ounces of blood were taken from a boy about ten years of age, and immediately after the cup was put into water heated to 150°. A similar quantity was taken in another cup from the same boy, at the same time, which was put into water heated only to 48°. The first coagulated completely in five minutes, but the latter remained quite fluid for twenty minutes, and then began to coagulate, but was not completely coagulated for five minutes more. When looking at each portion of blood an hour afterwards, it appeared that the blood which coagulated in the warmest manner had the greatest proportion of serum, and the least of crassamentum; but by next morning the serum in each was equal in quantity, and the crassamentum of equal size.

This experiment shows that heat above the natural standard acts as stimulus upon the blood, and makes it coagulate considerably sooner than cold does, though not more firmly. This heat did not act as heat upon the blood, but only as the stimulus; for heat acting as heat would also have coagulated the serum, which was not the case.

This experiment, or a similar one, is brought forwards as one of the proofs of the living principle of the blood, where it is contrasted with a similar experiment on living muscles.

To see whether blood, when mixed with different substances in strong solution, and which appeared to prevent coagulation, would, when diluted with water, admit of coagulation:

In December half an ounce of blood, immediately after it was taken from the arm, was mixed with one pound of water. This was intended as a standard to judge of the others. More blood was taken from the same person at the same time, to which a strong solution of Glauber's salts [sodæ sulphas] was added; this altered its colour to a florid red, and was found to prevent it from coagulating. A strong solution of Glauber's salts, therefore, has the power of preventing the coagulation of the blood. Ten minutes after this mixture half an ounce of it was mixed with one pound of water; half an hour after, another half ounce was mixed with one pound of water; at the end of an hour the same was done, and also after two hours: all these were allowed to stand twenty-four hours, when the pure blood and water had deposited a considerable dark-coloured sediment, and a light-coloured blood was suspended, which had begun to subside, leaving the fluid above perfectly transparent, and of a beautiful red colour. The different portions of blood which had been first mixed with the salt, and afterwards with water, had the cloud exactly like that of the pure blood, but there was no sediment whatever at the bottom of the vessel: this cloud gradually subsided, and left the fluid above of a beautiful red colour, and also quite transparent. At this time (viz. twenty-four hours after the mixture of the salt with the blood,) another half ounce was mixed with one pound of water, and next day the appearances were exactly similar to what have been already described. The sediment in the pure blood was most probably the coagulating lymph; and as there was none in the others, it is most likely that the lymph in them did not now coagulate.

As medicines, when taken into the circulation, whether by the stomach or by the skin, produce considerable effects on the constitution, I wished to know what effect such substances would have upon the blood with regard to the act and power of its coagulation.

Two ounces of blood were received from the arm into a vessel, as a standard of natural coagulation. Two ounces more were taken in another vessel, to which one ounce of water was added. The intention of this addition was to put this blood in the same circumstances with blood in other comparative trials respecting water, so that the difference, if there was any, must belong to the substance mixed with the blood, independent of the water. Two ounces more blood were received in another vessel, to which was added one ounce of the decoction of bark.

These different quantities were taken from one person, one after the other, in the same order in which they are here set down. After six minutes, the blood mixed with water was quite coagulated; after nine minutes, that mixed with the decoction of Peruvian bark formed a loose coagulum; after twelve minutes, the blood first drawn coagulated: the coagula of the first- and second-drawn blood were equally firm, the water in the second having been squeezed out along with the serum; but that mixed with the decoction of bark was much less so. It appears from these experiments that water rather hastened coagulation, but made it neither firmer nor looser in the texture.

In the following experiments the blood was first all received into one vessel, and stirred before it was mixed with the different substances. The intention of this was, that the three portions of blood might all be exactly under the same circumstances.

Two ounces were poured into a vessel as a standard of natural coagulation. Two ounces more of blood were poured into another vessel, to which were added two ounces of water, as in the former experiment. Two ounces more were mixed with two ounces of the decoction of bark. After twelve minutes, the two first were coagulated, and the coagula were equally firm; after fourteen minutes, that with the decoction of bark coagulated, but the coagulum was very loose. Upon comparing the three coagula next day, that which had the decoction of bark mixed with it was by much the least firm.

This experiment was repeated, and the result was nearly the same; and it shows that even putting equal parts of water and blood together did not alter the time or the firmness of coagulation, but that the decoction of bark evidently did [a].

Some blood was taken from the arm into a bason, stirred, and then mixed with different infusions, as follows:

Two ounces were mixed with the same quantity of the infusion of columba root; two ounces with the same quantity of the infusion of gentian; two more with two ounces of the watery solution of opium; and two ounces were kept in a vessel by themselves. The blood which had been mixed with the bitter infusions, and the simple blood, all coagulated at the same time, viz. in six minutes; but that which had been mixed with the infusion of gentian was firmer than with the infusion of columba root, but was not more firm than the coagulum of the simple blood. The blood which had been mixed with the solution of opium did not coagulate for twelve minutes, and then the coagulum was very loose.

This experiment with the opium was repeated, and the result was exactly the same.

Of extraneous matter in the blood.—Whatever is dissolved in the blood must be only diffused through it, not chemically combined with it, otherwise the nature of the blood itself would be altered, and the effect of medicine destroyed. The blood can receive and retain extraneous matter, capable of destroying the solids, by stimulating to action so as to destroy them [b].

---

[a] [Scudamore obtained a different result. In two experiments in which three or four parts of water at 80° were mixed with fresh-drawn blood, coagulation was retarded till nine and fourteen minutes, acquiring then only the consistence of a tremulous jelly; whereas similar portions of the same blood, to which no water was added, coagulated firmly in five! (*Op. cit.*, p. 38.) The effect of water, however, on coagulation depends on the quantity employed: equal parts, and all proportions under that, were uniformly found to hasten coagulation, although thirty or forty parts of water retarded the deposition of the fibrin at least a full hour. (*Prater*, pp. 17. 80.) When considerable quantities of water are employed, it is probable that coagulation is delayed by the coagulating particles being removed to a greater distance from each other.]

[b] See vol. i. p. 355, *note*.

Extraneous matter in the blood is capable of altering the chemical properties of the solids in those who work in lead, as is evident in the following case.

Morgan, a house-painter, who had been paralytic in his hands and legs for a considerable time, was thrown down, and had his thigh-bone broken just below the little trochanter. The upper end of the inferior portion had passed over the outside of the other, and moved with the knee, so that the end of the lower bone was taken for the great trochanter; but I discovered the fracture by extending the leg, and got the portions of bone in their places, and bound up the limb with a roller. It went on well for nearly a fortnight, only his hands swelling at times, which gave way to fomentations: in the third week he grew very ill, became low, had a kind of lethargy, a great deal of blood came out of his mouth, he sunk still lower, and died about three weeks after the accident.

On examining the body after death, the muscles, particularly those of the arms, had lost their natural colour; but instead of being ligamentous and semitransparent, as happens in common paralysis, they were opake, resembling exactly in appearance parts steeped in a solution of Goulard's extract. From this case it appears the lead had been evidently carried along with the blood, even into the muscles themselves*.

* [Dr. Christison has shown not only that particular poisons physiologically affect particular structures, or, in the language of Hunter, "take their different seats in the body as if they were allotted to them," but that they have also a disposition to accumulate substantially in particular organs. (*On Poisons*, p. 15, *et passim.*) It is doubtful, I think, whether Hunter was correct in supposing that the lead actually combines with the muscular fibre in the living body. In the dead body this certainly happens; that is, the oxide of the metal enters into direct combination with the animal fibre; but it is scarcely conceivable that this can happen in the living body. (*Trans. Col. of Phys.*, i. 317.)

With respect to the effect of various reagents on the blood, I have but little to say. Dr. Davy (*Edin. Med. and Surg. Journ.*, xx. 257.), Dr. Scudamore, Mr. Prater, and a number of other writers on the blood, have dwelt largely on this branch of the subject; but, as far as I understand the experiments which have been made, they do not seem to me to warrant any general conclusions respecting the physiology of this fluid. The extreme proneness of all organic bodies to undergo changes of constitution, and to assume new states of existence, in consequence of slight external causes, is an objection *in limine* to all such inquiries; but, in addition to these circumstances, the blood possesses a principle of life, so that it is neither possible to separate the physiological from the chemical effects, nor to arrange these effects upon any general principle derived from the nature of the agents employed. The most inert substances produce effects of the most marked kind, while bodies of the most destructive and virulent nature are almost totally inoperative.

Some bodies, as the concentrated mineral acids, act from a purely chemical effect, decomposing and consolidating the blood, and entirely destroying its colour and contractility; others, as many of the metallic oxides, induce coagulation, partly from a physiological, and partly from a chemical, effect,—precipitating and combining with the albumen. The caustic alkalis dissolve the fibrin, and keep the blood permanently fluid;

most of the neutral salts and vegetable extracts also retard, or entirely prevent, coagulation; although this effect is not permanent, for coagulation may subsequently be induced, by dilution with water, in the great majority of instances. The extracts of sarsaparilla, bark, and gentian, render the blood permanently fluid, although little or no effect is produced by arsenic, tobacco, extract of belladonna, or hydrocyanic acid. A long-continued temperature of 32°, a heat varying from 140° to 150°, the citric and tartaric acids, and a great variety of physiological causes, all produce the same effect, viz. that of gelatinizing the blood. Now it is impossible, in the present state of science, to refer these incongruous effects to any general principle, because we are entirely ignorant of the mode by which the generality of these agents operate. It is possible that bulky powders and extracts may prevent coagulation, in consequence of the interposition of their particles between the coagulating particles of fibrin; but then these are only a few instances out of a great number; besides that, on this supposition, the retarding effect ought always to be in proportion to the bulk of the substance employed, which is far from being the case. Dilution with water, as I have before observed, seems to operate in this way. The explanation of the incoagulability of the blood, when the neutral salts are added, upon the principle of the expansion or contraction of the globular particles, appears to me totally inadequate to explain the phenomenon, even though we should admit the fact that the globules of the blood do actually contract and expand in the manner supposed; for if the opinion formerly given (*note*, p. 20.) be correct, that the fibrin of the blood is quite independent of the red globules, it will be a matter of perfect indifference of course in what manner the globules may be affected. It is remarkable that blood kept fluid by means of salt retains its florid colour for years, and also its property of coagulating when diluted with water. Dr. Davy has made the curious remark, that when coagulation is prevented by a foreign admixture, the blood does not putrefy, although this effect is produced as usual by dilution with water.

It is also deserving of remark, that most substances which, when added in quantity, retard or prevent coagulation, accelerate this process when added only in small proportions; thus, electricity, hard running, and even the neutral salts, which are so powerful for keeping the blood fluid, manifestly hasten its concretion, if not carried to excess, agreeably to a general physiological law, that stimuli universally become sedatives when carried to their utmost point.

BIBLIOGRAPHY OF THE BLOOD.

Ackermann, J. F. Comment. de Combustionis lentæ Phænomenis, quæ, Vitam organicam constituunt. 1805.——*Adams, J., M.D.* An Illustration of Mr. Hunter's Doctrine of the Blood. 1814.——*Adelon, N. P.* Physiologie, 2ème édit. 1829. iii. 110.——*Albinus, B.* Dissert. de Massæ Sang. Corpusculis. 1688; et Dissert. de Pravitate Sang. 1689.——**Alison, M. P., M.D.* Physiology, 2nd edit. 1833. p. 62; and Supplement. 1836.——*Amici, Professor.* Edin. Med. and Surg. Journ., xv. 120. On the Shape of the Globules.——**Andral, G.* Précis d'Anat. Pathol. 1829. i. 11. *tr.* by *Drs. Townsend* and *West*; et Clin. Méd. 2ème édit. 1829–35. iv. 683. et passim. Sur les Lésions de Circulation.——*Anon.* An Essay on the Transmutation of Blood. 1725.——*Autenrieth, J. H. F.* Dissert. de Sang. 1792.

* Those authors which appear to possess the best claim to the *student's* attention are indicated by an asterisk; many other names, however, of scarcely inferior excellence, are passed over, in consequence of the necessity of stopping somewhere.

Babington, B. G., M.D.* Med. and Chir. Tr. xvi. 46. (1830.) On a concrete Oil, &c., as a Principle of Healthy Blood; and *ib.* p. 293. Considerations with respect to the Blood.——*Bader, J. H. L.* Exper. circa Sang. 1788.——*Baerts.* Diss. de Nat. Sang. inflamm. 1782.——*Barbatus, H.* Tractatus de Sang. 1667.——*Barruel, M.* Ann. d'Hyg. pub. i. 267. (1829.) Sur un Principe propre à caractériser le Sang de l'Homme et des Animaux.——*Bartholinus, J.* Misc. Acad. Nat. Cur. 1671. p. 23. Observ. de Sang. verminoso.——*Bastays, M. de la.* Sur les Mal. chron. qui proviennent de la Comp. du Sang. 1780.——*Bauer, F.* Phil. Tr. 1818. p. 173. On the Form and Size of the Globules.——*Beale, B.* On vicious Blood as a Cause of Disease. 1706.——*Bell, J.* Anat. and Phys., 4th edit. 1816. i. 503. On the Properties of the Blood, containing a refutation of Mr. Hunter's doctrine of the vitality of this fluid.——*Bellingeri, C. F. J.* Experimenta in Electricitatem Sang., &c. 1826; also in Annali Univ. di Med. 1827; and Lancet, xiii. 810. ——*Bennet, C., M.D.* Exerc. Diagn. (Sang. vitiis.) 1654.——*Berdoe, M., M.D.* An Essay on the Nature, &c. of the Blood. 1772.——*Berthold, A. A.* Beiträge zur Anat. Zool. und Phys. 1831. p. 259.——Berzelius, J. J.* Med. and Chir. Tr., iii. 198. (1812.) On the Chemical Properties of the Animal Fluids, and particularly of the Blood; also Traité de Chim., *tr.* par *A. J. L. Jourdan* et *M. Esslinger.* 1829–33. vii. 27. Le Sang.——**Bichat, X.* Anat. Gén. 1801. ii. 1. *tr.* by *C. Coffyn.* 1824; and additions, par *P. A. Béclard.* 1821. p. 72.—Rech. Phys. sur la Vie et la Mort, 3ème édit. 1805. p. 170. et passim. *tr.* by *F. Gold.*—Journ. de Santé de Bordeaux, ii. 61.——*Blainville, D.* Phys. Gén. et Comp. 1829–30. i. ——*Blundell, J., M.D.* Med. and Chir. Tr. ix. 56. (1818.) On the Transfusion of Blood.——*Blumenbach, J. F.* Medicin-Bibliothek. 1783. i. 177.—Comm. de Vi vitali Sang. 1788; et Comm. Soc. Gotting. ix. 3.—Inst. Phys. edit. 4tâ, 1821. *tr.* and greatly augmented by *J. Elliotson, M.D.* 5th edit. pt. i. 1835. p. 143.——*Boerhavii, H.* Praxis Medica. 1728. Aph. 58–144. et Præl. Acad. à *Haller.* 1740. §123. et nota.——*Bordeu, T.* (Th.) De Analy. Méd. du Sang. 1775.——*Bornholt.* Dissert. de Sang. Pravitate. 1702.——*Borelli, J. A.* De Motu Animalium. 1680. ii. prop. 132. Anal. Sang. et Forma ejus Comp.——*Borelli, P.* Hist. et Observ. Med.-Phy. Centuria. 1553. Cent. iii. obs. 4.——**Bostock, J., M.D.* Med. and Chir. Tr., i. 47. (1809.) On the Gelatine of the Blood.—Physiology, 2nd edit. 1828. i. 428.—Edin. Med. and Surg. Journ., xxxi. 114. (1829.) Obs. on the Coag. of the Blood.——*Boudet, F.* Arch. Gén. de Méd. 2de sér. ii. 128.——*Bouillaud, Professor.* Journ. Hebd. de Prog. des Sc. Méd. iii. 353. (1835.) Reflexions sur les Altér. des Liquides et sur l'état du Sang dans les Inflam. putrides.——*Bouillon la Grange, E. J. B.* Manuel d'un Cours de Chim. 1812. ii. 469.——*Boulton, R.* Of the Heat of the Blood, &c. 1698.——*Boyle, Hon. R.* Mem. for the Nat. Hist. of the Blood, &c. 1684.; and Phil. Tr. 1665. pp. 100. 117. 139.——*Bowerbank, J.* Entom. Journ., i. Micros. Observ. on the Blood of Insects.——**Brande, W. T.* Phil. Tr. 1809. p. 373. Obs. on Albumen and some other Animal Fluids;—*ib.* 1812. p. 90. Chem. Researches on the Blood, &c.:—*ib.* 1818. p. 181. On the existence of Carbonic Acid in the Blood. ——*Brandt.* Encyc. Wörterb., art. Blut. bde. v. (1830.)——*Bretschneider, F. F.* Comm. de Gener. Crustæ Inflam. 1788.——*Browne, J.* Essay on the Fundamentals in Physic, and upon the Structure of the Blood. 1709.——*Bruner.* Dissert. de Malâ Sang. Temperie. 1707.——*Bright, R., M.D.* Rep. of Med. Cases. 1828. ii. 63. et passim.——**Burrows, G., M.D.* Med. Gaz. xiv. 502. et seq. (1834.), and xvi. 647, et. seq. (1835.) Gulstonian and Croonian Lect. on the Blood and Urine.—— *Butt, J. M.* (Th.) De Sang. spont. Separ. 1760.; reprinted in *Sandiford's* Thesaurus Dissert. 1768–78. ii. 501.——**Burdach, K. L.* Die Physiologie. 1826–35. bde. iv. vom Blute.——*Burthart, J. R.* Ueber das Blut und das Albumen, &c. 1828.—— *Bushnan, J. B.* Hist. of a case in which Animals were found in the Blood. 1833.

Caldani, L. M. A. Mem. di Padova, v. 1. Osserv. Micros. sulla Figura delle Molecole rosse del Sangue. ——**Caldwell, C., M.D.* On the Vitality of the Blood. 1805.—— *Carminati, B.* Risult. di Sperienze ed Osserv. su il Sangue. 1783.——*Carradori, M.* Annali di Chimica, xiv. 86. (1797.) Exp. on the Coag. of Albumen.——*Carvinus.* De Sanguine, &c. 1562.——*Carswell, R., M.D.* Path. Anat. 1833–6. Art. Pus et passim.——*Cavallo, T.* Essay on Factitious Airs, with an App. on the Nature of the Blood. 1798.——*Chaillon, J.* Rech. de l'Origine du Sang. 1675.—— *Chevallier, A.* Ann. d'Hyg. pub. iv. 433. (1830.) Examen des Taches du Sang, &c. See *Burruel.*——*Chevreul, M.* Journ. de Phys. par Majendie, iv. 119. (1824.) Consid. sur la Nature du Sang; et Ann. du Muséum, x. 445.——*Chomel.* Dict. de Méd., art. ANÉMIE. 1821.——*Christison, R., M.D.* On Poisons. 2nd edit. 1832. p. 586. et passim.—Edin. Med. and Surg. Journ., Oct. 1829. On Milky Serum:— *ib.* xxx. 94. (1831.) On the mutual Action of Blood and Atmosph. Air.—— *Clander, G.* Misc. Acad. Nat. Cur. 1688. p. 326. Sanguis fere albus sine damno aliquot annos durans.——*Clanny, W. R., M.D.* Lectures on Typhus, and the Changes of the Blood in it. 1828.——*Coleman, E.* On Respir. and the Changes the Blood undergoes. 2nd edit. 1802.——*Collard de Martigny.* Journ. de Phys. par Majendie, viii. 152. (1828.) Recher. Exp. sur les Effets de l'Abstinence sur la Comp. et sur la Quantité du Sang; et *ib.* x. 111. Rech. Exp. sur la Respir., &c. ——*Copland, J., M.D.* Dict. of Med. 1835. art. BLOOD.——*Couerbe, M.* Ann. d'Hyg. pub. iv. 479. (1830.) Reflexions sur le Principe Volatil du Sang.—— *Courten, W.* Phil. Tr., xxvii. 485. Exp. and Obs. on several sorts of Poisons on Animals.——*Cruveilhier, J.* Anat. Path. 1828. passim.——*Crawford, A., M.D.* Exp. and Observ. on Animal Heat. 2nd edit. 1788.——*Currie, J., M.D.* Essay on the Vitality of the Blood. 1791.

Dance, M. Arch. Gén. de Méd., xviii. pp. 289, 473; and xix. pp. 5, 161. Changemens que subit le Sang dans le Fièvre continue et dans la Phlébite.——*Davies, R.* Essays to promote the exp. analyses of the Human Blood. 1760.——*Davy, Sir H.* Researches on Nit. Oxide Gas. 1800.——**Davy, J., M.D.* (Th.) De Sang. 1815.—Phil. Trans. 1822. p. 271. Observ. on the Buffy Coat of Blood.—Edin. Med. and Surg. Journ., xxix. 244. (1828.) On the Spec. Grav. of Blood and Serum:—*ib.* p. 254. On the Carb. Acid in the Blood:—*ib.* xxx. 248, (1829.) On the circumstances which affect Coagulation:—*ib.* xxxi. 21. (1829.) Is the Blood a living Fluid?—*ib.* p. 287. On the Nature of the Blood:—*ib.* xxxiv. 243. (1830.) On the Action of Atmospheric Air on the Blood.——*De Haen.* Ratio Med., pars i. c. 6 et 25; et iii. c. 33 –34.——**Denis, P. S.* Rech. Exp. sur le Sang, &c. 1830; et Journ. de Phys. par Majendie, ix. 176. (1829.)——*De Sandris, J.* De Nat. et Præternat. Sang. Statu. 1696.——*Deyeux, N.* Mém. sur les Altér. du Sang. 1797.—Journ. de Physique, xliv. 438. (1804.)—Consid. Chim. et Méd. sur le Sang des Ictériques.——*Diest, I.* An sui Sanguinis solus Opifex Fœtus? 1735.——*Dieffenbach, J. F.* Die Transfusion des Blutes, &c. 1828.——*Doemling, J. J.* Giebt es ursprüngliche Krankheiten der Säfte? 1800.——*Döllinger, J.* Was ist absonderung, und wie geschieht sie? 1819; and Denkschriften der Koniglichen Acad. der Wissenschaften zu Munchen, vii. 184.——*Doné.* Lecture faite à l'Acad. des Sc. 1834.——*Dowles, T.* Med. and Chir. Tr. xii. 86. (1823.) On the Products of acute Inflam.——*Duplay, A.* Arch. Gén. de Méd. 2nd sér. vi. 223. (1824.) Obs. d'une Altér. très-grande du Sang. ——*Dupuy, M.* Arch. Gén. de Méd., xiv. 289. (1827.) De l'Effet de la Ligature et du Section des Nerfs de la 8ème paire sur le Sang.——*Dumas, C. L.* Physiologie. 1800-3. iii. 377.—Recueil Périod. de la Soc. de Méd. de Paris. xxxiii. 353. Exp. à déterminer l'influence des 8 Nerfs sur le Color. du Sang.—See *Prevost.*

Edwards, H. M., M.D. Répert. Gén. iii. part 1. p. 25. (1827.) Sur la Struct. intime des Tissus.——*Eller, J. T.* Mem. de Berlin. 1751. p. 3. Nouvelles Exp. sur le Sang humain.——*Ellis, D.* An Inquiry into the Changes produced on Atmospheric Air. 1807.—Further Inquiries. 1811.——**Engelhart, J. F.* Comm. de vera Materiæ Sanguini purpureum Colorem impertientes naturâ. 1825.—Edin. Med. and Surg. Journ. xxvii. 94. (1827.)——*Everts, B. H.* Dissert. Phy.-Med. de Hæmatosi.

Falconer, M. Exper. Enquiries concerning the Blood. 1777.——*Fontana, F.* Nuove Osserv. sopra i Glob. rossi del Sangue. 1766.——*Fontana, G.* Atti di Siena. vi. 161. De Sang. Restitutione.——*Forget, C.* Journ. Hebd. de Prog. des Sc. Méd. 1834, 1835. p. 353. De l'Humorisme rationale.——**Fourcroy, A. F.* Syst. des Connoiss. de Chim. 1801. ix. 185. Sur le Sang.—Ann. de Chim. vi. 182. vii. 147; et Mém. de l'Acad. des Sc. 1789. p. 297. Sur les Altér. du Sang par l'Infl. de l'Air.——*Fracassinus, A.* Osserv. del Sangue. 1766.

Gaber. De Humoribus Anim.——*Galen.* Opera. 1679. iii. De Elementis.——*Gatti, E. A.* Saggio sul Sangue e sul Salasso. 1824.——*Gaspard, G.* Journ. de Phys. par Majendie, ii. 1. (1822.) iv. 1. (1824.) Mém. Phys. et Méd. sur les Maladies Putrides, &c.——*Gaubius.* Instit. Pathol. 1763. § 339 et seq.——*Gendrin, A. N.* Hist. Anat. des Inflam. 1826 passim.——*Gigna, J. F.* Misc. Societ. Taurin. (1758.) i. 68. De Colore Sang.——*Gordon, J., M.D.* Ann. of Phil. iv. 139. (1814.) On the Extrication of Caloric during the Coagulation of the Blood.——*Grant, R. E., M.D.* Lect. on Comp. Anat. in Lancet. (1833–4.) ii. 865 et seq.——*Gruithuisen, F. P.* Beitrage zur Physiognosie et Tautognosie. 1812. § 89.——*Gruner, C. G.* Dissert. Path. Sang. 1791.——*Guglielmini, D.* Opera. 1701. ii. § 44. De Sang. Naturâ et Constitutione.

Hall, M., M.D. Med. and Chir. Tr. xiii. 121. (1827.) On the Effects of loss of Blood; and also separately. 1830.—Encyc. of Med. 1832. art. Blood.——*Haller, A.* Elem. Phys. 1757–66. ii. lib. 5.—Deux Mém. sur le Sang, &c. 1756. *tr. anon.* 1757. ——*Hammerschmidt, J. A.* Discrimen inter Sang. Arter. et Ven. 1753.——*Harles, J. C. F.* Hist. Sang. 1794.——*Hartman.* Diss. super crustæ Inflamm. origine.——*Harwood, Dr.* Phil. Trans. abr. i. 185, note. Exp. on Transfusion.——*Harveii, G.* Opera. 1766. De Gener. Exerc. 52.——*Helwich, C.* Misc. Acad. Nat. Cur. 1697–8. p. 446. De Copiâ Ferri Sanguinis, &c.——*Herbst, E. F. G.* Commentatio, &c. De Quantitate Sang. 1822.——*Hermann, Professor.* Arch. de la Méd. Homæop. ii. 255; et Ann. d'Hyg. pub. vi. 342. (1831.) De l'Anal. du Sang des Cholériques. ——*Henke, U.* Ueber die Vitalitat des Blutes und Säfte Krankheiten. 1806.——**Hewson, W.* An Exp. Enquiry into the Properties of the Blood. 1772–7; and Phil. Trans. 1770. pp. 384, 398. On Coagulation:—*ib.* 1773. p. 303. On the Figure of the Red Globules.——*Hey, W.* Observ. on the Blood. 1779.——**Hodgkin, J.* Phil. Mag. ii. 130; and Appendix to *tr.* of *Edwards's* work Sur l'Infl. des Agens Phys. sur la Vie. On the Size and Form of the Globules of the Blood and animal Tissues.——*Hodgson, J.* On the Diseases of Arteries and Veins. 1815. p. 83 et passim.——*Hoffmann, F.* Med. Ration. Syst. lib. i. § 1. c. 5.——*Hoffman, M.* Dissert. de Sang. 1660.——**Hoffman, G. H.* Lond. Med. Gaz. xi. 881. (1833.) Exp. on the Colour of the Blood, and on the Gases which it contains.——*Hoffman, J. M.* Acta Acad. Nat. Cur. i. 466. De Sang. lacteo.——*Home, Sir E.* Phil. Trans. 1818. pp. 172, 185; and 1820. p. 1. On the changes the Blood undergoes in the act of Coagulation:—*ib.* 1826. p. 189. On the Coagulation of the Blood by Heat.

Jennings, E. A. Trans. of the Prov. Med. and Surg. Ass. iii. 43. A Report on the Chemistry of the Blood.——*Junker, J.* Chymia. p. 75; et Conspectus Path. 1736 passim.——*Jurin, J.* Phil. Trans. 1719. p. 1000. Exp. relating to the Spec. Grav. of the Blood.

Kater, Capt. Phil. Trans. 1818. p. 187. On the Size of the Globules.——*Kaltenbrunner, G.* Exp. circa statum Sang. in Inflam., &c. 1826: see also Répert. Gén., iv. 201. (1827.); et Journ. de Phys. par Majendie, viii. 81. (1828.)——*Kay, J. P., M.D.* On Asphyxia. 1834.——*Keill, J., M.D.* Phil. Trans. 1706 and 1708. On the Quantity of the Blood in the Body.——*Klein.* Dissert. de Sang., &c. 1737.——*Knight, T., M.D.* A Vindication of the late Essay on the Transmutation of Blood. 1731.——**Kolck Schröder van der, J. L. C.* Diss. sistens Sang. Coag. Historiam cum Exp., &c. 1820.——*König, G.* Exper. circa Sang. Inflam. et Sanit. 1824.——*Krimer, W.* Versuch einer Phys. des Blutes. 1823.——*Krouaner, J. H.* Dissert. de Sang. Hum. 1762.

Lamure, F. Rech. sur la Couënne du Sang.——*Lancisi, J. M.* De Motu Cordis. 1728. § 44. (Opera. 1745. iv.)——*Langrish, B., M.D.* Modern Practice of Physick. 1735. p. 67.——*Langswaert, G.* De Causa Rubedinis Sang. 1762.——*Leacock, J. H.* (Th.) De Hæmorrhagia et Transfusione. 1816.——**Le Canu.* Journ. de Pharm., Nos. ix. and x. (1831.) Sur l'Analyse du Sang.—Journ. de Chim. Med., June 1835. On Milky Serum.——*Le Gallois.* Le Sang est-il identique dans tous les vaisseaux qu'il parcourt? An xi.——*Lee, R., M.D.* Cyclop. of Med., art. PHLEBITIS and PHLEBOLITE.——**Leeuwenhoeck, A. van.* Phil. Trans. 1674. pp. 22, 121; 1723. p. 436. Micros. Obs. on the Blood.—De Globilis in Sang., &c. in Epist. Posth. 1723. p. 436.——*Leveling, H. P.* Disquisitio crustæ Inflam. 1772.——*Levison, G., M.D.* An Essay on the Blood, &c. 1776.——*Leuret.* (Th.) Sur l'Altér. du Sang: and Arch. Gén. de Méd., xi. 683.——*Leuret et Lassaigne.* Rech. Phys. et Chim. sur la Digestion. 1825.——*Lister.* See *Hodgkin.*

Macaire et Marcet. Mém. de la Soc. Phys. et Hist. Nat. de Génève, v. 400.——**Majendie, F.* Précis Elém. de Phys. 4ème édit. 1834. p. 233; et *Delille,* Journ. de Phys. 1821.——*Malpighi, M.* De Viscerum Structura et de Polypo Cordis. 1678.——**Marcet, C., M.D.* Med. Chir. Tr. ii. 342. Anal. of various Animal Fluids.——*Martini, S.* Edin. Med. Essays. 1748. ii. 79.——*Mayer, Professor.* Zeitschrift für Phys., erstes Heft. 1826. On the Coag. of the Blood in the Pulm. Vessels when the 8th pair of Nerves is divided.——**Mayo, H.* Physiology, 3rd edit. 1833. p. 17.——*Menghini, V.* Bonon. Comment. (1747.) ii. pp. 11. 244; and iii. 475. De ferrearum particulis in Sang., &c.——*Méry, J.* Acad. des Sc. de Paris, ii. 209. Obs. sur la Couleur du Sang.——*Metzger, J. D.* De Rubedine Sang. 1781.——*Meyen, F. J. F.* Diss. de primis Vitæ Phenom. et de Circ. Sang. in Parenchymata. 1826; and Isis, by L. Oken. 1828. p. 407.——**Michaëlis, F.* De partibus constitutivis Sang. 1827; and Journ. für Physiol. und Phys., by S. C. Schweigger. (1828.) iii. 94.——*Moises, H.* A Treatise on the Blood. 1746.——*Monfalcon.* Dict. des Sc. Méd. (1820.) art. SANG.——*Montault.* Journ. de Prog. des Sc. Méd. i. 138. (1836.) Ant.-Path. du Sang.——*Morgagni, J. B.* De Sed. et Causis Morb. Epist. i. v. and xxxi.——*Moscati, P.* Osserv. ed Esper. sul Sangue. 1776.——*Moulin, A.* Phil. Trans. 1687. p. 433. On the Quantity of Blood in Men, and on the Celerity of its Circulation.——**Muller, J.* De Respir. Fœtus. (de Sang., pp. 41, 142.) 1823.—Isis, by L. Oken. 1824.—Ann. des Sc. Nat. (1832.) xxvii.—Lettre addressée à l'Acad. des Sc. (1832.) On the Buffy Coat.

Nitzschke, C. Misc. Acad. Nat. Cur. 1670. p. 258. Lac ex vasa profluens.—*Nysten, P. H.* Rech. de Phys. et de Chim. Path. 1811.

Orfila et Andral. Dict. de Méd. (1827.) art. SANG.—Arch. Gén. de Méd. xvi. 16. (1828.) Nouveaux Mém. sur le Sang consid. sous le rapport Méd.-legale.——*O'Shaughnessy, Dr.* Report on the Chemical Path. of Cholera, p. 22.

Parent, A. Mém. de Paris. 1711. p. 24. Obs. sur les Cellules Poligones du Sang nouvellement tiré.——*Parmentier* et *Deyeux.* Journ. de Phys. et de Chim. 1794.——*Pasta, A.* De Sang. &c. 1786.——*Pitcairne, A., M.D.* Dissert. de Sang. (Opera. ii.) 1722.——*Piorry.* Collect. des Mémoires. 1831; et Traité de Méd. Prat. July, 1835. Sur l'Hémite ou l'Inflam. du Sang.——*Piorry* et *Mondezert.* Journ. Hebd. (1834.) ii. 281. On the Buffy Coat.——*Plenk.* Hydrologia, &c. 1794. p. 42 et passim.——**Prevost, J. L.* et *L. A. Dumas.* Bibl. Univ. des Sc. xvii. 302; and Ann. de Chim. et Phys. xviii. 280. (1821.) xxiii. 50, 90. (1823.) Examen du Sang et de son action dans les divers phénom. de la vie.—Ann. de Sc. Nat. 1824–5. Sur le Sang du Fœtus.——*Prater, H.* On the Blood. 1832.——*Priestley, J., LL.D.* On Air. 1774. iii. 357 et passim.—Phil. Trans. 1776. p. 226. On Respir. and the Use of the Blood.——*Prochaska, G.* Disq. Anat.-Phys. Organismi Corporis ejusque processus vitalis. 1812.——*Prout, W., M.D.* Ann. of Philos. xiii. 12. 265. (1819.) On the Phenomena of Sanguification, and on the Blood in general.——*Pyl, J. T.* Dissert. de Rubedinis Sang. 1775.

Rayger, C. Misc. Acad. Nat. Cur. 1675–6. p. 313. De sero lacteo V. S. extracto.——**Raspail.* Répert. Gén. iv. parte 2. p. 148. (1827.) vi. parte 1. p. 135. (1828.) Sur la Struct. intime des Tissus et du Sang.—Syst. de Chim. Organ. 1833.——*Rees, G. O.* Analysis of the Blood and Urine, &c. 1836.——*Reichel, G. G.* De Sang. ejusque Motu Exp. 1767.——*Reichelm.* Dissert. de Sang, &c. 1702.——*Reynaud.* Journ. Hebd. de Méd. ii. 84. (1834.)——*Rhades, J. J.* Diss. de Ferro Sang. &c. 1753.——*Ribes, F.* Mém. de la Soc. d'Emul. viii. 604.——*Richerand, A.* Physiologie, 9ème édit., *tr.* by *J. Copland, M.D.* 2nd edit. 1829. p. 232 et passim.—Mém. de la Soc. d'Emul. an iii. p. 296. Sur le Connex. de la Vie avec la Circulation.——*Rivinus.* Dissert. de Sang. Pravitate. 1702.——*Roche, L. C.* Nouvelle Elem. de Path. Méd.-Chir. v.; et Journ. Hebd. de Méd. 1833. Consid. sur les Altér. du Sang dans les Maladies.——*Rochoux, M.* Dict. des Sc. Méd. xvii. 123; and Dict. de Méd. (1826.) art. PATHOGÉNIE.—Nouv. Bibl. Méd. 1823; et Arch. Gén. de Méd. xiii. 160. (1827.) Maladies avec ou par Altér. du Sang; also Journ. Hebd. ii. 530.——*Rosa, M.* Lettere Philos. in Giornale della Medicina. (1783–91.) i. 185.——**Rose, H.* Gilbert's Ann. der Physik und Chemie. 1826.—Ann. de Chem. et Phys. xxxiv. 268.—Edin. Med. and Surg. Journ. xxvii. 96. (1827.) On the Presence of Iron in the Blood, &c.——*Rose, L. G.* De Motu Sang., &c. [Haller. Disput. Anat. ii. 567.] 1668.——*Rouelle.* Journ. de Méd. xl. et xlvi. and Med. and Phil. Comment. by a Soc. of Phys. in Edin. iii. 214. On the Nature of the Saline parts of the Blood.——*Rudolphi, C. A.* Gundriss der Physiologie, 1821–9. Bde. 1. p. 159; and *tr.* by *Dr. W. D. How.* 1825. i. 132.

Sabatier, J. C. (Th.) Des Métastèses purul. 1832.——*Scheel, P.* Die Transfusion des Blutes, &c. 1802–3. ii. bde.——*Schmiet, J.* Misc. Acad. Nat. Cur. 1672. p. 166. De Lacte ex V. S. profluenti.——*Schaper, J. E.* De massæ Sang. corpusculis. 1688.——*Schroeck, L.* Misc. Acad. Nat. Cur. 1690. p. 452. De Sang. Albo.——**Schultz, K. H.* Rev. Méd. i. 136 et seq.; Archiv für Anat. by J. F. Meckel. 1826; et Journ. de Prog. des Sc. Méd. v. On the Spontaneity of Motion in the Globules of the Blood.—Der Lebensprocess im Blute, &c. 1822.—Microsc. Untersuchungen über des Herrn R. Brown, &c. 1828.——*Schuz, G. F.* (Th.) Exp. circa Calor. Fœtus et Sang. ipsius, 1799; et præs. Autenrieth. 1799.——*Schneider, C. V.*

Dissert. de Sang. 1679.——*Schroeder*. See *Kolck*.——*Schurig, M.* Hæmatologia, &c. 1741.——*Schmidt, J. C.* Ueber die Blutcorner. 1822.——*Schwencke, T.* Hæmatologia, &c. 1743.——**Scudamore, C., M.D.* Essay on the Blood. 1824.——*Segalas d'Etchepare*. Arch. Gén. de Méd. xii. 103. (1826.)—Exp. sur le Sang, &c. ——*Sénac, P.* Traité du Cœur. 1749. l. 3. c. 4.——*Smith, H., M.D.* Essays Path. and Pract. on the Nature and Circulation of the Blood. 1761.——*Spitta, G. H.* De Sang. Dignitate in Path. restituenda. 1825.——**Stevens, W.* On the Blood. 1832; —Lond. Med. Gaz. (1834.) xiv. 49; and Phil. Trans. 1835. p. 348. Observ. on the Theory of Respiration.——*Stahl, G. E.* Dissert. de Sang. &c. 1706.——*Stoker, W., M.D.* Path. Obs. pt. i. 27. (1823.) ii. p. xiv. (1829.) Exp. on the Blood.——*Sturm, J. N.* Dissert. de Sang. Colore. 1762.——*Soubeyan*. Ann. des Sc. d'Observ. ii. 133. 465.——*Sydenham, T.* Opera. 1726. § 6. c. 3.

Taylor, J. R. Lond. Med. and Phys. Journ. lxvii. 187. (1831.) On the Buffy Coat of Blood.——**Thackrah, C. T.* On the Blood. 2nd edit., by Dr. T. G. Wright. 1834. ——*Thénard, L. J.* Traité de Chim. 2ème édit. 1817–8. iii. et iv. and *tr.* by *Mr. Children*.——*Thomson, J.* Lectures on Inflammation. 1813 passim.——*Thompson, T.* Syst of Chem. 3rd edit. 1807. v.——*Thouvenal, P.* Sur le Méchanisme et les Produits de la Sanguification. 1777.——*Tiedemann, F.* Physiologie. 1830. *tr.* by *Drs. Gully* and *Lane*. 1834.——*Torré, Abbé.* Phil. Trans. 1765. p. 252. Microsc. Observ. on the Blood.——*Traill, T. S.* Edin. Med. and Surg. Journ. xvii. 235. 637. (1823.); and xxiv. 421. (1825.) On Milky Serum.——*Treviranus, G. R.* Die Ercheinungen und Gesetze des organischen Lebens, &c. 1831.——*Treviranus, L. C.* Vermischte Schriften, anat. und phys. Inhalts. 1817. Bde. i. 122.——*Trousseau* et *Rigot*. Arch. Gén. de Méd. xii. (1826.) xiv. 321. (1827.) Sur la Color. cadavériques des Artères et des Veines.——**Turner, E., M.D.* Elem. of Chemistry. 4th edit. 1833. p. 887.

Valli, E. Discorso sop. il Sangue, &c. 1782.——*Vauquelin*. Ann. de Chim. i. 9. (1816.) Sur le principe Col. du Sang.——*Velpeau, A. L. M.* Arch. Gén. viii. 306. (1825.) ——*Verhelst, T.* Essai Phys. sur la Sanguification. 1820.——*Vieussens, R.* Phil. Trans. 1698. p. 224. On the Human Blood.——*Villermé, L. R.* Dict. des Sc. Méd. art. SÉROSITÉ. (1821.)——*Vines*. Lancet. xi. 294. 423. (1826–7.) On the Buffy Coat. ——*Vogel*. Ann. de Chim. et Phys. lxxxvii. 215. (1813.) De l'Exist. du Soufre dans le Sang:—*ib.* xciii. 71. (1815.) De l'Exist. de l'Acid Carb. dans le Sang.

Waldschmidt, J. J. Misc. Acad. Nat. Cur. 1671. p. 312. Ex Venâ Sanguis albus eductus.——*Waller, C.* Obs. on Transfusion. 1825.——*Wedel, G. W.* Misc. Acad. Nat. Cur. 1675–6. p. 1. De Conquassatione Sang.—*ib.* 1686. p. 323. Sanguis per micros. examinatus, ramosus.——*Wedemeyer, V. G.* Ueber das Nervensystem und die Respiration. 1817: and Archiv für Anat. und Phys. by T. F. Meckel. 1818. p. 356.——*Weiss, E.* Acta Helvet. iv. 351. (1760.) Obs. sur les Glob. du Sang. ——*Wells, W. C., M.D.* Phil. Trans. 1797. p. 416. Obs. and Exp. on the Colour of the Blood.——*Whiting*. Dissert. Med. de Sang. Ægrorum.——*Whytt, R., M.D.* Works. 1768. p. 26. On the Blood, et passim.——**Williams, C. J. B., M.D.* Med. Gazette. xvi. 718 et seq. (1835.) Obs. on the Blood, &c.——*Willis, R., M.D.* Opera. 1676. passim.——*Wilson, J.* Lect. on the Blood. 1819.——*Wollaston, W. H., M.D.* Phil. Trans. 1811. On the want of Sugar in Diabetic Urine.

**Young, T., M.D.* Med. Lit. 2nd edit. 1823. p. 571. On the Blood.

Zetzell, P. Svenske. Veten. Acad. Handl. 1770. p. 235. Phys. Undersoekning om tre arter Blod-watten.

CHAPTER II.

OF THE VASCULAR SYSTEM.

§. 1. *General Observations on Muscular Contraction and Elasticity.*

IT is not my present intention to explain all the circumstances connected with muscular contraction and relaxation, nor that other power of action introduced into an animal body, called elasticity[a] I propose only to state a few of the facts which throw some light upon the vascular system, by showing that there is in vessels a power of muscular action, and that the cooperation of elasticity is also necessary to their function. These may likewise assist in explaining the manner in which the two powers are combined. I may, however, occasionally be led to mention causes and effects which cannot be immediately considered as applicable to the vessels themselves, though they will render many of the phenomena in the vascular system more easy to be understood.

The common action of a muscle, from which its immediate use is derived, is its contraction; and the effect produced by it is that of bringing the origin and insertion, or the parts which it is fitted to move, nearer to each other *; which is universally the case whether the muscle is straight, hollow, or circular. It is likewise necessary that a muscle should relax, or be capable of relaxation; a condition which allows it to be stretched, by permitting the parts acted upon to recede from each other. Muscles, in common, probably, with every other part of the body, have a power of adapting themselves to the necessary distance between origin and insertion, in case an alteration has taken place in the natural distance; and I have reason to believe that, under certain circumstances, they have a power of becoming longer, almost immediately, than they are in the natural relaxed, or even the natural elongated state of their fibres. This opinion will be best illustrated in inflammation.

* I do not here consider the circumflex tendons; for, by the origin and insertion, I mean the muscular ends of the fibres.

[a] [See Croonian Lectures on Muscular Motion, &c. in Vol. IV. of this edition.]

Muscular contraction has been generally supposed to arise from some impression, which is commonly called a stimulus: I doubt, however, of an impression being always necessary; and I believe that in many cases the cessation of an accustomed impulse may become the cause of contraction in a muscle. The sphincter iridis of the eye contracts when there is too much light, but the radii contract when there is little or no light [a]. I can even conceive that a cessation of action requires its stimulus to produce it, which may be called the stimulus of cessation; for relaxation is not the state into which a muscle will naturally fall upon the removal of a continued stimulus; a muscle remaining contracted after absolute death, when the stimulus of relaxation cannot be applied; so that a muscle can as little relax after death as it can contract [b]. If a stone is raised, and the raising power removed, it falls; but it would not fall if not acted upon. When it has fallen it lies at rest; but so it would have done when raised, if gravitation would have allowed it. The stone is passive, and must be acted upon. Whatever becomes a stimulus to one set of muscles, becomes a cause of relaxation to those which act in a contrary direction*; and whatever becomes a stimulus to one part of a muscular canal, where a succession of actions is to take place, becomes also a cause of relaxation in the part beyond it, as in an intestine.

Muscular contraction, in some of the involuntary muscles, does not constantly arise from immediate stimuli, as in the sphincters; for the

* This might be called a sympathetic stimulus, and is that which regulates the actions of the whole machine, and which I have called, in another place, the stimulus of necessity.

---

[a] [Dr. Parry objects to this illustration, and thinks that the radii of the iris restore themselves by their simple tonicity, in the same manner as other muscles. It may be observed, that the fact of the muscularity of the iris, which is here presumed from anaogy by Mr. Hunter, has been since directly proved by the observations of Bauer and Jacob (*Phil. Trans.* 1822), and indirectly by Berzelius, who found that the iris possesses all the chemical properties of muscle. Dr. Roget also has informed us that the iris of his eye is partly under the influence of the will; and Mr. Mayo, that in some animals it instantaneously contracts on any mechanical irritation of the third pair of nerves (*op. cit.*, p. 291.): phenomena which are obviously only referrible to a muscular structure.]

[b] [Muscles which have long been contracted lose all disposition to relax, as may be observed in Fakirs and other religious visionaries, who compel themselves to remain in constrained positions of the body for a long time together, and in the contractions which follow diseases of the joints. Even a powerful grasp of the hand, continued only for a few minutes, is recovered from with difficulty. That peculiar tetanic spasm of the lower extremities which is induced by injecting a solution of opium into the stomach of a frog, is not relaxed by a division of the spinal marrow above the origin of the lumbar nerves.]

sphincter ani contracts whenever the stimulus of relaxation is removed, which may be said to produce the stimulus for contraction.

Muscular actions have been divided into the voluntary, involuntary, and mixed, which is only dividing them according to the different natural modes of stimuli, or causes of their action: to these a fourth might be added, where the actions are in consequence of accidental stimuli or impressions, to which both the voluntary and involuntary muscles are subject, viz. such as arise from affections of the mind *, or are the immediate effects of violence.

The involuntary contraction should be first considered, as the more necessary operations of the machine are carried on by it; for the machine could even exist independent of any voluntary contraction: but it could not go on if left wholly to the voluntary contraction of the muscles, unless we were endued with innate ideas capable of producing a will. This involuntary contraction is very extensive in the system, and is employed in carrying on a number of operations, of which the circulation is one; and which may be said to be, in a great measure, the œconomy of the animal within itself.

The mixed kind of contraction is most to our present purpose, and is of two kinds, though it has been in general supposed to be of one kind only, and that belonging solely to the muscles of respiration, as being in them the most conspicuous. But, in fact, we find another mode of involuntary actions in other muscles of the body, where it answers very useful purposes. In these the involuntary contraction may be reckoned the natural state; and it is a kind of permanent contraction, these muscles only relaxing occasionally, by which means parts are sustained or supported: the voluntary contraction of such muscles is also only occasional. All sphincter muscles in some degree partake of this power, and therefore should be called muscles with power of occasional relaxation. For although many circular muscles may not have these mixed contractions, as the orbicularis palpebrarum, yet that muscle has a disposition to contract peculiar to itself. Its relaxation is to be reckoned of the active kind, which may be called the relaxation of watchfulness; and it is when tired of this species of action that it contracts, which, on the contrary, may be called the contraction of sleep: or it may be considered as an elongator muscle to the levator palpebræ, with a disposition to remain relaxed while that muscle is contracted, but contracting when the elevator is tired. The natural contraction of the orbicularis muscle is involuntary, the relaxation, both natural and occasional, is involuntary; but it has likewise a voluntary contraction and relaxa-

* Mind and will are often blended together, but will has nothing to do here.

tion, which can be made to exceed the involuntary, resembling what is inherent in all the sphincters [a].

Sphincter muscles, as those of the anus and urethra; and probably the expulsatores seminis, and crura of the diaphragm, have both a voluntary and involuntary contraction. In the two sphincters of the anus and urethra this is evident; and the involuntary contraction in these muscles I have called sphinctoric. The sphincter ani possesses it to a degree just sufficient to resist the pressure of the air and fæces, while the parts above are inactive, preventing the escape of these, till they give the stimulus for expulsion, and then an involuntary relaxation naturally takes place, similar to what happens in muscular canals.

The sphinctoric contraction resembles in its effects that produced by elastic ligaments in other parts of the body, which action may be called contractile elasticity, as bringing back the parts to a certain necessary state, and retaining them there. But elasticity would not here have answered all the purposes, since, as it has no relaxing power, more force would have been required to overcome its resistance in the expulsion of the fæces than the gut above could have been able to exert. But the sustaining power being muscular contraction, a relaxation or cessation of that contraction during the time of expulsion leaves nothing for the fæces to do, but, by means of the action above, simply to dilate the relaxed parts. There is, likewise, in these muscles a still further power of contraction, which is produced by the will, and for the purpose of giving, on particular occasions, greater force than what is commonly necessary. The voluntary action of these muscles is therefore, we find, more powerful than the involuntary; but upon the whole I think we have reason to suppose that the involuntary muscles are much stronger

---

[a] [I see no reason for supposing that the orbicularis is different from the other sphincters, or that it has a disposition to contract peculiar to itself: it is only peculiar in being antagonized by the levator palpebrarum, which is a common voluntary muscle. The tone of muscles, to which may probably be referred the ordinary contraction of the sphincters, is that slight tendency to contract in the longitudinal direction of the fibres by which they adapt themselves to the variety of their situation. Now this tone is in great part lost in the extremities and common sphincters when the nervous supply is cut off, although it seems doubtful in what degree it is dependent on the nerves in common cases, so as to relax when an antagonist muscle comes into play. The tonic retraction of a divided muscle is equally energetic when the nerves which supply that muscle are divided as when they are entire; and fish are more effectually crimped when they are first knocked on the head. The heart of a turtle, recently plucked from the chest and deprived of blood, *actively* dilates and contracts; which would lead us to believe that the same action more or less takes place in all the muscles,—the relaxation of a muscle being not merely a cessation of action, but an active dilatation, requiring a stimulus for its production.]

than the voluntary. Can we believe that so thin a muscle as the colon of a horse could squeeze out its contents, consisting of a column of dung about eight inches diameter, if those involuntary muscles had no more strength than the muscles of an extremity? When we see the bladder of urine throwing out its contents through a large tube, to a distance, perhaps two yards beyond its extreme end, we must suppose a much greater force exerted than could belong to any such quantity of voluntary muscle. For I believe that by grasping the bladder with both hands we could not make the water flow out to an equal distance[a]. It may be here observed, that the power of involuntary contraction commonly remains longer than that of the voluntary, though I believe not in all instances; which difference produces a greater variety in the former than in the latter. Thus the muscular action of the arteries is longer retained than that of the heart.

Elasticity is a property of matter (whether animal or not) which renders it capable of restoring itself to its natural position, after having been acted upon by some mechanical power, but having no power of action arising out of itself. This is exactly the reverse of muscular contraction. Muscles, as has been already observed, have the power of contraction and of cessation, which last is called relaxation, but not the power of elongation, which would be an act of restoration, such as exists in elasticity. A muscle, therefore, has the power of action within itself, by which it produces its effects, but is obliged to other powers for its restoration, so as to be able to act again; whereas elasticity is obliged to other powers to alter the position of the parts, so as to require recovery or restoration: but this it is capable of doing itself; and by this power it produces its effects, becoming a cause of motion in other bodies. A body possessed of this property, when brought from the state of rest, is always endeavouring to arrive at this state, which it also endeavours to preserve; and it is capable of supporting itself in this state in proportion to the degree of elasticity which may belong to it.

---

[a] [It may be doubted whether the colon or the bladder ever act alone. Certainly the diaphragm and abdominal muscles cooperate in all ordinary cases. In injuries of the back, the rectum is frequently able to retain and expel the fæces, although the bladder is perfectly incapable of evacuating the urine. Now they both derive their nerves from the same part, but there is this difference between them,—the sphincter ani being relaxed, the fibres of the rectum have no difficulty in expelling its contents, but the urine has to be forced through a long and narrow canal at the same time that the bladder is generally much distended before the *nisus* arises, in consequence of which the muscle of the bladder acts to the greatest possible disadvantage; for the aperture and compressing force being given, the rapidity and projection of the stream will be inversely as the superficies of the containing vessel.]

The action of elasticity is continual, and its immediate effects are produced whenever the resistance is removed, by which it may be distinguished from other powers. Elastic matter can either be extended beyond its state of rest, or brought within it. Thus a spring being bent, its concave side is brought within this state, and the convex side is carried beyond it: when under these circumstances it is left to itself, both sides endeavour to restore themselves. The power of an elastic body is permanent, always acting with a force proportioned to the power applied, and therefore reacts as the body is elongated, bent, or compressed; but this is very different from the action of a muscle, as this last may act with its full force, or only part, or not at all, according to circumstances. Elasticity *, which has the power of resisting the action of other parts, as well as of restoring the substance endowed with it, when forcibly removed from a state of rest, is introduced into an animal body, in order to cooperate in many respects with the muscles, and so to act as to restore or fit them for a new action, becoming in many cases antagonists to the muscles, which will be described when we speak of the combination of the two.

§. 2. *General Observations on the Elongation of relaxed Muscles.*

Everything in nature that has the power of action has two kinds of motion exerted alternately, and a state of rest. Of the former, the one may be called the active, the other the state of recovery. In a muscle, the active is the state of contraction, the other the state of relaxation: the state of rest is merely the state of inaction. The contractile state of a muscle, as well as the relaxed, arises from a power inherent in itself; but the recovery or elongation must depend on some other power.

Simple relaxation of a contracted muscle is not sufficient to enable it to produce another requisite effect; it is, therefore, necessary that there should be an elongator equal to the quantity of contraction intended to be produced: and as no muscle has the power of extending itself into what I shall call the state of recovery, an elongator of some kind or other is required, to enable every muscle to produce its effect, by a renewal of contraction. This, although in some respects similar to the

* It is to be observed, that elasticity in animals does not, like muscular contraction, depend on life, an elastic body possessing that quality as perfectly after death as before. Elasticity admits of two actions; a contraction when the substance is extended beyond the natural state, and an extension when it is compressed within it: both these are possessed by the elastic parts which compose the vascular system; whereas muscles have but one action, or, at least, but one which can produce an immediate effect, and that is contraction.

winding up of a clock, in others differs materially from it. For the muscle being capable of relaxing itself, there is no resistance to overcome, except the vis inertiæ and friction of the matter to be removed: whereas in the clock, the power that winds it up must be greater than the spring or weight, to be capable of overcoming the gravity of the weight, or the elasticity of the spring, together with the vis inertiæ.

The elongation of muscles is not the immediate cause of their relaxation, but the effect of a contrary and necessary motion of the elongators, by which they are recovered so as to be enabled to renew their action with effect.

The elongators, or powers which enable muscles to recover themselves, are not always muscular, for when simple elongation is required, it is effected by other means, as elasticity, which is the case in part in the blood-vessels; and sometimes by motion in matter foreign to the body, yet propelled either by muscles or elasticity, as is also the case in blood-vessels. The elongators may be divided into three kinds, with their compounds.

The first kind is muscular, and these may either act immediately, or they may act on some other substance, by which action that substance becomes the immediate cause of the elongation. Those which act immediately, and become elongators to other muscles by their contraction, are in turn elongated by the contraction of these very muscles, to which they served as elongators, the two sets thus becoming reciprocally elongators to each other. This is the case with the greater part of the muscles in the body, and in some muscles, as the occipito-frontalis, two different portions are reciprocally elongators; yet these may strictly be considered as two muscles; for although there is no interruption, in the tendon they move the same part in two opposite directions, like distinct antagonist muscles.

These reciprocal elongators, by their mutual action on each other, bring out a middle state between the extremes of contraction and elongation, which is the state of ease or tone in both. This appears not to be so much required for the ease of the part moved, as for that of the relaxed muscle[a], either extreme of motion leaving the muscle in an uneasy state. We find, therefore, that as soon as any set of muscles cease to act, the elongators, which were stretched during their action, are stimulated either by this cessation, or by the uneasy state into which the parts moved have been put, to act in order to bring these parts into

[a The reading of this passage in all the editions, is "for the ease of the relaxed muscles, as for that the part moved," the reverse of which seems to have been intended by the author.]

a state the furthest removed from the extremes which were uneasy, and by which the stimulus arising from both is equally balanced.

This however, can only happen in such parts of the body as are furnished with muscular elongators; where these are wanting, the muscles of the part having but one office, their state of ease is that of simple relaxation, as they can have no middle state from the action of antagonists; but such are commonly muscular parts, or so constructed as not to be thrown into an uneasy position by the action of their muscles. I suppose, however that the elongated state of a muscle is an uneasy state: a muscle, therefore, that is stretched, although in a relaxed state, is uneasy, and will contract a certain length, to what is probably the middle state.

Still it is necessary that such parts as are simply muscular, and have no antagonist muscles appropriated immediately for such purposes, should have their muscles elongated; this is still performed by muscles, but in a secondary way; for instance, by a succession of actions in different parts, each performing the same effect, and the last action becoming an antagonist to the succeeding.

This second mode of elongation takes place in all the muscles which assist in forming canals. In them the muscles, if once contracted, cannot be elongated, or the part dilated again, unless by the contraction of some other part of the canal, propelling its contents into the relaxed part, and by that means serving as an elongator. This, in some instances, goes on in regular succession, as we know the dilatation of the fauces to be occasioned by the action of the mouth and tongue; that of the œsophagus, by the contraction of the fauces; of the stomach, by that of the œsophagus; the upper part of the intestines, by the stomach, and so on; the successive contractions of the last dilated parts pushing on the contents, and in that manner becoming elongators of the muscles next in succession of action. A first propelling power, such as a heart, could in these instances have had but little effect, and would even have been unnecessary; for as there must be a succession of contractions and dilatations, its power would soon have been lost. This mode of propelling substances through canals, as stated above, would probably have been too slow for the circulation in many animals, but I believe it is very much the case in others.

The elongation of the muscles of the bladder, from the distention of urine, becomes the means by which they are excited to recover themselves so as to renew their action, and may be referred to the same general head.

The third kind is by means of elastic substances, which render the combined actions produced by muscular contraction and elasticity more complicated. Elasticity we find to be introduced both as an assistant to the contraction of the muscles, and as an antagonist or elongator; the natural position being that which is produced by the elasticity. Thus we see elasticity combined with muscular action assisting in the contraction of muscles on one side, and likewise performing the office of elongators or antagonists on the opposite, by bringing parts which have been moved by muscles back into their natural position. Such parts too as have yielded to the action of some other power, as gravitation, are brought back into what may be called a natural state, and are retained there by elasticity, till that power is again overcome by another, as in the necks of some animals. We may hence see that the application of those powers is twofold; one, where the muscles and elastic substances assist each other; the second, where they are antagonists, the elastic being neither assisted by the muscular parts, nor the muscular by the elastic; for many parts of the body are so constructed as to admit of but one kind of muscular action, the other action arising from elasticity alone; it being necessary that such parts should have a determined or middle state, though not intended as a state of ease.

Of this kind are the blood-vessels, trachea, bronchia, the ears of animals, etc., in which, therefore, elasticity is introduced to procure that determined state, and is chiefly employed where the middle state is much limited. For it is to be observed, that the middle state, when produced by muscular action, has not commonly a determined point of rest, but admits of considerable latitude between the two extremes, except in the sphincters. Where it is produced by elasticity, it is always more determined, provided the elasticity has sufficient power to overcome the natural or accidental resistance; and where that is the case, we must suppose that a state, in some degree determined, was necessary to such parts. But where the elastic power is not sufficient to overcome the natural, or accidental resistance, then it is assisted by the muscular, which forms one of the compounds of the three modes of elongation, instances of which we have in many joints.

The relaxed state of a muscle would appear in general to be the most natural; but to this there are exceptions, a degree of contraction appearing natural to some muscles[a].

The face, for instance, is a part where the action of the muscles on one side influences the position of the parts on the other side, a circumstance, perhaps, peculiar to the face; here, therefore, the muscles bring and keep the skin in one position, till altered by an increased action in

---

[a] [I apprehend that all muscles, without exception, are endued with a tonic power of contraction, but in very different degrees. In the involuntary muscles, as the stomach and heart, it is scarcely at all visible; but it is highly developed in most of the sphincters.]

some other muscle; and when this increased action ceases, the constant and natural contraction of the whole (similar to that of the sphincter) immediately takes place*.

Sphincter muscles are the most remarkable instances of this, being always above three parts contracted†.

The constant and regular degree of contraction in those sphincter muscles, serves the purposes of elasticity, and may have superior advantages, as we know that they have a power of relaxing when their elongators act, which no elastic substance can have. Hence we see, that where a continued action only is wanted, there is elasticity; where an alternate action and relaxation, there is the action of muscles; where only an occasional relaxing power is required, there are muscles under certain restrictions; and where a constant power of contraction is necessary, but which is occasionally to be overcome by muscles, there are introduced both elasticity and muscular powers, cooperating with each other in their actions.

Where constant action is not necessary, muscles alone are employed, as in the greater number of moving parts in most animals; and where any position is required to be constant, and the motion only occasional, from being seldom wanted, there elasticity alone is employed for the purpose of constant position, and muscles for the occasional action‡.

When a position is to be pretty constant, and yet elastic substances are not employed, we have then muscles endowed with the power of constant contraction to a certain degree, but capable of either relaxation, or greater contraction, as in the sphincters.

We find, therefore, that in many parts of an animal body fitted for motion, a tolerably constant position is necessary, at the same time that an occasional self-moving power is also wanted, to serve as a sort of auxiliary to the performance of the necessary action. For such occasional actions, muscles, assisted by elastic substances, are employed, the elastic power easing the muscles in the fixed position, and the muscular giving the increased occasional action; and in other parts of the body, where a more constant action was wanted, and could not be

* As a proof that this is muscular contraction, and not elasticity, we find that the face in a dead body does not keep its natural form, nor resume it when lost.

† The parts supplied with sphincters do not contract after being dilated in the dead body, which they certainly would do if the contraction in the living body had arisen from elasticity.

‡ Some bivalves (as the oyster) have a strong muscle passing between the shells for closing them occasionally; but for opening them no muscles are made use of, as this is performed by an elastic ligament in the joint of the two shells, which is squeezed, when shut, by the contraction of the muscle; and when the muscle ceases to contract, the elasticity of the ligament expands it, so that the shell is opened.

completely obtained by elasticity, there are to be found muscles endowed with the property of both permanent and occasional contraction.

The elastic power is very remarkable in such parts of an animal body as require a constant effort to support them, elasticity being introduced to act against the power of gravitation, as in the necks of animals whose heads are held horizontally, or beyond the centre of gravity. This is effected by an elastic ligament, and is strikingly illustrated in the camel, whose neck is long. Between the vertebræ of the neck and backs of fowls are placed elastic ligaments for the same purpose; the wings of birds and bats are also furnished with them, by which means they are retained close to the body when not used in flying. On the abdomen of most quadrupeds are likewise to be found elastic ligaments, especially on that of the elephant, which affords a constant support to the parts in their horizontal position; and even the cellular membrane of the elephant has a degree of elasticity much above what is generally met with in cellular membranes. Hence there is less expense of muscular contraction in such parts. The trachea and its branches are instances of these two powers, being composed of cartilages, muscles, and membranes; the proportion of muscular substance, however, is small, the muscles which act principally upon this part being those of respiration; but the tendency of the action of the proper muscles of the trachea is to compress and alter the size of the trachea; this is counteracted by the elasticity of the cartilages and membranes exerting a constant and regular endeavour to keep it of one certain size.

The external ears of many animals furnish us with another instance of the joint application of these two powers, for being chiefly composed of elastic cartilage, they retain a general uniformity of shape, although that is capable of being altered occasionally by the action of muscles.

It is however to be observed, that in all cases where these two powers are joined, the muscular, as it can always act in opposition to the elastic, must be the strongest, and capable of being carried further than the other; it therefore must always be proportionably stronger than it otherwise need to have been.

Parts in which these two powers are employed are capable of being in either of three states,—the natural, the stretched, and the contracted; but in some parts the natural state may coincide either with the stretched or contracted, and consequently such parts are only capable of being in two states. The natural state is produced by the elastic power simply; the contracted is the effect of the muscular power alone; and the stretched is produced either by some foreign force, or body protruded, which may be effected by a muscular power.

§. 3. *Of the Structure of Arteries.*

The arteries in an animal, as far as we can examine them, are endowed with the property of elasticity, the use of which we perceive in the action of those parts; and this power is at all times demonstrable, while the muscular has been by some overlooked, by others denied, and has only been asserted by others as appearing necessary by reasoning from analogy.

The quantity of elasticity in any artery on which an experiment can be made is easily ascertained, as it only requires the application of an opposing force to prove both its power and extent. But it will appear from experiment, that the power varies according to the distance from the heart, being greatest at the heart; while probably the extent may be the same in every artery.

To endeavour to ascertain the elasticity of arteries, I made comparative experiments on the aorta and pulmonary artery. Having cut off a portion, of about an inch in length, from the ascending aorta, at half an inch above the valves, and having slit it up, it measured, transversely, two inches and three quarters, but when stretched to its full length, three inches and three quarters, having gained rather more than one third, and having required a force equal to the weight of one pound ten ounces to produce this effect. A similar section was made of the pulmonary artery in the same subject, which measured two inches and a half, transversely; and when subjected to trial in the same manner, was stretched to three inches and a half, being rather more in proportion than the aorta; so that the pulmonary artery appears to have rather more elasticity than the aorta. It is not impossible that this difference might have arisen from the aorta having lost some of its elasticity by use; for although I chose for my experiment the arteries of a young man, where I conceived them to be perfectly sound, yet if there could have been any diminution of the elasticity from use, it would be most considerable in the aorta.

These experiments were made on different arteries with nearly the same result, and seemed to prove that there was almost the same extent of elasticity, though not the same powers.

An artery being composed of an elastic and inelastic substance, its elasticity is not altogether similar to that of a body which is wholly elastic. There is an effect produced from stretching it that is expressive of the nature of both these substances, till it gives way or breaks; for an artery has a check to its yielding to so great a degree, and is stopt at once, when stretched to a certain point*, which check is occasioned probably by the muscular, together with the internal inelastic coat[a].

To prove the muscularity of an artery, it is only necessary to compare its action with that of elastic substances. Action in an elastic body can only be produced by a mechanical power; but muscles acting upon another principle can act quickly or slowly, much or little, according to the stimulus applied; though all muscles do not act alike in this respect. If an artery is cut through, or laid bare, it will be found that it contracts by degrees till the whole cavity is closed; but if it be allowed to remain in this contracted state till after the death of the animal, and be then dilated beyond the state of rest of elastic substances, it will only contract to the degree of that state; this it will do immediately, but the contraction will not be equal to that of which it was capable while alive. The posterior tibial artery of a dog being laid bare, and its size attended to, it was observed to be so much contracted in a short time as almost to prevent the blood from passing through it, and when divided the blood only oozed out from the orifice. On laying bare the carotid and crural arteries, and observing what took place in them while the animal was allowed to bleed to death, these arteries very evidently became smaller and smaller.

When the various uses of arteries are considered, such as their forming different parts of the body out of the blood, their performing the different secretions, their allowing at one time the blood to pass readily into the smaller branches, as in blushing, and at another preventing it altogether, as in paleness from fear: and if to these we add the power of producing a diseased increase of any or every part of the body, we cannot but conclude that they are possessed of muscular powers.

The influence of the heart in the body, like that of the sun in the planetary system, we know extends to every part; all the parts of the vascular system being supplied according to the necessity it has; though every part is not equally endowed with power, or disposition to make use of that power.

The arteries, upon the whole, may be said to possess considerable living powers, and to retain them for a long time. This is evident when we observe what must happen in transplanting a living part of

* This gives a determined size to an artery.

[a] [Thus Poiseuille, by direct experiment, proved that the force of reaction excited by the distension of a recent artery was greater than the force used to distend it, and greater also than an artery could exert some time after death, before decomposition had commenced. This is only to be accounted for by its muscularity. (*Journ. de Phys., par M. Majendie*, viii. 272.)]

one body with an intention that it should unite with another body and become a part of it: the part transplanted must retain life till it can unite so as to receive its nourishment from that into which it has been inserted. It is, however, to be supposed that in such situations life can be retained longer than in others, although it is well known that it is preserved in the vascular system, even when there is no collateral assistance. I found in the uterus of a cow, which had been separated from the animal above twenty-four hours, that after it had been injected and allowed to stand another day, the larger vessels had become much more turgid than when I first injected them, and that the smaller arteries had contracted so as to force the injection back into the larger[a]. This contraction was so obvious that it could not but be observed at the time, which was forty-eight hours after the separation from the body of the animal. This shows too the muscular power of the smaller arteries to be superior to that of the larger, and that it is probably continued longer after the separation from the body; a property which the involuntary muscles possess to a degree greater than the voluntary, in the former of which classes the muscular structure of the arteries is to be considered.

To ascertain how long the living power existed in any artery after separation from the body, or perhaps, to speak more properly, after that communication with the body was cut off, by which we have reason to suppose life to be continued in a part, I made the following experiments, for which I chose the umbilical arteries, because I could confine the blood in them, and keep them distended for any length of time. In a woman delivered on the Thursday afternoon, the navel-string was separated from the fœtus; it was first tied in two places and cut between, so that the blood contained in the cord and placenta was confined in them. The placenta came away full of blood; and on Friday morning, the day after, I tied a string round the cord about an inch below the other ligature, that the blood might still be confined in the placenta and remaining cord. Having cut off this piece, the blood immediately gushed out, and, by examining the cut ends of the cord, I attentively observed to what degree the ends of the arteries were open; and the blood having now all escaped from this portion, the vessels were left to contract with the whole of their elastic power, the effect of which is immediate. Saturday morning, the day after this last part of the ex-

---

[a] [The same fact is also proved by the great difficulty of thoroughly injecting the capillaries in a recently killed animal, so as to make the injection pass forwards into the veins. Thus also Wedemeyer found a much greater force requisite to force an irritating fluid, such as dilute alcohol or vinegar, through the capillaries of the living animal than when he employed a bland fluid.]

periment, having examined the mouths of the arteries, I found them closed up, so that the muscular coat had contracted in the twenty-four hours to such a degree as to close entirely the area of the artery. That same morning I repeated the experiment of Friday, and on Sunday morning observed the result of this second experiment to be similar to that of the former. On this morning (Sunday) I repeated this experiment the third time, and on Monday observed that the result had not been the same as before, the mouths of the arteries remaining open; which showed that the artery had become dead. There was but little alteration perceived in the orifices of the veins in all the experiments.

These experiments show that the vessels of the cord have the power of contraction above two days after separation from the body.

Having given a general idea of muscular action, including muscular relaxation, together with the union of the muscular and elastic power in an animal, I shall now apply them to the arteries.

There are three states in which an artery is found, viz. 1st, the natural pervious state; 2nd, the stretched; and, 3rd, the contracted state, which may or may not be pervious. The natural pervious state is that to which the elastic power naturally brings a vessel which has been stretched beyond or contracted within the extent which it held in a state of rest. The stretched is that state produced by the impulse of the blood in consequence of the contraction of the heart; from which it is again brought back to the natural state by the elastic power, perhaps assisted by the muscular. The contracted state of an artery arises from the action of the muscular power, and is again restored to the natural state by the elastic.

It has been shown that certain muscles have both a voluntary and involuntary contraction, and that in some of these the involuntary action having brought the part to a necessary position, supports it in that state till it be either necessary for the muscle to relax, or for the voluntary action to take place: instances of which I have given in the sphincter muscles. I shall now endeavour to show that the arteries have a middle state, but that in them the power of bringing the coats into a certain position, and sustaining them in it, is not the effect of a muscular but of an elastic power: and that the muscular action, both in contraction and relaxation, is involuntary.

In parts endowed with considerable elastic powers, although not apparently muscular, as many arteries, but which we yet know, from other modes of information, to be possessed of muscular power, elasticity is so combined as to produce a middle or natural state, by acting to a certain degree only as an elongator of the muscular part in some of its actions*. These two powers, muscular and elastic, are probably introduced into the vascular system of all animals, the parts themselves being composed of substances of this description, together with a fine inner membrane, which I believe to be but little elastic, and this membrane is more apparent in the larger than in the smaller ramifications. When we consider the construction and use of the arteries, we must at once see the necessity of their having these two powers, although in the greatest number it is impossible to give clear ocular demonstration of the existence of distinct muscular fibres. But still, as arteries are evidently composed of two distinct substances, one of which is demonstrably elastic, and we know them likewise to be certainly endowed with the power of contraction peculiar to a muscle, it is reasonable to suppose the other substance to be muscular; I shall endeavour also to prove its existence in such vessels, from their having a power of contraction in the action of death.

As the human body is always alluded to in this account, I shall found my experiments and observations on such animals only as have a similar structure; for in other animals, as the turtle, alligator, &c., we can plainly discern muscular fibres, the insides of the arteries and veins in these animals being evidently fasciculated.

Every part of the vascular system is not equally furnished with muscular fibres; some parts being almost wholly composed of the elastic substance, such as the larger vessels, especially the arteries, in which, were they equally muscular with the smaller vessels, the existence of muscular fibres might be more easily proved. Neither does the elastic substance equally prevail in every part, for many, especially the smaller arteries, or what have been called the capillary vessels, appear to be almost entirely muscular; at least I am led to think so from my own observations and experiments on this subject. From these experiments I have also discovered that the larger arteries possess little muscular powers; but that as they recede from the heart towards the extremities, the muscular power is gradually increased, and the elastic diminished. Hence I imagine there may exist a size of vessels totally void of elasticity: but this I should conceive to be in the very extreme parts only. For it is to be observed that every portion of an artery, of a considerable size, is capable of assuming the middle state, which state must be referred to the elastic power.

The greatest part of the arterial system evidently appears to be composed of two substances, which structure is most remarkable in the

* We can hardly suppose that the muscular coat of the artery assists the elastic in bringing it to the middle state when already contracted within it.

middle-sized arteries, where the two substances are more equally divided, and where the size admits of a visible distinction of parts. The best method to see this is to cut the vessels either across or longitudinally, and to look upon the edges that have been cut[a].

If the aorta be treated in this way, we shall find that though it appears to be composed of one substance, yet towards the inner surface it is darker in colour, and of a structure which differs, although but in a small degree, from that of the outer surface. If we proceed by this mode of investigation, following the course of the circulation, we shall find that the internal and external parts become evidently more distinguishable from each other: the internal part, which is darker, but with a degree of transparency, begins almost insensibly in the larger vessels, and increases proportionably in thickness as the arteries divide, and of course become smaller, while the external, being of a white colour, is gradually diminishing, but in a greater degree, according to the diminution of size in the artery, and of the increased thickness of the other coat, so that the two do not bear the same proportion to each other in the small arteries as in the larger. The disproportion, however, between them appears greater than it really is, some deception arising from the greater muscular power possessed by the smaller arteries, in consequence of which the inner coat will be more contracted, and therefore seem thicker. This circumstance alone makes the difference of thickness between the whole coats of a large artery and those of a small one

[a] [The reader is probably aware that the nature of the proper arterial tissue has formed one of the most contested points in all physiology. The fibrous coat of arteries, according to Meckel, is easily separable into different transverse slightly oblique layers, which resemble one another precisely in structure, but differ from true muscular fibre in possessing greater elasticity and hardness, and from being closer, firmer, more compact, and more brittle than muscles. They are also drier and flatter than the true muscular fibre, and contain no cellular tissue in their interstices. Hence some anatomists have been led to class this as a particular tissue (*tissue jaune ou élastique*) which enters into the composition of the air-passages, excretory ducts, intervertebral substances, coverings of the corpora cavernosa, &c., although it must be quite clear, from the preceding observations of the author, that it possesses a truly contractile as well as an elastic power. The decision of this question will probably depend on the idea which we affix to the term muscle; for if we limit the definition of this structure to such substances as possess a fibrous appearance, a peculiar chemical composition, and a power of alternate contraction and relaxation, I know not how we shall substantiate the affirmative of the question. The arteries, it is true, are fibrous, like many other dissimilar structures, but the appearance of these fibres is wholly different from that of muscles; upon chemical analysis they are not found to contain fibrin, and when subjected to stimuli of different kinds they behave in a manner totally different from that of muscles, their contraction being continuous and permanent, and resembling much more that of the skin and excretory ducts than that of true muscular structure.]

appear less than it really is; accordingly we find the coats of the humeral artery in the horse apparently thicker than the coats of the axillary, the coats of the radial as thick as those of the humeral, and the artery near the hoof as thick in its coats as any of the others.

There is yet another circumstance which also deserves attention in comparing the two coats, namely, that in many places, but especially at the surfaces of contact in the elastic and muscular substances of the middle-sized arteries, the fibres of the muscular and elastic are very much blended or intermixed. I mention this, because otherwise we might be led to draw false conclusions with regard to the comparative quantity of each substance, and because it explains by what means both these coats are made elastic. The external coat, however, is more so than the internal, being composed almost entirely of elastic substance, while the internal has a mixture of muscular with its elastic fibres.

As there is, therefore, a difference in the elastic power of the two coats, there must be a difference in their powers of contraction after death, the external coat, for instance, contracting more than the internal, and also, as there is a difference between the muscular and elastic powers of contraction, the muscular having the greatest, there must be a difference between the contracting powers of these two coats during life, but the reverse of that which takes place after death.

In those arteries which are evidently composed of two distinct substances, especially the smaller, we may observe two very opposite appearances, according as the elastic or muscular coats have contracted most. In the one, when we make a transverse section, and look upon the cut end, we may observe that the inner surface has been thrown into rugæ, so as to fill up the whole cavity; and if such an artery be slit up longitudinally, so as to expose its inner surface, we shall find that inner surface forming wrinkles, which are principally longitudinal. If the finger is passed over that surface, it feels hard, while the external is soft; but if the artery be stretched, and allowed to recover itself by its elasticity, which is the only power it now has, it will be felt equally soft on both surfaces, and its coats will be found to have become thinner than before[a]. On the contrary, I have observed in many of the smaller arteries, when the muscular contraction has been considerable, the external or elastic coat to be thrown into longitudinal inequalities, from not having an equal power of contraction with the

[a] [The internal surface is thrown into rugæ in consequence of the elasticity of the external coat being greater than the muscularity of the internal coat. How then can stretching smooth these rugæ, when it ought rather to increase them?]

muscular; an artery under such circumstances being to the touch as hard as a cord. But if the muscular contraction be destroyed by stretching, or passing something through the artery, then it becomes very soft and pliant, and the muscular coat having once been stretched, without having the power of contracting again, is thrown into irregularities by the action of the elastic.

The elastic coat of an artery is fibrous, and the direction of its fibres is principally transverse or circular; but where a branch is going off, or at the division of an artery into two, the direction of the fibres is very irregular. I cannot say that I have found any fibres which are to a great degree oblique or longitudinal, a circumstance that shows their simple elasticity to be equal to the intention or use, a transverse or circular direction of fibres not being the most advantageous for producing the greatest effect*. They are also elastic laterally [longitudinally?], from the direction of their fibres, which property shortens the artery when elongated by the blood, and I believe the muscles have little share in this action; the whole of which tends to show that the elastic power is equal to the task of producing, and really does produce, the natural state of the artery. What the direction of the muscular fibres may be I never could discover, but should suppose them oblique, because the degree of contraction appears greater than a straight muscle could produce, in which light a circular muscle is to be considered, as its effects are in the direction of its fibres; for either the diameter or the circumference of the artery will decrease in the same proportion, but not the area, which will decrease in proportion to the square of the diameter.

We should naturally suppose that, where the action of the heart is strong, elasticity is the best property to sustain its force; and that where the force and elasticity are well proportioned, no mischief can ensue. Where the force, therefore, of the heart is greatest there is the greatest degree of elasticity, which yields with reluctance, and constantly endeavours to oppose and counteract that force.

From these active powers of an artery, together with a foreign power, viz. the blood, acting upon them and distending their parietes, in a manner somewhat similar to the common action of fluids in canals, we may perceive that there are three actions which take place, all of which operate in concert with each other, and produce one ultimate effect.

As the filling of the cavity of an artery produces an extension of its coats in every direction, the arteries are endowed with the elastic power,

* This is a principle in mechanics so well known that it need not here be explained: we find it happily introduced in the disposition of muscles in various parts of the body.

which, by contracting in all directions, brings them back again to their natural state.

The action of the muscular power, being principally in a transverse direction, tends, when the artery is extended, to lessen its diameter, and assist the elastic power; but as its quantity of contraction is superior to that of the elastic power, it does or may contract the artery beyond what the latter could effect. When the muscular action ceases, elasticity will be exerted to dilate the vessel and restore it to a middle state again, becoming the elongator or antagonist of the muscular coat, and by that means fitting it for a new action as described in other parts of the body. This will be most evident in the middle-sized vessels; for in the smaller, the proportion of elastic substance is not so considerable, and therefore it will contribute less to the dilatation of the vessel when the muscular coat relaxes. Yet we must suppose that no vessel even to its very extremity, is ever entirely collapsed; but that it possesses an elastic power sufficient to give it a middle state. Although these different structures do not always bear the same proportion to each other in arteries of the same size, yet we must conclude there is in these vessels a certain regular proportion preserved, and I am inclined to believe that the elasticity is in some degree in an inverse proportion to the decrease of size, presuming at the same time that the muscular power increases in the same proportion. A vessel is stretched beyond its natural state, first by the force of the heart, and in succession by the first order of vessels; then it is that the elastic power is exerted to contract the vessel, and restore it to the natural size; and in the performance of this it will be more or less assisted by the muscular power, according to the size of the vessels; least in the larger, and most in the smaller vessels, as was observed above. There appears to be no muscular power capable of contracting an artery in its length, the whole of that contraction being produced by the elasticity. For in a transverse section of an artery, made when the muscles of the vessels are in a contracted state, it may always be observed, that the external or elastic coat immediately contracts longitudinally, and leaves the internal or muscular coat projecting; which would not be the case if there was a longitudinal muscular contraction equal to the elastic, and were not the quantity of muscular contraction greater than the elastic there would be no occasion for muscles. Another proof of this is, that if a piece of contracted artery be stretched transversely, or have its area increased, and be allowed to recover itself, it loses a part of its length. To understand this it will be necessary to know that muscular fibres by contraction become thicker, and in proportion corresponding with the degree of contraction in the muscle.

The thickening in the muscle of a horse was found to be an increase of one fourth part of thickness to one third of a contraction *; from which it follows that the more the muscular fibres of any vessel contract, the more the vessel is lengthened; but destroy the muscular contraction by dilating the artery, and the elastic power, which acts in all directions, will immediately take place, and restore the vessel to its proper size; which is a proof that the effect of the lateral swell produced by the muscular contraction is greater than that of the longitudinal elasticity of the artery.

If we examine how much the vessel has lost of its length in this trial, we shall find it will amount to about one twelfth of the whole; a proof that the internal coat does not contract so much longitudinally by its muscular power as the external does by its elasticity. By multiplying such experiments we have further proofs that the power of muscular contraction acts chiefly in a circular direction; for in a longitudinal section of an artery in its contracted state, the internal coat does not project as in a transverse section, both coats remaining equal; or rather, indeed, the elastic coat projects beyond the other, from the internal muscular coat having contracted most. But if this section be stretched transversely, the external coat then contracts, and leaves the internal most projecting; because the internal or muscular has now no power of contraction. If the transverse extension be repeated, and to a greater degree, the artery, when allowed to recover itself, will have its inside turned outwards, as well as bent longitudinally, having the inside of the artery on the outside of the curve, and often bringing the two ends together: but this is easily accounted for; for as by the transverse extension of the artery its muscular contraction is destroyed, it becomes pliant; and the only resistance to the elastic power on this side being now removed, it is allowed to exert itself to its utmost extent. In doing this it bends the section in a longitudinal direction, which also inclines us to believe that the external part of the elastic coat is the most elastic.

* This calculation is not accurate; for in the experiments made to discover if the muscle lost of its size in the whole when contracted, I found it hardly did: therefore, what it lost in length it must have acquired in thickness [a].

---

[a] [The fact that muscles, when they contract, acquire in thickness exactly what they lose in length, may easily be proved by observing the effect which the contraction of the ventricles of the heart, or live eels, have on a vessel of water, to which has previously been affixed a narrow graduated tube. We cannot, however, infer from this fact that the arteries are muscular, since precisely the same effect would follow from the contraction of any purely elastic body as follows from the contraction of a muscle.]

These experiments not only prove that the muscular power of an artery acts chiefly in a transverse direction, but also that the elastic power exists almost entirely in the external coat, and therefore that the internal coat must be the seat of the muscular power.

Experiments on the arteries of a horse bled to death.—To ascertain the muscular power of contraction in the arteries, and determine the proportions which it bears to their elasticity, I made the following experiments upon the aorta, iliac, axillary, carotid, crural, humeral, and radial arteries of a horse. In this animal the muscles were all allowed to contract equally, and therefore we might reasonably presume that the vessels (at least such of them as were furnished with muscles) would also be contracted, the stimulus of death acting equally upon muscles in every form and every situation. The animal had also been bled to death, so that the vessels had an additional stimulus to produce contraction in them, as we know that all vessels in animals endeavour as much as possible to adapt themselves to the quantity of fluid circulating through them.

As I supposed the larger arteries had less of this power than the smaller, and that perhaps in an inverse proportion to their size, in order to ascertain that fact, and also to contrast the two powers, I made my first experiments upon the aorta and its nearest branches, continuing them on the other branches as these became smaller and smaller. The arteries were taken out of the body with great care, so as not in the least to alter their texture or state of contraction. The experiments were made in the following manner: I took short sections of the different arteries, slit them up in a longitudinal direction, and in that state measured the breadth of each, by which means, as I conceived, I could ascertain their muscular contraction; then taking the same sections, and stretching them transversely, I measured them in that state, which gave me the greatest elongation their muscular and elastic powers were capable of. As by this extension I had entirely destroyed their muscular contraction, whatever degree of contraction they exerted afterwards must, I believe, have been owing to elasticity. Having allowed them to contract, I again measured them a third time in that state, and thus ascertained three different states of vessels, between which I could compare the difference either in the same or different sections, so as from the result to deduce with some degree of certainty the extent of these powers in every size of vessel. I say only with some degree of certainty; for I do not pretend to affirm that these experiments will always be exact; circumstances often happening in the body which prevent the stimulus of death from taking place with equal effect in every part. I have accordingly seen in the same artery some parts wider than others, even when the more contracted parts were nearest the heart, and this merely from the difference of action in the muscular power; for when that was destroyed by stretching, the parts contracted equally in both.

Exp. 1. A circular section of the aorta ascendens, when slit up and opened into a plane, measured 5½ inches transversely; on being stretched, it lengthened to 10½; the stretching power being removed, it contracted again to six inches, which we must suppose to be the middle state of the vessel. Hence the vessel appeared to have gained by stretching ½ an inch in width or rather circumference, which may be attributed to the relaxation of its muscular fibres, whose contraction must have been equal to $\frac{1}{12}$; 6 inches being the natural size, or most contracted state of the elastic power.

Exp. 2. A circular section of the aorta at the origin of the first intercostal artery, measuring 4¼ inches, extended by stretching to 7½ inches; it contracted again to 4 inches, and therefore gained $\frac{1}{17}$.

Exp. 3. A circular section of the aorta at the lower part of the thorax, on being stretched, and being allowed to contract again, gained $\frac{1}{16}$.

Exp. 4. A circular section of the iliac artery, measuring 2 inches, when stretched and allowed to contract again, measured 2$\frac{4}{12}$ inches, and therefore gained $\frac{1}{6}$.

Exp. 5. A circular section of the axillary artery, measuring 1 inch, when stretched and contracted again, measured 1⅛ inch, therefore gained ⅛.

Exp. 6. A circular section of the carotid artery, measuring $\frac{9}{12}$ of an inch, when stretched, measured $\frac{10}{12}$ and one half; and when contracted again, $\frac{10}{12}$; therefore had gained $\frac{1}{9}$.

Exp. 7. A circular section of the crural artery, measuring $\frac{10}{12}$, when contracted after being stretched, measured 1$\frac{2}{12}$ inch, therefore gained $\frac{1}{5}$.

Exp. 8. The humeral artery, near the joint of the elbow, in a contracted state, was thicker in its coats than the axillary; the circumference of the artery in that state being $\frac{7}{12}$ and one half; after being stretched and contracted again, it measured $\frac{9}{12}$, therefore gained $\frac{1}{7}$ and one half.

Exp. 9. A circular section of the radial artery being taken, was found so contracted as hardly to be at all pervious; and the coats, especially the inner, much thicker than even the humeral: when slit up it scarcely measured $\frac{3}{12}$ of an inch; and when stretched and allowed to contract again, $\frac{6}{12}$; it therefore gained $\frac{3}{12}$, which was about the whole contraction of the artery.

To see how far this power of recovery in the same artery took place at different distances from the source of the circulation, I made the following experiments on the spermatic artery of a bull, and likewise on the artery of the fore leg and penis. The spermatic artery, near the aorta, when stretched longitudinally, recovered perfectly the former length; when stretched transversely it likewise recovered perfectly. About the middle, when stretched transversely, it gained $\frac{1}{17}$. Upon the testicle when stretched transversely, it gained $\frac{1}{4}$, which was its muscular power.

The humeral portion of the artery of the fore leg, when stretched transversely, and also longitudinally, recovered entirely.

The artery of one hoof, or rather finger, when stretched transversely, gained $\frac{1}{70}$, which was the muscular power: when stretched longitudinally it recovered perfectly.

The artery of the penis, when stretched longitudinally or transversely, recovered itself perfectly. This artery is considerably more elastic longitudinally than the others, but not so transversely. This increased elasticity in the longitudinal direction may be intended to allow of the difference in the length of the penis at different times.

From these experiments we see that the power of recovery in a vessel is greater in proportion as it is nearer to the heart; but as it becomes more distant it lessens, which shows the decrease of the elastic and the increase of the muscular power.

Tabular View of the preceding Experiments[a].

	Measuring.	Stretched to.	Recovered to.	Contracted by death.
Aorta ascendens	$5\frac{6}{12}$ inches	$10\frac{6}{12}$	6	$\frac{1}{11}$ part.
Aorta descendens at first intercostal	$4\frac{1}{4}$	$7\frac{6}{12}$	$4\frac{6}{12}$	$\frac{1}{17}$
Aorta descendens at the lowest part				$\frac{1}{10}$
Iliac artery	2		$2\frac{4}{12}$	$\frac{1}{6}$
Axillary	1		$1\frac{1}{8}$	$\frac{1}{8}$
Carotid	$\frac{6}{12}$	$\frac{33}{24}$	$\frac{10}{12}$	$\frac{2}{3}$
Crural	$\frac{10}{12}$		$1\frac{2}{12}$	$\frac{1}{3}$
Humeral	$\frac{16}{24}$		$\frac{9}{12}$	$\frac{3}{14}$
Radial	$\frac{3}{12}$		$\frac{6}{12}$	equal to the whole.

Experiments on the power of Arteries to contract longitudinally.

To prove that arteries do not produce the same power of muscular con-

a [It may be proper to observe that the proportional rates of contraction by death, as set down in the above table, are deduced from the contracted instead of from the natural or middle state of the vessels; independently of which the numbers themselves are not correctly deduced. The following fractions represent the respective degrees of contraction in each case (omitting the 3rd, for which there are no data,) calculated for the natural state of the vessel, viz. $\frac{1}{12}$, $\frac{1}{18}$, $\frac{1}{7}$, $\frac{1}{9}$, $\frac{2}{5}$, $\frac{2}{7}$, $\frac{1}{6}$, and $\frac{1}{3}$.

traction in a longitudinal which they do in a transverse direction, the following experiments were made.

Exp. 1. A longitudinal section of the aorta ascendens, measuring two inches, when stretched and allowed again to contract measured the same length.

Exp. 2. A longitudinal section of the aorta descendens at the lower part of the thorax, of a given length, after having been stretched, contracted exactly the same length.

Exp. 3. Two inches of the same carotid artery used in the sixth experiment, when stretched longitudinally, recovered itself, so as not to be longer than before the experiment.

Exp. 4. A portion of that humeral artery used in the eighth of the former experiments was not altered in its original length, when it recovered itself after being stretched.

These experiments appear to be decisive, and prove that the muscular power acts chiefly in a transverse direction; yet it is to be observed that the elastic power of arteries is greater in a longitudinal than in a transverse direction. This appears to be intended to counteract the lengthening effect of the heart, as well as that arising from the action of the muscular coat; for the transverse contraction of that coat lengthens the artery, and therefore stretches the elastic, which again contracts upon the diastole of the artery.

From the account we have given of those substances which compose an artery, we may perceive it has two powers, the one elastic and the other muscular. We see also that the larger arteries are principally endowed with the elastic power, and the smaller with the muscular; that the elastic is always gradually diminishing in the smaller, and the muscular increasing, till, at last, probably, the action of an artery is almost wholly muscular; yet I think it is not to be supposed but that some degree of elasticity is continued to the extremity of an artery, for the middle state cannot be procured without it, and I conceive the middle state to be essential to every part of an artery. Let us now apply these two powers of action, or, to speak more properly, of reaction, with their different proportions in the different parts of the arterial system. From these different proportions we must suppose the elastic to be best fitted for sustaining a force applied to it, (such as the motion of the blood given by the heart,) and propelling it along the vessel; the muscular power, most probably, is required to assist in continuing that motion, the force of the heart being partly spent, but certainly was intended to dispose of the blood when arrived at its place of destination; for elasticity can neither assist in the one nor the other, although it is still of use, through the whole, to preserve the middle state. Elasticity is better adapted to sustain a force than muscular power: for an elastic body recovers itself again, whenever the stretching cause suspends its action, while muscles endeavour to adapt themselves to circumstances as they arise. This is verified by different sorts of engines whose pipes are made of different metals. A pipe made of lead, for instance, will in time dilate and become useless*; whereas a pipe of iron will react on the fluid, if the force of the fluid be in proportion to the elastic power of the iron: but the lead having little or no elasticity, whenever it is stretched it will remain so, and every new force will stretch it more and more. We are therefore to suppose that the force of the heart is not capable of stretching the artery so much as to destroy its elasticity; or, in other words, the force of the heart is not able to dilate the artery beyond the contracting power.

As the motion of the blood is mechanical, elasticity is best adapted to take off the immediate force of the heart; and as we go from the heart this property becomes less necessary, because in this course the influence of the heart is gradually lessened, by which means a more equal motion of the blood is immediately produced, and even in the first artery a continued stream is at all times obtained, although it is considerably increased by each contraction of the heart. Without this power the motion of the blood in the aorta would have been similar to what it is in its passage out of the heart, and would have been nearly the same in every part of the arterial system. For though the motion of the blood out of the heart be by interrupted jerks, yet the whole arterial tube being more or less elastic, the motion of the blood becomes gradually more uniform from this cause. Elasticity in arteries acts like a pair of double bellows: although their motion be alternate, the stream of air is continued; and if it were to pass through a long elastic pipe, resembling an artery, the current of air would be still more uniform[a]. The advantage arising from elasticity in the arterial system will be more complete in the young subject than in the old: for in the latter, the

* This accounts for the size of aneurisms in arteries whose coats must have lost their elasticity before they could be dilated.

---

[a] [The application of this principle in the construction of water-pumps and fire-engines is extremely simple. It consists in making the water pass through a chamber of condensed air, the elasticity of which causes the water to issue forth in a continued and uniform stream, instead of by jerks. This transformation of an alternating into a continued action may be expressed in the following proposition of mechanics. Every intermitting motion may be converted into a continued one, by employing the original force to compress a reservoir or spring, which keeps up a constant reaction.]

elasticity of the arteries being very considerably diminished, more especially in the larger trunks, where the force of the heart requires to be broken, the blood will be thrown into the second and third order of vessels with increased velocity. In the young the current is slower, from the reaction of the elastic power during the relaxed state of the heart; whereas at the heart the motion is equal to the contraction of the heart; and as the heart is probably twice the time in relaxing that it is in contracting, from this cause alone we may suppose the whole is two thirds less in the smaller vessels. As elastic bodies have a middle state, or state of rest, to which they return after having been dilated or contracted by any other power, and as they must always be acted upon before they can react, the use of elasticity in the arterial system will be very evident. It is by this means that the vessels adapt themselves to the different motions of the body, as flexion and extension; so that one side of an artery contracts while the other is elongated, and the canal is always open for the reception of blood in the curved, stretched, or relaxed state.

The muscular power of an artery renders a smaller force of the heart sufficient for the purposes of circulation; for the heart need only to act with such force as will be sufficient to carry the blood through the larger arteries, and then the muscular power of the arteries takes it up, and, as it were, removes the load of blood while the heart is dilating. In confirmation of this remark, it is observable in animals whose arteries are very muscular, that the heart is proportionably weaker, so that the muscular portion of the vessels becomes a second part to the heart, acting where the power of the heart begins to fail, and increasing in strength as that decreases in power. Besides this, it disposes of such part of the blood as is necessary for the animal œconomy, principally in growth, repair, and secretions. At the extreme ends of the arteries, therefore, we must suppose that their actions are varied from that of simply conveying blood, except those arteries which are continued into veins.

§. 4. *Of the Vasa Arteriarum.*

The arteries are furnished with both arteries and veins, although it cannot be said that they are to appearance very vascular. Their arteries come from neighbouring vessels, and not from the artery itself which they supply. This we see in dissection; and I found by filling an artery, such as the carotid, with fine injection, that still the arteries of the artery were not injected. On laying the coats of arteries bare in the living body, we can disc^rn their vessels more evidently some little time after the exposure, for then they become vessels conveying red blood, as in a beginning inflammation, growing turgid, when the arteries may be easily discerned from the veins by the difference of colour of the blood in each: these observations will also generally apply to the corresponding veins.

Perhaps arteries afford the most striking instance of animal substance furnished with two powers existing in the same part, one to resist mechanical impulse, the other to produce action. The first of these powers is greatest where there is the most impulse to resist; therefore we find it particularly in the arteries nearest to the heart, the better to support the force of that organ; but in those parts where gravitation is gradually increasing, the diminution of power in the artery is not in proportion to the diminution of the force of the heart.

In the veins the allotment of strength is commonly the reverse, for as they have nothing mechanical to resist, but the effect of gravitation, their principal strength is at the extremities.

We are to suppose that the power of the heart, and the mechanical strength of the arteries, bear a just proportion to each other; and therefore by ascertaining the last we may give a tolerable good guess with respect to the other. In this view, to determine the strength of the ventricles, so far as I was able, I made comparative trials of the strength of the aorta and pulmonary arteries of a healthy young man.

I separated a circular section of each, and on being slit, they measured $3\frac{3}{8}$ inches, their breadths being also equal. On trial, I found the aorta, being stretched to near 5 inches, broke with a weight of eight pounds. The pulmonary artery stretched to near $5\frac{1}{4}$ inches, and then broke with four pounds twelve ounces. This experiment I have repeated, but with very different results; for in one experiment, although the aorta took one pound ten ounces to stretch it, while the pulmonary artery took only six ounces, yet to break this pulmonary artery required eleven pounds three ounces, while the aorta broke with ten pounds four ounces; but this difference I impute to the aorta having lost its elasticity, which is very apt to happen in that vessel. There is nearly the same proportion of elasticity in both arteries; but the strength of the aorta in the first experiment appeared to be nearly double that of the pulmonary artery, while in the second it was less; yet we must suppose the result of the first experiment nearer the truth, for we seldom find the pulmonary artery diseased, while the aorta is seldom otherwise.

The mechanical strength of arteries is much greater in the trunk than in the branches, which is evident from accidents and from injections in dead bodies; for when we inject arteries with too much force, the first extravasation takes place in the smaller vessels. This can only be proved by subtle injections, which do not become solid by cold, such injections keeping up an equal pressure throughout the arterial system. In such cases the smaller arteries are found to give way first, viz. those of the muscles, pia-mater, and the cellular membrane; which contradicts Haller's theory of the relative strength of the coats of the vessels.

I am however inclined to suppose that they are even weaker in proportion to their size, viz. in proportion to the diminished force of the heart, or motion of the blood; but how far this is the case I will not venture to determine, as mechanical strength is not so much wanted in the smaller arteries as muscular; and as the mechanical strength of muscles appears to be less than the power of their own contraction, experiments made on the dead body upon parts whose uses arise from an action within themselves when active, are not conclusive. The flexor policis longus, being one of the most detached muscles in the body respecting structure and use, has been selected for experiments on this subject, and is found to raise by its action a greater weight than it can sustain after death. This, however, is liable to fallacy, as the two experiments are made on different muscles, one certainly healthy, the other most probably weakened by the disease preceding death.

The coats of arteries are not equally strong on all sides of the same artery; at the bending of a joint they are strongest on the convex side through the whole length of the curve; this is most evident in the permanent curves, such as in the great curvature of the aorta. Arteries are likewise strongest at the sharp angles made by a trunk and its branch, and at the angle formed by a trunk divided into two. These parts have the blood, as it were, dashing against them. Those likewise are the parts which first lose their elasticity and soonest ossify, being generally more stretched than the other parts of an artery, and making a kind of bag. These circumstances are chiefly observable in the curvature of the aorta and of the internal carotids, and at the division of the aorta into the two iliacs.

§. 5. *Of the Heart.*

The heart is an organ which is the great agent in the motion of the blood; but it is not essential to animals of every class, nor for the motion of the blood in every part where it is perfect; it is less so than the nerves, and many even possess the organs of generation, that have no heart. Its actions in health are regular, and characteristic of that state; and in disease its actions are in some degree characteristic of the disease; but although there is that connexion between the body and the heart, yet there seems not to be such a connexion between the heart and the body[a], for the heart may be in some degree disordered in its action, yet the body but little affected: it is therefore only to be considered as a local agent very little affecting the constitution sympathetically, except by means of the failure in its duty.

The heart in the more perfect animals is double, answerable to the two circulations,—the one through the lungs, the other over the body; but many that have only single hearts, have what is analogous to a double circulation; and this is performed in very different ways in different animals, so that one of the circulations in these is performed without a heart. A large class of animals, well known and pretty perfect in their construction, namely, all the class of fish, have no heart for the motion of the blood in the great circulation, or that over the whole body, having only a heart for the lungs or branchiæ, while the snail has only a heart for the great circulation, and none for the lungs; in the liver also of the most perfect animals, the motion of the blood in the vena portæ and vena cava hepatica is carried on without a heart. The absorbing system in every animal has no immediate propelling power; therefore this propelling power is not universally necessary.

The heart varies in its structure in different orders of animals, principally with respect to the number of cavities and their communications with each other, yet in all nearly the same purpose is answered. I shall here observe, that in the bird and quadruped there is a double circulalation, which requires a double heart, namely, a heart for each circulation, each heart consisting of an auricle and ventricle, called the right and the left; and from their forming but one body among them, they are all included in one heart; the right side, or heart, may be called the pulmonary, and the left may be called the corporeal. In many classes of animals there is to be found only one of these hearts; and according to the class, it is either the pulmonary or corporeal. In the fish, as was observed, the heart is the pulmonary; and in the snail the heart is the corporeal; so that the corporeal motion of the blood in the fish is carried on without a heart; and in the snail the pulmonary motion is carried on without a heart. In the winged insects, which have but one heart, as also but one circulation, there is this heart, answering both purposes; and in all these varieties breathing is the principal object.

The heart in most animals is composed principally of a strong muscle, thrown into the form of a cavity or cavities; but it is not wholly mus-

---

[a] [I apprehend that a reversal of the terms of this proposition is required, in order that the sense may agree with the context.]

cular, being in part tendinous or ligamentous, which last parts have neither action nor reaction within themselves, but are only acted upon; they are therefore made inelastic and rigid, to support the force of the acting parts in this action without varying in themselves.

In all animals which have red blood the heart is the reddest muscle in the body. Thus, in the bird, whose muscles are mostly white, the heart is red: we find it the same in the white fish.

As it differs in the different orders of animals respecting the number of cavities, it may admit of dispute what are to be reckoned truly hearts, and what only appendages; for some of its cavities may only be considered as reservoirs peculiar to some hearts.

The most simple form of heart is composed of one cavity only, and the most complicated has no more than two; it would seem indeed to increase progressively in the number of cavities from one to four, which includes the mixed; yet two of these ought not to be called parts of the heart, although they belong to it. The single cavity of the heart in the most simple class, or the two in the most complicated, are called ventricles. The other cavities belonging to it are called auricles. Many of those which have one ventricle only, have no auricle, such as insects; but there are others which have both a ventricle and auricle, such as fish, the snail, and many shell-fish; some of the last class have indeed two auricles, with only one ventricle, which shows that the number of auricles is not fixed under the same mode of circulation. Those animals which have two distinct ventricles, constituting four cavities, are what are called quadrupeds or mammalia, and birds. If the auricles are considered as parts of the heart, we might class animals which have hearts according to the number of their cavities, viz. monocoilia, dicoilia, tricoilia, tetracoilia; the tricoilia is a mixture of the dicoilia and tetracoilia. This is the case in distinct classes of animals; but it also takes place in other classes at different stages of life, for the fœtus of the class possessing four cavities may be classed with the mixed, having but one auricle, in consequence of the communication which exists in the fœtus between the two; and also but one ventricle, by means of the union which exists between the two arteries, which produces an union of blood, although not in the same way. Those passages, however, are shut up almost immediately after birth, or at least the canalis arteriosus*, which immediately prevents the foramen ovale from producing its former effects; therefore it is not so necessary it should be shut up in the adult. I have seen it, to common appearance, as much open as in a fœtus.

* There have been instances of the canalis arteriosus being open in the adult.

The heart may be considered as a truly mechanical engine; for although muscles are the powers in an animal, yet these powers are themselves often converted into a machine, of which the heart is a strong instance; for from the disposition of its muscular fibres, tendons, ligaments, and valves, it is adapted to mechanical purposes; and this construction makes it a complete organ or machine in itself. It is most probable that by means of this viscus a quicker supply of blood is furnished than otherwise could be effected.

In birds and quadrupeds, the heart, by its action, first throws out the blood, both that which is fit for the purposes of life, and that which requires to be prepared, the last having lost those salutary powers in the growth, repairs, secretion, etc. in the machine.

It may be said to give the first impulse to the blood, producing a greater velocity where the blood is simply conveyed to the parts for whose use it is destined. This velocity is alternately greater and less, and from the construction of the arteries alone, is gradually diminished, becoming more uniform where slowness and evenness of motion is necessary. This velocity of the blood in those parts where it is to be considered as passing only, allows a much larger quantity to flow through the part to which it is destined than otherwise could be transmitted.

The heart is placed in the vascular system, to be ready to receive the blood from the body, and to propel it back on the body again, although not in the centre of the whole; but it is reasonable to suppose that its situation is such as to be best suited to the various parts of the body; some parts requiring a brisk, others a more languid circulation. Some also require a greater supply of blood than others. We may suppose that the parts near the heart will receive more blood than those at a greater distance, because the resistance will be less if the vessels are of equal size in proportion to the size of the part.

The situation of the heart in the body varies in different animals. One would imagine when the animal was divided into its several portions, appropriated for the different purposes, that the situation of the heart would be nearly the same in all; but we find this not to be the case; its situation depends upon the organs of respiration more than any other part. It is placed in what is called the chest in the quadruped, bird, amphibia, fish, and in the aquatic and terrestrial insect: but not in what may be called the chest in the flying insect. The chest in the aquatic insect seems best suited to contain the lungs and branchiæ, and therefore the heart is placed there; but as the lungs of the flying insect are placed through the whole body, the heart is more diffused, extending through the whole length of the animal. The situation, therefore, of the heart is chiefly connected with that of the lungs; and when it is united with the body at large, it is because the lungs are also so disposed. We must suppose that these two have a relation to each other.

A heart is composed of an auricle and ventricle, and it is the ventricle which sends the blood through its course in the circulation; so that, from what has been said, it must appear that the ventricle is the true heart, the other parts having only secondary uses. As the ventricle is the part which propels the blood to the different parts of the body, its muscular power must be adequate to that purpose, and therefore it has a very strong muscular coat. Much more pains than were necessary have been taken to dissect and describe the course and arrangement of the muscular fibres of the heart, as if the knowledge of the course of its fibres could in the least account for its action. But as the heart can, in its contracted state, almost throw out its whole contents, to produce this effect its fibres must pass obliquely.

Its red colour arises probably from its being at the fountain head of the circulation, for those animals that have but little red blood, have it only in those parts near the heart; and the heart being nearest to its own powers, receives the blood before the vessels can so act as to dispose of the red blood, or allow of a kind of separation by distance; its constant action, too, renders it more red, as happens in other muscles.

The ventricles in the quadruped, bird, and amphibia, are called right and left, and this accords very well with the situation in such animals; but where there is only one ventricle, and that in some acting the part of the right, as in fish, and in others acting the part of the left, as in the snail, we ought to have some term expressive of their immediate use, and such as would apply to all animals that have such a viscus[a].

The auricles of the heart are to be considered only as reservoirs for the blood, to be ready to supply the ventricles; for an auricle is not to be found in all the animals which have a ventricle; nor does the number of auricles always correspond to that of the ventricles. Where the veins entering into the heart are small, in comparison to the quantity of blood which is wanted in the ventricles, there we have an auricle; but where the veins near to the heart are large, there is no auricle, as in the lobster, and generally in insects. In the snail, where the veins in common

[a] [The epithets pulmonary and systemic sufficiently express this difference of function.]

are large, yet as they are small where they enter the heart, there is an auricle; and as its office is somewhat similar to a large vein, it has some of its properties, viz. being in some degree both elastic and muscular.

The name sinus venosus is a very proper one; and as a proof that it is only such in the circulation, there are no valves placed between it and the veins[a].

As the heart is an engine formed to keep up the motion of the blood, and as it is necessary that this motion should be determined in a particular direction, it is adapted, as are also the other parts of the vascular system, to this purpose.

The heart is formed into a cavity, through which the blood must pass, receiving at once a considerable quantity of this fluid, upon which it immediately acts with equal force, although not progressively, as an intestine; and that this motion of the blood may be regulated, and a retrograde motion prevented, we find the valves constructed.

A valve, I believe, is in general understood to be a part in every machine calculated to allow whatever is to pass to move in one direction only, and the valves in the vascular system are intended for this purpose. They are of two kinds, having two modes of attachment, which is suited to the action of the part to which they are attached, and making a very essential difference in their formation. They are thin

---

[a] [In fish, as well as in several other animals, there are commonly placed two crescentic-shaped valves at the entrance into the auricle, between it and the sinus venosus, or bulbous enlargement of the venæ cavæ, which fact the author must have been well acquainted with, as several preparations are set up in the Hunterian Museum illustrative of this point. The observation, however, of the author in other respects is perfectly correct, and might be illustrated by numerous examples from comparative anatomy. Thus, in most of the batrachian animals the auricles are remarkable for their large size and the weakness of their parietes, which unite to give them an appearance much more resembling a great venous sinus than a true auricle. This conformation is particularly conspicuous in the *Siren lacertina*, where the number of fimbriated follicular processes sent off from the auricle give it the appearance of the branchial divisions of the vena cava in the cephalopods. In the gallery, or physiological department of the museum (Nos. 873–974.), there are numerous examples of these superadded sinuses, together with every variety of cardiac construction. In the chameleon the auricles are provided with two very large venous receptacles, twice as large as the auricles themselves, and extending the whole length of the chest; the object of which plainly is, to provide a receptacle for the superfluous blood when the tongue, which is a large erectile organ, and the only one assigned to this animal for the prehension of its prey, is not in action. (*See Houston in Trs. of R. I. Acad.*, xvi. 177.) Indeed this species of construction seems to be connected with the varying conditions of the circulation in most of those animals in which it occurs, whose habits of eating, diving, breathing, or exerting themselves are generally extremely irregular.]

inelastic membranes, having no action within themselves, with one edge fixed, the other loose in some, but not entirely so in others; they are either attached in a circular form, or in an oblique one. The circular attachment belongs to those of the ventricles, and the oblique to those of the arteries and veins. The circular are the most complex, requiring an additional apparatus to make them answer the intended purpose; for it is necessary that their loose floating edges should be restrained from inverting themselves into the auricle upon the contraction of the ventricles.

This is done by tendons, which are fixed at one extremity along the edge of the valves, and at the other to some part upon the inside of the ventricle. The tendons which are longest are inserted into columns of muscle, the intention of which is very evident: for if they had gone the whole length in form of a tendon, they would have been too long when the heart contracted, and the valves in such a case would have allowed of being pushed into the auricles, so far as to admit of the blood escaping back again into the cavity; but the carneæ columnæ keep the valves within the ventricle, in the contracted state of the ventricles; and the dilatation of the ventricles counteracts them, and places the valves in their proper situation in that state.

If the valves in this cavity had been placed obliquely along the inner sides of the ventricle, as in the beginning of the arteries and in the veins, the attachment then would not have been permanent; for it would have varied according to the relaxed or contracted state of the heart: it would have been short in the contracted state, and longer in the relaxed; therefore, to have a fixed base, it was necessary for them to be attached all round the mouth of the ventricles. I have reason to believe that the valves on the right side of the heart do not so perfectly do their duty as those of the left, therefore we may suppose it was not so necessary.

The vessels of the heart are called coronary arteries and veins. In quadrupeds and birds there are two coronary arteries, which arise from the aorta just at its beginning, behind two of the valves of the artery. From this circumstance a theory respecting the action of the heart was raised; but in the amphibia they arise at some distance, and not always from the same artery in the same species, often from the subclavian, and often from the anterior surface of the ascending aorta, which is reflected back. In the fish they arise from the artery as they are coming from the gills. The veins pass into the right auricle.

In all animals which have an auricle and ventricle, so far as I know, there is a bag (unattached) in which they are placed, called a pericardium*; but the insect tribe, whether aerial, aquatic, or terrestrial, have none, their heart being attached to the surrounding parts by the cellular membrane, or some other mode of attachment. In those animals which have this bag it is not a smooth termination of the cellular membrane, as the peritonæum may be supposed to be, but a distinct bag, as in man and all quadrupeds.

The use of this bag is probably that the heart may move with more ease and facility; the two parts, to wit, the contained and containing, acting as a kind of joint with a capsular ligament, and like such joints it contains a fluid, but not a synovia, as the two surfaces are not hard like cartilage; besides, the heart is kept very much in its place, which we must suppose is of use. I have conceived it also to be possible, as it is a pretty strong membrane, that it might in some degree preserve the heart from too great distension; for I have observed, by injections, that a little force will distend it beyond its natural size, if a part of the pericardium be taken off; but in the heart mentioned by Dr. Baillie there was no particular increase of bulk.

This bag, like most others, has a fluid which moistens the two surfaces. In every other cavity of the body the fluid is no more in quantity than what is simply sufficient to moisten the parts. In this bag, however, it is more, from whence it has acquired the name of liquor pericardii. There may be about a tea-spoonful in the whole. This fluid appears to be serum, and is commonly a little tinged with blood, which arises from the transudation of the red blood after death. That this cavity has more water in it than most other cavities of the body, may arise from there being a greater action of those parts on one another than takes place in others; it may also fill up the interstices formed between two round bodies, so that when the pulmonary artery and aorta are filled they may more easily assume a round figure.

The size of a heart we should naturally suppose is proportioned to the size of the animal and the natural quantity of blood, which last is, we might conceive, ever in proportion to the size of the animal; but I believe these modes of calculation will not be found to be just, for certainly some animals have much more blood in proportion to their size than others; and I believe the heart is not in size proportioned to the size of the animal, but bears a compound proportion or ratio to the quantity of blood

* There have been instances where the pericardium has been wanting in the human subject: a case of this kind is published by Dr. Baillie, in a periodical work entitled "Transactions of a Society instituted for promoting Medical and Chirurgical Knowledge."

to be moved and the frequency of the stroke it has to make; for when the quantity of blood is decreased, the frequency of the stroke must be increased; and as a proof of this we find when an animal loses a considerable quantity of blood, the heart increases in its frequency of stroke, as also in its violence. That it principally bears proportion to the quantity of blood is evident; for the right ventricle is equal in size to the left, if not larger, although it sends its blood to the lungs only, which are infinitely small when compared with the whole body; and the hearts of those animals which have but one ventricle, as fish for instance, which is similar in use to our right, are perhaps made as large in proportion to the size of the body as both ventricles in the quadruped[a].

The strength of a heart is commonly, if not always, in proportion to the size of the parts to which the blood is carried and the velocity with which it is propelled; which becomes a collateral proof that it is a universal agent in the circulation. In the complete heart this is not equal in every part of the same heart; the right ventricle being much weaker than the left, but still in the above proportions. The proportion between the two will be best known by ascertaining the difference in the strength of the two arteries, and this again will differ according to the whole parts the blood is sent to by the heart. In the fish, for instance, it is only necessary it should bear the proportion in strength to the whole fish that our right ventricle bears to our lungs, which is not in the least equal to that of the left ventricle; or, in other words, its strength should be commensurate with the size of the lungs. However, it is most probable that the right ventricle in the quadruped is stronger than in this proportion, because it is obliged to move a larger quantity of blood than is contained in any other part of the body of the same size, and with greater velocity: in the double heart, therefore, such as the human, the two cavities are not of equal strength, each being nearly in proportion to the size of the parts, or rather to the distance the blood is to go; the right ventricle only throwing it into the lungs, the left into the body. As a proof of this doctrine, we find that

---

a [The heart in animals of large dimensions is singularly small as compared with the bulk of the whole body, at the same time that its action is remarkably slow. In the fœtus, on the contrary, the heart is proportionably large, and its action in the same degree rapid. It would appear from the investigations of Treviranus, that the size of the heart as compared with the whole body decreases in proportion as the animal descends in the zoological scale. The following were the respective weights of the heart in different animals: mammalia, $\frac{1}{80}$ to $\frac{1}{160}$; birds, $\frac{1}{50}$ to $\frac{1}{122}$; amphibia, $\frac{1}{240}$ to $\frac{1}{278}$ fishes, $\frac{1}{350}$ to $\frac{1}{760}$. The rate of pulsation seems to diminish nearly in the same proportion as the size.]

in the fœtal state of this class of animals the two ventricles and the two large arteries are equal in strength. Indeed, from reasoning we should expect this, and even that the right ventricle should rather be the strongest, for at this period it sends the blood to the lower extremities; but since both the arteries unite into one canal, we must suppose it to be necessary that the velocities of the blood in both should be equal; and upon examination we find the two ventricles to be nearly equal in thickness in this young state of the animal. The mixed kind of heart, as that of the turtle, &c., is under the same predicament. The two ventricles are to be considered as joint agents in the circulation; and as the pulmonary artery and aorta are equally strong, it becomes a proof that the strength of the heart must be equal everywhere.

If we were to estimate the strength of the ventricles in those possessed of four cavities, by the strength of the aorta and pulmonary arteries, either by their absolute strength or elasticity, we might come pretty near the truth.

Dr. Hales made an experiment on a horse to ascertain the strength of the arteries, which gives us the power of the left ventricle; but all this explains nothing, for its power is equal to the use wanted.

The power of contraction of the ventricle must be within the strength of the artery; but it is hardly possible to ascertain what is the strength of an artery; nor, if we could, would it enable us to ascertain the strength of the ventricle, for the force of the heart is in part immediately lost by the blood being allowed to pass on, although not so freely as if the artery was open at the other end: in proportion, therefore, to the retardment, the artery is affected. We can ascertain the elastic power of a given section of an artery, and also its absolute strength; but we are not acquainted with the size of a section that will give the strength of the artery to which it belonged when the whole was in a perfect state or form.

Exp. 1. A section of a sound aorta, close to the valves, three quarters of an inch long, was stretched transversely to its greatest extent, which state was ascertained by measuring it with a pair of compasses, and the artery was allowed to contract. The weight required to stretch it again to the same degree was one pound ten ounces. To break the artery required ten pounds and a quarter.

Exp. 2. A section of the pulmonary artery, similar to the former in length and situation, required six ounces two drachms to stretch it to its full extent. To break it required eleven pounds three quarters.

The use of this viscus is in general very well known; however, its use has been frequently supposed to be more universal than it really is.

It gives to the blood its motion in most animals, and in all it sends the blood to the organs of respiration: in the flying insect it sends the blood both to those organs and to the body at large; but in fish to those organs only, the body at large in them having no heart. In the amphibia there is an attempt towards a heart both for the lungs and body, but not two distinct hearts. In the bird and quadruped there is a distinct heart for each. We may say, therefore, that there is one heart for respiration and another for the life, nourishment, &c. of the animal: these constitute the two ventricles.

As the extent of these two circulations is different, the two hearts, or, in other words, the two ventricles, are suited in their strength to the different extents of each circulation, as was observed above in treating of the strength of the heart.

How far the heart is alone capable of carrying on the circulation is not to be ascertained; for although the circulation is carried on in paralytic cases, yet this does not exclude the involuntary nervous influence of the part: this, however, varies very much in different classes of animals; for I have already observed, concerning the structure of the arteries, that their muscularity assisted in the circulation, and that in proportion as the vessels in general were endowed with this power the heart was weaker. I believe that the quadruped has the strongest heart of any class of animals; and I believe that their vessels have the least muscular power, more especially near the heart.

The immediate use of the heart in an animal would seem to be generally subject to as little variety as that of any other viscus; but perhaps the heart is subject to more variety than any other part in its construction. I have observed that it is either single, double, or mixed; that it is single without an auricle, single with one auricle, single with two auricles, double with a union of the two, making the mixed, and double with two auricles. With respect to its use, it is, in the most simple kind of single heart, to propel the blood through the body, immediately from the veins; which blood is to receive its purification in this passage, when the lungs are disposed throughout the body, as in the flying insect. In another single heart it is intended to mix both the purified and the adulterated blood, and of course to throw it out to the body and lungs equally in this mixed state, as in the lobster. In the single heart, with an auricle, its use is, in one class, to throw the blood throughout the body, after being purified, as in the snail; and in another single kind, with an auricle, it is to receive the blood from the body, and send it to the lungs only, as in all fish. In the single heart with two auricles it is formed to receive the blood both purified and unpurified, and dispose of it to both body and lungs in that state, as was observed in the lobster: the same thing happens, in some degree, in the turtle, snake, fœtus, etc. In the double heart with two auricles it acts like an union of the heart of the snail with that of the fish, one heart receiving the blood purified from the lungs, and sending it over the body, as in the snail; and the other receiving the blood from the body, and sending it into the lungs to be purified, as in the fish. From the above account we must see that the immediate use arising from the heart in one class of animals will not agree with its immediate use in another; but still, in all it is the engine employed to throw the blood to those parts into which the arteries conduct it[a].

It is impossible to say what the quantity of blood is that is thrown out of the heart at each contraction. The size of a relaxed heart in the dead body of any animal gives us the size of the cavity, or what it is capable of holding; but muscles seldom or ever are obliged to relax themselves to their full extent in common actions, although they often are when extensive effects are to be produced. The heart, like every part constructed for action, has its times of action beyond, and also within, its natural limit of action; but it is its natural action which should be ascertained. If we compare the actions of the heart with those of the body, we may suppose that the common quantity of motion in the heart is about half what it can perform; that is, it relaxes three fourths, and contracts one half; therefore a ventricle which contains four ounces, will, in common, only dilate so as to contain three, and will only contract so as to throw out two.

The question is, when the heart acts with more frequency, as from

---

[a] [I have already noticed a remarkable instance of the reach of Hunter's genius in regard to the different phases which the higher orders of animals undergo in the process of their development, corresponding to the different types of inferior organization (see i. 264, *note*). Perhaps the most striking exemplification of this truth is to be found in the vascular system, the different conditions of which, presented by different classes of vertebrate animals, during the different periods of their development, represent each link of a continuous chain of developments, extending from the lowest animalcules up through the invertebrate genera, to fish, tadpoles, amphibia, and finally to man. As it would be impossible, however, in the brief compass of a note, to trace these various and highly curious transformations through all their stages, and the means by which they are effected, I beg leave to refer the curious reader to Prof. Carus's Comp. Anat., *tr.* by Mr. R. T. Gore; Prof. Grant's Lect. on Comp. Anat. (*Lancet*, 1833–4. vol. ii.); Rolando, Sur la formation du Cœur et des vaisseaux artériels, veineux et capillaires (*Journ. Compl. du Dict. des Sc. Méd.*, xi. 323. xii. 34.); Pander, Mém. sur le devel. du Poulet dans l'Œuf (*ib.* xiv. 306.); Rusconi's different works on the larva of the salamander and common frog; and also to the labours of Weber, Meckel, Martin St. Ange, and Cuvier. A brief description of these changes as they occur in man may be found in Meckel's Manuel d'Anatomie, *tr.* by Jourdan and Breschet, i. 143.]

exercise, does it, or does it not also dilate and contract more fully, and also act with greater velocity in its contraction? I believe that all these circumstances take place; for in exercise, the pulse not only becomes more frequent, but fuller, as if more was thrown out of the heart; and the heart is found to make a greater emotion in the chest, striking with its apex against the inside of the chest with greater force*, which can only arise from a greater quantity being thrown out, and with greater velocity. The breathing corresponds with the quantity of blood and the velocity, for if a larger quantity passes through the lungs in a given time, the breathing must be in the same proportion increased; if with a greater velocity, the same thing must necessarily take place; and if a greater quantity is thrown out, and with a greater velocity, then the arteries must relax in proportion, since the different parts must correspond with each other: we must suppose, therefore, that in health, whenever there is any exertion greater than common, (which always increases the pulse,) the heart dilates more, contracts more, and does both with greater velocity; this I conceive arises from a necessity, which begins first in the veins, for when the body is in action the blood in the veins is obliged to move with greater velocity than when at rest: how far there may be other reasons for this, I will not pretend to determine.

Another question naturally arises: as we find that the times of repetition of the pulse or the actions of the heart increase in many diseases, does the same thing happen, that is above supposed to arise, from exercise in health? viz. does the heart dilate more, contract more, and also contract with more velocity? I believe this case does not in the least correspond with our former position. The pulse in such circumstances, although frequent, is small and hard, showing the arteries to be too much contracted by their muscular power, and therefore unfit to

* The reason why the apex of the heart strikes against the chest in its actions was, I believe, first accounted for by the late Dr. William Hunter, in his lectures, as far back as the year 1746. The systole and diastole of the heart simply, could not produce such an effect; nor could it have been produced if it had thrown the blood into a straight tube, in the direction of the axis of the left ventricle, as is the case with the ventricles of fish, and some other classes of animals; but by its throwing the blood into a curved tube, viz. the aorta, that artery at its curve endeavours to throw itself into a straight line to increase its capacity; but the aorta being the fixed point against the back, and the heart in some degree loose or pendulous, the influence of its own action is thrown upon itself, and it is tilted forwards against the inside of the chest[a].

[a] [The above explanation is correct as far as it goes; but the cause assigned is not the only one why the heart strikes with its apex against the ribs at the moment of contraction. The direction of the mass of its fibres is also concerned, which tends to tilt the apex forwards, as may clearly be proved by placing the heart of any animal in a state of action on a plane surface, when it will be found that the apex moves forwards, although the base is comparatively stationary.]

receive a large quantity of blood from the heart in any given time. The breathing does not correspond with the frequency of the pulsations, as in the former instance; yet it is possible that nearly the same quantity of blood may pass as when in health, the velocity in the contracted state of the heart and vessels making up for the increased size of the artery. That it moves faster in such state of vessels is, I think, probable; for in bleeding, the blood in the veins during such a state of vessels is commonly more florid.

Observations upon the heart's motion while under the influence of artificial breathing.

1. I observed that the auricles contracted but very little, so that they did not nearly empty themselves.

2. That the ventricles were not turgid at the time of their diastole, for I could feel them soft, and could easily compress them.

3. That the ventricles became hard at the time of their systole.

4. That the heart, when it ceased to act, became nearly twice as large as when acting, and that it recovered its small size again whenever it began to act[a].

Observations on the above appearances.—From the *first* observation, it would appear that the auricles are only reservoirs, capable of holding a much larger quantity than is necessary for filling the ventricles at any one time, in order that the ventricles may always have blood ready to

---

[a] [I subjoin the following extract from my friend Dr. Hope's Treatise on Diseases of the Heart, p. 28, which places this subject in a clear point of view. The experiments from which the following conclusions were drawn were performed on an ass, and attested by competent witnesses:

"*Of the Motions of the Heart.*

1. "The auricles contract so immediately before the ventricles, that the one motion is propagated into the other, almost as if by continuity of action; yet the motion is not so quick that it cannot readily be traced by the eye.

2. "The extent of the auricular contraction is very inconsiderable, probably not amounting to one third of its volume. Hence the quantity of blood expelled by it into the ventricle is much less than its capacity would indicate.

3. "The ventricular contraction is the cause of the impulse against the side; first, because the auricular contraction is too inconsiderable to be capable of producing it; secondly, because the impulse occurs after the auricular contraction, and simultaneously with the ventricular, as ascertained by the sight and touch; thirdly, because the impulse coincides with the pulse so accurately as not to admit of being ascribed to any but the same cause.

4. "It is the apex of the heart which strikes the ribs.

5. "The ventricular contraction commences suddenly; but it is prolonged until an instant before the second sound, which instant is occupied by the ventricular diastole.

6. "The ventricles do not appear ever to empty themselves completely.

7. "The systole is followed by a diastole, which is an instantaneous motion, accom-

fill them. From observation the *fourth*, it would appear that any idea we form of the size of a heart, from those in dead bodies, must be far from the truth; for the blood coming from every part of the body to the heart, in some measure distends it while it is in a relaxed state, so that when the heart begins to contract (as muscles do some time after death), it is kept dilated by the contained blood[a]. However, it may be

---

panied with an influx of blood from the auricles, by which the ventricles re-expand, but the apex collapses and retires from the side.

8. "After the diastole the ventricles remain quiescent, and in a state of apparently natural fulness, until again stimulated by the succeeding auricular contraction.

"*Of the Sounds**.

9. "The first sound is caused by the systole of the ventricles.

10. "The second sound is occasioned by the diastole of the ventricles.

"*Of the Rhythm.*

11. "Order of succession:

"1. The auricular systole.

"2. The ventricular systole—pulse and impulse.

"3. The ventricular diastole.

"4. The interval of ventricular repose, towards the termination of which the auricular systole takes place.

"*Duration.*

12. "This is the same as indicated by Laennec, viz.

"The ventricular systole occupies half the time, or thereabout, of a whole beat.

"The ventricular diastole occupies one fourth, or at most one third.

"The interval of repose occupies one fourth, or rather less.

"The auricular systole occupies a portion of the interval of repose."

With regard to the double sound, which, it may be observed, is distinctly isochronous with the systole and diastole of the ventricles, various opinions have been entertained; nor indeed can the question be considered as perfectly decided at the present moment. Thus, the *first* sound has been variously ascribed to the rush of blood into the great arteries, to the closing of the auriculo-ventricular valves, to the muscular contraction of the heart, and to the collision of the particles of fluid in the ventricles. The *second* sound has also been ascribed to the reaction of the arterial columns of blood against the semilunar valves, thus suddenly tightening these bodies; and to the impulse of the blood from the auricles refilling the ventricles. (*See Path. and Diag. of Diseases of the Chest, 3rd edit.* p. 163., *by Dr. C. J. B. Williams; Mr. Turner in Med. Chir. Trs. of Edin.*, iii.*; Dr. Corrigan in Trs. of King's and Queen's Coll. of Phys. of Ireland* (*New Series*), i. 151.*; M. Majendie in Lancet*, 1834 5. i.*; and Mr. Carlile in Dubl. Journ. of Med. Sc.*, iv. 84.)]

a [This observation applies particularly to the right or pulmonic side of the heart, which was hence incorrectly concluded by Haller to be $\frac{2}{7}$ths more capacious than the left. The left cavities are generally found nearly empty after death; but during life it is probable that both ventricles have the same capacity. It is certain that they project the same quantity of blood in a given time, and therefore, if one is larger than another it must empty itself less perfectly at each systole.]

---

* The sound which is heard when the ear is applied to the region of the heart of a healthy person, is double, consisting of a dull slow sound, immediately followed by a short quick one.

observed, that the increased size of the heart would be less in the present case, than natural, for the very quick motion of this viscus, under this irritation, hindered a full diastole; but when I left off blowing, and the heart ceased acting, it became large; and on resuming my artificial breathing, it again became small, which I did three times in the course of this experiment. But I think I have observed in general that the heart is not so much affected by the stimulus of death as the other muscles of the body. We seldom see a dead body that is not stiff; but we very often find the heart large and flabby, and not in the least contracted; and I am not certain but this may be the case also with some of the other vital parts, as the stomach and intestines.

It is to be set down as a principle, that the action of every muscle is alternate contraction and relaxation; and it cannot be otherwise; but as there is a necessity for a more constant and regular motion in the heart than probably in any of the other muscles, more disputes have arisen about the cause of its regular alternate motion. Some have accounted for it from the position of the mouths of the coronary arteries respecting the valves of the aorta, supposing, erroneously, that the heart has its blood in the time of its relaxation*; but the circulation, whether existing or not, has not such immediate effect upon a muscle; nor would it account for the action of the auricle in the same animal, nor for the action of the heart in a fish; but from what we shall observe on the valves of the aorta, we shall find that this opinion immediately falls to the ground. An easy experiment may put this beyond a doubt; for if the heart of a dog be laid open, and the coronary artery wounded, it will be found to jet out its blood as the aorta distends. Others have accounted for the alternate motion of the heart, from the course of its nerves passing between the two great arteries, so as to be compressed when the arteries are dilated; but this could only produce relaxation. We know, too, that such immediate compression on a nerve has no such immediate effect upon a muscle, not to say that it would most probably make it contract; for when the nerves of the heart are cut, this does not stop its motion, but rather makes it contract for the instant. The heart's motion does not arise from an immediate impulse from the brain, as it does in the voluntary muscles; and as it is only in the quadruped and bird that the nerves can be influenced in their passage to it, it does not account for this alternate motion in other classes of animals. The flowing of the blood into the heart has been assigned as a cause of its contraction; but even that will not account for it, although it will

* This will be readily understood when I come to explain the mode of action in the valves of the arteries.

for many of its phenomena, yet not for all, for a local stimulus merely is too mechanical to produce all the variety attending the action of this viscus; it would not be attended with that regularity which it has in health, nor that irregularity which we find in disease; neither could it ever stop, unless when absolute death took place; nor resume its action if it ever did stop. We find that those parts which have occasion for the immediate stimulus to produce action, have that action very irregular, as, for instance, the bladder of urine and intestines. The bladder is taking up its action as simply for itself, and not secondarily, however beneficial that might be for the whole in a secondary degree; but the heart's actions arise from its being so much part of the whole, as that the whole immediately depends upon it; therefore we must look out for another cause of this regular alternate action of the heart than that arising from mechanism or mechanical impression; something more immediately connected with the general laws of the animal œconomy.

The alternate contraction and relaxation of the heart constitutes a part of the circulation; and the whole takes place in consequence of a necessity, the constitution demanding it, and becoming the stimulus. It is rather, therefore, the want of repletion, which makes a negative impression on the constitution, which becomes the stimulus, than the immediate impression of something applied to the heart.

This we see to be the case wherever a constant supply, or some kind of aid, is wanted in consequence of some action; we have as regularly the stimulus for respiration, the moment one is finished, an immediate demand taking place; and if prevented (as this action is under the influence of the will), the stimulus of want is increased. We have the stimulus of want of food, which takes place regularly in health; and so it is with the circulation. The heart, we find, cannot rest one stroke, but the constitution feels it; even the mind and the heart is thereby stimulated to action. The constant want in the constitution of this action in the heart, is as much as the constant action of the spring of a clock is to its pendulum, all hanging or depending on each other[a].

[a] [This is another of those instances in which the author has mistaken the final for the proximate cause. The feeling of hunger is obviously not the cause of the action of the muscles of deglutition, nor the sense of present danger the cause of a man's changing his position; neither is "want of repletion" the immediate cause of the heart's action. The final cause it may be, but it cannot be the immediate.

In treating the question of the heart's action, two points require consideration: 1st, what is the source whence the muscular fibres of this organ derive their susceptibility of alternate contraction and relaxation; 2nd, what is the immediate cause which excites them to action.

I. With regard to the first of these points, though physiologists have, with few exceptions, attributed this susceptibility to nervous influence, they have differed greatly

The nearest dependence of the heart is upon the lungs, and probably they have the same upon the heart. The two together become, in their

---

respecting the portion of that system under the controul of which they have supposed the heart to be placed.

The most ancient opinion was, that the heart, like the other muscles of the body, was under the dominion of the brain; but the well-known facts, that acephalous fœtuses continue to live and grow, that the circulation may be kept up by the aid of artificial respiration for several hours after decapitation, and that in some reptiles the whole brain may be removed in successive layers without affecting the heart's action, have caused this opinion to be now generally abandoned.

According to a second opinion, which originated with Legallois, the actions of the heart depend on the brain and spinal chord, but with this difference in respect of common muscles, namely, "that the heart derives its power from *all* parts of the spinal chord, without exception; whilst on the other hand, each part of the body besides derives its power only from a *single* part of the chord,—that, namely, from which it receives its nerves." This conclusion was drawn from experiments on frogs, in which the brain and spinal marrow were wholly destroyed by means of a wire introduced through an opening into the cranium. In these experiments the heart's action was entirely suspended for a few seconds, and though it recovèred itself again after a short period, yet the rhythm was so altered, and the action so feeble, that no hæmorrhage ensued on decapitation, or amputation of the thighs, from which he hastily inferred, that this resumed action essentially differed from what occurs naturally, and in fact resembled the action of muscles which are irritated after death. If a part only of the brain or spinal marrow was destroyed or broken down, then the action of the heart was only enfeebled, and that in exact proportion to the amount of destruction.

Dr. Wilson Philip repeated and varied these experiments of Legallois, and ascertained that the spinal marrow may be cautiously removed without affecting the action of the heart; but that if this destruction be effected suddenly, as by crushing, then the action of the heart and vessels is immediately enfeebled, or else totally destroyed. He also found that the heart was highly susceptible of being affected by substances applied to the brain or spinal marrow, such as alcohol, opium, &c.; and hence concluded, that though there is no *necessary* connexion in the way of cause and effect between the influence of the nervous centres and the motions of the heart, yet that an intimate relation exists between them. Dr. Marshall Hall has however shown, that similar effects are produced on the heart when other parts of the body are subjected to similar treatment; that alcohol, or infusion of opium, affects the heart equally when applied to the external skin, as when applied to the brain, and that the heart's action is equally arrested by crushing the stomach, or even the extremities, as by crushing the brain or spinal marrow; and he therefore objects to Dr. W. Philip's conclusions. Examples, indeed, of this kind occur continually to the surgeon, in which the effect of a severe crushing injury to an extremity sinks the powers of the circulation beyond recovery, although amputation of the same part might have been performed with impunity.

M. Flourens admits that the spino-cerebral system, especially that part of it which administers to respiration, is necessary, to give energy and duration to the circulation; but he does not believe that this function is essentially and immediately dependent on the influence of these nerves, from the impossibility of reconciling such an opinion with the fact of the circulation going on in decapitated and acephalous animals.

The want, then, of such a connexion between the spino-cerebral system and heart as is found to subsist between the former and the system of voluntary muscles, has led to the adoption, by some physiologists, of a third opinion, namely, that the actions of

immediate use, interwoven with the whole, for a stoppage of respiration produces a stoppage of circulation, and a restoration of respiration pro-

---

the heart are dependent on the influence of the ganglionic system. This opinion is less capable of being proved or disproved than either of the others, in consequence of the extreme difficulty of separating the heart from its connexions, or at least all the nerves from the heart; so that though the heart of a turtle, apparently detached from its connexions, and completely removed from the body, will sometimes continue to beat for nearly an hour, yet we cannot be certain that this action does not depend more or less on the nervous filaments which enter into its substance.

Sir Charles Bell has moulded these various opinions in accordance with his own peculiar views of the nervous system, making the ordinary action of the heart to depend on the ganglionic system, but its connexion with the respiratory and sensorial functions to be derived through the cerebro-spinal nerves or par vagum; but it must be obvious that such an hypothesis is open to several of the objections urged against the opinions just stated.

Not satisfied with any of the above-mentioned views, Mr. Herbert Mayo has offered an entirely different explanation of the matter. Finding that the natural state of the voluntary muscles, in the absence of any special stimuli, is that of permanent relaxation or contraction,—that when irritated, they contract by a single and momentary effort, and when divided, instantly retract; that the involuntary muscles, on the contrary, retract slowly and gradually when divided, and when mechanically stimulated take on not one, but a series of actions,—he argues that the natural state of the latter class is that of alternate relaxation and contraction, and that consequently no special stimulus is required to induce a succession of actions in these parts. "For the brief period," he observes, "during which it is reasonable to suppose that the heart retains its perfect organization, no stimulus seems required to excite it to contract. The alternation of action and repose seems to be natural to its irritable fibre, or to be the immediate result of its structure; they appear not, like similar phenomena in the diaphragm, to depend upon a series of impressions transmitted from the brain or spinal chord."

There are some facts which seem to favour this view, and indeed to lead to the belief that incitability and contractility are properties inherent in and peculiar to muscular fibre totally independent of the nervous system, and that in fact the actual relation of this system to the muscular is that of supplying the stimulus to and regulating the actions of the latter in obedience to the necessities, exterior and organic, of the constitution; for, 1st, there is no proportion between the degree of contractility enjoyed by different muscles and the number and quantity of their nerves; while, 2nd, local forms of paralysis sometimes occur in which no agent, either electrical or galvanic, can induce contractions in the part, although the nerves going to that part are completely unchanged. In fact, those parts which possess the smallest number of nerves, as the heart, the intestines, the stomach, &c., are uniformly found to retain the power of spontaneous contraction after death for the longest period of time, while even the voluntary muscles are obedient to the same law, and retain their contractile property much longer where the animal has been stunned previously to the experiment being made.

The connexion, however, which exists between the due supply of nervous influence and the power of contraction in the muscles, is so intimate as scarcely to allow us on these grounds to consider them in any other light than as cause and effect; and one of the most weighty objections to Mr. Mayo's hypothesis is, that it obliges us either to consider the former as not essential to the latter in the case of the muscles generally, or to draw a stronger line of distinction between the causes of action of the voluntary and involuntary muscles than seems in nature to exist.

It appears to me that we have not yet a sufficient number of data on which to decide

duces a restoration of the circulation or heart's motion. Thus, in my experiments on artificial breathing, the heart soon ceased acting whenever I left off acting with my bellows; and upon renewing my artificial breathing, it, in a very short time, renewed its action, first by slow degrees, but became quicker and quicker till it came to its full action.

I believe this experiment cannot be reversed; we cannot make an

---

this question. The heart's action has been maintained by means of artificial respiration for upwards of two hours and a half after decapitation; and even acephalous fœtuses have survived their birth several days: yet the experiments of Dr. Marshall Hall seem to warrant the conclusion that the heart's actions ultimately derive their energy from the cerebral masses, and cannot be maintained for any permanency after their removal, the circulation gradually failing from the periphery to the centre. Although, therefore, the heart is first in the order of development, and undoubtedly ranks supreme among the vital organs in complete life—so that we should not expect it to be essentially dependent on any other—yet we have reason for believing that it is governed by all the laws which regulate the relations of similarly important organs, as well as all the laws which preside over the actions of similarly constructed parts.

To whatever opinion we may come respecting the dependence of the muscular fibres of the heart on the nervous system for their power of contraction, we can scarcely doubt that the nerves are the immediate agents through which the appropriate stimulus of the heart, namely, the blood, operates on these fibres, and excites them to action; and it may be, that this is their chief use in the ordinary actions of the heart.

II. The second point to determine is, what is the immediate stimulus of the heart's action? We have seen that the turtle's or frog's heart may continue to beat for a full hour after it is detached from the body and entirely deprived of blood, and that a sturgeon's heart pulsated regularly for ten hours under the same circumstances (p. 123, *note*); but is it not probable that these actions depended on habit operating on a class of animals whose tenacity of life is extraordinary? Under common circumstances it cannot be doubted that the heart, like every other organ, requires a special stimulus conveyed through the nerves to continue its action. Incitability and stimulus are correlative terms in physiological argument, and necessarily imply one another; and therefore to ascribe with Hunter the action of the heart to a negative impression, arising from a want of repletion in the constitution, appears to me to be perfectly contrary to the spirit of sound philosophy. There can, I think, be no doubt that arterial blood, circulating among the fibres of the heart, is necessary to maintain the incitability of this organ; but it is the *distension* produced by the returning blood, irrespective altogether of its quality, which is the sole stimulus of its action. The experiments of Bichat sufficiently established this fact; which is I think still further confirmed by the observation of Laennec, viz. that the ventricles during their state of repose and fulness (which occupies one third of the time between one beat and another) do not take on their action until the auricular systole commences, or in other words until the utmost degree of distension is produced in the ventricles. See *note*, p. 78;—also *An Essay on the Circulation, by Marshall Hall, M.D.;—Expériences sur la Circulation, by Spallanzani, tr. par J. Tourdes;—On the Vital and Involuntary Motions, &c., by R. Whytt, M.D.;—On the Vital Functions, by Wilson Philip, M.D.;—Du Système Nerveux, par M. Flourens;—Mém. de l'Institut, tom.* x.*;—Expériences sur le Principe de la Vie, par M. Le Gallois;—On the Influence of the Brain on the Action of the Heart, by Sir B. C. Brodie, Phil. Trans.* 1811. *p.* 36;—*Sur la Vie et la Mort, par X. Bichat;*—and *Outlines of Physiology, by H. Mayo.*]

artificial circulation, so as to know, that if we stopped the heart's motion, we should so readily stop respiration; and on producing the heart's motion, respiration would again take place; but if we could do this, I doubt very much its being attended with equal success, because I believe that in all deaths respiration stops first; however, it must be supposed, that if the heart stopped for any length of time, respiration would also stop; and if I were to take the following case as proof, it would appear that respiration would not go on without the heart's motion.

A gentleman[a] was attacked with a pain in the situation of the pylorus. The pain was such as indicated its seat to be in the nerves of the stomach and its connexions. It was such as he could hardly bear. The other attending symptom was a total stoppage in the actions of the heart, and of course the face was pale and ghastly. Not the least signs of motion in the heart could be felt. In this state he was about three quarters of an hour. He was attended by Dr. Hunter, Sir George Baker, Sir William Fordyce, and Dr. Huck Saunders. As he was perfectly sensible at the time, and could perform every voluntary action, he observed that he was not breathing, which astonished him; and at first conceiving he must die if he did not breathe, he performed the act of breathing voluntarily. This shows that breathing depends on the actions of the heart; and it also shows, that under certain circumstances the actions of both may be suspended, and yet death not be the consequence: as he spoke while in this fit, without attending to his breathing, it shows that the breathing which produces sound is voluntary; and if we had only the power of involuntary breathing, then probably we could not speak, for it is probable we could not regulate the action of the glottis and tongue (which are voluntary) to so regular an action of the lungs; for in speaking it is the one acting so as to correspond with the other, both becoming voluntary. A gentleman had a singular asthmatic affection, and his breathing gradually stopt and again gradually recovered, but became violent, and this constantly and alternately held two or three minutes; and when the breathing ceased yet he spoke, although but faintly.

In those animals which have two ventricles, it has been asserted by some that their actions are alternate; but observation and experiment show us that the two auricles contract together, and that the two ventricles also contract together. This can be observed by simply looking on the heart in its actions, and if we in that state make a puncture into the pulmonary artery and the aorta, we shall find the jet in both at the same instant, corresponding with the contractions of the ventricles.

---

[a] [The author here refers to what happened to himself. See *Life*, i. 44.]

Indeed the circulation in the fœtus is a proof of it, for in the child there would otherwise be two pulsations instead of one.

This alternate motion of the heart is quicker in some classes of animals than others, in some being extremely quick, in others very slow. In all the more inferior orders of animals I believe it is the slowest; and this may probably be in some degree in proportion to their imperfection. It is also slower probably in each class in proportion to the size, and we know it is slower in each species in some degree in proportion to the size, although not nearly exactly so. The pulse is also found to be quicker in the young than in the old of each species, in greater proportion than what we find arising from size only. Thus the motion of the heart of a caterpillar is extremely slow, and also of a snail. The motion of the heart in fish is not frequent; and we know it is extremely slow in the amphibia; but in those possessed of two ventricles, as in birds and quadrupeds, the motion of this viscus is much quicker: in them, too, it differs very much, in proportion to their size, although not nearly in the same proportion. Thus, a horse's pulse is about thirty-six in a minute, while a man's is about seventy. In the same species it is nearly of equal quickness; for in a man three feet high the pulse was eighty, while a man above eight feet high had a pulse about seventy.

§. 6. *General Observations on Blood-vessels.*

By the vessels in an animal are commonly understood those canals which carry the juices of the body, called the blood of the animal, to and from the heart, for the immediate purposes of the animal œconomy; and in those animals where no heart is to be found, yet vessels are found, though their uses are not so demonstrable; and in some of a still more inferior order, where no vessels can be demonstrated, yet, from analogy, canals may be supposed to exist, and those should still be called vessels*.

* Of this I am not certain. I have an idea that some animals absorb their nourishment, even without action, somewhat similar to a sponge, but dispose of it immediately by converting it into their own increase[a]

---

[a] [Ellis, the celebrated zoophytologist and a contemporary of Hunter, believed that he saw motions or actions in the mouths of the sponge analogous to those in the mouths of polypes; but it is now generally believed that he was deceived and that the ingestive orifices are passive, and that so far as they are concerned the nourishment is absorbed in the sponge, as Hunter states, without action. By what mechanism within the nutrient canals of the sponge the currents which perpetually traverse them are produced has never been determined: analogy points to the vibratile action of extremely minute

The vascular system in an animal is, in some degree, to be considered as the efficient part of the whole animal respecting itself, every other part of the body being more or less subservient to it, and depending upon it for existence and support; and therefore the greatest attention should be paid to every circumstance that can possibly explain the various uses of the vessels, for there is no operation respecting the internal œconomy of the animal but is performed by them, insomuch, that for the convenience of the vessels in performing those peculiar actions, they seem to constitute various combinations, which are called organs*. And although many parts have actions independent of the vessels, yet these are not for the purposes of growth, support, etc. So that the vessels are constructed for the immediate use of the machine, and may be called labourers in the machine. This naturally implies something that is not vessel or vessels, a something that constitutes the different parts of the body, and is only more or less vascular. The vessels are probably the very first active parts in the system, for we find them in action before they have formed themselves into a heart, and in such a state of parts we find them the only part that has any strength, while the other parts are only preparing for action: this is so remarkable, that we can dissect the vessels of a chicken in the egg without injection, the other parts easily giving way. These parts are formed of living animal matter, so composed as to constitute the different structures, fitted for their different uses, in the machine; yet some parts are so vascular as to appear almost to consist wholly of vessels, as if vessels were formed into such structures; but this we cannot conceive, for then they must lose the action of vessels.

In those animals where the vascular system is connected with a heart, which may be called the termination as well as origin of the vessels, we find that viscus to make so material a part of this system

* Perhaps it may be difficult to give a definition of an organ that will meet every one's ideas, or will distinguish those bodies accurately from what may be said not to be an organ. A muscle may be called an organ, but I would only consider it among the materials of which an organ is composed. I have the same idea of elastic substances, cellular membrane, bone, cartilage, etc.

I would, at present, define an organ to be a part of a particular construction, composed of a variety of substances, [elementary structures,] which are combined together to answer some particular purpose, which is the result of the actions of the whole.

---

cilia as the cause. With respect to the canals which are continued from the stomach, and which convey by their ramifications the alimentary fluid directly to the parenchyma of the animal, these are beautifully exhibited by means of coloured injections in some of the parenchymatous Entozoa and the Medusæ in the preparations Nos. 843—848 in the Gallery of the Hunterian Collection.]

as to require particular attention. In many of these animals we find two systems of vessels, the arteries and veins, and most probably they exist in all of them; there is also a third, which consists of the absorbents. The heart is the source of the arteries, and the termination of the veins and absorbents. The two first, depending on each other, form the circulation; and the third is essential to both, bringing the materials which are to circulate*.

The arteries are to be considered as the acting part of the vascular system, since they perform a variety of actions the uses of which are very important in the animal œconomy. They may be called universal or constitutional, for their actions are immediately productive of health or disease in the constitution; and if they could be diseased as a system, that disease would of course be universal: as their actions are expressive of health or disease, they become also one means of discovering either.

There is no internal operation in the machine, respecting growth, natural repair, and secretion, that is not performed by them. No new part is formed, nor additional alteration made in the structure of natural parts, nor repair for the loss of natural substances, either by disease or accident, but is made by the arteries, although of all these operations we know nothing but from the effect produced. These operations are performed by the termination of the arteries, which may be supposed to be of three kinds: one may be called arterial, conveying debilitated blood into the veins, and through their whole length may be called arteries; another kind consists of the separaters from the blood, performing the different secretions; and the third contains the formers and supporters of the body: the two latter kinds I should not call arteries; they are the workers, or labourers[a].

* This system is too extensive to be described in the present work, although it will be necessary to describe one use not hitherto attributed to it, as it explains one part of my system of disease.

[The only evident termination of arteries is into capillaries, carrying red blood, which are plainly distinguishable from any other set of vessels, as well by their uniformity of size as by the peculiarity of their mode of division and reunion. The arteries pursue a straight course, and up to a certain period are observed to divide and redivide in a regular series of bifurcating divisions; the blood always flowing from trunk to branch, and the branch being uniformly found to be smaller than the trunk. After a certain period, however, the artery is observed to break abruptly into an irregular network of vessels, consisting of an intricate interlacement of capillary tubes of uniform cylindrical diameter, which divide and redivide, unite and reunite by an infinite number of anastomoses, presenting, especially in the pulmonic circulation of some of the batrachian animals, a beautiful and splendid device. The current of blood in these vessels is probably more than twice as slow as in the smallest arteries, but in

The absorbing system also takes a very active part in the animal œconomy, whether natural or diseased, and seems in many actions to

---

consequence of the extremely devious and intricate course which it takes, it is next to impossible to follow any single globule through the mazes of its route into the veins: which veins again, I may observe, are formed by a re-collection of these tubes into the venous radicles, which uniting by twos and twos, in the reverse order of the arteries, ultimately form the venous trunks.

The venous radicles are not unfrequently observed to anastomose with each other, but rarely or never the minute arteries; neither is it ever observed that these latter terminate directly in the veins, but the transition is uniformly effected through the interposition of a capillary structure, which is proportionally more developed in the lungs than in the other parts of the body. In the arteries the blood is of a lighter colour than in the veins, and has a much greater velocity of motion; but in the capillaries the colour and velocity of the blood are uniformly the same, although the slightest disturbing causes are sufficient to make it flow faster or slower, or even to take a retrograde course where before it took a forward direction. In an unimpeded state of the circulation the pulsation is barely visible in the arteries, and not very distinctly so in the capillaries; but it may be rendered distinctly so in both, as well as in the veins, by impeding the course of the blood, by which the tension is increased so as even to produce a remarkable oscillation of the globules. I have seen the globules advance and retire over a space at least twenty times their own length at each pulsation of the heart, and this for an unlimited length of time. One reason, I imagine, that the pulsation is not more visible in the minute vessels in the natural state of the circulation is, that our senses are unable to appreciate the differences of velocity of bodies in very rapid or very slow motion; a cannon ball passing before our eyes at the rate of twenty miles an hour appears to go at the same rate as one at sixty miles, just as the hour-hand of a watch would still appear to go at the same rate as if it went twice as slow. Now as the actual area of the artery comprised in the focus of a high magnifying power is extremely small, at the same time that the apparent rapidity of the current is proportionally increased, the difference between the velocities in the systole and diastole of the heart is not perceptible. The difference in the degree of tension is certainly not the only cause of the difference in the degree of pulsation.

I have said that the arteries never directly communicate with the veins, but always through a vascular network; and this is strictly true in all warm-blooded animals, in which the systems of black and scarlet blood are preserved distinct. In inferior animals, however, as fish, the Batrachia, and even in the embryos of warm-blooded animals, as, *e.g.*, in the chick during the first days of incubation, such communications are found to exist, because in these instances it is not of the same importance to keep these systems apart. The term capillary therefore ought exclusively to be applied to this intermediate system of vessels, which appears essentially to differ both in function and distribution from any other parts of the vascular system. See *Schultz, in Journ. de Progrès des Sc. Méd.*, vii. 1828, and *Dr. Marshall Hall's Essay on the Circulation*, 1831.

Besides this visible system of capillaries, there can scarcely be any doubt that another system (invisible in consequence of its not admitting red globules) also exists. It is impossible otherwise to explain the nutrition of white structures, such as cartilage, the tunics of the eye, &c., or the phenomena of inflammation, when these structures become inflamed. The appearance which these colourless vessels assume when they become enlarged leads us to believe that they are similarly arranged as the coloured capillaries, and it is not improbable that all the processes of nutrition are carried on in these vessels. Haller and Bichat, and indeed most other physiological authorities, have superbe the antagonist of the arteries; while the veins are much more passive, being principally employed in returning the blood to the heart.

It is probable that every part of the body is equally vascular, although they may not all have equal quantities of blood passing through them, which must arise from the smallness of the vessels, and not from their being fewer in number. When we say that a part is very vascular, we can only mean that it is visibly so, by having a large vessel or vessels going to it, and ramifying in it; from which circumstance it contains a certain proportion of red blood, rendering the vessels visible, which may also easily be made conspicuous by injections. Where the vessels are smaller this is not the case. When we say, therefore, that a part is not vascular, we mean it is not visibly so; but still we must suppose such parts to be equally vascular, so far as respects their œconomy within themselves; but in such parts I conceive the blood to be more languid in its motion. Many parts appear to be much more vascular than they really are, from their vessels dividing and anastomosing, and taking a winding course before they terminate*; for it is by the number of terminations of an artery in a given space that a part is made vascular or not vascular: muscles appear to be more vascular than they really are. When parts have another use, in which blood furnishes the materials to be disposed of, as in secretion and respiration, where vessels fitted for such purposes are superadded, then parts become proportionably more vascular. When blood does not seem to be the matter to be disposed of, yet, if there are other operations continually carried on in a part, besides its simple support, as in a muscle, which has both the power of contraction and considerable sensation, &c., then the vessels are larger, and of course appear in great numbers. This is evident in the living body, for if a muscle is hardly allowed to act, its vessels become small, and it becomes pale; but if thrown into more violent action for a continuance, it becomes red: we cannot here suppose an increase of vessels, but only an increase of size. Thus we have parts vascular in proportion to the quantity of action they are capable

* By simply cutting into the spermatic artery [chord ?] of a bull it appears to be extremely vascular, though, according to our idea of vascularity, it is as little so as any part.

---

added two other terminations to the arteries, viz. the exhalant and excreting vessels; especially as in the liver, kidneys, and some other glands, injections may be made to pass from the arteries or veins into the excretory ducts. I am not aware, however, of any single fact to show that there is more reason in favour of the exhalant and excreting vessels of Bichat than of the lateral porosities of Mascagni. This doctrine may be true, or it may not be true; but it certainly cannot be recognised at present as one of the undoubted facts of science. The same may be said of the "workers, or labourers," of Mr. Hunter.]

of or under the necessity of performing: and this particularly in parts whose uses may be called double, as the organs of secretion in general, brain, and muscles; even in inflammation, and in proportion as these parts are employed in their peculiar actions, they become to appearance more vascular.

Some animals have naturally red muscles, without its being the effect of considerable action: this is very remarkable in the hare; but the redness in the muscles of this animal may be intended to adapt its muscles naturally for violent exertions at all times. Muscles are of different colours, respecting red and white, in the same animal; but that I believe is also in proportion to the quantity of action the parts are put to. This effect the epicure is well acquainted with: he knows that the wing of a partridge is whiter than the leg, and that the leg of a woodcock is whiter than the wing. The veal of this country is a remarkable instance of this: for the calf is hardly allowed to stir, and the muscles are white; but when the calf is allowed to follow its mother, the muscles are of a reddish colour. It may be, however, remarked that white meat is commonly the least juicy; and we find it remarkably so in those animals which are fed for this purpose, because they require nothing but their simple support, and, having little or no action within themselves, they have but little waste. Such change of appearance we find carried to a considerable extent in the uterus at the time of the menses; but much more particularly at the time of uterine gestation, where the vessels increase both in size and length, in proportion to the actions required. But parts whose use in the machine may be said to be passive, as tendon, cellular membrane, ligaments, investing membrane, bone, and cartilage (which last is probably the most passive), have all small vessels, and of course but few that are visible. As bone, however, is composed of two parts, viz. animal substance and earth, it is probable there may be more action required to form the latter than either tendon or cartilage, and therefore there will be more vessels.

As a further proof that this is a general principle, we find that all growing parts are much more vascular than those that are come to their full growth; because growth is an operation beyond the simple support of the part. This is the reason why young animals are more vascular than those that are full-grown. This is not peculiar to the natural operation of growth, but applies also to disease and restoration. Parts become vascular in inflammation: the callus, granulations, and new-formed cutis are much more vascular in the growing state, or when just formed, than afterwards; for we see them crowded with blood-vessels when growing, but when full-grown they begin to lose their visible vessels, and become not even so vascular as in the neighbouring original parts, only retaining a sufficient number of vessels to carry on the simple œconomy of the part, which would now seem to be less than in an original part. This is known by injections, when parts are in the growing state, or are just grown, and for some time after. We may observe when the smallpox is cured that the remains of the pustules are red and continue so for some time, which is owing to those parts being visibly more vascular than common; and those who have had the smallpox severely are in general afterwards more pale than others, when those parts have arrived at their permanent state. If we cut into a part that has had a wound or sore upon it which has been healed for a considerable time, we shall find that the cicatrix and the new-formed parts are not nearly so vascular as the original, which corresponds with what has been advanced, for we know that those parts are not equal in power to original parts. In short, whenever Nature has considerable operations going on, and those are rapid, then we find the vascular system in a proportionable degree enlarged.

The number of vessels in a part, and also the circulation of the blood through them, appear to keep pace with its sensibility; for first we find that most probably all parts endowed with vessels are sensible, and all sensible parts are to appearance very vascular. Where any increased action is going on, requiring increased sensibility, there is also an increased circulation through those vessels, as in the parts of generation during the time of coition, more especially in the female; and this increase of vessels, circulation, and sensibility in a part takes place in disease; as is well illustrated in inflammation, where the whole seems to be increased in the same proportion, especially the two last, viz. circulation and sensibility.

These observations can only be made in animals which have red blood, and best in those which have the most red blood; but it is not possible to ascertain with accuracy the proportion that one blood-vessel bears to another, so as to know the exact quantity of blood each part may possess, which would better ascertain the action of the part; for they may be said not to be measurable with any degree of accuracy, and therefore such calculations must be taken in the gross.

Vessels have a power of increase within themselves both in diameter and length, which is according to the necessity, whether natural or diseased. The necessity appears to arise from an increase of the part to which the artery is going, the formation of a new part, or an irritation. The *first* may be reckoned the natural increase of the body: the *second*, the occasional increase of parts, as of the uterus in uterine-gestation, where the vessels are increased in width in proportion to the whole solid contents, including the young; besides this, they are considerably increased in length before they reach the uterus, which obliges the spermatic artery in particular to be thrown into a serpentine form; this is more remarkable in some animals than in the human species. Instances of new-formed parts where the vessels are increased, are to be found in the stag, or all those of the deer kind which cast their horns, such animals having the arteries considerably increased at the time the young horn is growing, so that the carotid arteries, which before had only to supply the head and the external carotid, which before had only to supply the sides of the head, now become larger, and are continued into the horn, which is extremely vascular. After the separation of the fœtus, or the full growth of the horn, the vessels naturally lessen, to adapt themselves to the diminished size of the parts. It is curious to observe how vessels become enlarged upon any irritation, not only the arteries, but the veins, and not only the smaller branches, but the larger trunks. This was evident in the following case: I applied a caustic to the ball of the great toe of a patient every other day for more than a month, and after each application the surrounding parts put on a blush, and all the veins on the top of the foot, as well as up the leg, immediately began to swell, and became large and full. This was so remarkable that the patient watched for this effect on the days on which the caustic was applied, from its happening only on those days.

In diseases where there is an increased size of the part, as in tumours, etc., the increase of vessels is no less conspicuous, and they have the power of dilatation and increase of strength, in proportion to the size of the vessels, which are now endowed with new dispositions and actions, different from those they had before.

The arteries often perform diseased operations in the body, which become symptoms both of local and constitutional actions, as in inflammation, fever, etc., for they are not only active in local disease, but their action often becomes a symptom of a constitutional disease, whether original, or arising from a local cause; but these symptoms become mostly sensible to us in those arteries whose actions we can feel, because they have a peculiar action in their diastole as well as in their systole, which is sensible to the touch, from which sensation we in many cases judge of the state of the body at the time, as also of the state of the cause, when it is local and out of sight. The heart, the source of the circulation, is also affected from the same cause, so that its motion and the motions of the arteries commonly if not always correspond.

§. 7. *Valves of Arteries.*

The arteries arising from the heart, I believe in all animals, have valves, which are so many flood-gates, to hinder a return of the blood into the cavities; and as there are two main arteries in the human body, so there are two sets of valves, viz. one belonging to each artery. These are situated at the beginning of the artery, and, from their shape, are called semilunar. Veins have similar valves almost through their whole course. The valves are inelastic, being similar to the inner coat of an artery; but the difference in the properties of the valves and the arteries themselves (which are elastic) will be further considered in treating of the use and mode of action of the valves. Each of these sets is made up of three valves*, but in veins there are commonly only two. This difference in the valves of the arteries and veins is perhaps to bring the artery into a more rounded figure than could have taken place by two valves only: each of these valves is of a semilunar form, having one convex edge, and the other nearly straight. These valves are attached to the insides of the artery, at its very beginning, by their semicircular edge, which is oblique, the points, as it were, running a little way into the artery. These terminations in each valve come close to one another, but the loose edges, which constitute the diameter, are not cut straight off, but rounded. There is, besides, a small body on each, attached to or near the edge, between the two points, called corpora sesamoidea. These bodies are not placed exactly on the edge, but rather on that side next to the artery, leaving the edge of the valve loose: this situation is best adapted to their intended use; the reason of the loose edge being a little rounded, and of the bodies called corpora sesamoidea being placed there, arises from there being three valves to each artery. Each of these valves, with its artery, forms a pouch, whose mouth or cavity opens towards the artery; and the convexity of each of the valves, when the artery is dilated, makes nearly the third of a circle, which is turned inwards towards the centre of the artery, as well as towards the heart. It is from this oblique direction in the attachment that the valves perform their office, simply from the action of the heart upon the blood, and the blood upon the artery. This is entirely mechanical, depending on mechanical principles alone, as much as the action of a joint.

I have above observed, that the area described by the valves is the

* I have found in the human subject only two valves to the aorta; but this is very rare. [Mr. Mayo has figured a similar case in his Outlines of Physiology, 3rd Edit. p. 51.]

same with the artery when that vessel is in its systole, their outer surface lining the inner surface of the artery; but the artery being elastic, its diameter becomes larger when the blood flows into it; and the valves being inelastic, their loose margins or edges are brought more into straight lines across the area of the mouth of the artery, and nearer to each other, so as to make an equilateral triangle. Thus they are fitted to catch the returning blood, and the artery, reacting with considerable force on the blood, presses it on the valves, so as to push them inwards; these, having no pressure on the side next the heart, become convex on this side, shutting up entirely the mouth of the artery. Here then is an effect arising naturally out of a variety of causes, viz. the oblique direction of the valves, their want of elasticity, the elasticity of the artery, and the dilatation of the artery; so that the return of the blood does not open the mouths of the valves, and in that way shut up the mouths of the artery. To demonstrate this, let us suppose the extreme length of each of these valves to be an inch; then the circumference of the artery, when in its systole, will be three inches: in that case the valves lie close to the sides of the artery, and describe a circle of three inches circumference (as in Pl. XXI. f. 3.); but if you dilate this artery as far as the valves will allow, which will be rather more than one fifth, the valves will run nearly into straight lines, and make an equilateral triangle (as in Pl. XXI. f. 4.), whose sides are a little curved inwards. As the artery is filled from the contraction of the heart, it is distended; and as it is distended, the valves do more and more their duty, till at length, by the full distension of the artery, they are made to bulge inwards, and the loose edges, with the corpora sesamoidea, are pushed further towards one another, by all of which positions the area of the artery is entirely shut up[a].

---

[a] [If so great a dilatation of the artery, as is supposed, actually takes place during the systole of the ventricle, the effect upon the artery and valves would be different, I conceive, from what is represented in the text; for taking the extreme length of the valves to be one inch, and the circumference of the artery, in its systole, as three inches, and in its diastole as three inches + $\frac{1}{5}$ (which is the case supposed by the author), then would the artery, during its systole, dilate unequally, in the same manner as is observed in regard to veins; and instead of a circle, as in fig. 4. Pl. XXI., would be thrown into a form exhibited in fig. 6.; that is, the dilatation of the artery would take place at all points, excepting where the valves are attached; but there, in consequence of the inextensibility of these bodies on the one hand and the impossibility of their assuming a straight direction on the other, while the pressure from behind remains, the artery would bulge out in the intermediate spaces. The use of this arrangement is very evident, as it tends to keep the edges of the valves (*a a a* fig. 5.) partly patent, in readiness to catch the returning current of blood the moment the systole of the artery commences. According to the explanation of the author, the area of the artery would be partially closed, as may be observed by inspection of fig. 6., and thus offer a consi-

Pl. XXI. f. 3. shows the artery in its systole, with the three valves, nearly close to its sides. The two black dots are designed to represent the mouths of the coronary arteries, now covered by the valves.

Fig. 4. shows the artery in its diastole, where the three valves run nearly into straight lines, making an equilateral triangle of the area of the aorta. But as their edges are rounded, and the bodies of the valves make a curve inwards, they by these means fill up in part this triangular space, as is seen at *d d d*; and the corpora sesamoidea fill up the remaining other part at *e e e*. In this way the whole of the area of the artery is filled up.

The foregoing account is proved by injections against the valves; but it is still more clearly proved that the diastole of the arteries makes the valves do their duty, when it is injected with the current of blood; for in proportion as the artery is distended, the valves recede from the sides of the artery; and if the artery is fully distended, the communication is entirely cut off between the two pieces of injection, viz. that which is within the heart and that which is within the artery[a]. It may be objected here, that it will require a certain quantity of blood to make these valves do their office; and when there is not that quantity, it must be done by regurgitation. To this it may be answered, that nature always keeps a due proportion, and all the parts depend on one another; so that the quantity of blood that is just sufficient to keep the animal alive is sufficient to distend the artery so as to shut the valves*.

The valves of the pulmonary artery do not do their duty so completely as those of the aorta, for in them we do not find the corpora sesamoidea; and if we inject a pulmonary artery towards the right ventricle, it does not so completely hinder the injection passing into that cavity; nor are the two portions of injection completely separated when the artery is

* As people advance in life, especially men, we find the aorta losing its elasticity; and as it is acted upon with great force by the impetus of the blood, it loses that elasticity in the state of its diastole, which throws the valves continually across the area of the vessels; and as the valves in those cases commonly become thicker, and are often very irregular and bony, we find that they neither recede from the sides of the aorta, during the contraction of the heart, nor towards it during the systole of the artery; so that more blood is allowed to regurgitate into the ventricle, than in a regular circulation.

derable obstruction to the complete evacuation of the ventricle; besides, the degree of dilatation necessary to make the valves form an equilateral triangle is probably greater than ever takes place, particularly in debilitated states of the circulation.]

[a] [This is very far from being conclusive. The reaction of the elastic parietes, which have been previously distended by the injection, drives the blood back again upon the valves, and closes them. I may observe, that the semilunar valves are not, generally, so perfectly formed as accurately to close up the area of the artery, while the tricuspid and mitral valves are still less perfect.]

injected from the ventricle, as in the left side. So far as respects injections, the same observations are applicable to the valvulæ tricuspides; therefore I believe the valves of the right side of the heart are not so perfect as those of the left; and from hence we may suppose that the universal circulation requires to be more perfect than that through the lungs. We must see from this account of the action of the valves, that the mouths of the coronary arteries are opened by the action of the heart; for as the arteries dilate, they become more and more exposed.

§. 8. *Of the Division, or Branching, of Arteries.*

As all the arteries in animals possessed of a heart arise from or begin at that heart by one or two trunks only, they are obliged to divide into or send off branches or smaller trunks, which again divide into still smaller, till at last the whole body is supplied by the ultimate divisions. This is called the branching or ramification of arteries, and is somewhat similar to the branching of a tree. This branching of an artery does not depend on the artery itself, or on the powers propelling the blood, as in a tree, but is governed by the formation of the body; that is, according as a greater or less quantity of blood, or a greater or less velocity is necessary to different parts.

Various modes of branching are made use of to answer the above purposes. In general the most favourable mode for the free passage of the blood is adopted, viz. branching with acute angles, more especially those which are to carry the blood some considerable way; and still more so in those which are at a great distance from the propelling impulse of the heart, which I shall now more particularly consider.

As the force of the blood in the artery is stronger the nearer it is to the heart, the difference in the velocity of the blood, near and at a distance from the heart, if there was nothing to retard it, would be too great for the difference in parts; the near and the distant parts being in many instances of the same kind. To keep up a velocity sufficient for the parts, and no more, nature has varied the angle of the origin of arteries, at different distances from the source of the circulation. Thus we find that near the heart the arteries arise by obtuse angles; some of them being reflected, and the angles become less and less, till at length they are very sharp. The most remarkable instances of this are the intercostal and lumbar arteries: for these being a set of branches whose length and uses in the body are nearly the same, the difference is made in the greater obtuseness of the angles at which they arise in proportion as they are nearer the heart, as well as in the greater distance which they have to traverse in a retrograde direction from their origin to the parts supplied[a]. We find a difference even in the arteries which arise from the intercostals; for they are much more obtuse at the beginning of the intercostals than at their termination. The reason why this is not so evident in all the arteries of the body is, that there are so few arteries on the same side of the body which take the same course, go to the same distance, and have the same office: for some parts require a greater velocity than others, which will make a difference in the origin of the two arteries, supposing they should go the same length and take the same course. We see the same thing in the secondary arteries, such as the subclavian; for it sends off its branches near its origin at much more obtuse angles than it does further on. Haller, in his Physiology, says that the arteries arise at an angle of forty-five degrees, which is the greatest angle in projection; but he did not consider that in projection there are two powers, viz. gravitation and the force applied, while the blood in the arteries has only one.

It may be asked whether the blood in an artery of a given size, arising from a large one, is sent with the same force as if the artery had arisen from a much smaller trunk, or from an artery of the same size with itself, whose blood passed with the same velocity as in the large one. We find small arteries coming off at once from large ones, instead of being a third, fourth, or fifth from the large one. Arteries send off their branches at a longer or shorter distance, according to circumstances; or, in other words, they divide and subdivide more quickly in some places than in others. I believe this quick division is more peculiar to glands than most other parts, though it does not take place in all, as in the testicle. They divide also quickly in the substance of the brain. In the kidney this is also remarkable: they would seem in that gland to be hurrying to their termination. The same happens as soon as the arteries enter the substance of the brain. Other parts appear to have the arteries elongated before they enter the part, as the spermatic artery; more especially in some animals, as the bull, boar, &c.; and in the female, in the time of uterine-gestation, where we should expect the quickest circulation, we find the arteries elongated very considerably, which throws them into a serpentine course: all of which must retard

[a] [This passage I have ventured to alter. In *1st Edit.* it stands thus: "The most remarkable instance of this is in the intercostal and lumbar arteries; because, since they are a set of branches in the body whose length and uses are so much the same, if there be any difference in the angles, at the origin of the arteries, at equal distances from the heart, it must be made with regard to their length, from the origin to the part supplied."]

the blood's motion in the part. We also find arteries playing in the parts, ramifying and anastomosing, which diminishes the velocity of the blood, such as those of muscles, membranes, &c. We may suppose, from the foregoing instances, that in some a quick supply of blood was necessary in such parts; in one for the drain, in another for the support of the living powers; while in others a more regular, slow, and even motion answered the purpose better.

Arteries in common pass in as direct lines from their origin to their destination as possible; but this is not universally the case, for in many parts they run in a serpentine manner, so much so in some as to form a body of themselves. Thus, the spermatic artery in the male of many animals, more especially the bull, is so convoluted as to form a body. In the female also the spermatic artery increases its serpentine course in the state of uterine gestation. The internal carotid artery in man and many other animals, as the horse, where it passes through the skull, runs in a serpentine direction; and in the lion, bull, &c. it forms a plexus. This would appear to answer two purposes: one to lessen the impulse of the blood, as in the vertebral and internal carotid, spermatic artery, &c.: the other to allow of the stretching of the parts upon which the artery passes, as the mouth or lips, the uterus, and other parts of the body which admit of being stretched or relaxed, as the bladder, stomach, intestines, &c., independently of their elasticity.

We find not only the different systems of vessels communicating with each other, as the arteries with the veins, the veins with the heart to be continued into the artery again, and the absorbents with the veins to communicate in the end with the whole, but also the branches of each system communicating with one another, which is called anastomosis.

Anastomosing of vessels is the opening of one vessel into another; so that if one of them be prevented from carrying its contents, the office can be performed by the other. The most common mode of anastomosing is when two vessels run into one, or are continued into each other, or one vessel opens into another, from which others arise; but there is a peculiar communication between the two carotids, as well as between them and the vertebral, where a canal of communication passes directly between them; and this mode of communication takes place between the two descending aortas of some of the amphibia[a].

[a] [A similar construction is sometimes observed in the human subject, and has been figured by Tiedemann in his *Tabulæ Arteriarum*, Pl. iv. fig. 7.

I may observe, by the way, that the arch of the aorta, or rather the great trunks

This anastomosing is much more frequent in the smaller than the larger arteries. We seldom find trunks anastomose with one another. One reason for this is the great disproportion in number between the larger and smaller arteries; but the anastomosis is much more frequent in the smaller, in proportion to their number. The use of this is to give freedom to the circulation, as the chance of a stop being put to it is greatest in the smaller arteries, the circulation in them not being so strong, and passing through parts liable to be pressed upon. This is readily seen in the transparent parts of the living body, when viewed through a microscope.

In some parts of the body we find anastomoses in pretty large trunks; but these are in parts essential to life, very liable to be compressed, or both. The mesenteric artery anastomoses by large trunks; the mesentery being a part essential to life, and very liable to compression, from indurated fæces compressing the artery. In this case, if they only anastomosed by the small branches, on the intestines, the circulation might not be kept up sufficiently to preserve the gut. We observe the same thing in the brain; for there the arteries anastomose by large trunks, before they are distributed to the brain. The use of this is that all parts of the brain might have an equal quantity of blood at all times, even where accident had put a stop to the circulation in any one vessel; for the small anastomoses on the pia mater would not be sufficient to keep up a due circulation everywhere in the brain; as I believe the arteries do not anastomose in the substance of the brain itself. There are large anastomoses in the hand and foot, for the same reason as in the intestines.

All the uses arising from the anastomosing of the vessels, are, perhaps, not yet perfectly understood: general reasons can, I think, be assigned for them; but these will not apply to all cases: there is something, therefore, more than we are yet acquainted with. The absorbents and the veins, upon the whole, anastomose more frequently than the arteries; yet that circumstance is reversed respecting the veins in

---

which arise from the arch, are subject to more variations from the normal type than perhaps any other artery in the body.

It has generally been thought that the venous system presents greater and more numerous anomalies in its distribution than the arterial; and this observation is undoubtedly true as far as regards the superficial and smaller vessels, but not as regards the deep-seated and more considerable trunks. The aorta, for instance, is subject to at least twenty-nine varieties, in regard to the vessels which arise from its arch, whereas only one has been observed with respect to the vena cava superior, viz. when the right and left subclavians do not join previously to their reaching the heart. So likewise the renal and brachial arteries are much more irregular than the corresponding veins.]

some places, and in these instances the uses of these systems of vessels are also in some measure reversed. Where all the three systems of vessels have nearly the same mode of action, we find that their manner of anastomosing is somewhat similar, and probably the differences might be easily accounted for. Wherever they appear to be simply carriers, then their mode of anastomosing is somewhat similar: however, the absorbents anastomose more frequently than the veins, and the veins more than the arteries, and probably the absorbents anastomose everywhere. This is not so much the case with the veins, and not in the least so in some parts with the arteries.

Let us see if we can assign reasons for all this variety in the different systems of vessels. The absorbents, from the office of absorbing, are to be considered only as carriers; and as they have no propelling force applied to their contents, and their coats are not strong, it is very probable that a free communication between vessel and vessel should take place; upon the same general principle, the veins also anastomose, although perhaps not so frequently, and this difference may be because they have in some degree a propelling power applied to their contents, namely, the action of the heart. The arteries having a very strong propelling power applied to their contents, it was in them not necessary as a general principle; but where they are placed in similar circumstances we find them similar in this respect.

Although the anastomosing of vessels is upon a general principle very proper, yet in many cases it would appear to be very improper, as in the following parts. The arteries do not anastomose in the kidneys. This cannot arise simply from there being no occasion for it, on account of there being no lateral mechanical obstruction: since, from the same mode of reasoning, the veins should not anastomose, which they do very freely. This want of anastomosis in the arteries, therefore, answers some purpose in the œconomy of the part. In the liver, the branches of the vena portæ do not anastomose, although the arteries do in their smaller branches: we may therefore suppose some particular purpose answered besides free communication; and I believe the arteries do not anastomose in the substance of the brain, which makes the brain appear less vascular than it really is. We may observe, perhaps, as a general principle, that arteries near to their destination, where they are to perform their particular functions, do not anastomose. Thus the artery of the kidneys, the vena portæ*, the arteries in the substance of the brain, do not anastomose; nor do the arteries on the villous coat of the intestines.

* This vessel should be considered as an artery.

If it be questioned whether anastomoses are a means of retarding or accelerating the circulation, I should answer that they appear to me to retard the blood's motion[a], although we find vessels anastomosing as freely with one another at the greatest distance from the heart as near to it; but at the same time we may observe, that where we should suppose it was necessary for the circulation to be brisk we find no anastomoses in the arteries, as in the lungs, the kidneys, and I believe hardly in the liver, except on the peritoneal coat, whose arteries are continuations of the hepatic artery.

I believe that the anastomosing of vessels increases their volume on the whole, and therefore allows a greater quantity of blood to be in them than if they did not. That kind of net-work too which they make increases the magnitude of the vascular system; for to answer this purpose they take lateral and circular courses, which give them greater length than if they had simply passed between origin and destination in straight lines.

The better to ascertain the velocity[b] of the blood in the arteries at the different distances from the heart, it will be necessary to know whether an artery be a cylinder or a cone; and, when it divides into any number of branches, whether the whole of these taken together be less, equal, or greater than the vessel or vessels from which they arose; and therefore whether they hold less, the same, or more blood. It may be observed that arteries keep a pretty exact proportion with each other, the branches with the trunk, &c., through the whole system; and therefore, whatever may be their shape, they preserve it pretty regular: viz. if they are cylindrical, they are so regularly; if conical, the same. I should suspect, however, that the anastomosing of the arteries, in some degree, interferes with this regularity; but it is probable that the ultimate branches may come back again and correspond with the original trunk. To ascertain this, it is necessary to make choice of arteries which for some length either send off no branches, or at least such as are very

---

[a] [There can, I think, be no doubt that anastomoses retard the circulation, on the same principle as the current is retarded in passing from a smaller into a larger tube; also by opposing currents. See note on capillaries.]

[b] [Dr. Young estimated the mean velocity of the blood in the aorta at 8 inches per second; but less in the smaller vessels, in proportion to the gradually increasing area of the vascular cone (*Med. Lit.*, p. 609, and *note*, p. 38.). The velocity, however, will necessarily differ in different vessels, according to the obstruction which it meets with, although this is scarcely at all found to affect the arterial tension, which, according to the experiments of Poiseuille, is almost exactly the same in all parts of the body. The ventricles are estimated to throw out about one ounce and a half to two ounces at every contraction, and the whole blood to perform about twenty complete revolutions in every hour.]

small when compared with the trunk : for it is impossible to measure with any degree of accuracy the size of branches, and then calculate their different capacity, in comparison with that of the trunk from whence they are derived ; and I think it is reasonable to suppose that, whether an artery divides or not, the size must be the same in both, for it is necessary that the ultimate effect should be the same.

The arteries which are best adapted for this experiment are those of the placenta and of the testicles, particularly in the bull. The carotid arteries in some animals are tolerably well formed for experiments of this kind; for though these do not give us the exact proportions which the one end bears to another, yet they plainly demonstrate which end is the largest.

The arteries of the placenta evidently increase in size the nearer they approach to the placenta; and this so very considerably as to require no experiment unless it be intended to ascertain the difference correctly. In the spermatic artery of the bull it is equally evident ; but as these arteries are much longer than the distance between their origin and the parts which they are to supply, it may be supposed that this increase is peculiar to them, in order to answer some particular purpose. But the carotid arteries in some animals afford sufficient proof that the arteries in common become larger as they pass on and ramify; for the carotids may be reckoned ramifying arteries, as they send off branches.

The carotid artery of the camel among quadrupeds, and of the swan among birds, are very proper arteries for such experiments.

To be as accurate as possible, I injected the arteries of two camels and the arteries of a swan ; and, that one end might not be more distended than the other, the artery was well warmed and placed in a perfectly horizontal position. The pipe was fixed into the lower end*, and the injection made so warm as to keep fluid some time after having been injected : in this position it was allowed to cool. I made sections from each end ; and, that they might be perfectly equal, I took a hard piece of wood, an inch thick, and bored a hole through it of the size of the artery, so as to contain a section exactly of that length, having a moveable button fixed at one end, which could be turned upon the hole, or off, at discretion. The artery being introduced through the hole, a projecting part was cut through by a thin knife, in order that the artery might be divided at right angles to itself. After doing this, the artery was withdrawn, and the button was then turned upon the hole, so as

* The fixing the pipe into the lower end was rather in favour of increasing the size of this end.

to stop that end, and the cut end of the artery introduced to the bottom or button; this piece so inclosed was separated in the same manner.

Having taken a piece of the carotid artery from each end, which were of course exactly of equal lengths, I weighed them, and found that the section of the upper end was one grain and a half heavier than that of the lower.

The carotid artery of another camel, measuring three feet and a half in length, was found to send off forty-four small branches, about the size of the human intercostal arteries, with one as large as the ulnar. Of this artery a transverse section, of one inch in length, being taken from each end and weighed, that from the lower end was found to weigh two scruples sixteen grains and a half, while that from the upper end weighed only two scruples fourteen grains and a half. In similar sections of the opposite carotid, which sent off forty-seven branches, the difference in weight between the upper and lower section was five grains. Similar sections from carotid arteries of a swan being weighed, the lower sections were found to be three grains and a half heavier than the upper: the lower section weighing thirteen grains and a half.

Had the lateral branches been preserved an inch long, being the length of the sections of the trunk, I believe each might have weighed above a grain; and, in that case, the forty-four would have been nearly equal in weight to the trunk. Should this be true, the arteries increase very considerably, not only in their ramifications but in their trunks. I imagine if the carotid artery in the camel did not send off any branch in its course, it would increase in size, nearly in the same proportion with the umbilical artery, or the spermatic in the bull.

It is to be observed that as arteries divide they increase in size much faster than if they did not. For instance, if a section of an artery two inches long is equally divided into two, the section that is the further from the heart shall be heavier than the other, perhaps by one grain; but if the most distant section had divided into two branches, the two, taken together, would have been a grain and a half heavier; if three branches, two grains heavier, &c. The increase of size in the arteries as they ramify is an effect of the numerous ramifications[a].

From what has been already said it must appear that arteries form a cone, whose apex is at the heart; and, if this be the case in the adult, we shall find that it must be more so in the young subject, and will every day become less as the child increases in growth.

---

[a] [A part of this increase in weight must be laid to the account of the increased superficies of the coats of the vessels. The solid contents only should have been weighed in order to have rendered these experiments perfectly accurate.]

The capillary arteries in the fœtus are probably as numerous as in an adult; perhaps more so, for we know that there is the same number of principal arteries in each; as far as we can trace them, they seem to send off the same number of smaller branches; and in many parts we find a great many more small vessels in the fœtus than in the adult. In the eye, the membrane of the ear, &c., in all growing parts, such as callus, granulations, &c., we find a great many more vessels than in similar-grown parts, or in the same parts when completely formed; not in proportion to the size of the part, but more in number. These are strong proofs that many arteries are obliterated in the adult. How much more vascular, therefore, must a child be than an adult, in proportion to its size, when in a much smaller compass a greater number of arteries are accumulated[a]!

From this it would appear that the only great change in the vascular system is elongation [and enlargement] of the vessels: for, as we find very little difference between the blood of a fœtus and of an adult, it is natural to infer that the smallest vessels are nearly of the same size in both; for the termination of the arteries, or what may be called the operative part of the arterial system, being intended to perform the same functions in the fœtus as in the adult, it is reasonable to suppose that the increase is in the length [and diameter] of the whole vascular system; and that the increase in the size of the trunks is in a uniform gradation from the capillaries towards the heart, but never [in their aggregate capacity] becoming equal to the capillaries.

If the preceding account be true or nearly so, we see that there must be a great proportional difference between the size of the two extremes of the arteries in the young subject and the adult. We may venture to say that the aorta in the child is not one fourth of the size of that vessel in the adult, and that the capillaries are rather larger than those in the adult, which would of itself make the whole capillaries in the fœtus more than four times the size of the aorta in the same; and as these arteries are very short, the cone of course increases very fast.

In the fœtus in utero we are to consider that the aorta, at the beginning from the ventricle, is larger than in the adult, in proportion to the quantity of blood that passes through the foramen ovale: and beyond the entrance of the canalis arteriosus the aorta is increased in proportion to the size of the canalis arteriosus; and it is at this part its size is to be

[a] [It should not be forgotten, however, that there are other parts which become developed and require a large supply of blood in the adult. We may instance the muscular system, which can scarcely be supposed actually to contain an equal number of capillary vessels in the infant as in the adult. Some organs also, as the genital, must surely have a larger supply of vessels in the adult than in the infant.]

estimated. This probably makes the aorta, beyond the entrance of the canalis arteriosus, twice as large as in the adult in proportion to their size; but the drawback upon this, from the body, is the placenta; for the placenta is to be considered as part of the body, disposing of the blood that afterwards circulates through the lungs: however, when it is separated, it may take away with it nearly its own proportion of blood, although I rather suspect it does not. But I do not suppose it is equal to the quantity passing through the foramen ovale and canalis arteriosus; and if so, then the body has the overplus.

The aorta of a fœtus is, therefore, not only larger than that of an adult, but larger than in that proportion which the size of the fœtus bears to the size of the placenta. Or it may be put in this view: that, besides the difference in the size of the aorta in a young subject (as before observed) and in an adult, the size of the aorta in the fœtus is still larger, viz. more than in that proportion which the circulation in the lungs of the adult bears to the circulation in the lungs of the fœtus, which is probably much more than that of the placenta[*].

Experiment on the Arteries of a Child.—I injected the descending aorta of a fœtus, just above the diaphragm, in the same manner as I did the carotids in the camel and swan, by which means I injected the mesenteric artery, the subject of experiment. This artery has a trunk, which at first does not put off branches, and then sends off several, which may be all called so many trunks. These again do not immediately give off branches, and are therefore measurable with the trunk from which they arise.

I first made a section of the trunk of the mesenteric artery, near its root, before it sends off any considerable branches, one third of an inch in length; and then another section of the same artery, having the same length, close to the origin of the first branch: all the branches arising from it being preserved of the same length with the trunk itself. When they were weighed in opposition to each other, the trunk without the branches was found to weigh thirteen grains and a half; while that with the branches weighed eighteen grains, that is, four grains and a half more than the trunk. A section of the aorta, near half an inch long, being made just above the origin of the inferior mesenteric artery, was weighed against a section of the same length, including the inferior

* [I apprehend the author's meaning to be simply that the excess of the adult pulmonary circulation over the fœtal (which excess must previously have passed through the aorta) is more than equal to what formerly went to supply the placenta. Consequently the body must have had the overplus.]

mesenteric, likewise of the same length; the last section weighed one grain more than the other, the highest amounting to six grains, the lowest to seven. A section of the lower end of the aorta, including a portion of the two iliacs, was weighed against a section of the two iliacs, which was equal in length, and these were found to weigh rather heavier.

By the above is confirmed what I formerly asserted, that an artery not giving off branches does not increase so fast as another which does if we include all the branches.

From all that has been said it appears that there must be a much greater quantity of blood in a fœtus than an adult in proportion to their difference of size; and that the heart must be larger and stronger, in proportion, to move this blood, which will probably still circulate in the smaller vessels with less velocity.

The whole of these differences between the fœtus and the adult must be intended for the purposes of growth: and indeed we may discern the necessity of it; for if a child was not more vascular in proportion to its size than the adult, its growth, we might conceive, would only be in proportion to the number of its vessels, which would be twelve times less than they are, for a new-born child is only one twelfth in size to that of an adult. A child would, therefore, grow faster and faster every year, for instance, in proportion to its size, as the vessels would become numerous in that proportion. But this is not really the case, for children grow less and less every year in proportion to their size, only adding their first year's growth to themselves every succeeding year; though, perhaps, not quite so much, as the vessels rather decrease in number.

That this is the case may be proved by taking the eye for an example, which grows more the first year after conception than it does any year afterwards; so that the disproportion between the vessels of this part, in those two states, is particularly great.

The growth of an animal is, therefore, in proportion to the number of its capillary vessels. As the body grows, the vessels elongate to keep pace with that growth, the capillary vessels at last come to a stand, and the arterial system is daily losing ground.

The heart grows in proportion to the increased length of arteries, that it may be able to throw the blood through the whole, but not in proportion to the size of the whole body, because the vessels do not increase in number or size in proportion to the size of the body. But as the heart increases only in proportion to the size of the whole vascular system, while the body increases faster and more, the heart cannot be in proportion to the size of the whole body, hence its action must in time lose the power of elongating the body; and become merely sufficient to nourish what is already formed. Perhaps it does not even continue to do so much; for it is not impossible that the body may begin to decline from the moment it ceases to grow, the heart having pushed the growth of the body even beyond its own powers to preserve it in that state.

§. 9. *Of the Action of the Arteries, and the Velocity of the Blood's Motion.*

Arteries, during their diastole, which arises from an increased quantity of blood being thrown into them, increase much more in length than width, being thrown into a serpentine course; therefore, instead of the term diastole, it should rather be called the elongated state. It is, however, the increased diameter that becomes sensible to the touch[a].

---

[a] [The question of the immediate cause of the impression of the pulse has been a subject of considerable dispute, respecting which modern physiologists are by no means perfectly agreed, particularly as to the degree which the vessel enlarges or lengthens at each systole of the heart. The diametrical enlargement of the artery was altogether denied by Parry, Laennec, and Bichat; but not apparently with good reason, for it is very visible in the immediate vicinity of the heart in several reptiles. Haller observed it in the chick, Majendie and Hastings in the thoracic aorta of the horse, and Meckel and Tiedemann in the smaller arteries. The reason why it is not generally more visible appears to me to be this. The carotid artery of an animal, measuring $\frac{1}{4}$, or $\frac{25}{100}$, of an inch in diameter, being exposed for six inches, the elongation which this length of vessel is supposed to undergo at each contraction of the ventricle is estimated at $\frac{1}{4}$, or $\frac{25}{100}$, of an inch; so that, supposing the diametrical enlargement to take place only in the same proportion, it would not amount to more than $\frac{1}{100}$ part of an inch, which it would be difficult under any circumstances to see, and still more difficult in a unilateral aspect of the vessel. When, however, we further reflect that the time required for the transmission of a wave of blood from the heart to the most remote part of the body does not exceed a half second, and then calculate the extreme velocity with which this wave passes over a few inches of vessel, we shall not be surprised at not being able to perceive it. Besides, the mere fact of exposing a vessel is sufficient of itself to induce the contraction of its coats, so as completely to obliterate the tube; from all which circumstances I conclude that very little reliance can be placed on these kinds of observations. The experiments of Poiseuille, which seemed to evince that an actual enlargement took place, are not perfectly conclusive.

The elongation of an artery is barely appreciable in an undisturbed state of the circulation, but may be rendered distinctly visible by holding the nostrils of an ass (whose carotids have previously been exposed) until the respiration becomes laborious. The artery may now be observed to leap from its bed, and to become elongated and tortuous at each stroke of the ventricle; effects which may be imitated in the dead body, or on dead tubes, by forcible injections, and which are also observed to occur naturally in many parts subject to violent periodical excitements, as the testicle and uterus.

It has been observed, however, that a tangible shock may be conveyed through a fluid

This probably arises from the muscular coat opposing the dilatation of the arteries, while it cannot the lengthening. The dilatation of the artery producing the stroke is either felt by the finger or may be seen, when superficial; but were we to judge of the real increase of the artery by this we should deceive ourselves, for when covered by the integuments the apparent effect is much greater than it really is in the artery itself: for in laying such an artery bare, the nearer we come to it the less visible is its pulsation, and when laid bare its motion is hardly to be either felt or seen.

The more an artery is covered, especially with solid bodies, the more is the pulsation to be felt or seen; thus tumours over large arteries have a considerable motion given to them, and have often been supposed to be aneurisms. The knowledge of this fact, arising more from experiment than common observation in the living body, may be a sufficient reason for keeping to the old expression, dilatation.

This circumstance, which has been but little taken notice of, produces an effect which has also been unobserved. If the arteries had been dilated by the force of the blood's motion, as has been supposed, its motion should be much less retarded than it is; for even supposing that the increased area of the artery is the same when elongated as if dilated, and therefore holds an equal quantity to a dilated one, it must appear evident that the blood will not arrive so quickly at the opposite end[a].

---

much in the same manner as sound, so that we may discover the working of a water-pump at a great distance merely through the pipes, whether iron or leathern, by which it is connected.

Others have ascribed the pulse to the forward rush, without tumefaction, which takes place when an additional quantity of blood is injected into elastic vessels. It may be observed, however, that any elastic vessel, as, for instance, an intestine, perfectly full of fluid is capable, on being gently tapped with the finger, of communicating a rapid and distinct pulse to a great distance, although no forward rush can take place, but only a gentle undulation. Dr. Parry, however, has justly observed, that the impression of the pulse may be rendered much more obvious by slightly pressing on the artery thus 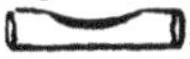 , so as to indent it, by which means the finger becomes directly opposed to the current of blood.

We occasionally hear of instances in which the pulse is said to vary, as well in its rhythm as in the number of its beats, in different parts of the body; but probably all such cases are resolvable into some irregularity of the heart's action: as when, for instance, it is partly intermittent, so as to give first a perfect and then an imperfect stroke —the perfect stroke only being sufficient to communicate the pulse to the extreme parts, although both may have this effect on those which are in the immediate vicinity of the heart. It is difficult, if not impossible, to assign specific causes for the numerous variations of the pulse which take place in disease. The sphygmometer, lately invented by M. Hérisson, is perfectly inefficient, and is not deserving of the least confidence.]

[a] [Sir C. Bell, in his "*Essay on the Forces which circulate the Blood*," has endeavoured, by an ingenious train of reasoning, to prove the reverse of this position; for, observing

The continual repetition of the cause of this serpentine course obliges the arteries in many places to retain this state, especially in parts that do not yield readily, as the skull, upon which the temporal artery is placed; and this retention of the serpentine course is still more obvious in those arteries which have lost a good deal of their elasticity. However, this increase[a] of the artery is so manifest as to be felt or seen, and produces what is called the pulse, which must gradually diminish in proportion as the arteries divide into smaller branches; for a small artery having a proportional pulse, and the arterial system increasing as it goes along, both of which causes diminish the velocity of the blood, and render the diastole less and its motions more uniform.

From the description I have given of the heart with its action, and the parts of which an artery is composed, it must appear that an artery is at all times full of blood, which is moving on with more or less velocity; because it receives it from the heart at interrupted periods, and when a given quantity is thrown in at one end, this will make a considerable difference between this part and the other, which part will of course be more upon the stretch; for although the artery dilates, yet as it is from the impulse of the blood, the blood must move much faster on in the diastole of the artery than its systole. This part of the artery will contract, and throw the blood into the remaining part; but not with the same force with which it was received; but still the artery beyond will receive it faster than it will give it. By these means, all the parts

---

that most organs which perform or are liable to be called upon suddenly to perform any extraordinary degree of action, as the uterus, brain, testicles, &c., are provided with highly tortuous vessels, he argues that this arrangement must be designed to give greater power to the local circulation, so as to increase the velocity of the blood in those parts, as occasion may require, without necessarily engaging the whole vascular system in this act; and this is supposed to be accomplished by the increased muscular superficies giving greater strength to the tortuous artery. We cannot, however, argue from final causes in such cases as this; neither can we at present, with any degree of precision, say how far the muscularity of the arteries is actually concerned in carrying on the ordinary circulation. We do, however, know, on physical principles, that the multiplication of angles, and the increased superficies of a tortuous vessel, must have the effect of retarding the current which passes through it; while, on the other hand, we know that the mere force of impulsion from behind is sufficient to produce a tortuosity of the vessel, as well of the arteries and veins as of inert tubes; but as it is not pretended that the veins assist the circulation by their muscularity, the tortuosity in them can neither arise from the cause assigned, nor be attended with the effect supposed. It is probable, therefore, that the tortuosity is produced by the same cause in both orders of vessels, and that it is attended with the same effect.]

[a] [Does the author mean by "this increase," the elongation or the diametrical enlargement of the artery? The preceding part of the paragraph would seem to point to the former meaning; but in the first paragraph of this section he says, "It is the increased diameter which becomes sensible to the touch."]

of the artery are brought to a more equal state; for this additional quantity of blood that was at first in one part only, is in some degree equally diffused through the whole arterial system; by which means, too, it is becoming proportionably slower in its motion: but all these circumstances will vary according as the arterial system consists of cylinders or cones; and if of cones, then according to the extremity which is the base; all of which may be conjectured, but cannot be exactly estimated. Yet that the force of the heart might not be lost, the elasticity of the great artery, over the smaller, is happily applied, because it propels the blood more forcibly on, between the strokes of the heart; for although we are to suppose that the heart, which was capable of distending a part, so as to make it re-act, and send the blood through any given length, was also capable of sending it through that length at once, yet we must see, that by an elastic power being applied at one end, while this is gradually lost towards the other, the elastic part acts with a superior force over the other, in the proportion as the other has less elasticity. This other being also less upon the stretch, is overcome by that which is more so, which is always the end next to the heart; for the muscular part relaxes, requiring hardly any force to distend it; and indeed, as the muscular power has contracted the artery within its middle or stationary state, and this more and more as we get into smaller vessels, the muscular coat is at first stretched by the recovery of the elastic power; so that the blood passes into the smaller branches with much less resistance than it would have done if the vessels had been elastic in proportion to their size. These proportions, however, in the blood's motion, arising from the elastic power of the arteries, will not be the same in the fœtus and adult, and will be still more different in the aged subject; for in this last the elastic power of the artery is diminishing as well as the muscular, the coats becoming more rigid; besides which, the vessels vary from a conical shape (whose apex is at the heart and basis at their extremities) towards a cylinder; and this change is also increased by the loss of many of the smaller vessels; so that as we grow up, the base of the cone is gradually diminished from two causes.

The elastic power will allow of a quantity of blood in the animal beyond the natural state of the artery, and the muscular power will allow of a smaller, without the animal being affected, although the muscular alone would have answered both these purposes. Arteries, then, are the conductors and disposers of the blood: as conductors they are, in every animal above fish, both passive and active; passive, in admitting of the propelling power of the heart; and active, in continuing that power to the extreme part.

Besides these reasons for a difference in the velocities of the blood at different distances from the heart, I conceive there is a material difference between the velocities of the blood in those vessels which carry red blood, and those which carry only the coagulable lymph and the serum; for where the red blood goes, there is a quicker return than where there is only the coagulable lymph and serum. For this there are two reasons, viz. that where the red blood passes, it is commonly nearer to the heart, while the other parts go to a greater distance: but besides this, the vessels which carry the red blood are larger, and, I believe, ramify more quickly; the velocity, therefore, of the blood is greater in them. Where the lymph and serum pass only, the velocity of the blood is languid, and it appears merely to carry nourishment, such as in tendons, ligaments, etc.

So far we are to consider the above as a general principle arising out of the construction of a blood-vessel; but there are secondary or collateral circumstances acting, so as to accelerate or retard the blood's motion.

Since the solids and fluids have a mutual dependence on each other, and since the solids answer various purposes, for which quantity, velocity, etc. are peculiarly necessary, we find that this intercourse between the two is with great exactness kept up. I have already observed that the angles at which the branches of an artery arise, either retard or allow of a freer motion in the blood; but Nature appears to have taken still more care in retarding the blood's motion where velocity might do mischief. She seems also to have taken more care about the blood's motion in some parts than in others; as, for example, in the brain, a part which probably cannot bear the same irregularity, in quantity or velocity of the blood, as many other parts of the body. I should suppose, that by sending four arteries to the brain, instead of one, or which would have been more regular, two, the force of the motion of the blood is broken, as well as by the winding course of the internal carotid arteries. The tortuosity of the vertebral arteries, likewise, are intended, we may suppose, to prevent a too great velocity of the blood, both because these arteries are longer than they need be, and the blood is hindered from moving in a straight line: but, besides the serpentine course of the arteries of the head, they pass through a bone (but principally the carotids), where the bony canal is closely applied to the coats of the artery; so that there can be no pulsation here, but a greater velocity of the blood in those parts, and probably less in the brain. This I should suppose retards also the motion of the blood in the brain, because the blood, passing through a smaller place than common, must meet with a greater resistance, and therefore a smaller quantity must pass through this part in a given time, so that the pulsation of the arteries in the brain should be less than anywhere else; for we may suppose that the motion is considerably lost by the blood coming into an elastic canal of the same diameter with that through which it passed before it came into the bony canal. If, then, this motion is lost, and the quantity of blood is really lessened in a given time, its motion must be more regular, and the pulsation less.

In some animals the carotid artery is found to divide and subdivide, forming a plexus, and the branches unite again before it goes to the brain. This is called rete mirabile, and in animals which have it will certainly break the force of the blood's motion; but since it is not universal, some peculiar purpose must be answered by it. It is not in the horse and ass, for instance; but it is in the lion. Where the vessels anastomose, there is also a considerable retardation to the blood's motion, and they are found to anastomose a good deal on the pia mater before they enter the brain, but I believe not within its substance.

§. 10. *Of Veins.*

The vessels* carrying the blood from any part of the body towards the heart are called the veins: they are more passive than the arteries, and seem to be, from their beginning to their termination in the heart, little more than conductors of the blood to the heart, that it may receive its salutary influence from the lungs. However, this is not unversally the case, for the vena portæ would seem to assume the office of an artery in the liver, and therefore becomes an active part; and we have many veins formed into plexuses, so as to answer some purpose, not at all subservient to the circulation; but still, in this respect, they are not to be reckoned active. They differ from the arteries in many of their properties, although in some they are very similar.

They do not compose so uniform or regular a system of vessels as the arteries, either in their form or use, being subject to considerable variety in their uses (which are, however, passive, not active), and often answering, from their construction, collateral purposes.

The coats of the veins, upon the whole, are not so thick as those of the arteries, but differ materially in different situations of the body. Thus, they become thinner and thinner, in proportion to their size, the nearer to the heart; however, this is not equally so through the whole venal system, but principally in the depending veins, as those of the ex-

* A vein is commonly a canal, especially that which carries red blood; but in many animals it is entirely cellular; yet I use the word as a general term when applied to the blood.

tremities, more especially the lower in man; and still more so, the nearer to the extreme parts. In such parts it is often difficult to distinguish the vein from the artery; yet this is not to be remarked in the veins of ascending parts, or those coming from the head, or such as are horizontal, especially in the human subject; and in animals which have a large portion of their body horizontal, there is little difference in the coats of such veins at different distances from the heart. I suspect the muscular powers are much greater in what may be called ascending veins, than either descending or horizontal; and I believe, in general, it is very considerable, for if we look at the back of our hand, and compare their size in a warm day or before a fire, and in a cold day, they hardly appear to be the same veins. They are not so strong in their coats as the arteries, and their strength is in an inverse proportion to their size in the extremities, and the reason is very obvious. They are more dense in their coats than the arteries, yet in the dead body they seem to admit the transudation of the blood; for when there is the least degree of putrefaction we can trace the veins with the eye on the skin, as if very large, the cellular membrane and the skin being tinged for some way on each side of the vein. In the liver we find injections escaping the vena cava hepatica, and getting into its substance in a peculiar manner.

They have nearly the same elasticity with the arteries; they are similar to the arteries in their structure, being composed of an elastic and muscular substance[a], the elastic in some degree preserving a middle state, although not so perfectly as in the arteries. The muscular power adapts the veins to the various circumstances which require the area to be within the middle state, and assists the blood in its motion towards the heart.

The coats of the veins themselves are vascular, although not very

---

[a] [The veins are less elastic, but much more extensible than the arteries; and in proportion to their substance, are capable of sustaining a much heavier weight without breaking. The *internal* coat of veins, besides being much thinner, more delicate, and less fragile than that of the arteries, is remarkably distinguished from the latter, by never becoming the seat of ossifications, which, in the arteries, take place so generally in rather advanced life as almost to be considered the normal state. It is remarkable that this disposition to ossification is, as Bichat remarked, strictly confined to the *arterial* portion of the system of red blood, commencing from the left auriculo-ventricular opening, through all the ramifications of the aorta; for the left auricle, and also the pulmonary veins, although they carry red blood, are rarely, if ever, affected in this manner. The *fibrous* coat of veins is principally seen in the depending and superficial veins of the body; but in general it is very obscurely developed, and in some veins cannot be said to exist. The fibres, according to Meckel, invariably run longitudinally, and from this circumstance are strikingly contradistinguished from those of the arteries.]

much so. The arteries arise from the nearest small ramifying arteries, and the corresponding veins do not terminate in the cavity of the vein to which they belong, but pass off from the body of the vein, and join some others from different parts, and at last terminate in the common trunk, some way higher. On laying open the jugular vein of a dog, and closing up the wound for some hours, and then opening it, I observed the vessels of this part very distinctly. They were becoming inflamed, therefore turgid, and I could easily distinguish between the arteries and veins by the colour of the blood in them.

Veins have interruptions in their cavities, called valves. They are thin inelastic membranes, of an exact semilunar form, their unattached edge being cut off straight, not curved, as in those of the arteries; and this is because there are only two of them whose semicircumference adheres to the sides of the vein. They are not placed in a transverse direction, so as to cut the axis of the vein perpendicularly, but obliquely, as the valves at the beginning of the arteries, making a pouch whose mouth is turned towards the heart. They are attached in pairs, the two making two pouches, whose edges come in contact. In the larger veins of many animals, as the jugular veins of a horse, &c., there are often three valves, as at the beginning of the aorta, but not so completely formed. These valves, as it were, cut the veins into two at this part. These two valves are not always of equal size. At this part there are always two swellings in this form, but I believe more in the adult than in the young subject. They are not formed from a doubling of the internal coat, as has been imagined, for the internal coat is elastic, but the valves are rather of a tendinous nature; from this circumstance, together with their shape and their mode of attachment to the sides of the vein, they always do their office whenever the vein is full, in the same manner as the valves of the arteries. The valves of the veins are chiefly in the extremities, jugular veins, and the veins on the exterior parts of the head, but never in the veins of the brain, heart, lungs, intestines, liver, spleen, nor kidneys. Where a smaller vein opens into a larger there is often a valvular structure at the acute angles, but this is not constant[a].

[a] [Single valves are often found to occur in veins of not more than a line in diameter, and occasionally also in the larger trunks; but sometimes three, four, or even five valves have been discovered where two only ordinarily exist. The valves are composed of a fibrous substance, lined by the internal membrane of the veins.

Valves very rarely occur in anastomosing or azygos vessels, for obvious reasons. Generally speaking, the number of valves is increased in the same ratio as the size of the vessels is diminished; but this extends only to a certain point, for after that the inverse ratio seems to be followed, so that in the smallest veins the valves disappear altogether. Valves are uniformly most numerous in depending and superficial parts,

The veins, taken altogether, are much larger than the arteries; but in the extremities the veins that attend an artery are sometimes less. Nevertheless, there are commonly two of them; but, besides these, there are superficial ones, which are much larger than those deeply seated. The best way, however, of judging is by comparing them with the corresponding arteries where there are no supernumerary veins, as in the intestines, kidneys, lungs, brain, &c. where we find that they are larger than the arteries: and this too where a considerable waste has taken place of the arterial blood in the different secretions. From this circumstance the blood's motion in them is slower, and they allow a greater quantity to be in the body at all times.

There is a greater number of trunks of veins in the body than of arteries, at least visible veins, for wherever there is an artery in common there is a vein, and in many places two, one on each side, which sometimes makes a kind of plexus round it; besides, there are many veins where there are no corresponding arteries, as on the surface of the body; for in the extremities many of the larger veins pass superficially, but those become fewer and fewer towards the trunk of the body. They are numerous also in the neck of the human subject; but in some of the viscera, as the intestines, the veins and arteries correspond in number very exactly. Dr. Hales, however, in his Statics, says that he has seen a number of arteries throw their blood into one vein; which, if true, shows that there are more small arteries than veins.

Although veins generally attend the arteries, there are some exceptions, even in corresponding veins, as in the pia mater; but they cannot all attend the arteries, there being more superficial veins on the extremities and neck, but the large trunks do. The supernumerary veins are not so regular as those that attend the arteries, being hardly alike in two people.

---

because in these parts the auxiliary aid of the valves is most needed to assist in carrying on the circulation of the blood. The following veins, in addition to those enumerated in the text, possess no valves, viz. the umbilical, vena cava inferior, vertebral, and veins of the spinal marrow. The uterine veins and also the spermatic veins in the female are not generally provided with valves, although they occasionally exist.

There is a remarkable deviation in the structure of the veins of the brain, adapted to the peculiar circumstances of that organ: for, in the first place, the sinuses are rendered incompressible, to guard against their being collapsed by any sudden increase of the arterial tension, which the inextensibility of the cranium would necessarily determine to these vessels, so as to compress their sides together; while, in the second place, this provision is rendered still more perfect, by the tributary veins of the pia mater being made to open into the sinuses in an oblique direction, opposite to the current of blood, so as effectually to oppose any reflux determination, upon the circulation being impeded.]

* [This, however, is more apparent than real in the dead body, in consequence of the continued action of the capillaries driving the blood into the dilatable veins.]

The veins may be said, upon the whole, to accompany the arteries, and it is most reasonable that this should be the case; since both perform the same office of conducting the blood, the same course must answer equally in both. This, however, is not universally the case, some veins being intended for particular purposes, as the vena portæ; some forming bodies, as the penis, plexus retiformis[a], and others varying their course for convenience, as in the brain. The veins of this viscus take in general a very different course from the arteries; but this is principally in the larger veins of the brain, for the smaller, which are in the substance, accompany the arteries. The intention of this seems to be that the largest veins, called the sinuses, should be so formed as not to be compressible, probably that there should be as little chance as possible of any stoppage to the circulation of the blood in this part. But in some parts of animals they vary their course from the arteries, where we do not so well see the intention, because it is not the case in others. Thus the veins in the kidneys of the cat kind and hyæna have the veins in part passing along the surface in the external membrane, like the sinuses in the brain. Veins seldom or ever take a serpentine course, because a retardment in the blood's motion in them answers no particular purpose in the œconomy of the parts, and the more readily the blood gets to the heart the better. However, the plexuses, although not intended to retard the motion of the blood, answer other purposes not immediately connected with the circulation.

Veins upon the whole anastomose more frequently than the arteries, especially by their larger trunks, and more particularly in the extremities; for we often see a canal of communication going between two trunks, and one trunk shall divide into two and then unite again. Where the veins and the arteries correspond, their anastomoses are nearly the same. I believe they do not anastomose in the lungs or liver; however, the veins corresponding to the arteries do not always follow this rule; for the veins in the spleen and kidneys anastomose in very large trunks, while the arteries do not at all. This anastomosing of the larger veins more frequently is because a vein is easily compressed and the blood has a ready passage into another; besides, the valves render it more necessary, for when the blood has got past a valve it cannot take a retrograde course, but may take a lateral: and indeed it is prin-

[a] [See Vol. I. p. 251, *note*. There can scarcely be any doubt that all the phenomena exhibited by the erectile tissues are due to the extreme extensibility of the venous tunics.]

cipally in those veins which have valves that we find those large anastomosing branches; by this means the blood gets freely to the heart.

As the area of all the veins is larger than that of the arteries, the blood will move more slowly through them; and this is evident from every observation that can be made. It may be observed in the large superficial veins in the extremities of the living body, and the difference of velocity in the blood flowing from a vein and artery in an operation is very great. The blood, however, moves with a good deal of velocity in a vein, for if we stop the circulation in the beginning of any of the superficial veins of an extremity, and empty the vein above, immediately upon removing the finger the blood will move along the vein faster than the eye can follow it: yet its motion is so slow as to allow the blood to lose its scarlet colour, and acquire the modena red; and this more so as it passes on to the heart.

The blood moves more slowly in the veins than in the arteries, that it may come into the right auricle more slowly; for if the two venæ cavæ were of the same size with the aorta, the blood would have the same velocity in them; which the auricle, as it is now constructed, could not have borne: but it may be probable, that the blood is assisted in its passage into the auricle by a kind of vacuum being produced by the decrease of the size of the ventricles in their contraction.

From the number of anastomosing branches, especially by larger trunks, from the blood being liable to temporary obstructions in many places, and also moving with little force, its course becomes often very irregular and undetermined, much more so than in the arteries.

The first cause of the blood's motion in a vein of a quadruped is the force of the heart, for I think we must suppose that the heart can and does carry on simple circulation; because, in paralytic limbs, where voluntary muscular action is totally lost, and where, I conceive, the involuntary is very weak, the circulation is continued, although, I believe, with much less velocity than in perfect and sound parts: besides, we have observed, that the arteries continue the motion of the blood in them where the heart either fails to do it, or where an increased motion may be wanted. The arteries, therefore, will assist the heart in propelling the blood through the veins; however, it is assisted by collateral causes. The second cause is their muscular contraction, which most probably is in the direction of the blood's motion, assisted by lateral pressure of all kinds; because the valves will favour this course wherever they are. However, as the valves are not universal, the motion of the blood in some veins must be carried on without them, and therefore they are not absolutely necessary.

Since we see the veins assuming the office of arteries in the liver of quadrupeds, birds, amphibia, and fish, and much more so in many of the inferior orders of animals, the motion of whose blood is first derived from the heart, we must suppose that veins have considerable power in carrying on the circulation; but the resistance being continually removed at their termination into the heart, will direct and assist the blood's motion in that direction, more especially when influenced by the action of the vessels themselves, or any lateral pressure. In those veins which are accompanied by the arteries, the pulsation of the artery assists in propelling the blood towards the heart, more especially where there are two or more attending an artery.

When treating of the motion of the blood in the arteries, I observed that its motion was not in a uniform stream, but interrupted, which arose from the heart's action; but as it receded from that viscus, that its motion gradually became more uniform, till at last it was nearly a continued stream. However it is not certain but an alternate accelerated motion is continued into the veins immediately from the heart, although it may not be an easy undertaking to ascertain this; for simply observing an accelerated motion in the blood of the veins, more especially the small ones, does not prove that this was an alternate increase immediately from the arteries.

Every artery has a pulsation in itself, immediately from the heart; but a secondary vein, or one that is a third or fourth in order of size, cannot, because it has more than one cause acting upon it; for such vein is receiving the impulse of the heart at very different times, owing to the larger trunk receiving blood by a number of smaller veins that come from a variety of parts: so that if the trunk was to receive it by starts from the smaller veins, it would only be a tremor or confused motion. This is a reason why this cause could produce none in the secondary veins[a]. The fact is, however, that there is a pulsation in the veins, for when we bleed a patient in the hand or foot we evidently see

[a] [The unintermittent continuity of the venous current arises *solely* from elasticity; for supposing the whole vascular system to consist of rigid tubes, the impulse would of course be instantaneous in every part of this system. It is not, therefore, the different lengths of the veins, but the great extensibility of these vessels which equalizes the current. This it is which gives to the veins the operation of an air-vessel (*note*, p. 170.) or compressed spring, the effect of which will be to transform the intermittent impulse of the heart into a continuous force. This may be proved by increasing the tension of the veins in a frog's leg, by partially retarding the circulation, when the pulsation immediately becomes visible in the small veins as well as arteries; although the reaction of the former soon equalizes the tension of the whole vessel, and thus prevents the propagation of the impulse to the larger trunks.

I think it probable that the pulsation which is sometimes perceived in veins of the

a strong jet, much more in some than in others, and much more here than in the bend of the arm. The query is, does this arise from the immediate stroke of the heart, or is it by the lateral pressure, occasioned by the swell of the arteries? To ascertain this the better, it is necessary to observe several things: we may remark that the pulsation in the veins is more in some parts than in others; thus, I should suppose it was more in the veins of the kidney, spleen, lungs, and brain, especially the last, than in many other parts; but this, from the lateral swell of the arteries, cannot, from the above observations, affect all parts alike, for the veins on the back of the hand being superficial, and not surrounded with vascular parts, could not be affected by arteries: but still it may arise from the lateral swell of the smaller arteries; and this acceleration, given to the blood's motion in the smaller veins, is carried to those on the back of the hand. But I think I have seen the difference in the projection so great, that it hardly could arise from that cause alone; and indeed, if this was the only cause, we should have it in some degree in every vein, for every vein is so far surrounded as to be in some measure affected from the swell of the arteries of the part; but we certainly do not perceive it in so great a degree in the bend of the arm. The larger veins near to the heart have a pulsation which arises from the contraction of the heart preventing the entrance of the blood at that time, and producing a stagnation.

This I saw very evidently in a dog whose chest I opened, and produced artificial breathing; but I could not say whether this arose from the contraction of the auricles, ventricles, or both: but the vena cava superior has a contraction in itself, in both dog and cat, and probably in the human subject. Even breathing produces a stagnation near the thorax, for during inspiration the veins readily empty themselves, but in expiration there is a degree of stagnation. Coughing, sneezing, or straining in any way where the thoracic and abdominal muscles are concerned, produces this effect.

I think it is probable, that where there is a universal action of the vascular system, the action of the arteries and veins is alternate. That

---

third or fourth class, as, for instance, in those of the arm, is due to a cause of this kind increasing the tension of the whole venous system, especially as a hard contracted pulse in the arteries is often associated with this appearance in the veins. In those cases where a pulsation is visible in the great veins, in the neighbourhood of the chest, it undoubtedly depends on the reflux of the blood on each systole of the auricle, or of the ventricle, if there should happen to be at the same time any disease of the heart, as, for instance, hypertrophy, attended with imperfect construction of the right auriculo-ventricular valves. The *respiratory* pulse is not synchronous with that of the arteries, and depends on too obvious a cause to require explanation.]

when the arteries contract, as in many fevers, the veins rather dilate, more especially the larger[a].

---

[a] [In order that the reader may perceive at one view the different relations in which the "circulation" may be viewed, I shall very briefly advert to the forces which are supposed to cooperate in this function.

1. *The heart* is undoubtedly the main agent of the circulation in all warm-blooded animals. According to Dr. Hales, the left ventricle ordinarily exerts a force of about 51·5 pounds, and propels the blood into the arteries with a force equivalent to about four pounds to each square inch of the arterial surface. The accuracy, however, of these deductions has lately been called in question by M. Poiseuille, and apparently with good reason. (*Journ. de Phys., par Majendie*, ix. 354.)

2. *The arteries* were regarded by Hunter as a sort of supplementary heart, scarcely less instrumental in the propulsion of the blood than the heart itself; although it is probable that in this estimate he was as much mistaken on the one hand as Dr. Arnott has lately been on the other in denying their agency altogether. (*Elem. of Physics, 5th edit.*, i. 555.) I shall not, however enter here into the controverted question respecting the muscularity of the arteries, which appears to me to be a dispute about words rather than facts, for that the arteries possess a power of varying their calibre, quite independently of the force *e tergo*, is proved by the most indisputable facts (see p. 161 *et seq.*). Admitting, therefore, the muscularity of the arteries as a fact, the question arises, in what manner is the circulation affected by it? It is objected to the author's explanation of the action of the arteries, 1st, that if the arteries were extensively elastic, the intermittent stream in the arteries would soon be converted into a continuous one; 2nd, that no vermicular or progressive motion in the arteries has yet been observed; 3rd, that no diametrical enlargement is visible in the living body; and 4th, that it is impossible to explain the almost perfect instantaneity of the pulse in all parts of the body, on the supposition that the tubes through which it is propagated are in a relaxed state. It is supposed, on the contrary, that the contractile fibres of the vessels operate at the same moment with the heart, so as to induce a rigidity of the whole arterial system, in order that the heart may produce its effect through all the vessels, almost as it would through tubes of metal. (*Arnott ut supra.*) Now the first of these objections does not apply, because such extensive elasticity as is supposed to exist does not occur, for even in the dead body the pulse may be imitated; neither does the second objection apply much better, because the very assumption that the pulse depends on the transmission of a wave of blood, presupposes a certain interval of time, and consequently a progressive dilatation. The third objection has been adverted to already (see *note*, p. 216.), to which I may add, that Poiseuille found, by direct and careful experiment, that the artery apparently dilated with each systole of the heart, that it reacted with a force superior to the impressing impulse, and that the arterial tension was nearly the same in all parts of the system at the same time. (*Journ. de Phys., par Majendie*, viii. 296. ix. 48, 50.) The fourth and last objection equally falls to the ground, when it is recollected that no such rigidity as is supposed to be necessary for the propagation of the pulse actually occurs, for the isochronism of the pulse is equally conspicuous in all states of the arterial tension, and is scarcely less remarkable in the dead body.

When the heart contracts, a wave of blood is impelled into the arterial system, already full of blood, and the phenomena which immediately follow are, 1st, an onward motion of the whole column of blood; and 2nd, a dilatation of the arteries in all directions, which dilatation can only take place at the expense of the force first exerted by the heart, but instantly reacts in the same proportion, so that no power is really lost, except what arises from friction, which is probably more than compensated for by the actively contractile properties of the arteries themselves. Now the rate at which a wave of blood is propagated is estimated at sixteen feet in a second, so that the contraction of the arterial system must be nearly instantaneous in all parts, although it must be apparent that the least deviation in this respect will be sufficient to give a vermicular character to the motion, and consequently a direction to the current.

It seems probable therefore that the arteries do actually cooperate with the heart in propelling the blood, although I am disposed to regard this effect rather as incidental than as one of the primary objects for which muscularity was introduced into the arterial structure. The primary objects seem to be, 1st, to enable the arteries to accommodate their capacity to the varying quantities of blood in the system; 2nd, to modify the velocity and quantity of blood sent to individual parts, without engaging the whole system in this act; and 3rd, to secure the temporary arrest of hæmorrhage.

3. *Adjacent muscular contraction* can only operate on that portion of the blood which has already passed the principal bar of the capillary circulation. It must materially tend, however, to accelerate the blood during active exercise, although it has probably little effect on the ordinary circulation. The alternate action and relaxation of the abdominal muscles in ordinary respiration will be attended with a similar effect.

4. *The pulsation of the arteries* against the adjoining veins must ultimately be referred to the force of the heart. Inconsiderable as this agency may appear, it is certainly deserving of being taken into account, for when we reflect on the force with which the foot is raised when one leg is laid in rest over the other, we may see how the same force, counteracted by the elastic tension of the skin, and thus brought to operate on the venous circulation, may have considerable effect; not to mention the fact that large arteries and veins are often bound together in a common sheath of fascia.

5. *The pressure of the external air* has been a good deal insisted on. A tendency to form a vacuum in the chest has been supposed to arise from four causes: 1, the active dilatation of the right auricle and ventricle; 2, the contraction of the ventricles; 3, the resiliency of the lungs; and 4, the enlargement of the chest during inspiration. Without, however, entering into the specific objections which may be urged against each of these views separately, I shall merely observe, in general, that the circulation goes on with quite as much celerity in the fœtus in utero as in the adult; that it goes on in birds, turtles, cetacea, &c., in which the lungs are adherent to the chest, and in fishes in which there are no lungs at all; and finally, that it goes on in artificial respiration, when the heart and chest are fairly exposed, as well as in persons who voluntarily hold their breath. Nothing, indeed, can be conceived less adapted for the office of a pump than the whole aspect of the venous system, which would infallibly collapse if any considerable external pressure was exerted upon it. It is probable that the utmost sugescent power of any of these causes, or all of them combined, in ordinary respiration is not sufficient to raise a column of blood of a single inch (*Arnott*, p. 572.); for although the force *e tergo* soon raises the tension of a vein on which a ligature has been placed nearly to the same degree as that of the arteries, yet the suction on the near side of the ligature is not sufficient to empty this portion of the vessel, provided it lies ever so little below the horizontal plane of the heart.

Poiseuille, in his experiments, found, that even in the arteries the flow of blood was sometimes entirely arrested during forced inspiration, and accelerated in the same proportion during expiration (*op. cit.*, viii. 298.); effects which are still more visible in the great veins in the immediate vicinity of the chest, as well as in those of the brain and spinal marrow, from these vessels, which are destitute of valves, allowing a regurgitation of blood: nothing, however, is gained to the circulation by this means, for one effect is exactly balanced by the other, the sugescent and repellent influences being exactly correspondent.

6. *Gravity.* The arch of the aorta rising several inches above the entrance of the vena

cava inferior into the auricle, the gravitating pressure of the descending column of blood in the arteries will of course be sufficient to lift the ascending column in the veins several inches beyond what is actually required. The reason that the tension of the veins is not equal to that in the arteries is that the blood in the former finds a ready escape into the auricle, so that unless some obstruction is found in the auricle, the venous tension can never exceed that which will be required simply to lift the column of blood to the heart, added to that required to overcome the friction. Dr. Hales found, that although the column of blood from the carotid artery of a horse rose ten feet in his experimental tube, the venous column did not exceed six inches; but "when from agitation of the animal, or any straining exertion, the passage of the blood into the breast was impeded, all the veins became tense, and a tube inserted into the returning jugular had blood running over, at a height of three feet above the heart." A similar increase of tension is shown in common venesection, so that the first jet of blood is often found to ascend to the top of a lofty bedstead, although a minute afterwards the stream may not project a single foot. Poiseuille found that the arterial tension of the carotid of a dog was just doubled when the aorta and its primary branches were previously tied.

7. *The Capillaries.*—It was Bichat's opinion that the influence of the heart did not extend beyond these vessels, but that "dans le système capillaire générale la contractilité insensible ou la tonicité reste seul pour cause de mouvement du sang;" and certainly, if we admit ever so little force to reside in this system, the extent of it is so great that the aggregate force of the whole would amount to something very considerable. I shall not do more than simply refer to plants, sponges, medusæ, entozoa, and many of the lower tribes of animals, in which the circulation of the nutritive fluids seems entirely to be dependent on the force of the capillaries; but as we ascend the animal series we still observe the influence of this system, the heart seeming to be, as in fishes, rather an appendage to respiration, to ensure the regularity of this function, than necessary to the general circulation. Hunter has remarked that the heart is proportionally small wherever the arteries are endowed with great muscular powers, examples of which may be found in fœtuses and hybernating animals: in both of which there is comparatively great tenacity of life, joined to an unusual development of the cutaneous capillary circulation. In the fœtus a double circulation is to be maintained through the placenta and the system, although the heart is found to be proportionally small as compared with the whole mass of blood, at the same time that it is placed under such circumstances that it cannot possibly receive any assistance from suction or muscular motion.

Another series of proofs is derived from diseases and malformations of the heart and great arteries. In many of these examples (See *Otto's Compend. of Path. Anat.*, pp. 262—269, and *Meckel's Man. d'Anat.*, ii. 109, 292.) it seems impossible to consider the heart as the prime agent of the circulation; not to mention that the fœtus has occasionally attained its full growth in the womb, and even lived for some days after expulsion, where not the smallest rudiment of a heart has been observable. (See *Brodie* in *Phil. Tr.* 1809, p. 161.) Now, as there is no pulsation in the vena cava of adults, in the trunk of the lymphatic system, nor in the aorta of fishes, but the fluid in these vessels is entirely propelled by the force *e tergo*, it seems reasonable to infer that probably the same principle operates in the fœtus, and that the organization in fact follows more or less the inferior type where the capillary circulation is totally independent of a central organ.

Many facts, however, might be stated which seem directly to prove the independent action of the capillaries: 1. The derivation of blood into the collateral cutaneous capillaries, and the increased warmth which ensues thereupon, in cases where a ligature has been placed on the main artery of a limb. 2. The united force of the capillaries, as evinced in the raising of the toe when one leg is placed over the other, as contrasted with the small force required to stop the current of blood in any large artery, seems only explicable on this principle. 3. Blushing, and partial determinations of blood in health and disease. In fevers the heart is observed to act with great energy at the same time that the whole capillary system is proportionably contracted, while, on the other hand, local determinations and excitements are perfectly compatible with a feeble action of their viscus. No fixed relation, in short, seems to exist between the activity of the central organ and the peripheral circulation. 4. Nearly allied to this is the derivation of blood to a wounded vessel or part after the extraction of the heart; and the generation, as it were, of new vessels capable of admitting red blood. 5. The liability of the capillary circulation to be retarded or entirely stopped by causes operating on the nervous system, notwithstanding that the heart's action continues unabated; for it must be evident that the power which can resist the impulse of the heart at one time, may assist it at another. 6. The different velocities of the blood in the same series of capillaries, and the liability of these velocities to be reversed from slight causes, is sufficient proof of the power of these vessels to control the local circulation. 7. The power of the capillaries to carry on the local circulation after the removal of the heart has been attested by numerous observers. Guillot remarked it in the frog's foot, when separated from the body, for nearly half an hour, (*Journ. de Phys., par Majendie*, xi. 170.) although the progression of the blood in such cases has generally been observed to be very irregular. 8. Hence the vacuity of the arterial system after death, and the gorged state of the veins; and hence also the disappearance of the blush of inflammation after death; but in deaths from lightning the arterial system is found full of blood, contrary to what generally happens; for the cause of death being such as to destroy the tonicity of the vessels, the capillary tubes are now no longer able to pump the blood from one system of vessels into the other. In asphyxia the right ventricle continues to act vigorously for some time after apparent death, although it is unable to propel its contents forward through the pulmonary capillaries, in consequence of these vessels being paralysed by the black blood (see *note*, p. 158.). 9. The experiments of Hunter and Wedemeyer before mentioned can only be explained on this hypothesis (p. 158); and, *lastly*, the analogy which arises from the foregoing phenomena, that the blood when it gets into the capillary structure falls more or less under the dominion of those laws which regulate the circulation of the inferior animals.

The inference which may fairly be drawn from the whole of these facts seems to be that the capillaries possess a *distributive* power over the blood, so as at least to regulate the local circulation independently of the central organ, in obedience to the necessities of each part. In the lower animals a slow circulation only of the blood is required, because the respiratory organs being here distributed over the whole body, and the systems of black and red blood being imperfectly preserved, a rapid circulation would answer no object: here, therefore, the capillaries suffice. In proportion, however, as the respiratory organs become more centralized so does the distinction between the two bloods become more definite and the necessity for arterial blood more imperative; so that here a heart becomes necessary, in order that the blood may be subjected to the influence of the air in a complete manner, and be supplied with due rapidity to the different organs of the body. It is possible that the capillaries may possess a *propellent* as well as a distributive power, and thus vicariously assist the heart under certain circumstances. I do not think it probable, however, that they concur to any great extent in the ordinary circulation.

8. *Vital attractions and repulsions*, existing either between the vessels and their contained fluids, or else between the different particles of the fluids themselves, is another agency to which many of the preceding phenomena have been ascribed. The following are the grounds for this opinion: 1. The capillaries appear as mere inert tubes under the microscope. 2. A determinate circulation or cyclosis is carried on in

the parenchyma of many animals and vegetables where no vessels exist. 3. A similar phenomenon is observed in the first days of embryonic life, the vessels being a result or consequence of these motions; and, lastly, the globules possess an inherent power of self-motion (see *notes*, pp. 63. 131), in virtue of which they move in determinate directions, agglomerate together in piles or rouleaux, traverse the substance of recently deposited lymph, ascend against the force of gravity when effused on the surfaces of living membranes, escape from the blood-vessels into the parenchyma of the surrounding textures, &c. &c. (*Haller, Döllinger, Gendrin, Rayer-Collard, Kaltenbrunner, and Marshall Hall.*) These attractions and repulsions are supposed by some to resemble the attractions and repulsions of similar particles united so as to compose muscular fibre, and by others to depend on the different electrical relations induced by respiration and nutrition altering the chemical constitution of the blood. Thus, according to this principle, attraction is supposed to draw the blood *to* a part being in action, and repulsion to drive it *from* it, and this in exact proportion to the energy of the action going on in that part; so that instead of the increased circulation being, as is commonly supposed, the cause of the increased action, the very reverse is the case. The vital action induced in a branch of a tree exclusively exposed to the sun, is the cause and not the effect of an increased flow of sap into it. (See *Alison's Physiology*, p. 32, and *Supp.*, p. 25.)

9. *Endosmose and Exosmose.*—Attempts have been made to refer the circulation of the blood to these sources, but it is difficult to conceive how such causes can give a determinate direction to the circulating fluids, or how the circulation thus carried on can be affected by physiological causes. (See *Raspail's Organic Chemistry, tr. by Dr. Henderson*, p. 400.)

BIBLIOGRAPHY OF THE VASCULAR SYSTEM*.

Adye, R. (Th.) De Sang. Circ. viribusque eundem facientibus. 1778.——*Albinus, B. S.* Acad. Adnot. 1754. l. iv. c. 8. De Arteriæ Memb. et Vasis.——*Alderson, J., M.D.* Quart. Journ., xviii. 223. Remarks on the Beating of the Heart.——*Alison**. loc. cit. and Fourth Report of Brit. Assoc., p. 674. On the Contractile Power of Arteries leading to Inflamed Parts.——*Andral.* l. c.——*Araldi, M.* Mem. delle Soc. Ital. (1804.) xi. 342. 383. (1810.) xv. 166. 196. Della Forza e dell' Influsso del Cuore sul Circolo del Sangue.——*Arnott*, N., M.D.* Elements of Physics. 5th edit. 1833. p. 543.

Baer, C. E. à De Ovi Mamm. et Hominis genesi. 1828.——*Barclay, J., M.D.* A Descrip. of the Arteries. 1812.——*Baron.* Bulletin des Sc. Méd. ii. 169. L'Usage des Anastomoses.——*Barry, Sir David.* Rech. Exp. sur les Causes de Mouvement du Sang dans les Veines. 1825. and *Transl.* 1826.——*Bassuel, C.* Mém. de Math. et de Phys. (1750.) i. 22–55. Diss. Hyd.-Anat. des Artères.——*Beclard.* Mém. de la Soc. Méd. d'Emul. (1817.) viii. Sur les Blessures des Artères.——*Behrends, J.* Diss. quâ demonstratur Cor Nervis carere, additâ Disquis. de Vi Nervorum Arterias cingentium. 1792.——*Bell, Sir C.* An Essay on the Forces which circulate the Blood. 1819.——*Bellieri, L.* De Urinis et Pulsibus, &c. 1698; et Opuscula. 1714. De Motu Cordis.——*Belmas, D.* Sur la Structure des Artères, &c. 1822.——*Berdoe.* l. c.——*Bertin, J. E.* Quæstio Med., An Causa Motus alterni Cordis multiplex? 1740. (*Haller.* Disp. Anat. ii. 429.)——*Bertin, R. T.* and *Bouillaud, J.* Traité

* See p. 138 for the explanation of the star and for the titles of those works which are here merely referred to.

des Maladies du Cœur, &c. 1824.——*Bernouilli.*—See *Passavant.*——*Berzelius, J. O.* A View of the Prog. of Anim. Chem. *tr.* by G. Brunnmark. 1813. pp. 24, 25. On the Chem. Constitution of the Arter. Tunics.——*Bichat**. l. c.——*Black, J., M.D.* On the Capill. Circ., &c. 1825.——*Blancardi, S.* Anat. Pract., &c. accedit item tractatus de Circ. Sang. &c. 1688.——*Bordeu, T.* Rech. sur le Pouls, &c. (ou Œuvres Comp. 1818. i.) 1754.——*Bourdon, Is.* Rech. sur le Méchan. de la Respir. et sur la Circ. du Sang. 1820.——*Borelli.* l. c.——*Breckelmann, M. L. R.* De Nervorum in Arteriis Imperio Dissert. 1744. (*Haller.* Disp. Anat. iv. 425.)——**Brodie, Sir Benj.* Phil. Trans. 1809. p. 161. Account of a Dissect. of a Human Fœtus in which the Circ. was carried on without a Heart.—*ib.* 1811. p. 36. On the Influence of the Brain on the Action of the Heart.——*Bosch, H. Van den.* Theor. und Prakt. Bemerkenger über das Muskelvermögen der Haargefaschench. 1792.——*Breschet.* Rech. Phys. et Path. sur le Système veineuse. 1819.——*Broussais, F. J. V.* Mém. de la Soc. Méd. d'Emul. vii. 1. and Ann. de la Soc. de Méd. de Montp. xx. 195. Sur la Circ. Capillaire.——*Brown, R.* Phil. Mag. et Ann. of Phil., Sep. 1828. p. 161. Micros. Obs. on the Self-movement of organic and inorganic Molecules.——*Buniva.* Recueil périod. de la Soc. de Méd. vii. 110. Exp. sur les Injections dans l'Anim. viv. et dans le Cadavre.——**Burdach.* l. c.——*Burns, A.* On the Diseases of the Heart. 1809.

Carlile, H. Third Report of Br. Association (1834), p. 454. Observ. on the Motions and Sounds of the Heart.——*Carlisle, Sir A.* Phil. Tr. 1805. p. 1. Croonian Lecture on Muscular Motion.—*ib.* 1800. p. 98; 1804. p. 17; and 1806. p. 1. On a Peculiarity in the Distrib. of the Arter. of slow-moving Animals.—— *Carson, J., M.D.* An Inquiry into the Causes of the Motion of the Blood, &c. 1815.——**Carus, C. E. G.* Lehrbuch der Zootomie, *tr.* Fr. by A. J. L. Jourdan, 2ème édit. 1835. ii. 298. Système Vasculaire, and *tr.* Eng. by R. T. Gore. ii. 263.——*Chirac, P.* De Motu Cordis, &c. 1698.——*Chassaignac, E.* De la Circulation Veineuse. ——*Clark, W., M.D.* Fourth Report of Br. Association (1835), pp. 95, 129. Report on Animal Physiology, comprising a Review of the Blood and Powers of Circulation.——*Clift, W.* Phil. Tr. 1815. p. 91. On the Influence of the Spinal Marrow on the Action of the Heart. ——*Cloquet, J.* De l'Influence des Efforts sur les Organes dans la Cavité thoracique. 1820.——*Corvisart, J. N.* Sur les Maladies du Cœur, &c., 3ème édit. 1818, and *tr.* by C. H. Hebb. 1813.——*Coxe, R.* An Enquiry into the Claims of Dr. William Harvey to the Discovery of the Circulation of the Blood, &c. 1834.——*Cranen, T.* Œcon. Anim. ad Circ. Sang., &c. 1703.——**Cuvier, le Baron, G.* Leçons d'Anat. Comp. an vii–xv. and Le Règne Animal. 1829.

Dennison, R., M.D. Disp. Inaug. Arter. omnes et Venarum Partem Irritabilitate præditas esse. (in Smellie's Thes. Med. iii. 394.) 1775.——**Döllinger.* l. c. et Journ. des Prog. des Sc. Méd. ix. Sur la Circ. Capill.——*Dutrochet, H.* Rech. Anat. et Phys. sur la Struct. intime des Anim. et des Vég. et sur leur Motilité. 1824.—De l'Agent immédiat de Mouvement Vital. 1826; and Ann. des Sc. Nat. xv.

Ehrmann, C. H. Struct. des Artères et leur Propriétés et leurs Fonctions, &c. 1822.—— *Ens, A.* (Th.) De Causâ Vices Cordis alternas producente. 1745. (*Haller.* Disp. Anat. ii. 409.).——*Entius, G.* Apol. pro Circ. Sang. 1689.

Falconer, W., M.D. Observ. respecting the Pulse. 1796.——*Fischer.* Dissertatio de Motu Sanguinis, 1720.——*Floerckius, G.* (Th.) Transitum Sang. per Vasa minima, &c. 1713.——*Flourens, P.* Rech. sur les Fonctions du Syst. Nerveux dans les Animaux vertébrés, 1824–5. and Supplément du précédent, 1825. and Mém. de l'Institut, tom. x.——*Formay, J. L.* Versuch einer Wurdigung der Pulsen. 1823.——*Fouquet, H.* Sur le Pouls (nouv. édit.). 1818.

Gardien. Bull. du Sc. Méd. iv. 31. Sur la Circ. Capill.——*Gayant, L.* Mém. de Paris. i. p. 36. Obs. sur les Valv. des Veines.——*Gendrin,* l. c.——*Gerdy, S. N.* Sur l'organ. du Cœur, dans le Journ. Comp. du Dic. des Sc. Méd.——*Giulo et Rossi.* Mém. de l'Acad. de Sc. de Turin. iv. 50. Dissert. de Excitabilitate Contract. Vi Partibus Musc. ope. Elect.——*Glass, C. P.* De Sang. Circ. 1736. (*Haller.* Disp. Anat. ii. 201.)——*Grant.* l. c. et Edin. Phil. Journ. xiii. and xiv.——*Gruner, C. J.* Semiotice Phys. et Pathol. 1775.——*Guillot, N.* Journ. de Phys. par Majendie. (1831.) xi. 145. Obs. sur quelques Phénom. de la Circ.

Hales, G., D.D.* Statical Essays. 4th edit. 1767.——Hall, M., M.D.* On the Circul. of the Blood. 1831.——**Haller, A.* l. c. et Mém. sur la Nat. Sens. et Irrit. des Parties. 1756. §. xi.—Opera Minora. i. 60–241. Sur la Circul. Capill.—Sur la Formation du Cœur dans le Poulet, &c. 1758.——Comm. Soc. Gotting. i. 263. Exp. de Cordis Motu; and *ib.* iv. 396. De Sang. Motu Exp. anat.——*Harrison, R.* On the Surgical Anat. of the Arteries. 1824-5.——**Harvey, G.* De Cordis et Sang. Motu. 1648.——**Hastings, C., M.D.* On Inflam. of the Mucous Mem. of the Lungs, with Exp. Inquiries respecting the contractile power of the Blood-vessels in Inflam. 1820.——*Hebenstreit, J. S.* De Vaginis Vasorum. 1740.——*Heberden, W., M.D.* Med. Trans. ii. 18. Remarks on the Pulse.——*Hering, Prof.* Zeitschrift für Physiologie, iii. and iv. part 1.—Journ. de Prog. des Sc. Méd. x. et Med. Gaz. (1834). xiv. 745. Exp. tending to show the Rapidity of the Circ.——*Hewson.* l. c.——*Hodgson,* l. c.——*Home, Sir E.* Lect. on Comp. Anat. 1814. p. 47. On the Mechan. of the Heart.——*Hope, J., M.D.* On the Diseases of the Heart, comprising a new View of the Physiology of the Heart's Action. 1832.——*Housset.* Mém. sur les Parties irrit. et sens. ii. 404.——*Humboldt, F. A.* Exp. sur l'Irrit. des Fibres Musc., &c. *tr.* from the German by *J. F. Jadelot.* 1799.——*Hunt, J.* Obs. on the Circ. of the Blood, &c. 1787.

**Jones, T. F.* On the Process employed by Nature in suppressing Hæmorrhage. 1805. ——*Jurin, J.* Phil. Trans. 1718. p. 863; 1719. pp. 929. 1039. Diss. de Potentia Cordis.

**Kaltenbrunner.* l. c.——*Keill, J.* Tentam. Med.-Phy. de Velocitate Sanguinis. 1718: and Phil. Tr. 1719. p. 995.——*Kerr, G.* Obs. on the Harveian Doct. of the Circ. of the Blood. 1819.——*Konrad, G. V.* De Arter. Fabricâ. 1814.——*Kramp, C.* De Vi vitali Arteriarum, &c. 1785–8.——*Kreysig.* Ueber die Herzkrankheiten. 1814.

Laennec, R. T. H. De l'Auscult. Médiate. 3ème édit. 1831. pp. 195, 445. *tr.* by J. Forbes, M.D. 4th edit. 1834. On the Action of the Heart.——*Lamure, F.* Mém. de Paris, 1749. p. 541; and 1765. p. 620. Rech. sur la Cause de la Pouls des Artères.——*Lancisi.* l. c.——*Langelott, A. C.* De Fabricâ et Usu Cordis. 1676.——*Lassone.* Mém. de Paris, 1756. p. 31. Rech. sur la Struct. des Artères.——*Leeuwenhoeck.* l. c.——*Le Gallois.* l. c. et Exp. sur le Principe de la Vie. 1812.—Nouv. Bull. de la Soc. Philom. (1812.) iii. 5. Sur la Force du Cœur; et Recueil périod. de la Soc. de Méd. xxxv. 425.——**Leuret.* Journ. des Prog. des Sc. Méd. v. Sur la Circ. Capill. ——*Lister.* Phil. Tr. 1834. p. 365. Obs. on the Struct. and Functions of tubular and cellular Polypi, showing the mode of circ. in these animals.——*Lorry.* Savans Etrangers. (1752.) iii.——*Lower, R., M.D.* Tractatus de Corde. 1728.——*Luca, S. E., M.D.* Quædam Obs. Anat. circa Nervos, Arterias adeuntes et comitantes. 1810. ——*Ludwig, C. G.* (Th.) De Arter. Tunicis. 1739. (*Haller.* Disp. Anat. ii. i.)

**Majendie.* l. c. et Journ. de Phys. (1821.) i. 97. 102. 132. and 190. Sur la Circ. et sur l'Action des Artères dans la Circ.; and Lectures on the Circ. in Lancet 1834–5. i. 310. et seq.——*Malpighi.* l. c.——*Martin-Saint-Ange.* Anatomie Analytique: Circulation du Sang, considérée chez le fœtus de l'homme, et comparativement des quatre classes d'animaux vertébrés. 1833.——*Marx, H.* Diatribe Anat.-Phys. de Structurâ atque Vitâ Venarum. 1819.——*Mauban, R.* Essai sur la Circul. 1808.——*Mayo, H.* l. c. and Anat. and Phys. Comm. 1822–3. p. 16.——*Mayer, J. C. A.* Anatomische Beschreibung der Blutgefasse des menschlichen Körpers. 1777–8. et Edit. 2de. 1788.——*Meckel, J. F.* Journ. Comp. du Dic. des Sc. Méd., i. 259. Sur le Développment du Cœur, et Man. d'Anat. Gén. *tr.* by *A. L. Jourdan* et *G. Breschet.* 1825. i. 125. Du Système Vasculaire.——*Meyen,* l. c.——*Mondini.* De Arteriarum Tunicis, in Opuscoli, &c. 1817.——*Moulin.* l. c.——*Munro, A.* (*Prim.*) Edin. Med. Ess. and Obs., ii. 264. Remarks on the Coats of Arteries.——*Murray, A.* Descrip. Arteriarum. 1783–98.

Nicolaus, H. A. De Directione Vasorum pro modificando Sang. Circ. 1725. (*Haller.* Disp. Anat., ii. 481.)——*Nysten.* l. c. et Nouv. Rech. Galv. sur les Org. musculaires, &c. An xi.

Paletta, J. B. Mem. dell' Instit. Ital., i. 34. Del Movimento retrog. de Sangue.——*Parry, C. H., M.D.* On the Arterial Pulse. 1816; and Add. Exp. 1819.——*Passavant, D.* (Th.) De Vi Cordis. 1748. (*Haller.* Disp. Anat., vii. 329.)——*Pasta, A.* De Motu Sang. post Mortem, &c. 1786.——*Pechlin, J. N.* De Fabricâ et Usu Cordis. 1676.——*Pelletan.* Clin. Chir. 1810. iii. Sur le Cœur.——**Philip, A. P. W., M.D.* Exper. Enquiry into the Laws of the Vital Functions. 2nd edit. 1818; and Phil. Tr. 1815. pp. 65, 424. On the Relations between the Nervous and Sanguiferous Systems.—See also Treatise on Sympt. Fevers. 4th edit. 1820. pp. 15, 17.; et Med. and Chir. Tr., xii. 401. On the Circulation, and particularly the Capillary.——*Piorry, P. A.* De l'Explor. des Organes par la Percussion, and Collect. de Mém. sur la Phys. 1831. 3ème. Sur la Circ.——*Plenk.* l. c.——**Poiseuille, J. L. M.* Journ. de Phys. par Majendie, (1828.) viii. 273. (1829.) ix. 341. Sur la Force du Cœur aortique:—*ib.* p. 44. Sur l'Action des Artères dans la Circ. artérielle:—*ib.* (1830.) x. 277. Rech. sur la Cause du Mouvement du Sang dans les Veines.——*Portal, A.* L'Anat. Méd. 1804. iii. 72; and Mém. de Paris. 1770. pp. 42, 244.——*Posewitz, J. F. S.* Phys. der Pulsadern des menschlichen Körpers. 1795.——*Prevost* and *Dumas.* Ann. des Sc. Nat. iii. 46. Développement du Cœur et Formation du Sang.—See also tom. xii.——*Prochaska.* l. c.

Raspail. l. c. et Bull. des Sc. Nat. xii. 193.——*Rayer-Collard.* Essai d'une Syst. de Zoonom., p. 80.——*Regis, J. C.* De Sang. in suo per vasa progressu, &c. (*Haller.* Disp. Anat., ii. 595.)——*Reichel.* l. c.——*Reisel, S.* Misc. Acad. Nat. Cur. 1673–4. p. 245. 1678. p. 91. 1682. p. 448. De Circul.——*Rezia, J.* De Ratione Sang. Motus in Arterias. (*Ræmer.* Dissert. Med. Ital.)——*Richelmann, J. E.* De Valvularum, &c. 1683.——*Richerand.* l. c. et Mém. de la Soc. d'Emul. an iii. 296.——*Riolan, J.* De Motu Cordis et ejus Circ. 1652.——*Rolando.* Journ. Comp. du Dic. des Sc. Méd., xv. 323. xvi. 34. Sur la Formation du Cœur et des Vaisseaux, &c.——*Rose, L. G.* l. c.

Sabatier, R. B. Traité d'Anat. 3ème édit. 1791. iii.; and Mém. de Paris. 1774. p. 51. Sur la Circ. du Sang du Fœtus et sur la Capacité du Cœur.——*Santorini, J. D.* Obs. Anat. 1724. cap. viii. De iis quæ in Thoracem sunt.——*Sauvages, F. L. B.* Mém. de Montp., ii. 140. 211. Théorie du Pouls and Mém. de Berlin. 1755. p. 34. Rech.

sur les Loix du Mouvement du Sang.——*Scarpa, A.* Tabulæ Neurol. ad illust. Hist. Anat. Cardiacorum Nervorum. 1794.——*Schedel, F. J.* Physiologia Pulsus. 1829. ——*Schliting.* Savans Etrangers, i.——*Schmidt, D. W.* (Th.) De Motu Sanguinis per Cor. 1737. (*Haller.* Disp. Anat., ii. 391.)——**Schultz, K. H.* l. c. et Journ. Comp. du Dic. des Sc. Méd., xix.——**Sénac.* l. c.——*Sharpey.* Edin. Med. and Surg. Journ., xxxiv.——*Smith.* l. c.——*Spallanzani, Z.* Exp. sur la Circ., &c. *tr.* par D.M.M. Tourdes. *An.* viii.——**Soemmerring, S. T.* De Corp. hum. Fabricâ. 1794–1801. v. Angiologia, and Lehre vom Barre des menschlichen Körpers, iv.——*Soutien, G.* Rec. périod. de la Soc. de Santé de Paris, iii. 402. Sur la Circul.——*Sprengel, K.* Beiträge zur Geschichte der Pulsen. 1787.——*Storer.* Trans. of a Soc. for the Improvement of Med. and Chir. Knowledge. 1812. On the Want of Pulsation in paralytic Limbs.——*Swieten, S. Van.* (Th.) De Arteriæ Fabrica, &c. 1725.

Testa, A. J. Delle Malattie del Cuore. 1810–3.——*Thomson, J.* l. c.——**Tiedemann, F.* l. c. et Tabulæ Arteriarum. 1822–4.——*Treviranus.* Erscheinungen, l. c.——*Turner, T.* On the Arterial System. 1825.——*Tyssot, P. F.* De Circ. Sang. 1743.

Vaust, J. F. Rech. sur le Struct. et les Mouvemens du Cœur. 1821.——**Vershuir, G.* De Arteriarum et Ven. Vi irritabili, &c. 1766.——*Vieussens.* l. c.et Novum Vasorum Corporis hum. Systema. 1705; and Traité de la Struct. et du Mouvement du Cœur. 1711.

Walter, F. A. Angiologisches Handbuch. 1789.——**Wedemeyer.* l. c. et Edin. Med. and Surg. Journ., xxxii. 10; and xxxiv. 89.——*Weitbrecht, J.* Comm. Acad. Petrop., vi. 276. vii. 283. viii. 334. De Circul. Sanguinis.——*Whytt.* l. c.——*Wilson, A., M.D.* On the Circul. of the Blood. 1774.——*Winslow, W.* Mém. de Paris. 1711. pp. 196, 201. Sur le Cœur.——**Wintringham, C., M.D.* An Inquiry into the Exility of the Vessels of the Human Body. 1743; or Works. 1752.——**Wolff, C. F.* Acta Acad. Petrop. 1780–7; et Nova Acta, i. and viii. Dissert. Octonovem de Cordis Fibris.——*Wrisberg, H. A.* De Nervis Arterias Venasque comitantes. 1800.

**Young.* l. c. et Phil. Tr. 1808. p. 164. Hydraulic Investigations concerning the Motion of the Blood.—1809. p. 1. On the Functions of the Heart and Arteries.

Zerrener, A. T. N. An Cor Nervis careat et iis carere possit? 1794.——*Zimmermann, J. G.* Diss. Phys. de Irritabilitate. 1751; and Das Leben des Herrn von Haller. 1755. ——*Zugenbuhler.* Diss. de Motu Sang. 1815.

N.B. For the Pathology of the Vascular System consult *Otto's* Compendium of Path. Anat., *tr.* by *J. F. South.* 1831. § xix.; *Ploucquet's* Repertorium Medicinæ Practicæ. 1808–9; and *Reuss's* Repertorium Commentationum a Societatibus Literariis. 1801–13. tom. x. and xii.

PART II.

CHAPTER I.

UNION BY THE FIRST INTENTION.

I MAY observe, that all alterations in the natural dispositions of a body are the result either of injury or disease; and that all deviations from its natural actions arise from a new disposition being formed[a]. Injury is commonly simple; disease more complicated. The dispositions arising from these are of three kinds: the *first* is the disposition of restoration, in consequence of some immediate mischief, and is the most simple. The *second* is the disposition arising from necessity; as, for instance, that which produces the action of thickening parts, of ulceration, &c. This is a little more complicated than the former, as it may arise both from accident and disease, and therefore becomes a compound of the two. The *third* is the disposition in consequence of disease; which is more complicated than either, as diseases are infinite. Yet many local diseases, although complex in their natures, are so simple in their extent as to allow the removal of the diseased part; becoming, when that is done, similar to many accidents[b].

As disease is a wrong action of the living parts, the restoration to health must first consist in stopping the diseased dispositions and actions, and then in a retrograde motion towards health.

---

[a] [This observation is probably correct as far as regards injuries, which necessitate a new disposition, and consequently new actions, in order to repair the injury. But with regard to disease, it is, I think, manifestly wrong. Disease is a disordered state of action of the living parts, which must have been preceded by a disposition to such state of action. How, then, can such an alteration in the disposition be considered as the result of disease? It should rather be, all alterations in the natural dispositions of the body are the result of injury or some other cause tending to disorder them.]

[b] [It would probably have been better to have divided these dispositions into two kinds, viz. healthy and unhealthy. The temporary thickening of the parts in the union of fractured bones and numberless other processes is as much a restorative action as union by the first intention, not to mention that this last action is invariably attended with some degree of thickening of the parts.]

In treating systematically of such complaints as are the objects of surgery, we should always begin with the most simple, and advance gradually to the more complicated, by which means we shall be more clearly understood.

There are many complaints requiring the attention of the surgeon which cannot be called disease; because, having been produced by something foreign to the body, as in accidents, they are to be considered as a violence committed upon it, altering in some degree the structure of parts, and consequently interrupting the natural operations already described. The parts so hurt not being able to pursue their original or natural mode of action, are obliged to deviate from it; and this deviation will vary according, [1.] to the nature of the violence, [2.] the nature of the part, and [3.] the state of the constitution at the time.

An alteration in structure requires a new mode of action for its restoration: as the act of restoration cannot be the same with what was natural to the parts before any alteration had taken place. The alteration of structure by violence requires only the most simple change in the natural action of the part to restore it, and of course the most simple method of treatment by art, if it be such as to require any assistance at all; for there are many accidents where none is necessary. It will be proper to observe here that there is a circumstance attending accidental injury which does not belong to disease, viz. that the injury done has in all cases a tendency to produce both the disposition and the means of cure.

The operations of restoration arise naturally out of the accident itself; for, when there is only a mechanical alteration in the structure, the stimulus of imperfection taking place immediately calls forth the action of restoration. But this is contrary to what happens in disease; for disease is a disposition producing a wrong action, and it must continue this wrong action till the disposition is stopped or wears itself out. When this salutary effect, however, has once taken place, the state of the body becomes similar to that in a simple accident, viz. a consciousness of imperfection is excited which produces the action of restoration.

In injuries arising from accident we have hitherto supposed that the parts have no tendency to any diseased action independently of the accident, for if they have, it is probable that such a tendency may be stronger than the disposition for restoration, and in that case they will fall into the peculiar diseased action, as was explained when treating of susceptibility. Let us take the scrofula and the cancer as examples, and we shall find, that if a part be hurt which has a strong tendency to scrofula, it will most probably run into the scrofulous mode of action in preference to that of restoration, and therefore we have many joints, when injured, assuming the scrofulous action, called white swelling; or if a woman beyond thirty years of age receives a blow on the breast, it is more likely to acquire the cancerous mode of action than that of restoration, which should be well distinguished from what is immediately consequent, viz. the inflammation; for on this depends a knowledge of diseases.

Although accident may be said to produce an effect on a part (whatever that effect may be,) which has a tendency to its own cure, yet there are often not only immediate consequences arising from that effect, as inflammation; and again, the consequences of this inflammation, as suppuration; but the bases of diseases are also frequently laid by it, not by producing them immediately or naturally, but by exciting some susceptibility of the constitution or of a part into a disposition for a disease which may be latent for a considerable time, and then come into action. Thus scrofula, cancer, &c. often arise from accident, even where the parts, in consequence of the injury, have gone through the immediate and the secondary stages of a cure.

Those effects of accident which arise from the nature of the parts hurt may be divided into such as take place in sound parts, and such as affect parts already diseased. The first is what I shall at present treat of; the second, being connected with disease, is not to our present purpose.

The injuries done to sound parts I shall divide into two sorts, according to the effects of the accident. The *first* kind consists of those in which the injured parts do not communicate externally, as concussions of the whole body or of particular parts, strains, bruises, and simple fractures, either of bone or of tendon, which form a large division. The *second* consists of those which have an external communication, comprehending wounds of all kinds, and compound fractures. Bruises which have destroyed the life of the part may be considered as a *third* division, partaking, at the beginning, of the nature of the first, but finally terminating like the second[a].

§. 1. *Of Injuries in which there is no external Communication.*

The injuries of the first division, in which the parts do not communicate externally, seldom inflame, while those of the second commonly

[a] [The greater violence of the inflammation succeeding to injuries which communicate externally may be a sufficient ground for the division of the text, although it should be remembered that the reparative processes are identically the same in both cases. Ruptured muscles and tendons, and many kinds of bruises, excite quite as much inflammation as clean incised wounds of the same parts.]

both inflame and suppurate. The same operations, however, very often take place in both, though the order in which they happen is reversed, the first becoming like the second, by inflaming and suppurating, and the second being in many cases, when properly treated, brought back to a resemblance of the first, and united by the first intention, by which inflammation and suppuration are prevented. But when the life of a part has been destroyed by the accident, it must necessarily suppurate; and therefore these injuries will be rendered similar, in this respect, to those which communicate immediately, and have not been united by the first intention.

That injury which in its nature is the most simple, and yet calls forth the actions of the part to recover from it, is a degree of concussion*, where the only effect produced is a debility of the actions or functions of the whole or part, similar to that occasioned by a bruise, in which the continuity of the substance is not interrupted: in such a state the parts have little to do but to expand and reinstate themselves in their natural position, actions, and feelings; and this is what happens in concussion of the brain[a].

The rupture of a small blood-vessel is, perhaps, the next in order of simplicity. Where the continuity of the part is broken, extravasation takes place, and the blood is diffused into the common cellular membrane, into the interstices of some part, or into a circumscribed cavity. But should the vessel be either very large, or essential to life, such as the femoral, brachial, or coronary arteries; or should the rupture take place in a vital part, as the brain, or into interstices or cavities belonging to a vital part, as into the cavities of the brain or pericardium, in all such cases the injury may kill from the extravasation alone, however inconsiderable may be the original mischief.

The operation of restoration in this case, when the vital parts are not concerned or disturbed, consists, first, in the coagulation of the extravasated blood between the ruptured parts, laying, as it were, the foundation of union; next, in closing the ruptured vessel or in promoting its inosculation; and some time after in bringing about an absorption of the superfluous extravasated blood. If the vessel close, that effect is produced by the muscular contraction of its coats; but in what way it

* Here I mean concussion as a general term, not confining it to the brain.

[a] [Concussion of the brain is not unfrequently attended with an extravasation of blood in minute specks over an extended surface of the interior of the organ, as if arising from a rupture of a multitude of minute vessels: (See *Bright's Medical Reports*, vol. i. p. 405, and plates.) Probably some organic derangement takes place in all cases of concussion, although, from the extreme delicacy and minuteness of the ultimate structure, such changes are not always cognizable by our senses.]

inosculates, whether by the two orifices when opposed having a mutual attraction, and, instead of contracting the two portions of the ruptured vessel elongating, so as to approach each other reciprocally, and unite*, or whether by a new piece of vessel being formed in the intermediate coagulable lymph, is not easily determined[a].

Inosculation, however, can only take place where the extent of the parts divided is not great, and the opposite surfaces remain near each other; but even then it is most probable that we must in part ascribe to another mode of union the communication of vessels which takes

* Inosculation is a term commonly used by writers, but whether it was derived from theory or observation is not material. The very few instances where it can be observed, together with the want of accuracy in those who first introduced the term, would incline me to think that it arose from theory or opinion only. I never could get an opportunity of observing it in all my experiments and observations on inflammation, except in the coats of the eye. In many inflammations of that organ we find an artery or arteries passing from the tunica conjunctiva to the cornea, and ramifying on that part. These have been often cut across to prevent the influx of blood; the two ends are seen to shrink, but in a little time they are again perceived to unite, and the circulation to be carried on as before. In this there can be no deception; and to perform, therefore, such an operation effectually a part of the vessel should be removed[1].

---

[1] [Nothing certainly is known respecting the mode in which vessels inosculate. According to Professor Thomson, Mr. Hunter was deceived respecting the direct inosculation of the vessels of the sclerotic coat of the eye. "An attentive examination," he says, "of the phenomena will show that it is not the divided extremities that unite again, but the folds of small branches that are prolonged into the intermediate space, which become channels of communication between the larger trunks, which had been divided, but the extremities of which had been previously closed." (*Lect. on Inflam.*, p. 213.) This account, however, does not appear to me to render the matter at all more clear.

With regard to the means employed by nature for arresting hæmorrhage, see *note*, i. 359.]

[a] [Arteries of considerable size are sometimes regenerated in the lower animals. Dr. Parry tied the carotid artery of a young ram in two places, and removed two inches and a half of the intermediate portion, but in twenty-seven days the vessel was completely restored, so that scarcely any evidence appeared of the operation having been performed. In another case the right and left carotids of a young ram were tied with single ligatures, but the continuity of these arteries was also completely restored in the course of eight weeks, although not in so perfect a manner as in the former experiment.

The process by which this is accomplished seems to be as follows. Coagulable lymph is first poured out by the inflamed vessels in the intermediate space between the two ligatures, which soon becomes organized, when a number of minute vessels may be observed extending in parallel lines between the two extremities of the artery, and thus making a communication between them. After a time one of these vessels is observed to enlarge, till at length it acquires the full size of the original vessel; but, in proportion as this takes place, the others dwindle away, and the superfluous lymph becomes absorbed. Such at least seems to be the process in brute animals where a portion of a large artery has been removed. I am not aware that anything similar has been observed in man.]

place between the two divided surfaces; for where inosculation does not or cannot take place, the union of the ruptured vessels is produced by the coagulation of the extravasated blood of this part, which becomes vascular. That the blood becomes vascular is clearly shown in the case of the blood extravasated on the testicle. [Pl. XVIII. and XIX.] The superfluous extravasated blood is taken up by the absorbents, by which means the whole is reinstated as much as it is in the power of the parts to do it.

I may observe here that the power of recovery in the arteries is greater nearly in proportion to the smallness of their size, which is combined with several causes, viz. their distance from the heart, their elasticity, their division into smaller branches, and their accumulated diameters becoming larger, which allows them to recover. Secondly, there is an increased power within the smaller artery itself, abstracted from the above circumstances[a].

This includes a great variety of cases, and the most simple difference which can happen between them will be owing to the magnitude of the ruptured parts, or to a difference in the parts themselves, or to the magnitude of the injury, or to a difference in the effects. It will comprehend simple fractures of all kinds, broken tendons, (as is often the case with the tendo Achillis,) and even many injuries of the brain, producing extravasations of blood, which is probably the only way in which the brain can be torn when there is no fracture[b].

Some of these will often require art to reinstate them in the natural position, out of which they may have been put by the accident, or by some peculiar circumstance attending the nature of the part, as we see in a fracture of the patella, or broken tendon, where the upper part being too far pulled up by the muscles, it must be reinstated by the hand of the surgeon, to bring the parts into a situation more favourable to their recovery.

But extravasations, even from the most simple accidents, are often so situated as to obstruct the actions of life; as, for instance, in that affec-

[a] [The arteries become more muscular in proportion as the impetus of the blood becomes less powerful; both which circumstances must combine to render the obliteration of a bleeding vessel more effectual and speedy. Is this, however, the author's drift? or does he mean by "the power of recovery" that the small arteries, which are "the formers and supporters of the body," or "the efficient part of the whole animal respecting itself," are capable of reinstating themselves after injury sooner than other parts?

[b] [Concussion of the brain may be in three degrees: 1. It may occasion an extensive rupture of the substance of the brain; 2. it may occasion rupture of the minute vessels only, giving rise to an effusion of blood from a multitude of minute points; and, 3. it may only strain the organ, without producing any visible rupture. These last cases, however, are not unfrequently fatal. See *note*, i. 488.]

tion of the brain which is called apoplexy. The same thing happens in extravasations into the pericardium, or into any of the other vital parts, where little can be done although much is wanted. In many other parts, where the actions of life cannot be affected, yet the extravasations are often too considerable to allow the parts to go through their proper modes of restoration. The quantity of extravasated blood being often so large as to distend the parts, and form a kind of tumour called ecchymosis, of which I shall now treat. The extravasated blood in such cases being the only visible complaint, to remove it is the cure; which may be effected by absorption, or, if necessary, by an operation.

An ecchymosis we may consider as of two kinds, one in which the blood coagulates when extravasated, the other where it remains fluid; but this distinction makes little difference in the disease itself, and of course little in the mode of treatment. It should be observed, however, that the first kind for the most part terminates well, while the second sometimes inflames and suppurates.

When these injuries get well by the absorption of the blood, the cure is gradual, and often takes a considerable time; but if the tumours become less and do not inflame, they should be allowed to go on to perform their own cure: and even where inflammation takes place, that should be permitted to advance to suppuration, and the tumours to threaten bursting before they are opened by art, or, what I believe would be still better practice, they should be left to open of themselves altogether.

In some instances, a blow, the cause of the ecchymosis, may have injured the superficial parts or skin so much as to produce inflammation; and under such circumstances I should recommend the case to be treated as an inflammation arising from any other cause, without paying attention to the blood underneath. It often happens that the blow has deadened the skin over this blood, which deadened part, as is usual in such cases, must, in a certain time afterwards, separate from the living. Where this has taken place, and the extravasated blood has coagulated, it has often been found to remain in the cavity as a mere extraneous body, without acting, and without even allowing the stimulus of an exposed surface or of an imperfect cavity to take place. The edges of the skin all round showing the disposition to contract over this blood, as if it was a living part to be preserved, nothing has seemed to be wanting to finish the cure but the blood being alive with due powers of action.

In these cases the common practice has been to scoop out the blood and distend the internal surface with warm dressings, to stimulate it to inflammation, &c., and, a sore being the consequence of this method, it goes on as sores commonly do. But in other cases, where the opening leading to the coagulated blood has been very small, I have seen that, without any other means being used, the blood has been gradually squeezed out of the orifice by the contraction of the surrounding parts, till the whole cavity became so much contracted as to contain no more than what seemed to serve as a bond of union to the parts; and thus the cure has been completed without further trouble. The following case was treated in this way.

Mrs. B—t fell backwards and pitched upon a pail which was behind her, and the left labium pudendi struck against its handle with the whole weight of her body. Within five minutes after the accident the bruised part swelled to as great a degree as the skin would allow; from which sudden appearance of the swelling, and the feeling of fluctuation, I concluded that blood had been extravasated by the rupture of some small artery. I bled her, and desired a poultice to be applied to the part, in order to keep the skin as easy as possible under such distention. Believing the tumour to arise from extravasated blood, I did not choose to open it, that the bleeding might be sooner stopped by the pressure of the extravasated blood against the sides of the cavity. Some hours after the accident the skin burst, and a good deal of blood came away. On examining the wound, I found the opening of considerable size, leading into a cavity as large as the egg of a goose, and filled with coagulated blood, which I did not remove, for the reason given above, that it might assist in stopping the vessels which were still bleeding. The poultice was continued, the bleeding gradually became less, and every time I examined the part I found the cavity diminished, but still filled with coagulated blood, which continued to be pushed out of the wound, and after some time a slough came off from the bruised skin, which enlarged the size of the wound. About a fortnight after the accident the parts were all so much collapsed as to have forced out the blood entirely, and there seemed only a superficial sore, not above an inch long and half an inch wide.

What may it be supposed would have been the consequence if I had enlarged the opening, scooped out the blood, and dressed the part with lint, or any other application I might think proper? The effect of such treatment would certainly have been a large sore, nearly of the same size with the cavity; and the sides of the cavity would have inflamed and suppurated. Is there not reason to believe that the coagulated blood, by remaining in the wound, prevented inflammation over the whole surface, and allowed the parts to contract to their natural position, so as to leave no other sore than that where the skin had burst and sloughed? This practice should be generally followed in such cases of ecchymosis

The second species of ecchymosis is that in which the blood has not coagulated but remains fluid. This case, although it also frequently occurs, does not always terminate so well as the former, nor allow of such a salutary termination, where an opening has been made, either by the accident or by art, for then suppuration will be produced all over the cavity; more caution is, therefore, necessary to prevent an opening. It has often the appearance of an encysted tumour; but, being an immediate consequence of some accident upon the part, its nature becomes readily understood, though sometimes from its situation it has the symptoms of an aneurism attending it, neither does the cause of it contradict this idea.

If formed over a large artery, the tumour will be attended with a pulsation; but when from this cause it cannot be made to subside by pressure, yet it is not, therefore, to be supposed harmless, as in fact it requires to be treated with great caution. If the pulsation should arise from the real influx of blood, this will soon be shown by the increase of the tumour, and will lead to the proper treatment, viz. opening it and stopping the bleeding vessel[a]. This seldom happens from contusion, the kind of accident destroying in some degree [the texture of the parts, and] the free exit of the blood out of the artery; and if the tumour should not increase after a certain period, even if there be a pretty evident pulsation, we may then be certain that it assumes this symptom from some neighbouring artery or arteries. The ecchymosis which is produced on the head of a child during birth has sometimes a pulsation, arising from that of the brain, as the sutures are still open; and every tumour of the scalp, whether from a blow or any other cause, may be mistaken for aneurism, if it appears before the fontanel be closed, and should it be opened without proper examination may disconcert the ignorant surgeon.

That the blood does not coagulate in this species of ecchymosis, must arise from some peculiar mode of action in the vessels, occasioned by the effects of the injury; for I apprehend that in such cases the blood dies in the act of extravasation, in the same manner as the blood of the menstrual discharge whenever it is effused.

The ecchymosis which we have mentioned as happening very commonly to children in the birth, particularly under the scalp, requires nothing to be done, as by waiting with patience the whole will in general be absorbed; but although this is commonly the event in new-born

[a] [This constitutes the false diffused aneurism of authors, which always requires that the vessel should be secured both above and below the wound with as little delay as possible. The pressure of the effused blood on the superior portion of the artery often prevents any pulsation from being perceptible.]

infants, yet ecchymosis does not terminate alike favourably in other cases, the tumour often remaining for a considerable time without undergoing any change, and after months sometimes disappearing, but at other times inflaming and suppurating.

When an extravasation of blood takes place between the scalp and head, in consequence of a blow, which is very common, and continues fluid, we find a kind of ridge all round the bag, and by pressing all round the edge of the bag the finger sinks, so as to give distinctly (as we conceive) the feeling of a depressed bone; but this feeling of depression following the edge of the ecchymosis all round, is a proof that it cannot be depression of the bone, because no depression could be so regular, nor would any depression be of the same extent with the ecchymosis. The edge of the scalp surrounding the ecchymosis seems to be raised, and I believe it is; if so, then something similar to the adhesive inflammation must have taken place to set bounds to the extent of the bag, and to hinder the blood from getting into the cellular membrane. It might, perhaps, be the best practice to make a small opening into such tumours with a lancet, and by letting out the blood, get the sides of the cavity to heal by the first intention[a]. When the parts inflame and suppurate, the case is to be treated as an abscess.

This sometimes disappears by resolution; but this being seldom permitted, the ecchymosis is reduced either to the state of a fresh wound, which is allowed to suppurate, or an abscess; for surgeons are induced to open early by seeing an inflammation and feeling a fluctuation, two strong motives when every circumstance is not well attended to; but in such cases I should wait till I observed evident signs of suppuration, viz. the thinning of the skin over the matter, and pointing of the contents, which are the only true marks of the formation of matter, as well as of its coming near the skin.

If the blow should have deadened a part of the skin, then a separation of the slough will take place, and expose this cavity so as to produce suppuration. And this is to be considered as a step still further removed from the most simple species of injury than where the blood coagulates. I am not able, under such circumstances, decidedly to say which is the best practice, whether to leave the slough to separate, or to make a small opening and allow the blood to escape slowly from the cavity.

In both kinds of ecchymosis, when inflammation has taken place in

---

[a] [It can rarely be necessary to interfere with these cases, which generally do well under a simple treatment. The liability of the scalp to erysipelatous inflammation renders it particularly inexpedient to make any breach of the surface.]

the skin from the violence, if it has not advanced to suppuration, the object of the surgeon should be to bring about the resolution of the tumour: when he finds there is no further increase of the tumour, he may conclude that resolution is beginning to take place, which being clearly ascertained, he is then to assist in exciting the absorbents to do their duty, in order to take up the extravasated blood. I believe the best stimulus is pressure, which, if urged beyond the point of ease, sets the absorbents of the part to work, for the purpose of removing the substance which presses, or the part that is pressed; but most commonly the body pressing, if it be subject to the laws or powers of absorption; and in this case the extraneous substance pressing on the inner surface of the cavity is the extravasated blood which we wish to have removed. The following cases explain this.

A lady fell and struck her shin against a stone; a considerable ecchymosis came on almost immediately, and the skin over it inflamed to a considerable degree. The blood had not coagulated; there was therefore a perceptible fluctuation underneath, and her physician recommended an opening to be made. I was sent for, and on examining the part, was rather of opinion, from the surface being a regular curve, and no part pointing, that matter had not formed; I therefore recommended patience; the subsiding of the inflammation, and the application of such pressure as she could bear without uneasiness, caused the whole tumour to be absorbed.

A man was brought into St. George's Hospital whose thigh had been run over by the wheel of a cart; a very large ecchymosis was formed on its inside, and a considerable inflammation of the skin had taken place. The blood had not coagulated, therefore a fluctuation could easily be felt; but as there was no appearance of pointing, similar to that of matter coming to the skin, I was in hopes that suppuration was not coming on; and although the inflammation was considerable, I supposed that it might arise rather from the violence of the accident than from the extravasation: I waited, therefore, the event; saw the inflammation gradually go off, and as that subsided I observed the tumour diminish, although it was very slow in its decrease. I then directed a slight compress to be applied, after which the tumour evidently diminished much faster than before, till the whole was absorbed.

The union by the first intention usually takes place so soon after the injury that it may be said to be almost immediate, for when the blood has coagulated in such a situation as to adhere to both surfaces, and so as to keep them together, it may be said that the union is begun. It is not, however, immediately secure from mechanical violence, and the blood itself, by losing its power of retaining life, may likewise be rendered unfit to preserve the communication with the adhering surface, by which it is connected with the body at large, and thus the union be of course prevented. If there be no such impediment, then the union of the parts may be very quick; but it will be in some degree according to the quantity of extravasated blood interposed, for if that be large, the whole blood will not become vascular, but the surface only which is in contact with surrounding parts, and the rest will be absorbed as in the ecchymosis. Where the quantity is small, as in a slight wound without laceration, and where all the divided surfaces can be brought into almost absolute contact, their union will be firm in twenty-four hours, as happens in a hare-lip or wounds of the scalp.

Although under such circumstances the blood seems to change into a solid form very quickly, yet when the situation of the wound particularly subjects the parts to mechanical violence, we should not trust to this union being completed in so short a time. In the hare-lip, for instance, perhaps forty-eight hours may be required to make it perfectly secure, and except when the stitches, by producing ulceration, might make scars, there can be no harm in allowing such parts even a longer time for their union. But in wounds of the scalp this caution is not necessary, and indeed in such cases it is scarcely required to make stitches at all.

In cases of accidental injury, whether they be in themselves slight or considerable, in whatever situation or part they may have happened, if the salutary processes, above described, go on readily, no other effect of injury, or irritation, or pain, in consequence of Nature's operations, is felt. No universal sympathy or fever takes place, except what arises from the mere injury done, but all is quiet as if nothing had happened. This is sometimes the case even in a simple fracture of the bones of the leg, in fissures of the skull, etc. However, the magnitude of the accident often produces effects which are alarming, and more particularly when they happen to parts essential to life. These effects are often the cause of much danger, the constitution becoming affected according to the nature and importance of the parts injured. Thus concussion and extravasation affecting the brain, must likewise affect the constitution, from the natural action and influence of this organ on the body being diminished, increased, or otherwise disturbed. The same thing happens from an injury done to any other vital part of the body, and the effects will be according to the use of such parts, or the influence which they have on the system.

However, these immediate and salutary operations do not always take place simply, for they are often altered by other circumstances, as the accident sometimes becomes the cause of irritation, and produces another operation of the parts, called inflammation, which is often of singular service, by increasing the power of union in the broken parts.

This inflammation will generally be in proportion to the degree of injury done, the nature of the parts injured, and the state of the constitution at the time, which, in other words, is in proportion to what is requisite for the first powers of union. But it sometimes happens that inflammation goes further than is required, and produces a variety of actions succeeding each other in regular progression[a]. This may occasionally be observed in certain simple fractures, in which the extravasated blood acting as an extraneous body, becomes the cause of the suppurative inflammation; and the simple is in this way brought to a state resembling the compound fracture. The inflammation, however, does not extend over all the lacerated parts, as when they are exposed at the time of the injury, many of these having united by the first intention.

We may here observe, that accidents of the most simple kind may produce effects which do not allow the common operations of nature to take place, as when a large blood-vessel is broken, or when a fractured rib penetrates into the lungs, or a compression of the brain arises from a fracture of the skull. But none of these accidents admit of the modes of cure above mentioned, as they each require particular treatment, and therefore are not to our present purpose.

---

[a] [Among the conditions necessary to ensure the success of union by the first intention, those which refer to the constitutional peculiarities of the individual are most deserving of attention; as, for instance, a predisposition to gout, scrofula, rheumatism, or erysipelas, which will often be excited into action by the merest breach of surface, and thus frustate the designs of the surgeon. The same thing will also happen from internal organic disease, from what is called the inflammatory diathesis, arising from over nutrition; from long-protracted disorders of the digestive organs; and above all, from a peculiar and unnatural excitability of the nervous system, induced by debilitating causes, especially by the abuse of spirits, and accompanied as it usually is by a weakly frame of body. It is extraordinary how slight a cause will be sufficient in such cases to excite inflammation of a dangerous character, accompanied with local gangrenous tendency and all the worst symptoms of typhoid fever. To this head may also be referred the important fact noticed by Mr. Travers, viz. that the inflammation and fever which follow injuries and operations, severely affecting the nervous system, and through it the circulation, are generally found to be modified by the preceding state of the system, so as to assume in their progress a low or typhoid character. Inflammations occurring in such states of the body are apt at once to run into suppuration, without previously passing through the adhesive stage. The propriety of paying attention to these circumstances previously to undertaking operations, especially those of convenience, is too obvious to be insisted on.]

§. 2. *Of Injuries where the Wound communicates externally.*

The second division of injury arising from accident is where the ruptured parts communicate externally, producing effects different from the former. These may be divided into two kinds, viz. wounds made by a sharp-cutting instrument, and contusions producing death in the parts injured. Wounds are subject to as great a variety as anything in surgery.

A wound is a breach made in the continuity of the solids of a part, beginning most commonly on the external surface, and proceeding inwards, although sometimes its direction is from the inside outwards, as in compound fractures. A gun-shot wound may be said to partake of both circumstances, as it passes through a part: wounds often admit of the same mode of cure with accidents which do not communicate externally; but then it requires the art of the surgeon to place them in the same situation, or under the same circumstances. A wound is either simple or compound; the simple is what I have now to explain, and is of such a nature as to admit of union by the first intention. Of this description we may likewise consider wounds which are the consequence of certain surgical operations.

The form of the instrument by which wounds have been inflicted will also make a difference in their nature: for if it be sharp it will make a clean-cut wound; if obtuse in its shape a bruised one, and may also deaden a part, and the parts may likewise be torn after having been cut; all of which varieties will render a different treatment necessary towards effecting a cure.

In the most simple cases of wounds, a number of blood-vessels being divided, there is an effusion of blood, which escaping by the wound, the internal parts are left exposed, especially the cellular membrane; and these, if not brought into contact with corresponding living parts immediately, or by means of the coagulated blood, will inflame and suppurate. Accidents of this kind differ from those of the first division by communicating externally, a circumstance which makes them often require very different modes of treatment. In cases where parts have been forced out of their natural situation, they should be reduced, that when cured they may answer their natural purposes, as in fracture, dislocation, &c.

Wounds admit of three modes of treatment, arising from their size, situation, and the nature of the parts wounded. One mode is artificial, two are natural: in which last the constitution is allowed to perform the cure in its own way, which will be explained when we speak of scabbing.

These being different from the former and from each other, it might be thought that I should have considered them first as being natural processes; but the first can be put into the same state with the two others, and therefore ought to precede them. For this purpose art must be employed by the surgeon to bring the separated surfaces into contact; that, by retaining them there till union shall have taken place, the injury may be removed from the state of an exposed wound. This treatment of fresh wounds, with a view to cure them by the first intention, is equally proper after many operations as in accidental injuries. Instances of this often occur after dissecting out tumours, scalping when no fracture is found, and when trepanning has not been performed; and it has been put in practice even where the trepan has been applied. It has been employed also after amputations; in short, wherever a clean-cut wound is made in sound parts, and when the surfaces can be brought into contact, or where there is sufficient skin to cover the part, this practice may and should be followed.

In no case, however, of a breach of continuity can we entirely prevent the parts from retaining the appearance of a wound; for the breach in the skin will more or less remain, and the blood will coagulate, become dry, and form a scab. But this operation of nature reduces the injury to the state of a mere superficial wound, and the blood, which is continued from the scab to the more deeply-seated parts, retaining its living principle, just as the natural parts do at the bottom of a superficial wound, the skin is formed under this scab in the one case as in the other; yet if the scab should either irritate, or a part underneath lose its uniting powers, then inflammation, and even sometimes suppuration, may be produced. It is often, however, only inflammation that is produced; the scab here preventing the further progress of mischief in the same manner as the scabbing of the pus on a sore prevents the process of suppuration, which becomes one of the uses of pus.

In many of the cases in which we mean to produce union by the first intention, it is not necessary to be very nice in sponging out the blood, with a view to make the two surfaces of the flesh come entirely into contact, the blood itself answering a similar purpose[a]. In several cases, having brought the two portions of loose skin together, I have seen the two cut edges unite almost immediately; and though the cavity underneath was distended with blood, yet it did well, the tumour gradually decreasing as the blood was absorbed: this is to be considered in the same light as an ecchymosis.

When the portion of skin is not sufficient to cover the whole wound, and the cut edges cannot be brought together, still the skin should be made to cover as much as it can, in order to diminish the size of the parts that must otherwise suppurate and form a sore; as, in consequence

[a] [The impropriety of this advice will appear from the note at the end of this chapter.]

of this mode of treatment, the living extravasated blood is confined in the wound, and coagulating there unites the two surfaces together.

The mouths of the vessels are soon shut, either by inosculation or their own power of contraction, and by the blood becoming vascular, as in the former stated case of union by the first intention; and if there should be any superfluous extravasated blood, we know that it will be afterwards absorbed. The blood being alive, this uniting medium becomes immediately a part of ourselves, and the parts not being offended by it no irritation is produced. The red particles are absorbed, and nothing but the coagulating lymph is retained, which being the true living bond of union, afterwards becomes vascular, nervous, &c.

This mode of treatment by art, though an imitation of the former, can seldom be supposed equally complete; perhaps we ought not to expect it to be so in any case, as there are circumstances often attending the artificial mode of treating wounds which do not occur in the natural. The ligature used for tying a blood-vessel leaves an extraneous body in the wound*; a part deprived of life by the instrument, &c. will become an extraneous substance, and the surfaces cannot always be brought into contact, so as to allow a perfect union to take place. In such cases, union is prevented by the blood losing in part its living principle, especially in those parts next to the external surface; and perhaps the art employed by the surgeon himself may assist in changing the original state of the wound, as the passing of needles and ligatures must always produce suppuration through the whole passage. These substances, so circumstanced, most probably become the cause of irritation, and consequently of inflammation. But if the position of the parts be such as in any sort to allow of union, although not readily, the inflammation will go no further than the first stage, and will even give assistance to the first mode of union.

The possibility of effecting a cure by this method is probably limited to some certain distance of time after the wound has been received, though that space may admit of some latitude; perhaps the sooner it is done the better; but while the blood continues to be extravasated it certainly may be attempted upon our first principles of union.

Where the former bond of union is lost in a part, to produce a new one a secondary operation takes place, namely, inflammation; and if this is likewise lost, then a third mode of union will arise, which is by means of granulation.

* If such a wound has a depending angle, and the vessels should even be tied nearer the upper angle than the lower, yet I would advise to bring the loose end of the thread out of the wound at the lower, for by that means the matter will flow much more easily.

If the divided parts are allowed to remain till the mouths of the divided vessels are entirely shut, inflammation will inevitably follow, and will furnish the same materials for union which are contained in extravasated blood, by throwing out the coagulated lymph; so that union may still take place, though some time later after the division of the parts. This inflammation I have called the adhesive; and the inflammation that precedes suppuration I have called the suppurative inflammation[a]. If the parts, however, continue too long asunder, suppuration must follow, and pus is unfriendly to union. We may here observe, that suppuration takes place on exposed surfaces with a much less degree of inflammation and in much less time than on those which are not exposed, and from their not being opposed by living surfaces, which tend to bring on the adhesive state, they continue it much longer.

Whether this coagulating lymph issues from the half-closed mouths of the vessels which were cut, or from the surface of the opened cells, is not easily determined, but most probably it is from the latter[b], as it

---

[a] [It is now generally considered that *union by the first intention* and *adhesive inflammation* are essentially the same processes, modified by the degree of inflammation. Union by the first intention is uniformly attended with some degree of pain and swelling, together with increased heat and vascularity, which, taken conjointly, constitute the definition of inflammation.

I may observe, that Mr. Hunter's language is doubly objectionable: *first*, because it implies two kinds of inflammation, instead of two stages of the same kind; for suppuration is invariably preceded by adhesion, or the effusion of coagulable lymph; while, on the other hand, adhesion may always be converted into suppuration by simply increasing the irritation: *secondly*, because the word termination implies that the inflammation ceases upon the occurrence of adhesion, suppuration, or mortification, which is by no means true in all cases, nor to the full import of the word in any case. Practically speaking, the language certainly expresses an important fact, which is, that the occurrence of either of these phenomena greatly mitigates the inflammatory action.]

[b] [This opinion is rendered probable from the analogy which exists between the cellular and serous structures. There cannot be any doubt, in respect of the latter, that the same vessels are capable of secreting a simple healthy serum, a turbid unhealthy serum, serum and lymph, lymph mixed with pus, or pure pus corresponding with the degrees of inflammation present, or irritation applied; but if this may happen to the pleura or peritoneum, why not also to the cellular membrane? which is similar in structure and function, and each cellule of which may be regarded as a small serous bag, in which all the phenomena of serous membranes are represented in miniature. Precisely the same phenomena are exhibited by serous membranes, cellular tissue, and recent wounds, under inflammation, and therefore it is probable that the lymph which in the two former cases is poured out without breach of surface, is also poured out from the same class of vessels in the latter case. The centre of a common phlegmon contains pus, because there the inflammation is greatest: the areola external to this is consolidated by the effusion of lymph; and still beyond this there is effusion of serum, producing simple œdema—exactly corresponding to the exudation, 1. of serum, 2. of coagulable lymph, and 3. of pus, from the surfaces of a recent wound or from the superficies of a serous membrane which has been irritated.]

comes on about the same time that the swelling of the surrounding parts begins to appear. There is reason to suppose it to be the same kind of discharge with that which causes the swelling, and which is continued through the whole course of this stage of inflammation; for on examining the dressings of such wounds as are allowed to suppurate, several days after the wounds have been made, the lint is generally adhering to the surface by means of the coagulating lymph, the suppuration not having yet sufficiently taken place to loosen it.

When these operations are completed in due order, the simple operations of the animal are entirely confined to the part, neither the mind nor the constitution seeming in such cases to be at all affected, except that there is a feeling of tenderness in the part. But whatever these sensations may be, they arise entirely from the injury done, and not from the operation of union, unless when the suppurative inflammation comes on.

The inflammation often runs so high, even where the parts have been brought into contact, as to destroy, by its violence, that union which the extravasated juices were intended to produce, the consequence of which is suppuration at last. Is it by this excess of inflammation that the extravasated juices lose their living principle, and become as it were extraneous bodies? or is it not possible that in these cases the inflammation may be the effect rather than the cause of the loss of the living principle, by the blood first losing its living principle, and inflammation arising from it as a consequence?

The time required to complete this union will be nearly the same as that required for union by the first intention, and probably less if there be no particular tendency to suppuration; but if there be, union may be suspended some time longer, for here the uniting medium will be thrown out in larger quantity; and where the union is most easily effected there is less of this medium: when two surfaces unite by inflammation, they are commonly in contact, or else most probably union from this cause would not so readily take place. We shall find in the description of the adhesive inflammation that the union of two sides of a circumscribed cavity is very soon effected, and soon becomes strong.

There is another mode of union, which, although upon the same principle, yet differs with regard to the parts which are to be united.

I have hitherto explained union as taking place only in the division of corresponding parts of the same living body, but it is equally possible to unite different parts of the same, or of different bodies, by bringing them into contact under certain circumstances. There is seldom occasion for such practice; but accident, or rather want of attention, has in some cases been the cause of union taking place between different parts of the body. The chin has been united to the breast, the tongue to the lips or cheek, etc., and when this happens it has commonly been through the medium of granulations. The attempt to unite parts of two different bodies has only been recommended by Taliacotius. The most extraordinary of all the circumstances respecting union is by removing a part of one body and afterwards uniting it to some part of another, where on one side there can be no assistance given to the union, as the divided or separated part is hardly able to do more than to preserve its own living principle, and accept of the union.

The possibility of this species of union shows how strong the uniting power must be. By it the spurs of the young cock can be made to grow on his comb, or on that of another cock; and its testicles, after having been removed, may be made to unite to the inside of any cavity of an animal. Teeth, after having been drawn and inserted into the sockets of another person, unite to the new socket, which is called transplanting[a]. Ingrafting and the inoculating of trees succeed upon the same principle*.

* That the living principles in two bodies which have a perfect affinity to one another should not only be a preservative, but a cause of union, is evident; but even in bodies which appear foreign to one another the stimulus of an extraneous body is not produced where union is not intended, and cannot take place, although we should at first suppose that the extraneous stimulus would be given, and suppuration succeed[b].

This is verified by the eggs of many insects, which are laid under the skin of different animals, producing only the adhesive inflammation in the surrounding parts, by which the skin is thickened and a nidus is formed for the eggs.

The Guinea worm, called vena medenensis [*Filaria Medinensis*, Rudolphi], is also a striking instance of this; for while the animal is endowed with the living principle, it gives but little trouble, yet if killed it gives the stimulus of an extraneous body, which produces suppuration through its whole length. Other instances of the same sort are,

---

[a] [See the ensuing chapter, and Vol. II. *On the Diseases of the Teeth*, p. 55; also Boronio, *Degli innesti Animali*, 1804, in which work an account is given of the transference of portions of the integuments from one part of an animal to another with perfect success—experiments, it may be observed, which strongly corroborate the testimony of Fiovaranti, Molinelli, Garengeot, Dionis, Makau, Balfour, Barthélemy, Piedagnel, &c. respecting the reapplication and subsequent growth of parts, as of the nose, tips of the fingers, lips, &c. which have been completely severed from the body.

The Rhinoplastic or Taliacotian operation has been revived of late years, and applied with considerable success to the cure of several species of disease and deformity. Thus, Sir Astley Cooper has applied it to the cure of fistulæ in perinæo attended with loss of substance; Mr. Lynn to the restoration of the under lip, upon whieh the beard afterwards grew; Mr. Earle to supply the place of the cicatrices of burns; and a great many other surgeons, particularly on the Continent, to the restoration of the nose, cheeks, lips, &c.]

[b] [The author, I apprehend, is mistaken in saying that no stimulus is given in those cases. Generally, if not always, sacs are formed for the lodgement of these ova, just in the same way as for bullets or other extraneous inert substances, by the effusion of lymph and consolidation of the neighbouring textures.]

§. 3. *Practical Observations respecting Union by the first Intention.*

It is with a view to this principle of union that it has been recommended to bring the sides or lips of wounds together; but as the natural elasticity of the parts makes them recede, it has been found necessary to employ art for that purpose. This necessity first suggested the practice of sewing wounds, and afterwards gave rise to various inventions in order to answer this end, such as bandages, sticking-plasters, and ligatures. Among these, the bandage commonly called the uniting bandage is preferable to all the rest, where it can be employed; but its application is very confined, from being only adapted to parts where a roller can be used. A piece of sticking-plaster, which has been called the dry suture, is more general in its application than the uniting bandage, and is therefore preferable to it on many occasions.

I can hardly suppose a wound, in any situation, where it may not be applied, excepting penetrating wounds, where we wish the inner portion of the wound to be closed equally with the outer, as in the case of hare-lip. But even in such wounds, if the parts are thick and the wound not large, the sides will seldom recede so far as to make any other means necessary. The dry suture has an advantage over stitches, by bringing a larger surface of the wound together, by not inflaming the parts to which it is applied, and by neither producing in them suppuration or ulceration, which stitches always do[a]. When parts, there-

the œstrum bovis [*Œstrus bovis*, Fabricius], which lays its eggs in the backs of cattle; the œstrum tarendi [*Œstrus tarandi* (both back and nose of reindeer), Fabricius], which lays its eggs in the back of the reindeer; the œstrum nasale [ibid.], which lays its eggs in the noses of reindeer; the œstrum hæmorrhoidale [*Œstrus equi*, or *Gasterophilus equi*, Leach], which lays its eggs in the rectum of horses; the œstrum ovis [*Œstrus ovi*, Fabricius], which lays its eggs in the nose and frontal sinuses of ruminating animals, particularly sheep; the little insect in Mexico called migna [*Acarus americanus*, Linnæus], which lays its eggs under the skin; and lastly, the cheggars [*Pulex penetrans*, Linnæus], which get into the feet of animals.

---

[a] [It is almost unnecessary to say that these different modes of keeping the sides of wounds in contact may be conveniently united, especially the interrupted suture and sticking-plaster. In operations upon the eyelids and other similar parts, where the use of sticking-plaster is inadmissible, from the difficulty of its application, the interrupted suture may be employed with the greatest advantage. At the end of from twenty-four to thirty-six hours the union by lymph will be accomplished, and the ligatures may then be withdrawn without producing either suppuration or ulceration, or leaving any permanent marks. Sutures may be employed in a multitude of other cases, concurrently with sticking-plaster and bandages, with the greatest advantage. The evils attributed to this practice by Pibrac and some of the French academicians are entirely visionary. Sutures, however, should always be confined to the skin, and ought never to be inserted in tendinous parts.]

fore, can be brought together, and especially where some force is required for that purpose, from the skin not being in large quantity, the sticking-plaster is certainly the best application. This happens frequently to be the case after the removal of tumours, in amputations, or where the sides of the wound are only to be brought together at one end, as in the hare-lip; and I think the difference between Mr. Sharp's cross-stitch, after amputation, as recommended in his Critical Enquiries, and Mr. Alison's practice, shows strongly the superiority of the sticking-plaster or dry suture. In those parts of the body where the skin recedes more than in others, this treatment becomes most necessary; and as the scalp probably recedes as little as any, it is therefore seldom necessary to apply anything in wounds of that part. The practice will certainly answer best in superficial wounds, because the bottom is in these cases more within its influence.

The sticking-plasters should be laid on in stripes, and these should be at small distances from each other, viz. about a quarter of an inch at most, if the part requires close confinement; but when it does not, they may be at greater distances. This precaution becomes more necessary if the bleeding is not quite stopped, for there should be passages left for the exit of blood, as its accumulation might prevent the union, although this does not always happen. If any extraneous body, such as a ligature, should have been left in the wound, suppuration will take place, and the matter should be allowed to vent at some of those openings or spaces between the slips of plaster. I have known a very considerable abscess formed in consequence of this precaution being neglected, by which the whole of the recently united parts has been separated.

The interrupted suture, which has generally been recommended in large wounds, is still in use, but seldom proves equal to the intention. This we may reckon to be the only one that deserves the name of suture; it was formerly used, but is now in a great measure laid aside in practice, not from the impropriety of uniting parts by this process, but from the ineffectual mode of attempting it. In what manner better methods could be contrived, I have not been able to suggest. It is to be understood that the above methods of bringing wounded parts together, in order to unite, are only to be put in practice in such cases as will admit of it; for if there was a method known, which in all cases would bring the wounded surfaces into contact, it would in many instances be improper, as some wounds are attended with contusion, by which the parts have been more or less deadened; in such cases, as was formerly observed, union cannot take place according to our first principle, and therefore it is improper to attempt it.

In many wounds which are not attended with contusion, when we either know or suspect that extraneous bodies have been introduced into the wound, union by the first intention should not be attempted, but they should be allowed to suppurate, in order that the extraneous matter may be expelled. Wounds which are attended with laceration, although free from contusion, cannot always be united by the first intention, because it must frequently be impossible to bring the external parts or skin so much in contact as to prevent that inflammation which is naturally produced by exposure But even in cases of simple laceration, where the external influence is but slight, or can be prevented (as we observed in treating of the compound simple fracture), we find that union by the first intention often takes place; the blood which fills up the interstices of the lacerated parts having prevented the stimulus of imperfection in them, and preventing suppuration, may afterwards be absorbed.

Many operations may be so performed as to admit of parts uniting by the first intention, but the practice should be adopted with great circumspection; the mode of operating with that view should in all cases be a secondary and not a primary consideration, which it has unluckily been too often among surgeons. In cases of cancer it is a most dangerous attempt at refinement in surgery[a].

In the union of wounded parts by the first intention, it is seldom or never possible to bring them so close together at the exposed edges as to unite them perfectly by these means; such edges are therefore obliged to take another method of healing. If kept moist, they will inflame as deep between the cut surfaces as the blood fails in the union, and there suppurate and granulate; but if the blood is allowed to dry and form a scab between and along the cut edges, then inflammation and suppuration of those edges will be prevented, and this will complete the union, as will be described by and by.

As those effects of accidental injury which can be cured by the first intention call up none of the powers of the constitution to assist in the reparation, it is not the least affected or disturbed by them; the parts

[a] [Where inflammation has already come on, so as to threaten suppuration, it is generally not advisable to attempt union by the first intention. In amputations also, where the parts are consolidated and thickened by previous inflammation, it generally answers better to allow the process of suppuration to unload the cellular tissue; and when granulations begin to appear, to draw the edges of the wound gradually together. In operations where, from the nature of the parts, the skin cannot be kept in contact with the subjacent parts, as in the removal of the testicle, tumours from the axilla, groin, &c., the cure will generally be effected more rapidly by inducing suppuration at once, by which the formation and accumulation of matter in inconvenient situations will be avoided. The surgeon will find many other occasions for putting in practice the excellent advice of our author, to consider the mode of union by the first intention as only of "*secondary*" importance.]

are united by the extravasated blood alone, which was thrown out by the injury, either from the divided vessels, or in consequence of inflammation, without a single action taking place, even in the part itself, except the closing or inosculation of the vessels, for the flowing of the blood is to be considered as entirely mechanical. Even in cases where a small degree of inflammation comes on, it is merely a local action, and so inconsiderable, that the constitution is not affected by it, because it is an operation to which the powers belonging to the parts themselves are fully equal. The inflammation may produce a small degree of pain, but the operation of union gives no sensation of any kind whatever.

The first and great requisite for the restoration of injured parts is rest, as it allows that action which is necessary for repairing injured parts to go on without interruption; and as injuries often excite more action than is required, rest becomes still more necessary. But rest may be thought to consist merely in abstaining from bodily exercise; this will in general be proper, as most parts of the body will be affected either immediately, as being engaged in the action itself, or intermediately by some connexion with the injured parts. Thus, if the injury be in the limbs, and not such as to prevent walking altogether, still persons should not be allowed to walk; and we find from the want of this caution, complaints in those parts are commonly longer in recovering than in others; for by keeping the limbs at rest the whole progressive motion is stopped, a thing more disagreeable to the mind than any prevention of motion in the body. If an arm be injured, it is not so; the want of its use is not so distressing to the patient, because he can enjoy locomotion, and may have no objection to keeping his hands quiet. Rest is often admitted from necessity, as in the fracture of a leg, but seldom where motion is only an inconvenience. But it must appear that the rupture of a vessel requires union as well as the fracture of a bone, although the vessel having more powers of restoration within itself than the bone, and having less occasional disturbance from other powers, especially than fractures of the lower extremities, yet the rest should be proportioned to the mischief which would follow from the want of it; and this will vary according to the situation of parts.

The same principle of rest should apply to every injury, although this is not often allowed to be the case. Thus where an injury produces inability to move a part, especially a joint, it is, from fear of the loss of motion, not only allowed to be moved by its own muscles, which would be the most proper mode, if motion at all was necessary, but is moved by the surgeon, or by his direction, who, not satisfied with mechanical violence, has recourse to stimulants, as warm applications, in order to rouse up the internal action of the parts, and at the very time when everything should be kept quiet till restoration of the injury has taken place. In many parts of the body this practice is not so injurious as in others, in which it may be attended with very serious consequences. Thus, when a man has suffered a concussion of the brain, and perhaps a blood-vessel has given way, the mind is deranged, becoming either defective or too acute; and if these symptoms should continue but a little while, the medical assistant applies blisters to remove the effect, either forgetting or not rightly judging the cause. This is even carried further: we hardly see a man taken with all the signs of an apoplexy where a paralysis in some part takes place, or hemiplegia*, but that he is immediately attacked with cordials, stimulants, electricity, etc. Upon a supposition that it is nervous, debility, etc., the poor body is also tortured, because it cannot act, the brain not being in a condition to influence the voluntary muscles: we might with exactly the same propriety stimulate the fingers when their muscles were torn to pieces. I must own I never saw one of them which had not an extravasation of blood in the brain when opened, excepting one, who died of a gouty affection in the brain, with symptoms similar to apoplexy†[a]. Such a case, most probably, would require a very different mode of treatment, therefore when it happens to a gouty man, blisters to the head, feet, etc. would probably be the best practice; but surely this would not be the proper practice in a rupture of a vessel: we ought to bleed at once very largely, especially from the temporal artery, till the patient begins to show signs of recovery, and to continue it till he begins to become faintish. We should give saline purges freely, to diminish impetus and promote absorption; then great quietness should be enjoined, and as little exercise of body as possible, and especially to avoid coughing and sneezing.

* It may be observed here, that the only difference between an apoplexy and hemiplegia is in degree, for they both arise from extravasations of blood.

† For many years I have been particularly attentive to those who have been attacked with a paralytic stroke, forming a hemiplegia. I have watched them while alive, that I might have an opportunity to open them when dead; and in all I found an injury done to the brain, in consequence of the extravasation of blood. I have examined them at all stages, when it was recent, some of weeks' standing, others of months', and a few of years', in which I saw the progress of reparation.

---

[a] [The fact which is here stated, as well as the condemnation of stimulants, although generally true, must be taken with some exceptions. Apoplexy and hemiplegia not unfrequently occur without the slightest trace of sanguineous or even of serous effusion, being discoverable after death, such cases seemingly depending on simple inanition, sudden congestion of the brain, narcotic poisons, or a highly exalted state of nervous irritability. In some of these cases common sense too plainly directs to a stimulant mode of treatment to make it doubtful, although this treatment is not necessarily exclusive of local depletion.]

Plain food should be directed, and but little of it; nor will such cases ever allow of being roused to action, when as much recovered in their texture as nature can accomplish, to the same degree that other parts will admit of or even require.

These observations lead us to consider the means of relief, for, besides rest, it often happens that the parts can be relieved from the secondary consequences of the injury, such as inflammation, etc. But this leads to constitutional and local treatment, and will be included in the history of inflammation.

I have already mentioned that when the salutary effects above described take place, the constitution is not in the least affected; yet it is proper in all cases where much mischief might arise from a failure, to pay a little attention to the constitution. The patient should eat plain food, drink weak liquors, and have the body kept open. This treatment, with rest suitable to the case, will in many instances prevent evils that might otherwise occur and prove troublesome.

§. 4. *Of Scabbing*.

The operations which I have described prevent inflammation, especially that sort of it which produces suppuration; but even where the parts are not brought together, so as to admit of union by the first intention, nature is always endeavouring to produce the same effect. The blood which is thrown out in consequence of the accident, and which would have united surfaces brought into contact, is in part allowed to escape, but by its coagulation on the surface a portion is there retained, which drying and forming a scab*, becomes an obstacle to suppuration. The inflammation in this case may be greater than where union can be effected, but not nearly so great as when suppuration takes place. The blood lying on the fresh surface, although not now alive, and therefore not fitted for union with the living parts underneath, yet precludes the necessity of any further discharge as a covering to the exposed surface, which is one of the uses of pus.

This might be considered as the first mode of healing a wound or sore, for it appears to be the natural one, requiring no art; and in the state of parts before mentioned, the complete union is in some degree indebted to this mode of healing, by uniting the edges that were not or could not be brought into close contact, by means of a scab; proper attention to this has, I believe, been too much neglected.

* A scab may be defined first, dried blood on a wound, dried pus on a sore, a slough from whatever cause allowed to dry, mucus from an inflamed surface, as in the nose.

Many wounds ought to be allowed to scab in which this process is now prevented; and this arises, I believe, from the conceit of surgeons who think themselves possessed of powers superior to nature, and therefore have introduced the practice of making sores of all wounds: as a scab, however, must always be on a surface, it is only on superficial wounds, or on superficial parts of deeper wounds, that scabs can form.

How far this practice may be extended I do not know: but there are cases in which it should be discouraged, as where deep-seated extraneous bodies have been introduced, as in gun-shot wounds, or where deeper-seated parts have been killed; but it will answer extremely well where the superficies only is deprived of life.

Superficial hurts are very common on parts opposite and near to some bone, as on the head, shin-bone, fingers, &c., but more especially on the shin. In all such cases it is better to let them scab, if they seem inclined, or will admit of it; and, if that should not succeed, they can but suppurate at last, and no harm is done.

In many deep-seated wounds, where all the parts have remained in contact, those underneath will unite much better if the surface be allowed to scab. Some compound fractures (more especially where the external wound is very small) should be allowed to heal in the same way; for by permitting the blood to scab upon the wound, either by itself or when soaked into lint, the parts underneath will unite, the blood under the scab will become vascular, and the union will be complete even where the parts are not in contact.

How far this practice may be extended is not yet ascertained. A small wound doing well under this treatment is a common case, and some examples of large wounds are mentioned[a], though these do not so generally succeed; but I do not know that there is any danger in the attempt. In many cases, therefore, which seem doubtful, where the external contusion is not very great, or not continued of the same size as in the deeper-seated parts, it may be tried. In some of those cases which have been allowed to scab, the parts injured have appeared ready to go into inflammation: a red circle has been seen all round, produced by the irritation of the scab. Suppuration takes place underneath the scab, and the pus makes its escape from under its edges; but even in such cases, I should be cautious of treating it as a suppurating sore. I

[a] [Mr. Wardrop, in his Lectures on Surgery, has related a very remarkable case, in which "the largest wounded surface" he ever beheld, arising from the ablation of a diseased breast, almost entirely healed under a crust of blood, which remained on the surface of the wound for upwards of thirty days,—the process of granulation, approximation of the edges, and cicatrization of the wounds going on underneath, with scarcely any irritation or inflammation of the adjacent integuments. See *Lancet*, 1832–3, ii. 653.]

should allow it to go on, and occasionally press the scab in order to squeeze out the pus; for it very often happens that the red circle surrounding the scab becomes of a dusky brown, which is the best sign of resolution, the suppuration diminishes, and the whole does well. But if inflammation should proceed further, and seem to be increased by the mode of treatment, it must not be urged further: the scab should be poulticed, in order to soften it, that it may come off easily, and the case should afterwards be treated according to the nature of the sore.

This practice succeeds wonderfully well in cases where we find applications of all kinds disagree with the skin. A person shall get a blow on the shin which shall probably deaden a part; a poultice is then often applied; that poultice brings out pimples on the surrounding skin; these pimples increase and become sores of some breadth; the poultice is increased in breadth to cover them; new pimples arise, and so on, till I have seen a whole leg full of those sores. In such cases I always allow the wound to scab; and, to accomplish this, the best way is to take off the dressings in the morning, and put on trowsers, without stockings, and by the evening the parts are scabbed; or we may powder them with lapis calaminaris, or chalk finely powdered, and desire the patient to go to bed, for the first night, with the trowsers on: where the sore has been only one, I have made a circular pad, and bound that on till the scab was formed.

The mode of assisting the cure of wounds by permitting a scab to form is likewise applicable, in some cases, to that species of accident where the parts have not only been lacerated, but deprived of life. If the deadened surface is not allowed to dry or scab, it must separate from the living parts, by which means these will be exposed, and suppuration brought on; but if the whole can be made to dry, the parts underneath the slough will cicatrize, and the dried slough will at last drop off. I have seen this take place after the application of a caustic, and many other sloughs. Where this can be effected it is the best practice, as it will preclude inflammation and suppuration, which in most cases should be avoided if possible. I have treated many cases in this way, and the living parts underneath have formed a skin as the slough separated. This will more readily take place where the cutis is not deprived of life through its whole substance; for it has a much stronger disposition and greater powers to restore itself than the cellular membrane has to form a new cutis; indeed the skin formed upon entire new flesh is very different from the original cutis; therefore, as the skin is the part most liable to these accidents, we have the best chance of succeeding in this way when the cutis alone is injured.

This practice is the very best for burns or scalds, after the inflammation has either been considerably prevented, or subdued by proper applications or by time, for which there probably are more remedies than for an inflammation arising from any other cause, as if there was something specific in such causes[a]. Whatever will abate an inflammation arising from accident will have the same effect upon a scald or a burn; and, from the diversities of applications, we have opportunities of knowing the best. Oil was long an application, but which has no virtue: spirits of wine has also been long applied, and with very good effect. The common application, which is a soap made with lime-water and oil, seemed to answer better; and now vinegar is strongly recommended, and I think with justice, as far as I have seen.

Cold lessens all inflammations, and is a very good application where it can be applied, but it cannot be applied so universally as many others; however, cold has this disadvantage, that the pain, although removed while under the application, occurs with double force when it is removed, much more than from any of the other applications, and the reason is evident, for, as the warmth returns, the pain is increased by the warmth, even in sound parts. On the contrary, it is recommended that when a part is burnt to hold it to the fire as close and as long as it can be held, which undoubtedly lessens the succeeding inflammation, and soon gives ease. This I have often seen, and probably it can only be accounted for on the principle of producing the act of contraction in the vessels. I have taken a bucket of cold spring water with me, when I have made an attempt on a wasp's nest, and put my hand into it after having been stung; and while my hand was in the water I felt no pain, but when I took it out the pain was greater than when I put it in. This is not the case with other applications, for their specific virtues are not counteracted by any natural circumstance attending the body, and then they can be applied with a continuance to any part where the skin is thin.

The blisters commonly break, and so much the better, as the application can come in contact with the inflamed surface; but as on the hand, foot, fingers, and toes, especially in working people and those who walk much, the blisters seldom break of themselves, they should be pricked with a needle to take off the tension .

---

[a] [The intractable suppurative disposition which sometimes ensues on these injuries, added to the peculiar tendency which is exhibited by the cicatrices of burns to contract and degenerate into a semicartilaginous structure, would seem to indicate a specific mode of irritation. In many of these cases granulations appear to be produced after cicatrization, so as to give rise to a tuberculated appearance of the surface of the cicatrix, which raises it above the surrounding parts.]

[b] [The advantage arising from the direct application of remedies can never compensate for the irritation which inevitably arises from exposure of the sensitive cutis to the atmosphere. The simple evacuation of the bullæ, by gently puncturing them, relieves the tension, which is all that is required to be done.]

When the inflammation has gone through its stages, then the parts should be allowed to dry. This in many parts is very awkward, as when a large surface of the body is scalded; for exposure is necessary, and in some parts it is almost impossible, as behind the ears, arm-pits, &c. To keep the cloths from sticking to the parts, it is necessary to powder them with some inoffensive powder, such as lapis calaminaris, very finely powdered chalk, &c.; this does not hinder evaporation, which is the principle of scabbing; and if the discharge should be so much at first as to moisten the first powdering, then strew more over the whole till it forms a hard crust. This is hardly necessary on the face, but it will rather dry sooner by being at first powdered. In such cases nature will go on infinitely further than if the parts had been disturbed by our applications.

§. 5. *Accidents attended with death in a superficial part.*

In the foregoing account of injuries done to the body, and of the modes of restoration, we have been so far from considering inflammation as one of them, that hitherto it has been inculcated to guard against it with the utmost care. It sometimes, however, takes place, and is one of the modes of restoration when the methods above mentioned fail, as well as a mode of restoring parts under disease. We shall therefore proceed to explain its principle; but as there are accidents, already mentioned, which often advance to suppuration, I shall now treat of them.

Among the divisions of accidents, one is where death is produced in the injured parts, and where inflammation and suppuration must take place, in consequence of the dead parts which separate not being within the power of the former treatment to produce a cure; but it should be remembered that the inflammation, which is the forerunner of suppuration in such cases, is not nearly so great as even the inflammation arising from a wound that suppurates. In many accidents, such as bruises, the skin preserves its living powers, while the cellular membrane underneath has become dead; this will afterwards produce an abscess, and must be treated as abscesses commonly are, remembering that in the present case the abscess, after being opened, will be later in acquiring the healing disposition than abscesses commonly are; the dead cellular membrane must separate, which will come away like wet dirty lint.

It sometimes happens that in one part the skin, in another the cellular membrane only, shall become dead; and in such cases I have often observed that the bruised skin sloughs much sooner than the cellular membrane. An abscess, therefore, is frequently forming under the sound skin while the other parts are healing: a circumstance which often disappoints both the patient and surgeon.

When the wound, or the dead part, is considerable, it is probable the treatment will in general be very proper; because the degree of mischief calling up the attention of the surgeon, and producing acquiescence in the patient, he will be induced to submit to whatever may be thought necessary. The best application, at first, will probably be a poultice, which should be either simple or medicated, according to the nature of the succeeding inflammation, and continued either till the inflammation has subsided and suppuration come on, sufficient to keep the parts moist, or till the slough has entirely separated, when the sore may be dressed according to its particular disposition. But such accidents as have a superficial part killed (when the slough would readily separate and the parts suppurate kindly) are often treated improperly at first, by the patients themselves applying Friar's balsam, or some such medicines; but these not being within the power of scabbing, inflammation comes on and alarms the patient. A poultice is then commonly applied, which removes the first dressing, and the slough appears, which gives a disagreeable appearance to the wound, and it is supposed to be a foul sore. From such an idea various methods are employed, and the application of red precipitate, &c. but with no good effect, and the patient becomes fretted from a sore apparently so trifling being so difficult to heal; but it is impossible that such a sore can heal while there is a slough to separate. It is therefore the surgeon's business to inform himself of the nature of the complaint, to explain it to his patient, who will then become better satisfied, and less uneasy about his own situation. When this piece of slough comes away, the sore will put on an appearance according to the nature of the constitution or of the part, and is to be treated accordingly[a].

---

[a] [According to the modern views the modes of union above detailed are always accompanied by adhesive inflammation, and should therefore have followed the ensuing chapter "on the fundamental principles of inflammation." The parts are united, not by the extravasated blood becoming vascular, but by the effusion and organization of coagulable lymph. There are two principal objections to the doctrine as laid down by Hunter and supported by some modern physiologists: the *first* of which is that it assigns two distinct causes for the production of the same phenomenon; and the *second* that there is an absolute deficiency of direct proof of the organization of the coagulum, notwithstanding the frequency of hæmorrhagic effusions and the easy manner in which this question may be brought to the test of experiment.

1. There seems not the slightest reason for believing that the mechanism essentially differs by which naturally contiguous parts morbidly adhere and that by which artificially divided parts unite from a principle of conservation, and yet all the phenomena of adhesion in disease uniformly point to the presence of inflammation and the effusion of coagulable lymph. Mr. Hunter indeed freely admits that blood is not necessary to union, but is only one of two modes, at the same time that he considers the coagulable lymph which is poured out in adhesive inflammation as different from the coagulable

CHAPTER II.

FUNDAMENTAL PRINCIPLES OF INFLAMMATION.

An animal in perfect health is to be considered as a perfect machine, no part of it appearing naturally weaker than another; yet this is not

---

lymph of the blood. "It must," he says, "have undergone some change arising from the action of the vessels," which renders it different from "the coagulating lymph with its common properties. We should infer that this coagulating matter is not simply coagulating lymph such as it is when circulating, but somewhat different, from having undergone a change in its passage through the inflamed vessels." When therefore we consider that the fibrin of the blood and the plastic coagulable lymph which is thrown out in inflammation are not the same substances, or at least not in the same state; that the coagulable lymph is the universal medium of adhesion in all cases of disease; that it is thrown out also in all instances of recent wounds; that it is sufficient of itself to effect their union; and that the presence of blood invariably impedes and very often completely prevents this event: when, I say, we consider these circumstances, and take them together, we can scarcely refuse our assent to the position that coagulable lymph is the invariable agent in all cases of adhesion; especially when we reflect,

2. That there is an absolute deficiency of direct proof on the other side; for, whatever some may say, Mr. Hunter always speaks hesitatingly on this point. "I *think*," he says, "that I have been able to inject what I *suspected* to be the beginning of a vascular formation of the coagulum when it could not receive any vessels from the surrounding parts;" and in one of his letters to Dr. Jenner, dated July 6, 1777, he says, "I do not remember Dr. Fordyce's ever supposing a polypus vascular. I should rather believe he supposed the contrary. You know it comes near my idea that the blood is the bond of union everywhere, but I should very much suspect that a polypus formed after death is not of that kind. I am pretty certain that I have injected them in arteries after amputations, and I have a preparation which shows and supports my theory." Now it is very remarkable, considering the frequency of extravasations of blood in the human body, that no unequivocal example of organized coagulum has yet been produced, and it is also material to observe that the examples of this kind which Hunter supposed he possessed were not calculated to carry conviction on such a point, for the injecting pipe being inserted at random into the substance of a coagulum of blood it could scarcely happen otherwise than that the injection should diffuse itself through the substance of the clot, as through a sponge, and thus present some obscure resemblance to organization. Experimentalists have been able to inject, from the adjoining vessels, the organized coagulable lymph within twenty-four hours after its effusion, but this has never been done in regard to the blood. Effusions of blood have been known to exist in the brain and cellular membrane, and in the cavities of the great vessels and aneurismal sacs, for months and even years, and yet so far from becoming organized or identified with the surrounding parts they have invariably acted as foreign bodies, producing either inflammation and consolidation of the surrounding textures into sacs for their protection, or suppuration for their speedy expulsion. The argument from tumours is much too unsatisfactory to be admitted to have any weight in this question (see *note*, I.

strictly true; but still if no relative action, with regard to external matter, was to take place, the machine would, in itself, be tolerably perfect for its own actions. As the animal, however, is employed upon common matter, and therefore liable to accidents, which interrupt the natural operations, it becomes absolutely necessary for its continuance that it should possess, within itself, the power of repair; we find it accordingly endowed with powers of repair upon many such occasions; but where parts give way from their own natural actions, this mischief cannot be repaired; because, if they are not able to sustain their own actions, they cannot recover when diseased or injured. It is found that some structures of parts more readily give way than others, and conse-

---

367); and the same may be observed of the facts referred to by the author, (pp. 119, 243, and I. 236 *et seq.*) in which coagula of blood were found adherent to the insides of the coats of veins, or to the tunica vaginalis of the testicle. Nothing can be concluded from observations made at so great a distance of time from the occurrence of the injuries, which are just as likely to have occasioned an effusion of lymph as an effusion of blood. Not to mention that if blood had been effused it would probably not have presented so defined an outline, and would have gravitated to the bottom of the sac.

Modern physiologists, however, have brought forward another series of proofs derived from the products of organization being found in the centre of recent clots, such as pus, encephaloid matter, the matter of cancer, scrofula, melanosis, &c. A vast variety of these apparent transformations or degenerations of sanguineous coagula into fibrous, osseous, or morbid growths, independently of any connexion with the surrounding parts, have been reported by modern pathologists, (*Andral, Clin. Méd.* iv. 683, and *Précis d'Anat. et Path.* i. 537. ii. 407 *et passim.—Gendrin, Histoire des Inflammations.—Reynaud, Journ. Hebd. de Méd.* ii. 84.—*Dr. Burrows in Med. Gazette*, xvi. 678.—*Arch. Générale de Méd.* Oct. 1834. p. 223, &c.) while others have not hesitated to ascribe the origin of phlebolites to the same source. (*Lee, in Cycl. of Pract. Med.*, art. VEINS.) I may observe, however, that these are doubtful explanations of obscure morbid phenomena, and cannot with any justice be applied to the establishment of a leading doctrine respecting the reparative processes of the healthy structure. We know enough of the proneness of all organic bodies to undergo various important transformations arising from slight changes of chemical constitution, independently of the actions of vitality, to make us hesitate in attributing such changes in the blood to the operations of life; especially when there is no single proof of the presence of organization by which this can be supposed to be effected. The delineations of vascular coagula given by Sir Everard Home, and his speculations on the subject of the formation of blood-vessels by the evolution of carbonic acid gas, are too vague to be formally combated: the permeation of loose coagula under the vacuum of an air-pump is not surely to be wondered at, and would equally take place in a deal board under similar circumstances. (See *Phil. Trans.* 1818. pp. 172. 185. and *Preparations in Museum*, Nos. 23 B, 23 C. 23 D, and *Catalogue of Physiological Series*, i. 4.)

The use of the blood seems to be entirely provisional, and intended merely to serve the purpose of agglutinating the edges of recent wounds, so as to defend them from the contact of the external air until the coagulable lymph is poured out. The lymph thus poured out incorporates with the blood, and in proportion as the former becomes organized the latter becomes absorbed. The reader is referred to Chapter III. on *Adhesive Inflammation* for a more particular account of this process.]

quently are much longer in repair, either when diseased or injured by accident. We also find that different situations, of similar parts, give them advantages or disadvantages with regard to their powers of restoration. This is principally known from injuries being done to them, or in consequence of those injuries from the attack of a disease. It is also shown in the common actions of the body or parts, of which, in health, we have comparative trials. We never can know what a thing is incapable of doing till it gives way, which giving way is either a disease, or that which is productive of disease: nor can we know the powers of restoration in the part till it is tried[a].

As a proof that parts cannot always be proportioned to the action or powers applied which have no action within themselves, but are only acted upon by external force, we adduce the instances of a broken patella or broken tendo Achillis, or a thickening of the valves of the heart. In the first, however, there is commonly another power superadded besides simply the actions of the parts, viz. the body falling and being stopped at once. In the valves of the aorta, however, and the valvula mitralis, we have the best examples, for they become thickened from

---

[a] [The author's meaning seems to be, that where derangements of the animal œconomy arise from injuries done by external bodies, or by the undue action of those parts on which depend the *animal* functions, as contradistinguished from the *organic*, that there we find the parts possess a power of repairing the injury, or at least show a disposition to repair it, for they do not always succeed; and this is certainly true. A blood-vessel may be ruptured in the lungs, or a bronchitis occasioned by too violent exertions of the voice; the eye may be inflamed by employing the organ too long on external objects, or the brain by too great mental exertion; and yet the innate resources of the œconomy may be found sufficient to right the system under these evils, just in the same manner as if they had arisen from external violence: but let these same derangements proceed from the natural actions of parts performing the organic functions, and then they will be irremediable, for the very spring and source of all power in the system is then vitiated at its fountain-head.

The above observations, however, must be taken with many limitations, for we are seldom able to say what diseases arise from the natural actions of parts, independently of external influences. In the instance adduced of thickening of the valves of the heart, we know that certain external actions tend to produce this lesion; whilst, again, we cannot say that it is one necessarily arising after a time, and therefore natural; for we do not always find it in old people. Scrofula, rickets, fever, inflammation, &c. frequently arise spontaneously, and, as we presume, from some fault in the ordinary organic functions, and yet the resources of the system prove adequate for the cure, and often increase with the increasing exigencies of the case. In gout, as in many of the exanthemata, the very evil, or *materies morbi*, which oppresses the system, and which is, at the same time, the product of systemic derangement, becomes the stimulus by which the constitution is enabled to throw it off. Morbid growths and degenerations of structure are probably the only cases really so situated as to be beyond the natural powers of recovery; and yet even here it sometimes happens that the parts get rid of the evil in another way, that is, by sloughing, as in cases of cancer.]

the actions of the parts themselves; while no such effect takes place in the valves of the pulmonary artery: even an aneurism proves the same.

Where there is a difference in structure there are comparative powers to resist the consequences of actions, attended with injury, such as their admitting more or less readily of thickening, ulceration, or mortification, and their comparative powers of restoration. When we compare the powers of restoration in muscle, nerve, cellular membrane, ligament, tendon, bone, etc. with each other, they are found to be very different. Muscles, skin, and probably nerves, possess the greatest powers of that kind; and the cellular membrane, ligament, tendon, bone, etc. the least; and are, in this respect, pretty equal among themselves. How far elastic ligaments have powers of resistance and repair I do not know, but I should suppose they have them in a very considerable degree, from the vessels not giving way so readily as in many of the others[a].

Their comparative powers become pretty evident in most of their diseases, but chiefly, I think, in mortification. As mortification is the most simple effect of debility, it gives the comparative powers of parts in the most simple manner. We find that muscles, skin, and often blood-vessels, stand their ground, while they are deprived of their con-

---

[a] [It is singular that Hunter should attribute to the cellular membrane so low a power of reparation, when in fact it would seem to possess this power in a higher degree than any other tissue of the body. Cruveilhier declares it to be the only self-repairing tissue, and that by means of which the actions of restoration are carried on in all the others; and accordingly, we find that as we descend the animal scale, and the other tissues disappear, leaving the animal more and more largely indebted to the cellular membrane for its composition, so does the power of reproducing mutilated parts increase. The power of reparation and reproduction enjoyed by this tissue, as compared with its other vital endowments (which seem to be of the lowest kind), is certainly not a little extraordinary, and seems to rank with the analogous fact of the superior tenacity of life in the lower animals, which obviously increases as the organization becomes more and more simple,—the powers of action not being in them, as our author supposed in regard to the higher animals, any indication of the powers of life (see pp. 3 and 229 *ante*), but seemingly the reverse; the energy and variety of action of any part or animal being generally inversely to the tenacity of life and the powers of reproduction and reparation. This fact affords some ground for the opinion of Blumenbach, that generation, reproduction, and reparation are merely to be regarded as modifications of the same process.

It may perhaps be stated in general terms, that the proneness of parts to fall into disease as well as to recover from it, when once they have deviated from the healthy action, are nearly in proportion to each other, and very nearly in proportion to their vascularity and complexity of organization. Thus the inflammation of bone, cartilage, and of the white tissues generally, is much more intractable and much slower in its progress than that of the more vascular parts; but then the former parts are much less disposed to become inflamed, being, as it were, wisely protected by their want of vascularity from those evils to which, from their situation and uses, they would otherwise be obnoxious.]

necting membrane, which has either sloughed off or ulcerated; tendons likewise slough off as far as these muscles, and stop there.

I have also observed, that difference in the situation of similar structures in the body makes a material difference both in the powers of resistance to injuries, and of reparation when injuries have taken place. This difference seems to arise in proportion to the distance of the parts from the heart, or source of the circulation. Thus we see muscles, skin, etc. becoming more readily diseased in the legs than anywhere else, and more slow in their progress towards a cure; but this is not wholly to be laid to the charge of situation or distance from the source of the circulation, some portion of it is to be attributed to position, the legs being depending parts, and those parts which are most distinct happen also to be the most dependent*. We find an horizontal position assist in the repair of such parts, but even then they are not equal in their powers to parts situated about the chest; the difference therefore is principally to be attributed to situation, or distance from the heart. The same disease that showed the comparative powers between the muscle and tendon, shows also that they are equally affected by position; thus we see ulceration and mortification taking place in the lower extremity, as such, more readily, and with less powers of repair, than happens in parts near the chest.

This is still more the case if the person be tall. This is seen by changing a limb from a horizontal position, in which it was easy, to a dependent one, wherein it feels pain; because the new position increases the length of the column of blood in the veins. I am inclined to believe that the retardation of the cure is more owing to a stagnation of the blood in the veins, from the length of the column, than from a deficiency in the motion of the blood in the arteries. As the readiness of a part to fall into disease, and its backwardness to admit of cure, arises from position, it is in some degree compensated by rest and a change of the position.

These differences in the structure, situation, and position of parts in the body, make, I believe, but little difference in the progress of specific diseases: the venereal disease, however, certainly does not make such progress in bone, tendon, etc. as in the skin; nor does the cure advance so rapidly in those parts; but both these effects may be attributed to another cause, which is, that bones and tendons are more deeply seated. I believe, however, that position makes no difference in the disease itself, although it may have some influence upon the power of cure, and perhaps in all specific diseases, in the progress towards a cure; for a

* We find in most authors the whole laid to this, which I shall more fully discuss in the history of opinions.

venereal sore is always approaching nearer and nearer to the nature of a common sore, and therefore is more and more readily influenced by what influences a common sore. But in diseases for which there is at present no cure, as the cancer, I believe it makes no difference where it is situated, or in what it is placed, except in the case of such parts as have a tendency to such diseases, which no one of the parts above mentioned has more than another.

I have so far considered, in the general way, the comparative powers of different structures, of different situations, and of different positions in some parts of the body when affected by disease. Disease is the only circumstance which exposes these principles to our view; but to see how far the same principle was carried in natural operations, of which the most remarkable is the growth of parts, I made several experiments on fowls. The first was the common experiment of transplanting the spur of a young chicken from its leg to its comb, in which experiment I always found that the spur on the comb, when it took root, grew much faster and became much larger than that left on the leg. This I attributed to the greater power of action in the comb than in the leg, although they are pretty nearly at equal distances from the source of the circulation; but probably position also favoured it, as there was no stagnation in the veins of the head. In the power of producing such effects in disease, as well as in the growth of parts, I was then desirous to know the comparative degrees between the male and the female. I wished also to ascertain if the parts peculiar to the male could grow on the female, and if the parts of a female, on the contrary, would grow on a male.

Although I had formerly transplanted the testicles of a cock into the abdomen of a hen, and they had sometimes taken root there, but not frequently, and then had never come to perfection, yet the experiment could not, from this cause, answer fully the intended purpose; there is, I believe, a natural reason to believe it could not, and the experiment was therefore disregarded*. I took the spur from the leg of a young cock, and placed it in the situation of the spur in the leg of a hen chicken; it took root, the chicken grew to a hen, but at first no spur grew, while the spur that was left on the other leg of the cock grew as usual. This experiment I have repeated several times in the same summer, with the same effects, which led me to conceive that the spur of a cock would not grow upon a hen, and that they were, therefore, to be considered as distinct animals, having very distinct powers. In order to ascertain this, I took the spurs of hen chickens and placed them on the legs of

* Vide p. 256, and book on Teeth, II. 55.

young cocks. I found that those which took root grew nearly as fast, and to as large a size as the natural spur on the other leg, which appeared to be a contradiction to my other experiments. Upon another examination of my hens, however, I found that the spurs had grown considerably, although they had taken several years to do it; for I found that the same quantity of growth in the spur of a cock, while on the cock, during one year, was as much as that of the cock's spur on the hen in the course of three or four years, or as three or four to one; whereas the growth of the hen's spur on the cock was to that of the proper spur of the cock as [one to two?] two to one.

These experiments show that there is an inequality of powers in different parts of the same animal, and that the legs have much less than the comb; they also show that there is a material difference in the powers of the male and the female. The spurs of a cock were found to possess powers beyond those of a hen, while at the same time, the one animal as a whole has more powers than the other; yet when I apply these principles to the powers of cure in local diseases of the two sexes in the human race, I can hardly say that I have observed any difference. It is to be observed, however, that women commonly live a much more temperate life than men, which certainly must have considerable influence both with regard to resisting and curing diseases.

In all complicated animals, among which man is the most complex, the parts are composed of different structures, and we find that in such animals the powers of action of those different structures within themselves are very different; when they are therefore excited to any common action, the varieties produced should be well known and particularly attended to. Besides, every similar structure in different animals does not always act in the same manner. Thus we cannot make a horse vomit; nor can we give many specific diseases which attack the human subject to any other animal, more particularly the morbid poisons. The mode therefore of action in one animal does not implicitly direct to the mode of action in another; nor does the same structure in the same animal always act in the same way at all times: it acts at various times in a way similar to the same structure in various animals; and, besides, the same structure varies its action in different situations in the same animal. Besides, the exterior actions of life make a very material difference in the internal actions of animals, or in the excitement of disease, either universally or locally; for there are parts which cannot bear one mode of life, while there are other parts which cannot bear another,—parts and mode of life being in opposition with each other. A great many of these varieties depend upon the difference in the natural strength and weakness of the parts; but as those vary very considerably in different habits, so the varieties are increased; and likewise, as many occurrences in life produce the principle of strength or weakness, we have those varieties still more increased, as well as disease.

These observations, as heads, I shall treat more fully, but not as my principal subject, attending to them only so far as they are connected with inflammation and may illustrate the varieties in that action.

§. 1. *Of the different Causes which increase and diminish the susceptibility for Inflammation either in the whole body or in parts.*

Susceptibility for inflammation may be said to have two causes, the one original, the other acquired. The original constitutes a part of the animal œconomy, and is probably inexplicable. Of the acquired it is probable that climate and modes of life may tend considerably either to diminish or increase the susceptibility for inflammation.

The influence, however, of climate may not be so great as it commonly appears to be, for it is generally accompanied by modes of life that are not suited to others; and if we consider how much less pernicious many climates are now than they were formerly, arising from the mode of living being different, we may be led to allow less influence to climate; and, on the other hand, if we consider how diseases become multiplied and varied in the same climate, we shall see that climate alone is not attended with so much variety as may have been supposed. It is observed by some of the ablest physicians of this day that the fever called inflammatory is now not so common in this country as it was formerly represented to have been; that it is now seldom that in fevers they are obliged to have recourse to the lancet, at least to that excess which is described by authors in former times. They are now more obliged to have recourse to cordials than evacuations, and indeed the disease called the putrid fever and putrid sore throat are but of late date. I remember when the last was called Fothergill's sore throat, because he first published upon it and altered the mode of practice. I remember when practitioners uniformly bled in putrid fevers; but signs of debility and want of success made them alter their practice.

Whether the same difference takes place in inflammation I do not know, but I suspect that it does in some degree, for I am inclined to believe that fever and inflammation are very nearly allied, that is, that either will be according to the constitution, which is not the case with specific diseases, excepting in their common modes of action, which consist either in fever or inflammation; but I believe we have much less occasion for evacuations in inflammation than there was formerly; the lancet therefore in inflammation, and also purgatives, are much more laid aside. How far climate varies the constitution, so as to alter the nature of diseases, I do not at present know; but it would appear from Dr. Blane's account that inflammation is hardly a disease in the West Indies.

How far an alteration in the mode of life is the cause of this difference I will not pretend to say, but certainly the way of life is very much altered. We certainly live now more fully than what they did formerly: we may be said to live above par. At the full stretch of living, therefore, when disease attacks us, our powers cannot be excited further, and we sink, so as to require being supported and kept up to that mode of life to which we have been accustomed.

A kind of constant state and variety of mind may often alter constitutions so much as to alter the mode of diseased action, which is much more common in some countries than others. We may be pretty certain that this state of mind often produces the inflammation of the gout.

Probably there is but little power in art to correct the susceptibility of inflammation; however, if the susceptibility of the body be similar to that of the mind it ought to be in some degree corrected by art. The mind is corrected by reason, together with habit, but the body can only have the last employed upon it: it might be made less susceptible by the immediate causes coming slowly upon it, or by avoiding those causes, and even acting in diametrical opposition to them. This will at least answer in the acquired susceptibilities. The acquired susceptibility for inflammation, or indeed for any other disease as it is acquired by art or habit, may be lessened simply by a cessation of those habits; and if the habit is of any particular kind, which is always ascertainable then the habit of the contrary is to be used, which must also be ascertainable.

Strength and weakness are the opposites of each other, and therefore must have very different effects in disease. They have very different powers in resisting disease, in their mode of action, and also in their readiness to terminate that action. Strength, probably, under every circumstance, produces good effects, or at least it is always more in the power of management by art than weakness. I can conceive, however, that too much strength might act with too much power, becoming unmanageable under disease that excites action.

In inflammation when the constitution is strong then it will be commonly the most manageable, for strength lessens irritability. But in every kind of constitution inflammation will be the most manageable where the power and the action are pretty well proportioned; but as every part of the body has not equal strength, these proportions cannot be the same in every part of the same constitution. According to this idea of strength, the following parts, viz. muscles, cellular membrane, and skin, and more so in proportion as they are nearer to the source of the circulation, will be most manageable in inflammation and its consequences, because they are stronger in their powers of action than the other parts of the body. The other parts, as bone, tendon, ligament, &c., fall into an inflammation which is less in the power of art to manage, because, though the constitution is good, yet they have less powers within themselves, and therefore are attended with the feeling of their own weakness; and I believe they affect the constitution more readily than the former, because the constitution is more affected by local disease when the parts have less power within themselves of doing well, and the effects, if bad, on the constitution reflect a backwardness on the little powers they have. Strength and weakness of the constitution, or of parts, are synonymous terms with a greater or less quantity of animal life, or living principle joined with powers of action[a].

---

[a] [See *note*, p. 271. It is not easy to fix the exact import of the words "too much strength" as used by our author. Properly, as applied to the constitution, strength should mean not only a vigorous but a well-balanced action of the various organs of the body amongst themselves; and, as applied to parts, a just equalization of the various functions carried on in individual parts, such as the nervous, vascular, secretive, absorbent, nutritive, &c. In this sense the strength can never be in excess; but probably our author simply intended to express a tendency to excess of action of some one function or organ over that of another, which forms no part of strength. It is an important practical truth, however, that persons who habitually live "above par" are the worst subjects to cope with any serious shock to the system; a tendency to diffuse cellular inflammation, gangrene, and low typhoid symptoms being a usual result of the effort made by the constitution under such circumstances to reestablish itself.

As to parts "having a feeling of their own weakness," it is obvious that such expressions explain nothing when examined into, but contribute to keep true knowledge out by deceiving us with the semblance of it. If we find that the constitution is more injured by a disease affecting some structures than others, it should be our business to inquire strictly into the various facts connected with the two cases, with a view of drawing some general deductions from them, and not be satisfied with allegorizing the vital powers. At present I believe we must be content to regard it as an ultimate fact that parts affect the constitution in proportion to the weakness of their reparative powers; the whole system being, as it were, called upon to cooperate and unite its strength in support of the feeble part when it comes to be diseased.

I would observe, by the way, that such cases as these mark more than any others the distinction between mere physiology and pathology. The most exact knowledge of the anatomical and physical properties of the tissues, of their morbid appearances after death, and of their functions in a state of health, would afford little or no clue to the actual relations which subsist between them and the constitution in a state of disease. The mere physiologist might predict with tolerable certainty the leading consequences of inflammation affecting the vital organs, but he would be totally at a loss to conjecture

The inflammation, if in vital parts, will be still less manageable; for although the parts themselves may have pretty strong powers, yet the constitution, and the natural operations of universal health, become so much affected that no salutary effect can so readily take place, and therefore the disease becomes less manageable. If the vital part is the stomach, or such as the stomach readily sympathises with, inflammation in such parts will be still less manageable, for no operation can go on well, either in the stomach, or in other parts where this viscus is affected, as the powers of restoration become weaker than ever.

In weak constitutions, although the inflammation be in parts which admit of the most salutary operations in the time of the disease, and in situations the most favourable to restoration after disease, yet the operations of inflammation are proportionably more backward as to their salutary effects in such constitutions, and more or less according to the nature of the parts affected, which I shall now consider more fully.

§. 2. *Effects of strength or weakness of Constitution, and of Parts, while under Inflammation.*

Whatever is to be the consequence of injuries, especially inflammation, is produced much more readily in a strong constitution than in a weak one. A wound, for instance, made upon a person of a healthy constitution and sound parts will unite almost at once: it admits readily of a union by the first intention. A greater strength of constitution and of parts admits of resolution, while in the adhesive state of inflammation, very readily, and therefore tends much to prevent the suppurative inflammation from taking place, for it gives a better disposition to heal by the adhesive; so that the union of parts by the first intention, the inflammation and resolution, as well as the readiness to change from the one to the other, according as the preceding is prevented, depends equally upon the strength and health of the constitution and parts inflamed. We may also observe that a greater strength and soundness of the constitution or parts inflamed, when the inflammation has got beyond the stage of resolution and has assumed the disposition for suppuration, hastens on inflammation and suppuration, and also brings it soon to a termination, while at the same time the matter is brought more quickly

the effects of disease affecting the different tissues (as, for example, the serous) without actual observation; a remark equally applicable to the therapeutic part of the art, and worthy of the attention of those who build the knowledge of their profession too exclusively on the investigation of diseased appearances and on mere anatomical aud physiological acquirements.]

to the skin by ulceration. Whatever therefore is the step which nature is to take, whenever an injury is done or a necessity for inflammation has taken place, it is performed with readiness and facility in strong constitutions and parts.

Weakness of constitution and weakness of parts are supposed to be the immediate cause of most tedious or chronic diseases. It appears to be often used as a general term, as have also nervous, bilious, to denote anything for which we cannot well account, and to which I am certain there has been affixed no precise meaning. Every action that is not acute, especially a mild continuation of some of the symptoms of a former violent disease, is called weakness. Thus a gleet is called a weakness, fluor albus is called a weakness, diarrhœa is called a weakness: none of which I conceive simply to arise from weakness, for I believe that weakness seldom or never becomes an immediate cause of disease or action of any kind; but it often becomes the predisposing cause of disease, many diseases not taking place except where weakness is an attendant, as agues, scrofula, nervous, &c., none of which are simple weakness; and it may continue many diseases when they have already taken place. This is, I think, very evident in many diseases which would terminate well if there was strength in the constitution to perform the right actions. However, where there is a strong susceptibility for any one disease, in which weakness might also become a predisposing cause, I can believe that in such cases weakness, especially if suddenly brought on, may become an immediate cause of that disease: as, for instance, a man may, from a wound or any other cause, have a strong tendency to a locked jaw. If you bleed that man freely it is a thousand to one but that a locked jaw comes on: weakness produces a consciousness of its own want of powers, or incapacity, which produces increased action, that even proceeds the length of unnatural actions, called nervous[a]. These effects are no less visible in acute diseases in

[a] [The author here seems to depart from the definition of strength and weakness given in p. 277. Weakness as opposed to strength should be considered merely as a less degree of energy of *all* the vital actions, while the balance between them is still equal, the degree of energy being generally in proportion to the vascularity, and activity of the circulation. In this view a weak constitution may be as healthy as a strong one, as in a man and a woman, and probably be even less exposed to attacks of disease; for a watch may last as long as a clock, provided it be taken equal care of, and keep the truest time of the two.

Weakness, however, is used in another sense to signify the loss of balance between the vital actions, as in the present paragraph. Thus the loss of blood, by weakening the energy of the *circulation* without proportionally diminishing the *innervation*, may predispose to locked jaw; and probably most predispositions, whether natural or acquired, are of this kind.]

such constitutions, which include accidents or violence of all kinds; for they run into too violent action which is not of a salutary kind, and therefore may be called unnatural diseased action.

When a wound is made in a person of a weak habit there is a great backwardness in the two cut surfaces to unite by the first intention, therefore inflammation takes place if there be strength of constitution to produce it, which is not always the case, so that in such habits inflammation is more likely to be a consequence; but this does not arise from a greater readiness to inflammation in the habit, but from a want of power and disposition to heal, which renders inflammation necessary. However, in this case the want of powers or disposition to unite may partly depend upon a different principle from that of weak parts or solids: it is probable that the blood of people of weak habits is weak in its living principle, which it therefore very soon loses upon extravasation, so as to become unfit for a bond of union, by which it degenerates into an extraneous body, and therefore the suppurative inflammation must take place if there be strength to produce it.

In weak habits and diseased parts inflammation is slow in any of its salutary effects, and is hardly capable of either producing the adhesive or suppurative inflammation. If they should take place, it is but imperfectly, and the inflamed parts surrounding the suppurative surfaces are hardly capable of resolution, but continue inflamed; we even find in many constitutions, where the animal powers are very much weakened, that, instead of their readily running into inflammation, it is hardly possible to promote it even from a breach of continuity in the solids, which in most other cases is surest of being followed by inflammation: such constitutions are in general those which are dropsical. I have seen several cases where the power has been so weak that the wound, after tapping, has not united by the first intention, nor has even acquired the adhesive state of inflammation, and has admitted water to pass through it from the abdomen for several weeks without the peritoneal inflammation being excited. In the same dropsical habits I have seen scarifications in the legs or feet not inflame, so that the cells were not united but continued to discharge the water for many weeks. In such cases of extreme weakness this total want of inflammation would appear to be a salutary effect; for in many dropsical cases, where the parts have powers to inflame, but not sufficient to go through the different stages of the inflammation, and at last resolve as in healthy constitutions, the inflammation generally produces a total loss of animal powers and the part mortifies, which often produces death in the whole, so that in such cases the parts only act to destroy themselves*. As a further proof

* Vide paper on the recovery of drowned people, in Vol. IV.

that debility is often the cause of increased inflammation, in consequence of any violence, and often the cause of mortification, is plainly shown in Mr. Dick's account of dropsies among the troops in the East Indies. (*Duncan's Edin. Med. Com.*, x. 207.) In the first year of the attack in any man he durst not venture to scarify the legs; but when they were attacked with the same disease the year following, which was often the case, whenever he attempted to scarify the legs a violent inflammation and mortification were the consequence. He was in this second attack obliged to have recourse to strengtheners; and we may observe that, in the case of tapping, if the constitution is irritable, the cavity of the abdomen commonly feels the effect, and inflammation of the peritoneum and death is the consequence.

As the effect which this inflammation has upon the constitution is by sympathy, it must be in proportion to the readiness with which the constitution assumes that action. This susceptibility is stronger in some constitutions than in others; and every constitution is more susceptible of sympathy with some parts of the body than with others. The kind of constitution which is least affected by this inflammation is that which is in general most healthy, where sympathy hardly takes place. This happens to be the case with such constitutions as can most readily perform all the different operations with ease; and when the parts inflamed are able to manage their own business they thereby affect the constitution less; for we shall find that a constitution may be affected by a local disease merely because it is beyond the power of the part to cure itself.

But it is to be observed that constitutions in full vigour, or which have not been in the smallest degree accustomed to local disease, take the alarm much more readily than those which are not in such full health, or which have been accustomed to local disease. Thus, if a man in perfect health gets a very bad compound fracture in the leg, or has his leg taken off, either for this fracture or in consequence of any other accident, he stands a much worse chance of recovery than one who has been accustomed to a local disease. Even the man with the compound fracture will do much better if his leg is not taken off till the first symptoms are over[a]; or at least we may be certain that the symptoms arising from the amputation will not be nearly so great as those that arise

[a] [The author, I apprehend, does not mean to advocate delay where the operation will certainly sooner or later become *unavoidable*, but only to state the fact that those who have long suffered from some local irritation generally bear operations the best. I may mention that the doctrine of delay is now universally disallowed by the best authorities, foreign and English, the most favourable time for operating being as soon after the constitution has rallied from the nervous impression caused by the accident as possible.]

at first from the fracture, or would have arisen from the immediate amputation. This would appear to be a contradiction to the above position; but, upon an accurate investigation, I think it may be accounted for; for, first, I do not look upon full health as the best condition to resist disease[a]. Disease is a state of body which requires a medium: health brooks disease ill, and full health is often above par; persons in full health are too often at the full stretch of action, and cannot bear an increase, especially when diseased; and, as I before observed, it is a new impression on the constitution, and till it be in some degree accustomed to local disease it is less able to bear such as is violent; besides, the removal of a diseased part which the constitution has been accustomed to, and which is rather fretting the constitution, is adding less violence than the removal of a sound part in perfect harmony with the constitution; the difference, however, is not wholly owing to that cause, for the circumstance of a constitution being accustomed to a mode of life, &c. which it is to continue, makes a considerable difference.

§. 3. *Of Parts of the Body most susceptible of the three different Inflammations to be treated of.*

All parts of the body are susceptible of inflammation, although not all equally so; nor will all parts of the body admit readily of the three different kinds of inflammation I mean to treat of, some parts admitting readily of one only, others of two, and others of all the three; which difference appears to be according to the situation of the inflamed parts in the body, and also the nature of the parts inflamed.

The cellular membrane the first. The cellular membrane free from the adipose appears to be more susceptible of the adhesive inflammation

---

[a] [Exemption from disease may be compatible to a certain extent with a predominating action of some one system over another, as of the vascular or nervous; yet such constitutions are ill adapted to contend with disease, and ought not in truth to be called healthy. The inhabitants of hot climates are prone to nervous diseases, as tetanus, &c., but are little obnoxious to inflammation; while during the Peninsular war it was found that the Portuguese, from being less disposed to inflammation, recovered from injuries which the English would certainly have died from, probably from the latter using a fuller and more stimulating diet, although both might previously have enjoyed equal apparent good health.

The justness of Hunter's observation is remarkably exemplified in the case of draymen, bargemen, and such class of persons, whose habits of severe labour lead them to the habitual excessive use of fermented liquors and an inordinate diet, the consequence of which generally is that they form the worst class of patients in our public hospitals, and speedily succumb under severe operations.]

than the adipose membrane, and much more readily passes into the suppurative. Whether this arises from surfaces inflaming more readily than other parts I will not pretend to say. Thus we see that the cellular membrane connecting parts together as muscles, and the cellular membrane connecting the adipose to muscles, easily inflames and runs readily into suppuration, and as it were separates the muscles from their lateral connexion, and even separates the adipose from the muscles, while the skin and adipose membrane shall only be highly inflamed, and the matter so formed must produce ulceration through all this adipose membrane to get to the skin, and then through the skin, in which last mentioned parts it is much more tedious; ulceration therefore does not so readily take place in those parts as it does in the common connecting membrane. Muscles, nerves, and blood-vessels are parts which nature wishes to retain, and the adipose membrane contains a substance which is properly no part of the animal, viz. oil: it may therefore be more difficult for this part to be absorbed than what are properly the parts of the animal itself[a].

As a deficiency in the power to heal becomes a stimulus or an incitement to inflammation, we find that similar parts, in proportion as they are removed from the source of the circulation, such as the lower extremities, are more ready to inflame than others not so circumstanced; and what adds to this backwardness is their being depending parts, which adds to the incitement.

The deeper-seated parts of the body, and more especially the vital,

---

[a] [I believe it may be laid down generally that parts are disposed to suppurate in proportion as they are lax in structure, by which the blood-vessels are deprived of their due support and distended and ruptured with great facility. A sort of scale marking the suppurative tendency might be formed on this principle, commencing with the mucous membranes, and passing on through cellular membrane, adipose membrane, skin, the free surfaces of serous membranes, the internal tunics of blood-vessels, the internal parenchymatous viscera, fibrous membranes, cartilage, bone, &c. The first step in the formation of an abscess seems to be the softening and breaking down of the tissues by the exudation of a mixture of serum, coagulable lymph, and blood; so that if an abscess be opened early it will be found to contain rather a grumous bloody serum, together with broken down cellular membrane, than pure pus such as would afterwards be formed; and therefore the more the natural structure of any part favours this exudation and vascular distension the more readily will it suppurate. This at least seems to be a nearer approach to the true proximate cause why the cellular membrane goes more easily into suppuration than muscles, nerves, and blood-vessels, than the ascription of a "desire of nature to retain them," which at most is only the final cause allegorically expressed; nor is it even this as regards the adipose matter, which is, in truth, very easily absorbed and redeposited, as we daily witness in alternate fatness and leanness. The gradual breaking up of the pulmonary tissue in inflammation of the lungs, and conversion of it into a diffuse suppurative mass as contrasted with the other firmer viscera, strongly favours the above view.]

very readily admit of the adhesive inflammation, which is proved by dissections; for we hardly ever open a human subject where there are not in the circumscribed cavities considerable adhesions; and most probably many in the common cellular membrane, if they were equally visible. The deeper-seated parts, however, do not in common so readily pass into the suppurative inflammation; and this readiness to accept of the adhesive most probably becomes a cause why the suppurative inflammation does not so readily take place. But if the inflammation comes on at once, with great violence, it would appear to pass almost at once over the adhesive immediately to the suppurative action; or perhaps where it may appear to have done this there may be an erysipelatous disposition; for although it is not the disposition of the erysipelatous inflammation to suppurate, yet it has a greater backwardness to produce adhesions. This effect we often find take place in the abdomen, in the thorax, &c., and I have already mentioned that I suspect the erysipelatous inflammation does, in some degree, reverse the common rules of the common inflammation, by being more ready to suppurate in deep-seated parts than in the superficial, and extend much further towards the centre of the body. I suspect too that the coverings of the brain, viz. pia and dura mater, have something of this disposition. They appear to suppurate very readily, or with very little inflammation; for from a slight blow on the head we find these membranes much oftener suppurate than we should from a similar blow on the shin-bone: for instance, a blow on this bone will only produce suppuration on the external surface, very seldom in its internal cavity; but a blow on the head that shall not even produce the adhesive inflammation in the scalp shall make those membranes suppurate[a].

Inflammation, wherever situated, is always more violent on that side of the point of inflammation next to the external surface. This effect we often find take place in the abdomen, in the thorax, &c., and I have already mentioned that I suspect inflammation, wherever situated, if there be a continuity of parts between it and the external surface, will be greater on that side next to the external surface of the part than towards the centre of the part. This also equally takes place in inflammation, although close to the different outlets of the body, and is probably most easily demonstrated in them. Thus, for instance, if an inflammation comes on in the socket of a tooth at its root, inflammation will not take place on the inside of the jaw, but towards the outside; and if it is be-

---

[a] [This may be accounted for by the jar which the cranium receives, which often leads to the immediate separation of the dura mater from its internal surface. A blow on the dead body will produce the same effect.]

yond the union of the lips with the gum it will attack the skin over the inflamed part, while all the internal parts, such as the gums on both sides, but principally on the inside and tongue, if in the lower jaw, shall be perfectly sound.

If an inflammation attacks the cellular membrane on the outside of the gut near the anus, although the gut is in contact with the inflamed part, yet the inflammation extends to the skin of the buttock, while the gut remains pretty free from inflammation.

If an inflammation attacks the peritonæum covering an intestine, and if adhesions between it and the peritonæum lining the abdomen are a consequence, the inflammation immediately passes through the abdominal muscles towards the skin, while the proper coats of the intestines shall in most cases remain sound; however, this is not always the case, although much more commonly so than the reverse. We see the same thing in the obstruction of the natural passage of the tears, called fistula lacrymalis, for there the sac and skin ulcerate on the inner angle of the eye, while the inside of the nose defends itself by becoming thicker, so much so in many cases as to stop the cavity of the nose and unite with the septum, which has been the cause of the failure of the operation for the fistula lacrymalis. We even find that if an abscess forms in a frontal sinus from an obstruction in its duct that the matter makes its way through the frontal bone externally, instead of getting into the nose. The same observations are applicable to abscesses in the antrum, which are common cases; and indeed, if we observe accurately, we shall find that nature rather defends such parts as are either deeper seated or on the inside of outlets, as will be explained hereafter.

The specific qualities in diseases also tend more rapidly to the skin than to the deeper-seated parts, except the cancer; although even in this disease the progress towards the superficies is more quick than its progress towards the centre. The venereal has something of the same disposition with the cancer, although not so much. In short, this is a law in nature, and it probably is upon the same principle by which vegetables always approach the surface of the earth.

That this is a general principle in vegetation requires no illustration, but what is the immediate cause is not so easily determined. I conceived it might be the light, not warmth, for the ground is often warmer than the air or surface into which vegetables are often growing. To ascertain this as far as I could by experiment, I took a tub, about eighteen inches deep, and about two wide, and filled it with fine mould, in which I planted some beans and peas; their eyes were placed in various directions, and over the surface was spread a close-meshed net. The mouth of this tub was turned down, was raised about three feet from the ground, and was suspended between two posts. Round the tub, and over its bottom, which was uppermost, were placed wet straw, mats, &c. to take off any influence the sun or air might have upon its contents, and a small hole was bored in its bottom, to which was fixed a small long tube that came through the straw. This was intended for pouring some water, if I found the earth get dry, into the tub. Under the mouth of the tub I placed looking-glasses, in such a way that the light was thrown upon the mouth of the tub, or surface of the earth. The weather was fine, so that through the whole day there was the reflection of the light from the looking-glasses upon the surface of the mould, which was much more powerful than daylight without the direct rays of the sun. This I continued till I conceived that the beans and peas had grown some length, but not finding their tops coming down through the surface of the mould, I examined the contents of the tub, and found that they had all grown upwards towards the bottom of the tub, and that in those whose eyes had been placed downwards the young shoot had turned round so as to arise up.

As one experiment leads to another, I wished to see how a bean would grow if kept in a constant rotatory motion. For this purpose I put some earth in a basket, having the shape of a cylinder, and about a foot diameter, with the two ends of wood for greater strength, through the centre of which I fixed an axis or spindle; in this earth I planted a bean, about half way between the surface and axis, with its eye to the surface. The basket was laid across the mouth of a large tub, with the ends of the spindle resting on the edges of the tub, which were fitted to one another so as to allow of easy motion. Round the basket was rolled some small cord, to the end of which was suspended a box, water tight; into this was put lead, so as almost to make it sink in water, and which was sufficient to turn the basket round in the open air. This large tub was filled with water, and the box placed upon it, and the spindle with the basket placed across the mouth of the tub; a very small hole was bored at the lower end of the tub, which allowed the water to escape, but very slowly; as the water sunk in the tub the box descended, and as the box descended the basket was turned round. This tub took about twelve hours in emptying, and during that time the spindle with the basket only turned about one and a half. The tub was repeatedly filled, and when I conceived the bean might have grown some inches, if it had grown at all, I examined it, and found it had grown as much as if it had been planted in the common ground, but it had no particular direction but that of passing in a straight line from the bean, which was at first towards the circumference, the direction in which it was planted; but in its course it had met with a small stone, which had turned it into the direction of the axis, and it had gone on in a straight line in that direction. Here, as there was no fixed inducement to grow in any one direction, the bean grew in a straight line, in that direction given it by chance[a].

This circumstance of the deeper-seated parts not so readily taking on the suppurative inflammation as those which are superficial, is shown in cases where extraneous bodies irritate any parts; for we find that extraneous bodies are in general capable of producing inflammation, but if these extraneous bodies are deeply seated, they may remain for years without doing more than producing the adhesive inflammation, by which means they are inclosed in a cyst, and only give some uneasiness; or if they are such as can be made to change their situation by the actions of the body upon them, as pins and needles, or from gravity, as is the case sometimes with bullets, then the parts through which they pass seem not to be much altered or disturbed*; but if the same body was nearer to the skin it would produce suppuration. This is proved by the cases that have occurred of people swallowing pins, needles, etc.: they have been found to travel almost over the whole body, without producing any effect, except in some situations exciting some sensation; but when they have come near to the skin, the very same substance has generally produced suppuration.

This principle shows itself very remarkably in the cattle which feed in bleaching fields; there is not one of these killed without having their stomachs, etc. stuck full of pins, and no seeming inconvenience takes place, for they appear to be healthy, and fatten as readily as other cattle. However, it is to be remarked that these pins are not found in the fourth or digesting stomach, therefore do not give that disturbance to the constitution that might be expected. It is probable that these cases of

* This circumstance of such bodies moving in various directions, and not towards the surface, is a proof of the truth of my principle, for their motion arises from a mechanical cause, and is ruled by it; whichever way it is directed they must move, whether by gravitation, as is the case with bullets, or by the mechanical pressure of the part upon the two ends of the pin, which will determine the motion towards the point.

---

[a] [The experiments of Mr. Knight render it probable that the directions taken by the plumula and radicle of seeds is referable alone to gravitation, and may always be counteracted by centrifugal force. When beans were planted on the circumference of a wheel, which was made to perform 150 vertical revolutions in a minute, the radicles invariably receded from the axis, whilst the germens sought the centre. The same thing also happened when the motion was horizontal, but with this difference, that when the number of revolutions was 250 in a minute the direction of the radicle was ten degrees below the horizon, but forty-five degrees below this line when the revolutions were reduced to 80, the germens always taking the opposite direction at a corresponding angle. (*Phil. Trans.* 1806, p. 99, and 1811, p. 209.) There seems, therefore, no ground for the analogy in the text.]

pins, etc. owe their want of power in producing suppuration, not entirely to situation but in some degree to the nature of the substance, metals perhaps not having the power of irritation beyond the adhesive, for when the adhesive has taken place the part appears to be satisfied. This appears also to be the case with the introduction of glass, even in superficial parts: a piece of glass shall enter the skin just deep enough to bury itself; inflammation shall come on; the wound in the skin, if brought together, shall heal by the first intention; and the inflammation shall not exceed the adhesive, but rather degenerate into the disposition for forming a sac, by which means a sac is formed round the glass, and no disturbance is given to the irritability of the parts. This was the case with Mr. Knight, apothecary, who had a piece of glass three fourths of an inch long run into the palm of his hand, and remained there for ten weeks, without any further inconvenience than retarding the motion of the hand, and sometimes giving a pricking pain, when the sac was made to press upon the points of the glass; this insensibility, however, arises from a sac being formed with such properties, but it cannot be assigned as a cause in the case of bodies moving as pins.

Whether this fact, of external parts assuming the suppurative inflammation more readily than the internal, arises from unknown properties in the parts themselves, or from circumstances which attend situation, such as heat, cold, etc., is not easily determined; but whatever be the cause, the effects are good, as many situations of inflammation, viz. the internal, would prove dangerous if the parts were always, or often to suppurate; of two evils, nature chooses the least; while, on the other hand, when near the external surface, it becomes the least evil to produce suppuration, in order to get rid of the extraneous matter. Accidents may be assigned as one cause of this frequency upon the external surfaces, but the cases of pins above mentioned (which is accident), show, that even when it arises from accident, the parts near the external surface much more readily suppurate; and in all cases arising from the constitution, or spontaneous, the external inflammations exceed the internal in number, violence, and extent.

§. 4. *Of the two Parts that have the Orders of Inflammation respecting Priority inverted.*

I formerly divided the surfaces capable of taking on inflammation into two; the first of these was the cellular membrane in general, together with the whole circumscribed cavities; the second was all the outlets in the body, commonly called mucous membranes; for instance, all the ducts of glands, and the alimentary canal. The first order of parts, I have already observed, generally, if not always, takes the adhesive first, in the true inflammation, and then all the three inflammations in succession; for the adhesive is immediately admitted in the cellular membrane and circumscribed cavities, to exclude, if possible, suppuration, where suppuration, and of course ulceration, would prove hurtful.

In the following parts the order of inflammation, with regard to its being adhesive or suppurative, appears to be inverted; as the ulcerative is a consequence either of the adhesive or of the suppurative inflammation, it is ruled equally by both. In internal canals*, where adhesions in most cases would prove hurtful, the parts run immediately into the suppurative inflammation, the adhesive inflammation in common being excluded; such parts are the internal surfaces of the eyelids, nose, mouth, trachea, air-cells of the lungs, œsophagus, stomach, intestines, pelvis of the kidneys, ureters, bladder, urethra, uterus, vagina, and indeed all the ducts and outlets of the organs of secretion, which all these parts mentioned may be in some degree reckoned, and which are commonly called mucous membranes. In such parts, if the inflammation is but slight, the suppurative in common takes place, which is almost immediate, as it is not retarded by the adhesive stage, which accounts for the quickness of suppuration of these parts in many cases. I have known a violent discharge of pus come on the surface of the urethra only a few hours after contamination. These facts are shown us every day in various inflammations of those parts, and particularly in the gonorrhœa, cold in the nose, lungs, intestines, etc. The matter from such is generally not called true matter, or purulent, but is often so, if not always, having all the characters of pus; however, this will be according to circumstances. Since those surfaces are, in general, secreting surfaces, suppuration would appear to be only a change in the secretion; and I think I have visibly seen, or could visibly trace, the one change gradually leading into the other: the different parts, therefore, of which the pus is composed will not always be in the same proportion, so that the matter will seem to vary from true matter towards that of the common secretion of the part, and *vice versâ*. But this does not alter the position, for it is common to matter from a sore; and even common to our ordinary secretions.

If this inflammation, which produced suppuration on those surfaces, becomes more violent, or has something of the erysipelatous disposition, we find that it moves from the suppurative to the adhesive, and throws out the coagulating lymph. I have seen this in the intestines, often

* I make a distinction between an internal cavity and a canal; they are very different in their construction; their uses, and also their mode of action in disease are very different.

on the inside of intestines that had been strangulated in a hernia. I have been able also to produce it on the inside of the vagina of an ass, by injecting a strong solution of corrosive sublimate. But if of the erysipelatous kind, these surfaces will take on the adhesive action immediately or at first. This is evidently the case in what is called the ulcerous sore throat; I have seen it in the trachea; I have seen it thrown up from the lungs in branches; I have seen it in the pelves of the kidneys, ureters, bladder, and urethra. This is contrary to the mode of action of the erysipelatous inflammation in the cellular membrane and circumscribed cavities, for there it hardly produces adhesions; and when it suppurates the suppuration takes place first.

The common inflammation and the erysipelatous would seem to change actions similar to the adhesive and the suppurative, according as they are changed to places of different dispositions, never acting in the same way under the same apparent circumstances, and, therefore, something specifically different. As the adhesive inflammation is commonly excluded from such surfaces in the true inflammation, so of course is the ulcerative in such cases; for it is in general only as a consequence of the adhesive and suppurative having previously taken place, with the confinement of pus, that ulceration becomes necessary; for the ulcerative in such cases is a consequence of a stimulus arising from pressure from within[a].

In inflammation we seldom pay attention to more than the continued and the universal sympathy; how far the contiguous takes place without

---

[a] [It may generally be concluded that the inflammation is of a specific or unhealthy kind, either when coagulable lymph is thrown out in the first instance on mucous canals, as in thrush, croup, diptherite, dysentery, &c., or when, in all other structures, the puriform secretion is not first preceded by an exudation of lymph, as in erysipelas, diffuse cellular inflammation, purulent depositions after severe accidents, &c. The employment of the term erysipelatous to designate every species of spreading inflammation and almost every deviation from the standard of health is extremely vague, and has been objected to with much propriety by the author (see *infra*). Whether erysipelas can take place indifferently in any of the structures of the body has been a much-mooted point: certainly the distinctive symptoms will generally if not always be wanting. Even in the mucous membranes, which exhibit so striking an analogy in structure and functions to the skin, there is a marked difference in the general characters of their inflammatory affections, not to mention that they evince no disposition whatever to travel from one to the other, but generally keep perfectly distinct. The membranes of the brain indeed are often more or less affected in extensive erysipelas of the head and face, but this is rather attributable in my opinion to the near proximity of the sympathizing organ to the scene of inflammatory excitement than to any proper extension of the inflammation itself. The retropulsion of erysipelas, like that of every other external inflammation, is apt to induce inflammation internally, but there is not the least proof to show that this new action has the specific character of the original disease.]

adhesions, further than sensation, I am not certain. I believe it never produces inflammation without them; for we may observe, that a testicle shall be considerably inflamed, and the scrotum not in the least affected. The scrotum shall even inflame and slough off, without the testicle being affected till death, or exposure takes place in the tuni.a vaginalis; then it becomes an exposed or imperfect surface, similar to the opening or application of a caustic in the hydrocele; but I know that contiguous sympathy produces a nervous tenderness or sensibility, expressed by the word sore. Thus I have seen complaints in the viscera of the abdomen produce a vast tenderness in the skin of the abdomen; and also complaints of the lungs produce a tenderness in the skin of the chest opposite to the complaint. The remote sympathy sometimes takes place when particular parts are inflamed.

The continued is that sympathy which increases the inflammatory space, by which means the inflammation spreads beyond the irritating point. This becomes more a subject of surgery than any of the sympathies, because it increases the local complaint, and it takes its peculiarities from the constitution at large, as well as from the nature of the parts inflamed; as much can be learned from it in an inflammation as from any other symptom.

The universal sympathy, or constitutional, is where the whole constitution feels the local diseased action.

§. 5. *The natural cause of the Adhesive Inflammation being limited.*

As the body is made up of dissimilar parts, whose construction and functions are peculiar to themselves, yet all tending to the benefit of the whole, we find them also keeping themselves distinct in many of their diseases as long as they can; and if it is a disease somewhat peculiar to the part it will be kept in proportion longer confined. Thus a cancer in the breast will spread faster in the glandular part of the breast than in the surrounding parts which may even be in contact with it. A disease taking place in any part of a lymphatic gland will communicate its disease to the whole of that gland much sooner than to the surrounding cellular membrane. Even a disease common to all parts alike, if it takes place in any dissimilar part, will keep distinct at first.

Thus an inflammation in a lymphatic gland is not taken up by the surrounding cellular membrane till the inflammation has made some considerable advancement, and then it begins to inflame. Thus a lymphatic gland shall inflame and the surrounding parts shall not, till other processes besides inflammation are going on, viz. suppuration; this, however, will be more or less, according to the constitution, for if it has a strong susceptibility for the erysipelatous, the dissimilar parts will more readily sympathize with the seat of the disease. Thus the investing membranes have not this sympathetic connexion with the parts which they either cover or line; nor have the parts either covering the investing membrane, or lined by it, any sympathizing affection with it in the adhesive stages of inflammation. Thus the peritoneum is both a lining and a covering, and so is the pleura. If the peritoneum which lines the cavity of the abdomen inflames, its inflammation does not affect the parietes of the abdomen; or if the peritoneum covering any of the viscera is inflamed, it does not affect the viscera. Thus the peritoneum shall be universally inflamed, as in the puerperal fever, yet the parietes of the abdomen and the proper coats of the intestines shall not be affected; on the other hand, if the parietes of the abdomen or the proper coats of the intestines are inflamed, the peritoneum shall not be affected.

The same principle will lead to distinctions between an inflammation of the lungs and that of the pleura; but I suspect that the reticular or connecting substance, which joins the air-cells of the lungs, has a greater sympathetic affection with the air-cells, or reciprocally with each other, than the before-mentioned parts; and this may arise from the thinness of the air-cells. And it is also upon the same principle that inflammation of the pia mater is seldom continued into the substance of the brain, although the pia mater may be in some degree considered as a continuation of the same vessels.

Contiguity of parts does not communicate inflammation. Thus when an intestine is inflamed the inflammation is not communicated to the peritoneum, lining the abdomen, although in contact; but I have already observed it produces somewhat of a soreness, even to the external touch; but if continuity by adhesions takes place, then inflammation will be continued from the one into the other.

The second cause of the limitation of inflammation is simple contact. I have already observed, that exposure of internal surfaces becomes an immediate cause of inflammation; and when it extends further than the surface of exposure, it is then by continued sympathy only, and that a whole cavity, if wholly exposed, will wholly acquire the inflammation; but we may now observe, that although a cavity is opened and so far rendered imperfect, yet simple contact of its sides renders it perfect again, and sets bounds to the immediate cause. To explain this further, we may observe that there is no such thing in an animal as empty space, exclusive of outlets or reservoirs, which cannot be reckoned internal or circumscribed cavities, for they are perfect by not being such. Every part of the body is either connected by a continuation of one part into that of another, or by simple contact. This takes place equally, either in the common cellular membrane, or in the circumscribed cavities; for if a wound is made either into the cellular membrane, or into a circumscribed cavity, we find that the surfaces of both, beyond the cut edges, are naturally and generally in contact with one another, for without this union by the first intention would not take place, either in circumscribed cavities, or in the common cellular membrane. To explain this position, let me suppose a case.

If we make a wound into the cavity of the belly, and in a sound state of those parts, we shall find that every viscus is in contact with some other viscus, and that the whole inside of the peritoneum is in contact with the viscera in general; so that no space is unfilled while this contact of parts remains. If this wound is not allowed to heal by the first intention, still we shall find that no inflammation will take place, or extend further than the attachment of those parts to the cut edges, except what is owing to continued sympathy. If this was not the case, every part of the same cavity must inflame, because every part would be equally imperfect; for if this contact was removed, upon the receiving of the wound, or at any time afterwards, the whole cavity must inflame, because every part is equally under the same predicament with regard to exposure. The same thing would take place in the common cellular membrane if those cells were not (in a natural state) in contact. Inflammation, in case of wounds, would as readily extend over the surface of each cell, as air does through the cavity of each cell when blown into it. Now this simple and natural contact of natural parts keeps off the inflammation beyond the cut edges of exposure; and inflammation only takes place at this part to preserve this contact, as also to serve as a basis for the future operations.

This, I apprehend, is upon the principle of contiguous sympathy, two surfaces being simply in contact, mutually agreeing not to inflame; or perhaps, more properly expressed, by being in contact there is a mutual harmony which prevents their being excited to inflammation. This circumstance is a reason why we should not attempt to bring circumscribed cavities to universal suppuration, by simply opening them and allowing them to collapse; for we may be pretty certain that union only will take place at the exposed edges of contact, which excludes the general cavity, and which is the reason why the operation for the radical cure in the hydrocele often fails. If, on the other hand, this natural contact of parts did not preserve the whole beyond the cut edges, then we must allow that the cavity is under the same predicament with the cut edges; and if the cut edges inflame, so must the whole.

In cases of spontaneous inflammation of circumscribed cavities, we find where this contact is completest, that the inflammation and its consequences are the least; for instance, in the abdomen, in the cases of the peritoneal inflammations, the inflammation is the greatest where the surfaces are not so well opposed to one another, viz. in the angle between any of the two viscera.

This fact of simple contact being sufficient to exclude the irritation for inflammation, was well illustrated in a woman who had the Cæsarian operation performed upon her, where a wound of eight inches long was made into the cavity of the abdomen to extract the child. After the child was extracted, the wound could not be brought exactly together; therefore, so far gave rise to a peritoneal inflammation; but the belly collapsing, and falling on its contents, they all came in contact as before, and the woman living twenty-six hours, gave time for the inflammatory irritation to take place. After death it was found that the intestines were united to the peritoneum all round the wound for about half an inch in breadth, and the surface of the intestines which lay unattached and exposed at the bottom of the wound were inflamed, while every other viscus, as well as the peritoneum, beyond the adhesions, were free from inflammation.

Ulceration does not seem to obey this law so much, and the reason is, that ulceration is a second operation, and is preceded by inflammation, so that pus is brought equally through every part, if equally susceptible of ulceration, which all parts are not, although not depending upon their being similar or dissimilar. Thus a muscle or artery will not ulcerate so readily as cellular membrane; but if pus was formed on the inside of an artery, or in the centre of a muscle, they would ulcerate very readily, and the ulceration would not stop, or remain stationary, when it came to the cellular membrane, but would go on; if pus, too, be formed in a lymphatic gland, ulceration would go on in the parts between it and the external surface as fast as it did in the gland, if not faster, because inflammation would have gone before, and, as it were, assimilated the parts, and all from this cause, viz. being equally disposed to ulcerate. The cause of the spreading of inflammation is sympathetic; but the cause of ulceration is immediate[a].

---

[a] [Difference of structure has nearly as marked an effect in many instances in resisting the extension of ulceration as it has that of inflammation. This is very little observed in the progress of an abscess towards the surface, because the extension of ulceration in this case depends on the continued presence of the immediate cause, viz. the distension or pressure from behind, and therefore takes place as it were necessarily; whereas, when it depends on sympathy alone, as in ulceration of the bowels, stomach, bladder, &c., nothing is more common than to see the muscular fibres clean dissected by the ulcera-

§. 6. *Of Inflammation—its Stages.*

I have given the most simple idea I can form of an injury done to a part, with the natural, immediate, and consequent means of restoration. I have also treated of cases where they become a little more complicated, requiring the aid of art as a substitute for the simplicity of the first. The action of the parts is not necessary in either of these, except that of the blood forming its vessels and other solid parts, and becoming of the nature of the parts in which it is extravasated. But I took notice, [1.] that the violence done was often so great, or that restoration did not take place so readily, as in all cases to exclude irritation; we had, therefore, an action in such cases taking place in the parts called inflammation; and [2.] that this action assisted in the restoration by producing an extravasation of the coagulating lymph, which became the second bond of union. I have also stated what may be called the natural tendency to inflammation, to serve as a kind of leading principle.

We shall find that inflammation may arise from very different causes, and often without any apparent cause, and that its operations are far more extensive than simply the act of producing union in parts divided by violence; for it more commonly produces union in whole parts or in natural separations, such as the common cellular membrane, large circumscribed cavities, joints, etc., because such surfaces are not naturally disposed to unite, but only in consequence of some uncommon action being produced; and although these adhesions are unnatural, yet that tendency of the parts to admit of this union becomes a species of cure. It is in consequence of the parts taking on, in some degree, the same mode of action which divided parts do when brought in contact, that in such cases suppuration is precluded.

As inflammation often arises from disease, its salutary purposes are in many instances not so evident, although they may finally take effect; as it likewise takes place in disease, or becomes the ultimate in disease where it did not begin in it, as in the scrofula, cancer, &c. and some indolent tumours; on these accounts too its salutary purposes are sometimes not obvious. However, upon the whole, as inflammation is an action

---

tive process, and pertinaciously resisting its further progress; or should these equally give way to the ulcerative action, still the peritoneal covering (not so thick, perhaps, as a piece of common writing-paper,) is interposed, to arrest its further progress, and prevent the fæcal contents escaping into the peritoneal cavity. The same fact is also observable in superficial ulcerations of the skin, in abscesses of the lungs, brain, &c. It is very unusual to find the dura mater or pleura perforated in such cases.]

produced for the restoration of the most simple injury in sound parts, which goes beyond the power of union by the first intention, we must look upon it in such instances as one of the most simple operations in nature, whatever it may be when arising from disease or in diseased parts. Inflammation is to be considered only as a disturbed state of parts, which requires a new but salutary mode of action to restore them to that state wherein a natural mode of action alone is necessary. From such a view of the subject therefore inflammation in itself is not to be considered as a disease, but as a salutary operation consequent either to some violence or some disease[a]. But this same operation can and does vary: it is often carried much further, even in sound parts, than to accomplish union, producing a very different effect, and forming a very different species of discharge from the former; instead of uniting and confining the parts, rather separating and exposing them, which process is called suppuration, and varies with circumstances. However, even this in sound parts leads to a cure, although in another or secondary way; and in disease, where it can alter the diseased mode of action, it likewise leads to a cure; but where it cannot accomplish that salutary purpose, as in the cancer, scrofula, venereal disease, &c., it does mischief.

This operation of the body, termed inflammation, requires our greatest attention, for it is one of the most common and most extensive in its effects of any in the animal body: it is both very extensive in its causes, and it becomes itself the cause of many local effects both salutary and diseased.

It has its different stages, in which it produces more immediately its different effects, which are local, such as adhesions, suppuration, and ulceration, and often death in the part inflamed, together with secondary complaints which are universal, as fever, nervous affections; and when in parts that cannot heal, or in constitutions which are too weak, the hectic fever, next dissolution, or universal death. However, by its forming those adhesions, it often precludes the necessity of suppuration; and also entirely prevents many local diseases where probably suppuration would be the consequence if such adhesions had not taken place, with all the train of consequences of suppuration, such as abscesses, fistulæ, diseased bones, &c., which are prevented by it. It is also one of the modes of action in many specific diseases, and in morbid affections proceeding from poisons.

Inflammation is not only occasionally the cause of diseases, but it is

---

[a] [This is too great refinement. The definition of disease ought certainly to include all such deviations from the natural state as either produce suffering or endanger life.]

often a mode of cure, since it frequently produces a resolution of indurated parts, by changing the diseased action into a salutary one, if capable of resolution.

By these extensive powers inflammation becomes the first principle in surgery. In one point of view it may be considered as a disease in itself, where it takes place without any visible cause, and it may be looked upon as an increase of the mischief when it is a consequence of some injury; but in either case it is a sign of powers, and of necessary powers: for if a part under the influence of such irritation as should naturally excite inflammation had either no powers, or no disposition to exert them, the consequences would be much worse, for mortification would probably take place. I intend at present to consider the most common causes and effects of inflammation, together with the end proposed by nature in producing it, and the use to which it can be applied in surgery. It becomes therefore necessary, first, to begin with describing its most simple forms, together with its general effects, and then to particularize as I proceed.

Inflammation has several well-marked local peculiarities by which it is distinguished. I shall call by the name of inflammation whatever produces the following local effects, viz. pain, swelling, and redness, in a given time, and these dependent on, or the effects of, one immediate cause.

Inflammation appears capable of arising from three causes, which may be called remote. *First*, from some accidental force applied to a part, making a wound or bruise which cannot recover itself unless by inflammation. Such violence at least is naturally capable of exciting it. *Secondly*, from some irritation which does not destroy the texture of parts, but simply the natural actions, as many irritations, such as pressure, friction, heat, cold, blisters, pungent applications, and often fevers of every kind. *Thirdly*, from a particular disposition in parts themselves, as boils arising spontaneously, without the constitution having been preconcerned; so little so, as to have given the idea that such inflammations were healthy. Each of these will be of a kind peculiar to the constitution; but from whatever cause inflammation arises, it appears to be nearly the same in all, for in all it is an effect intended to bring about a reinstatement of the parts nearly to their natural functions.

Inflammation may first be divided into two kinds as first principles, viz. the healthy and the unhealthy. The healthy probably consists only of one kind, not being divisible but into its different stages, and being that which will always attend a healthy constitution or part, is rather to be considered as a restorative action than a diseased one, and would rather appear to be an effect of a stimulus than an irritation. The unhealthy admits of vast variety, (diseases being almost numberless,) and is that which always attends an unhealthy constitution or part, and will be according to the kind of health in that constitution or part, but principally according to the constitution; however, many parts naturally have a tendency to run into inflammations of particular kinds. Most of those arising from the nature of the constitution are, I conceive, in most cases, if not in all, called, although erroneously, the erysipelatous inflammation; which will be further taken notice of.

The simple act of inflammation cannot be called specific, for it is a uniform or simple action in itself; but it may have peculiarities or specific actions superadded.

Inflammation is either single or compound: it may be called single when it has only one mode of action in the part inflamed, as in its first stages; compound, when attended with another mode of action, or when it produces other effects.

Inflammation is capable of producing three different effects, viz. adhesions of the parts inflamed, suppuration in the parts, and ulceration of those parts; which I have called the adhesive, the suppurative, and the ulcerative inflammation. The last, or ulcerative, is properly speaking, only a secondary effect of inflammation, not being performed by the same vessels; however, it is possible it may keep up inflammation, as it always keeps up a species of violence, viz. a destruction of the parts. The two first do not take place in the same vessels at the same time, but succeed one another, although all the three effects may exist at the same time in the different parts of the same inflammation.

I have placed the adhesive first in order, although it is not always so; for, with respect to the priority of those three actions of inflammation, it depends principally upon the nature of the parts, together with the degrees of violence of the inflammation.

To explain this more fully we shall first divide the body, respecting inflammation, into two parts, viz. the cellular membrane, or the body in general, together with the circumscribed cavities, as belonging to the first; and then all the outlets of the body, as the second. We shall treat of each according to the nature of the parts, and of the inflammation joined, and observe their effects, which will show that the common effects of one, as to priority, may be changed into those of the others, and become second or third, according to the nature of the parts, the inflammation, and its degree of violence.

We may observe that inflammation, but more especially the suppurative, in the first order of parts, more readily takes place nearer to the surface of the body than in parts more deeply seated; and as a proof of this observation it has been formerly observed that tumors, and even extraneous bodies, will make their way from some deeper-seated part to the skin, but no inflammation shall take place till they arrive near the skin. But this circumstance will be more fully described when I treat on suppuration.

It does not seem necessary that both surfaces which are to be united should be in a state of inflammation for the purpose of effecting a union: it appears only necessary that one should be in such a state, which is to furnish the materials, viz. to throw out the coagulating lymph, and the opposite uninflamed surface accepts simply of the union. Nor is it even necessary that either surface should be in a state of inflammation to admit of union; for I just observed that extravasated blood produces a union [union by the first intention] without inflammation, and we often find adhesions of parts which can hardly be called inflamed. Thus a truss applied to a rupture will produce adhesions, as has been observed, although it may sit very easily.

In describing inflammation it will be found that the principal theory of inflammation will be introduced in the adhesive stages; for in the first-stated parts it appears only preparatory to the suppurative either in preventing or promoting it.

When inflammation takes place in the first order of parts it is commonly the adhesive; but it will be according to circumstances whether the suppurative or the ulcerative follows first. That either the one or the other should follow seems to arise in many cases from an increase of the inflammation; but it sometimes happens that the suppurative takes place almost immediately, and probably from two causes: the first is the intensity of the inflammation, its exceeding the adhesive almost immediately; the second, an inflammation of a different kind, where the adhesive makes no part of the inflammation, and suppuration takes place in the first instance. I suspect that the erysipelatous inflammation has very little of the adhesive in its nature, and therefore probably these inflammations are in some degree of this nature, and go into suppuration without adhesions. In some cases ulcerations must take place prior to suppuration, as when an inflammation happens on a surface, viz. the skin, as, for instance, in a chancre, and with such violence as is necessary for suppuration to take place, then ulceration must begin first, so as to expose internal surfaces for suppuration; but in the parts of the second order, viz. internal canals or ducts, it is the suppurative inflammation which most readily takes place first; but if carried further the adhesive follows, as will be more fully explained hereafter. When it is an inflammation of the first order of parts, the suppurative succeeds the adhesive, and the ulcerative may be said to be an action superadded to the suppurative, arising out of effects produced by the first, now becoming new causes, the suppurative naturally taking place in the time of the first, and the ulcerative in consequence of the suppurative, which has called forth the action of another system of vessels, the absorbents; all of which may be reckoned as three different modes of action arising from the first irritation or cause.

The adhesive as also the suppurative inflammation, either in the first or second orders of parts, with their varieties, may have a principle superadded which does not in the least alter their inflammatory mode of action, which still continues to go on. This principle is some specific disposition from scrofula or poisons, as the venereal, smallpox, &c.

These three different modes of action, viz. the adhesive, the suppurative, and the ulcerative, when carried on perfectly, are generally the effects of a good constitution, seldom attending the unhealthy: they are what I would call common inflammation.

I have already observed that common inflammation either takes place in parts that constitute the largest part of an animal, which are all the circumscribed cavities, all the cellular membrane, and the substance of every part, the two last of which are the most universal; or upon internal canals or outlets, which are, in common, only excretory ducts.

I have also observed that whenever any extraneous matter is to be discharged, whether already existing, as matter already formed, or a ball lodged, &c., or only preparatory to its formation, such as inflammation that has a disposition to suppurate, the inflammation is always greatest and extends furthest on that side next to the skin: for instance, suppose that a man is shot in the thigh, that the ball passes through to within an inch or two of the opposite side, and that it has not deadened any part for an inch or two of the last part of its passage so as to allow this part to unite, we shall find if that ball excites inflammation it will not be along its passage, where we should (without knowing the principle) have mostly expected it, but the inflammation will commence on that side next to the opposite skin that has not in the least been hurt. If the ball passes quite through, and a piece of cloth is carried in, which lies in the middle between the two orifices; if the passage is pretty superficial, say only an inch distant from the skin where the cloth lies, but which is two or three inches from either orifice, we shall find that the inflammation for its exit will not lead to either orifice, but directly across to the skin[a].

---

[a] [That is, the ball or the piece of cloth produces the greatest inflammation in that part where the stimulus of its presence is most felt, which is in the immediate spot where it is lodged, while the external parts being more extensible than the internal, the inflammation and ulceration necessarily take the former direction. This fact of the greater extensibility of the external parts removes much of the mystery which has been gene-

As the adhesive inflammation precedes the suppurative in everv part of the body except the outlets, as was observed, and the suppurative commonly precedes the ulcerative, excepting on an external surface, the propriety of following likewise this order of nature in treating of them will appear evident, especially as each succeeding inflammation is in some measure illustrated by that which has gone before.

§. 7. *Of the different degrees and different kinds of Inflammation.*

Inflammation will in general be in proportion to the exciting cause (in which may be included the mischief done), the constitution, and the nature of the part; in all which, as there is great variety, so must there be in the inflammations. The degrees of inflammation will be more in the adhesive than in the suppurative, for the adhesive may have all the degrees of violence between the most slight inflammation and suppuration; but the suppurative is a more fixed or determined quantity, for when got to a certain point it takes a new action, and inflammation ceases. However, we have not always inflammation producing suppuration when it has arrived to a certain degree of violence, for in some it often goes beyond that point which would produce it in others, and in such cases there is no disposition for suppuration, and it seems to become stationary, for neither has it any disposition for resolution.

Spontaneous inflammations which are to suppurate are more violent than those inflammations arising in consequence of an operation or accident, which also must produce suppuration; and those inflammations from either operations or accidents, if they have not produced death in the part operated upon, are more violent and of greater extent than those where death in the part has been produced.

The inflammation of a boil or abscess is more violent, and commonly more extensive than that in consequence of a cut, or even an amputation of a leg. The inflammation in consequence of a cut or amputation of a leg will be more violent than that from a gun-shot wound, or from the application of a caustic, which produces death in the part, and even although more parts have been destroyed by these means; neither do specific diseases, except the gout, produce so violent inflammation,

---

rally thought to attach to the approach of abscesses or foreign bodies to the surface of the body Distension as pressure must produce very nearly the same mechanical state of parts.]

nor are they commonly so painful as what I have called the common inflammation.

It may appear not to be an easy matter to account for all those differences: however, it is possible that in the spontaneous inflammation there is more occasion for inflammation than suppuration; the inflammation being the only action which is necessary to produce the ultimate effect, as, for instance, in the gout: in this disease the inflammation is the only thing necessary for its action, and the inflammation runs much higher than many others do which produce suppuration*. The spontaneous inflammation arises often from disease, which probably makes the parts more susceptible of inflammation.

When inflammation arises from the irritation of death in a part, let the cause of that effect be what it will, whether mechanical, as in bruises, gun-shot wounds, &c., or by chemical means, as caustic, &c., the inflammation is late in coming on, and in comparison with the others gentle when come on. However, in many bruises, even where the death of parts has taken place, we have inflammation quick and violent; but then the living parts have also suffered, and have suffered much more than if simply wounded. In many bruises we also have inflammations quick and violent, even where death has been produced in a part; but then death does not take place in all the hurt parts, as in many gun-shot wounds, such as those attended with fractured bones, in which the surrounding parts were only hurt so far as to bring on irritation and not death. If caustics do not act with vigour they will irritate so as to bring on the inflammation sooner than if they had killed the part quickly[a].

Irritating substances, when of no specific kind, produce inflammation sooner than other visible causes of inflammation. If of a specific kind, then the time, sort, and violence [of inflammation] will be according to that kind. But irritating applications must be continued for some time to produce violent inflammation. These differences are easily accounted for; quick death does not irritate the part killed, and the contiguous living part, not being itself hurt, is only irritated to get rid of the dead

* It is a curious circumstance in the gout, that although it is attended with all the common effects of the adhesive inflammation, as considerable swelling, &c., which swelling must arise from extravasation of the coagulating lymph, yet adhesions do not seem to be the intention, for none are produced; the lymph is in general taken up, and chalkstone or tophaceous matter [urate of soda] put in its place.

---

[a] [This is also well exemplified in the application of ligatures for the removal of piles, nævi materni, enlarged tonsils, &c. The pain and inflammation consequent on such operations are immensely increased by not tightening the ligature with a degree of force sufficient entirely to cut off all vascular communication.]

part. A wound is a quick irritation of a living part, so that it inflames more readily and more violently according to the quantity of irritation; but that cannot be of long standing, as nature sets about procuring relief. But when irritating substances are applied, the part inflames quickly, according to their power of irritation; and if they are continued, nature is not allowed to relieve herself, but is constantly teazed, by which means the inflammation becomes also violent.

I need hardly mention that fever is often the cause of local inflammation: we see this happen every day. These causes, and of course the inflammation, are of two kinds: one which may be called accidental, as inflammation arising in consequence of common fever; the others are more determined, depending upon the species of fever, which may be called specific, as the smallpox, chickenpox, &c. These inflammations, in consequence of fever, are commonly supposed to be critical; but I very much doubt the truth of this opinion. The smallpox and chickenpox are, perhaps, the strongest instances of an appearance in proof of this opinion, and perhaps the measles as a critical inflammation might be produced as another; but I believe that it is peculiar to these diseases to form inflammation and sores. We must allow, however, it is not absolutely necessary, even in them, that abscesses should be formed, viz. the pock, to lessen or carry off the fever; for the specific fever in them cannot exist beyond a certain time, even although no eruption appears.

But I think that in the cases of the smallpox, chickenpox, and the measles, those diseases often prove the contrary to that which is supposed to be the case; for we have large abscesses as often formed after those diseases as after any other, which are commonly supposed to be the settling of the fever in this part, but which are equally accidental with those from common fever, and therefore we cannot suppose that those abscesses are critical in such diseases, because they are either common abscesses or scrofulous; for no one disease can have two distinct and different critical inflammations. In further confirmation of my opinion, those inflammations are found to be not in the least of the nature of the disease which produces them, so little so in most cases as to be truly specific of another kind, viz. the scrofulous. Now we certainly find it difficult to conceive one universal specific disease, as the smallpox, &c., producing a local one of another specific disposition to cure the first, or terminating in another disease, whose mode of action is totally different; and the more so when we see that the same local diseases can and do arise from every kind of fever. To ascertain this fact, therefore, we are to look out for that disposition, or that mode of action, common to all fevers which are capable of producing this effect, with the disposition of the constitution or of the part at the time; and we shall find that this kind of inflammation depends upon the constitution and part at the time, and not upon any peculiarity in the fever, as is also the case with the smallpox eruptions, viz. they partake of the constitution.

This common principle in fever, of producing local inflammation, is the simple fever itself abstracted from every peculiarity. A fever, in all cases or of all kinds, is a disturbed action, like inflammation itself, which may be joined with any specific mode of action, and this disturbed action will always be according to the constitution, even when joined with any specific quality. The inflammatory fever is, perhaps, the most simple, because it is a simple fever on a constitution having no peculiarity of disposition. The putrid fever (as it is called) is perhaps no more than the same fever upon a constitution that has a peculiarity of action under that disturbance, and therefore it proceeds according to that peculiarity. This is well illustrated in specific diseases; for instance, in the smallpox.

The smallpox produces a fever, viz. a disturbed action, joined with the specific; and although this action is produced by the same poison in two different persons, yet the one shall be the true inflammatory, and the other the putrid, the erysipelatous, &c. Now the same poison can have but one mode of irritating, abstracted from its poisonous quality, and this one mode produces fever; and it also can have but one mode of irritating in respect of its poisonous quality, but that fever, abstracted from its poisonous quality, will be according to the nature of the constitution at the time, the poison being capable of producing nothing but a fever joined with its specific poison, and that specific quality takes place equally on every kind of constitution, the poison itself having no power of affecting the constitution in one person differently from that of another; it can only act, in a greater or less degree, according to the susceptibility of the person for such irritation. Now since every fever, whether common or specific, is equally capable of producing local inflammation, which may be carried the length of suppuration, and as it cannot with any degree of reason be called critical in specific fevers, we have no reason for supposing that those suppurations are critical in the common fever, or in those fevers which are of no specific kind.

It was a leading doctrine of Boerhaave that inflammation consisted in an obstruction of the minute vessels, in consequence of too great a spissitude of the fluids, and his practice consisted in seeking for attenuants; but this theory seems to be almost entirely exploded. This was certainly too confined an idea of all the causes of inflammation, and reduced all inflammations to one species. The only distinction between inflammations must have arisen from the nature of the obstruction, if there could be any; but this could never account for the action of many specific diseases and poisons. It was also too mechanical. If they had said that any obstruction to the natural actions of a part which could stop the blood's motion in it became a cause of inflammation, they would not have been so materially wrong as to a possible cause of inflammation.

It has been as much laboured, on the other hand, to show that the cause cannot on any occasion be obstruction in the blood's motion through the small vessels; but I will venture to say that any cause which can obstruct the motion of the blood for a given time will become the cause of inflammation; for either the cause of the obstruction itself, or the blood being retained in the smaller vessels for a certain time, will either irritate or unite the parts; or where it irritates will throw the vessels into such actions as naturally arise out of an extraneous irritating cause, but not an increased motion of the blood behind, to drive on the obstructed blood through these vessels, as has been supposed. It will excite that action which in the end produces suppuration, in order to get rid of the extraneous matter which was the cause of the obstruction, such as pressure on external parts, or the obstructing matter itself, which is to be reckoned extraneous. But though pure inflammation is rather an effort of nature than a disease, yet it always implies disease or disturbance, in as much as there must be a previous morbid or disturbed state to make such effort necessary.

All inflammations attended with disease have some specific quality, which simple inflammation has not; and in such cases it is the specific quality which is the disease, and not the inflammation; for such constitutions or parts as are capable of falling into the true adhesive and suppurative inflammation are to be looked upon as the most healthy and the freest from diseases of all kinds. Indeed, even where there is a specific quality, it often can hardly be called disease; for in the smallpox, where the disorder goes through its different operations well, it is exactly similar to common healthy inflammation; for if such an irritation as above described were to attack a constitution or parts in another state than that of health, we should then not have either the adhesive or suppurative inflammation taking place, but most probably some other, such as the erysipelatous or scrofulous, according to the nature of the constitution or parts at the time.

This state of health in a constitution is so remarkable that we see in the time of the symptomatic fever, when nature would seem to be universally disturbed, a kindly or benign inflammation going on, and kindly suppuration; which shows that this fever has no specific tendency to wrong action, the constitution being only disturbed by sympathizing with a local injury, but not capable of giving or reflecting back upon the part inflamed a diseased disposition or action. And this is so remarkable that such inflammations as seem to affect the constitution by sympathy only, which is commonly either from extent, quantity, or the seat of it being a part essential to or connected with parts belonging to life, go on as kindly as they do in a small inflammation, as a boil, which does not affect the constitution in the least. Indeed fever is a good symptom when equal to the injury, and of the same kind with the local affection, when that kind is good.

Let us take an amputation of a leg as an example, which produces something more than a disturbed constitution, for there is a great loss of a substance to that constitution, which, abstracted from the violence, would probably produce considerable effects till the constitution became accustomed to the loss; but even with all this loss we often find that a healthy inflammation shall come upon the stump, and a kindly suppuration take place, while the symptomatic fever lasts. In many cases also it still keeps its ground even when affected by many specific irritations which are foreign to it; and nearly in the same manner as when affected by a common irritation, which will only rouse that constitution into action, but not alter it, having only the specific difference added, so that the parts will go readily through the adhesive or suppurative inflammation; the specific being only an attendant on this healthy action: this we see plainly to be the case in the healthy smallpox, and the lues venerea in its first stages. But, on the contrary, if the constitution is such at the time as would readily fall into an unhealthy inflammation, from common irritation or accidental violence, then it will also fall into that state when irritated by a specific irritation foreign to the constitution, such as the smallpox, which in this case will run into the confluent kind[a].

There are many constitutions which have a tendency to specific diseases that, when injured by fever or any constitutional complaint, readily produce the specific inflammation in such parts of the body as have the greatest susceptibility for any specific action; or if such parts are affected by any local violence, the parts affected will not go through the healthy adhesive inflammation, nor will they enter into the healthy sup-

---

[a] [Dr. Gregory has justly observed that the mildness or malignancy of smallpox does not depend so much on *badness* of constitution or differences in the contagion as on *idiosyncrasy* or *peculiarity* of habit; for as there are certain constitutions which suffer more than others from lead, mercury, and the venereal poison, so there are certain systems unusually irritable under the operation of the variolous virus. If this observation is just, and there seems no reason to doubt it, it will materially affect the soundness of Mr. Hunter's conclusions.]

purative inflammation, but will fall into the specific inflammation peculiar to the habit: such is the case with an erysipelatous habit. Or if a specific inflammation has already taken place, any violence done to it, when already begun, will increase that disposition and action, which we plainly see to be the case with the scrofula, because this disease can and often does arise from such a cause alone. Besides the constitution producing such effects, there are many parts of the body which have a greater tendency to some specific disease than the constitution in general; which particular parts will fall into these specific inflammations more readily than others, either upon the constitution being affected, or a violence committed upon themselves: for instance, many parts of the body have a greater tendency to fall into the scrofula than others, and these will fall into that mode of action when injured, either by means of the constitution or from accident; except the constitutional complaint is such as to be a specific for the scrofula, which I can easily conceive it may. In the cancer also, if the disease has previously taken place, then the tendency of an injury is to exasperate and increase it.

But there are specific irritations which do not affect either the part or the constitution, as a common irritation, but affect them in a way peculiar to the irritation, altering at the same time both the parts affected and the constitution from a healthy state to an unhealthy one of its own kind. This seems to be the case with the plague, perhaps with the putrid and jail distempers in a less degree; for, whatever be the kind of constitution which they attack, they always reduce that constitution to their own kind: it is not a healthy operation going on and the specific superadded, as in the healthy smallpox, &c. However, even the plague has its degrees of power over a constitution, some being much more easily, and of course more violently, affected than others. This change in these cases, especially in the first, is often so great that the constitution hardly ever recovers it, so that the patient dies; which we have observed above is not the case with many other specific diseases or poisons, as the smallpox, &c., for this disease makes no change in the constitution peculiar to itself.

From what has been said it must appear that the irritations which are capable of producing those inflammations may be either simple, as those which produce the adhesive, or producing with it other modes of action, as either suppuration or ulceration; and also either of the above modes of action may be joined with some of the specific actions.

Hence we may conclude that irritations, of whatever kind, either produce an inflammation peculiar to the constitution, or the nature of the parts, or according to the irritating cause, as in the plague; and where it is according to the constitution, that many specific irritations may be added without altering the nature of the inflammation itself, and that they only determine its situation, extent, duration, &c. according to the specific disposition added, provided the constitution be healthy; but if the constitution be unhealthy (whether affected with erysipelas, putrid fever, or plague), and the specific disease be superadded, it will be a mixture of both, that is, it will be a specific inflammation set down upon a constitution of a peculiar kind, and partaking of the character of both, and those specific properties will not be so distinct, or so well formed, as when they appear in a sound constitution.

If the constitution has a susceptibility to be putrid, and the smallpox attacks it, the inflammation will be the smallpox joined with the putrid mode of action of the constitution, which will affect the mode of action peculiar to the smallpox, and destroy the specific difference of the inflammation belonging to the smallpox: the pustules will spread, not suppurate, and look livid according to the putrid disposition. These constant effects, peculiar to the constitution, may be changed from the one to the other just as the constitution changes, for the smallpox may begin upon a healthy constitution, in which they will be distinct or circumscribed; but if the constitution becomes diseased, they will spread; and if the constitution takes a healthy turn again, they will begin to contract to their specific distance again*.

* The knowledge of these facts is of great service in the cure of many specific diseases; for, whatever the specific disease may be, we are always to treat the patient in one respect according to the general nature of the inflammation; and if we have a specific remedy we are also to join that with the other; but if we have not a specific remedy, we are then only to take up the disease according to the constitution.

Let us illustrate the foregoing propositions by example. The first case is explained by the venereal disease in the form of a chancre: the venereal matter produces an inflammation and ulceration according to the nature of the specific disease and the constitution; if the constitution is perfectly healthy, then the effects are the suppurative and specific disease joined; the limits of both are confined according to the constitution and the nature of the specific disease, for the inflammation and ulceration never extend beyond the specific affection; but if the constitution is such as readily to fall into the erysipelatous, then it becomes the erysipelatous and specific joined; and although the extent of the specific affection is limited, that of the erysipelatous is not: the consequence of which is that it spreads over the whole prepuce, and often the whole skin of the penis.

In this disease, under such circumstances, we are led to the method of cure: for although we have a medicine for the venereal inflammation, yet bark is to be given for the erysipelatous; the quantity to be given is according to the predominancy of the one or the other. The effects of this practice are very striking: for as the erysipelatous inflammation lessens it becomes more confined in its limits, and, as it were, drawn into the original point; and when it becomes truly suppurative and venereal, its limits then are brought within the specific distance.

The second case is explained by the smallpox. The variolous matter in healthy constitutions produces the suppurative and specific inflammations: the specific is limited,

Many people are much more susceptible of inflammation than others, even of the common kind, and those probably may be reckoned simply irritable. In such it is more violent, and in such it is more apt to spread, the surrounding parts being ready to act or sympathize with an action to which they are prone; continued sympathy more readily takes place in such cases*: but this is not universal, for we find many very considerable inflammations confined to the part irritated, and in such instances continued sympathy is not great; only the part irritated takes up the action violently.

The term or idea of inflammation may be too general, yet it is probable that it may form a genus in which there is a number of species, or it may be more confined in its classification, and be reckoned a species containing several varieties[a]. These are, however, so connected

and directs the suppurative; but if the erysipelatous comes on, the suppurative ceases; it then spreads along the surface, uniting inflammation with inflammation, and producing the confluent smallpox.

We have no specific remedy for the smallpox, nor can we readily have any for a disease which cures itself; our business then is to cure the erysipelatous, if possible, and leave the constitution to cure the specific.

* This one might illustrate by a piece of paper being either dry or damp. If dry, then ink will not spread, it will be confined to its point; but if damp it will spread, being attracted by the surrounding damp to which it has an affinity.

---

[a] [Many objections have been raised to the present treatise, on the score of its defective classification: but the fact is, the greater number of these have arisen from a mistaken apprehension of the author's object (see particularly *James on Inflammation*, 1st edit., p. 10), which seems to have been solely to explain the phenomena of *healthy* inflammation, and only so far to notice the specific varieties of this action as they served to illustrate the main subject. The author, consequently, setting out with the observation that the essential nature of inflammation always remains the same, however complicated the phenomena may be, first presents to his reader's view a general account of healthy inflammation, which is regarded as the type or primary form of all its varieties. Having done this, he proceeds to notice the different causes which give rise to those modifications of the primary form called varieties, and these he groups together under two general heads, viz. structure, position, climate, age, &c. on the one hand, and specific differences of constitution or of exciting cause, on the other; but as the latter necessarily imply a deviation from the healthy standard, they are only incidentally noticed: although it was impossible that the author, out of the fullness of his experience, should not occasionally expatiate on collateral points, when these happened to be of importance. By this method of procedure, which is the method of the crystallographer, the most complicated forms are gradually deduced out of the most simple; and it certainly appears to me that no other method would have served the purpose equally of consolidating the various and heterogeneous facts of this subject. We may regret that Mr. Hunter's scheme did not embrace the complete pathology of inflammation, but we cannot charge this as any defect of the present treatise.

I believe, further, that the subject of inflammation is incapable of any strict nosological classification, principally from the want of some fixed circumstance of leading importance to serve as the basis of a system. It may be very allowable to use such epithets as sthenic or asthenic, acute or chronic, phlegmonous or erysipelatous, scrofulous or carbunculous, because these terms serve to express a resemblance of the existing

among themselves that we cannot justly understand any one of the species or varieties without forming some idea of the whole, by which means, when treating of any one, we can better contrast it with the others, which gives us a clearer idea both of the one we are treating of and of the whole. So far as it appears to be necessary to take notice of the different inflammations, as illustrative, they may be comprehended in five divisions; although I must own that if we take in all the specific diseases which produce inflammation, such as the venereal disease in its different forms, the gout, &c., they may be without number. However, many of them produce very much the same appearance and effects with those which are of no specific kind. The specific is of no particular kind, but only the cause; and the specific effect is a something superadded. The present, viz. the adhesive, with its different effects, as suppuration, I shall consider as one. The œdematous, which comes nearest to the adhesive, forms a second division. The erysipelatous, [a third], the carbuncle [a fourth], and that which leads immediately to mortification [a fifth]. There is another inflammation, very like chilblains [*Erythema nodosum ?*], which is not very lively and is often in blotches, some the breadth of a shilling, others of the breadth of half-a-crown, and even broader, &c. This inflammation certainly arises from irritable debility; the blotches look more of a copper colour, and the skin over them is often diseased. All, except the first, have a kind of affinity to each other; although I think the œdematous has the least affinity to the three last, and many vary so as to make it difficult to say to which species the varieties belong. There are a great many other inflammations, but which arise from some specific cause, as the gout, scrofula, &c., or poisons; but as these do not explain, or illustrate by contrast, the adhesive or suppurative inflammation, I shall not give the

---

inflammation to some certain types which are well understood; but it would be in vain to attempt to arrange the *whole* of the varieties of inflammation under any two or more of these heads. Neither would the classification founded on difference of tissue, as first proposed by Dr. Carmichael Smith, be at all more practicable, because the same tissue is subject to different kinds of inflammation, and the same kind of inflammation may occur in different kinds of tissue, or be transferred by metastasis or otherwise from one to another. In fact there is no other practicable mode of viewing the subject but that of the author, which is to consider healthy inflammation as the standard, and the degree and kind of deviation from this standard as the specific and distinguishing characteristic of individual inflammations.

Of all the modifying circumstances, with the exception perhaps of specific causes, it must be admitted that none has greater and more permanent influence than that of texture: but constitutions will sometimes predominate over texture, and the specific nature of the cause over both. Mr. Hunter, in his own masterly manner, has traced the influence of these various circumstances, and especially of texture, in modifying inflammation, in which may be distinctly traced the germs of those brilliant views which were afterwards so successfully developed by the illustrious Bichat.]

outlines of them here, except just to mention the particulars of the gout as an inflammation.

The action of the complete gout has all the characters (while it lasts) of the true inflammation, and which may be called the inflammatory action of the gout; but it has many singularities attending it which attend no other inflammation, and which of course become some of its specific characters. The inflammation of the gout is very different from the adhesive and suppurative in its sensation. It seldom throbs; it is a pricking, cutting, and darting pain; besides which there is a pain which feels as if the inflamed parts were all moving, and in that motion there is pain; therefore the action, which is the cause of the pain, must be very different, and is most probably from the action of the vessels, not from their distention, as in the suppurative inflammation.

It probably comes on more quickly than any other. Its violence is probably greater, in duration it is probably the most uncertain, and its going off is quicker than of any other inflammation. Its shifting from one part of the body to another is probably in some degree peculiar to itself, and it leaves parts in a state which no other inflammation does. Without entering further into the nature of this disease than saying it is an act of the constitution, I shall describe some of its visible effects, which of course can only be observed when it falls on an external part, and when it does it is most commonly on an extremity, more especially on the lower, but sometimes on the upper, and still more commonly the extreme parts of the extremity in either the upper or the lower; and its principal seat in the extremity is a joint. When it falls on internal parts it is most commonly the stomach, which is only supposed by its effects or symptoms, from its being transferred, and from the mode of relief. It attacks also the brain, producing delirium, giddiness, the loss of the natural and accustomed feel of the body, incessant sleepiness, &c., which is also known by the above circumstances. When it falls on other parts, either externally or internally, it is not so much determined on what part it is most apt to fall. It sometimes falls either on the lungs or muscles of respiration, the throat, testicles, urethra, producing a discharge, &c., on the anus, forming piles; which can only be known to be gout by collateral circumstances.

Why the extremities, the stomach, and brain should be similar in susceptibility to take the gouty action from the constitution is not easily accounted for. I should be inclined to suppose that its effects on the stomach or brain are not similar to those on the extremity, or probably it does not advance so far in its effects there, because in that case it would certainly kill. Its effects on the extremities are, I believe, always more or less an inflammation, or at least it has the common visible or sensible effects of inflammation. It is most probably what may be called a true specific inflammation, for it produces the same immediate effects in every constitution, therefore does not produce an inflammation according to the constitution, having the specific action added, similar to poisons; but from its nature it produces the same effects in every constitution. I have seen constitutions whose extremities were attacked with the œdematous inflammation, attended with a purplish appearance; violent pain in such cases comes on, which creates some apprehensions of a tendency to mortification: upon looking at the part we may suspect suppuration, the inflammation to appearance being of that kind; but may think it odd that such healthy inflammation and suppuration should take place in the midst of inflammation of so contrary a kind, but shall find no suppuration; the inflammation shall continue its period and then leave the extremities in a much better state than it found them. Although the inflammatory action of the gout is attended with great pain, yet I think it is not so tender as the true inflammation is: a part may be violently inflamed, and yet it may be handled or squeezed; the nerves are not in such a state of irritation: its consequent effects are very different from that of the true inflammation, for instead of entire resolution it gives the disposition to the inflamed parts to fill the joint, or whatever parts have been affected, as, for instance, the cellular membrane with chalk[a].

However, chalk is not necessarily an effect of the gouty inflammation; for in a gouty habit we have chalk formed where there never had been any gouty inflammation, yet it is singular it should attack such dissimilar parts as the skin, ligaments, &c. It has not only no tendency to suppuration, as an immediate effect of inflammation, but it leaves the parts in a state not easily excited to inflammation: the chalk shall remain for years without producing inflammation, and seldom produces it at all but from quantity; and when the interior surfaces are exposed they hardly take on common inflammation and suppuration, healing more readily than a sore of the same magnitude from any other cause: even a joint shall be exposed, yet common inflammation shall not come on, nor shall it suppurate; only a watery fluid shall come out, bringing with it the chalk occasionally, and it shall heal up kindly. It is probable that the gout is not always an act of the constitution, but

---

[a] [The experiments of Wollaston have shown that these tophaceous depositions consist principally of urate of soda, combined with a little urate and phosphate of lime. The most remarkable fact, however, connected with the appearance of gouty concretions, is the coexistence or alternate deposition of uric acid from the urine: so that a paroxysm of gout is not unfrequently known to pass off by a copious secretion of this acid from the kidneys.]

that parts may be so susceptible, or rather disposed, for this action that they may immediately run into it when deranged. If this notion be well founded, then it may be a question whether this local affection relieves the constitution for the time from any susceptibility for such an action.

It may be disputed whether the following are all inflammations or not. They often arise from the same causes: accident, for instance, produces all of them. They have certainly many characters in common, although not always the same result. The vessels becoming enlarged, there is an extravasation, pain, and a separation of the cuticle, but seldom a formation of matter, although there sometimes is, which happens when they have at first more of the adhesive state; and there is a circumstance which I think is common to them, namely, a red streak passing from the inflamed part generally towards the trunk, although not always in this direction. In common language they are called erysipelatous, although very different, the erysipelatous being one of the best marked inflammations of any. I do not mean to treat of these but in a general way, not even when considering the method of cure. It is probable there is no specific distinction between any of these inflammations but what arises from the constitution or the parts, for we find them all proceeding from what may be called the same accidental cause, which therefore cannot produce anything specific; the distinctions in the mode of action of the inflamed parts being occasioned by a peculiarity in the constitution, or the nature of the part itself; but probably in the constitution.

It has been supposed that the different species or varieties of inflammation arise from the difference in the nature of the part inflamed; but this is certainly not the case[a]; for if it was, we should soon be made acquainted with all the different inflammations in the same person, at the same time, and even in the same wound: for instance, in an amputation of a leg, where we cut through skin, cellular membrane, muscle, tendon, periosteum, bone, and marrow, the skin should give us the inflammation of its kind, the cellular membrane of its kind, the muscles of theirs, the tendons of theirs, the periosteum, bone, marrow, &c. of theirs; but we find it is the same inflammation in them all: it is the adhesive in them all if the parts are brought together, it is the suppurative if the parts are exposed. I shall at present only take notice of the four last[b], as I mean to treat more fully of the first, which cannot be so completely understood without seeing the distinctions.

---

[a] [See *note*, p. 310.]

[b] [Namely, the species of inflammation referred to at p. 310, viz. the œdematous, erysipelatous, carbunculous, and sloughy inflammations.]

[1.] What I would call the œdematous inflammation is when the extravasated fluid is water; it has very much the appearance of the adhesive, and probably comes the nearest to it of any, being of a scarlet colour, but much more diffused. The fluid extravasated, being principally the serum, renders the swelling more diffused than even the inflammation itself; it is very painful, or rather sore, but there is not so much of the throbbing sensation as in the adhesive inflammation; it appears to be only on the surface, but most probably goes much deeper; for in such cases the extravasated fluid is in too large quantity to be furnished by the cells of the cutis alone; but in this we have not the same guide as in the adhesive, viz. the swelling and inflammation corresponding with each other. The difference between this inflammation and the adhesive arises, I conceive, from the principle of inflammation acting upon a dropsical disposition, which is always attended with weakness; whereas a greater degree of strength would have produced the adhesive inflammation under the same cause or irritation; and what makes me conceive this is, that in many cases of anasarcous legs we have exactly this inflammation come on from distention, which adds to the extravasation of the serum, as well as in most cases of scarifications of œdematous parts to evacuate the water. When this inflammation takes place it is much more lasting than the adhesive, and I believe seldom or never produces suppuration; but if it should run into this stage it is more general, and the whole cellular membrane in the interstices of parts is apt to mortify and slough, producing very extensive abscesses, which are not circumscribed.

[2.] The erysipelatous inflammation is very peculiar, and most inflammations that are not of the true adhesive and suppurative kinds are called so, although probably they do not in the least belong to it; and this may arise more from the want of terms than the want of discrimination. This inflammation often arises spontaneously, or in consequence of a low or debilitating fever. It often arises from accident, but then it is commonly a secondary inflammation, although not always: for the first shall have gone off, and when suppuration was to take place it shall have come kindly on, but afterwards the erysipelatous shall take place. This may be called a remote inflammation, and is in this respect somewhat similar to the locked jaw. It is more commonly a cutaneous inflammation than situated in the deeper-seated parts, although in some constitutions every inflammation, wherever it exists, will most probably be of this kind; however, the skin appears to be most susceptible of it, because it will spread over a prodigious surface of skin, while it does not affect even the cellular membrane underneath, at least not commonly. There is an inflammation which attacks internal canals which is classed with the erysipelatous, but how far it is the same I do not know; it is certainly not the suppurative, and as almost every other inflammation was formerly called erysipelatous, this has been supposed to belong to this kind of inflammation. The inflammation I am speaking of is more common to the throat than any other part, often going down the trachea. Whatever it is, it may be considered in some of its effects to be in direct opposition to the adhesive and the suppurative inflammations; for where the adhesive most readily produces adhesions, there the erysipelatous does not, as in the common cellular membrane; and where the adhesive seldom takes place, excepting from extreme violence, there this inflammation (if erysipelatous) has a tendency to produce adhesions, as in canals or outlets; it also opposes, in some degree, the suppurative, in being backward in producing suppuration even in those places where suppuration most readily takes place, such as canals and outlets, for there, as above observed, it more readily throws out the coagulating lymph.

Whatever the inflammation may be, it is certainly attended with nearly the same kind of constitutional affection. The fever in both appears to be the same, viz. accompanied with debility, languor, &c. The extravasation in consequence of the erysipelatous inflammation is not so great as in either the adhesive or the œdematous; nor is it of that kind which produces adhesions between the parts inflamed, which in this inflammation would commonly be unnecessary, as it seldom produces suppuration, but is attended with very bad consequences when it does. It appears to support itself by continued sympathy, for it commonly begins at a point and spreads, while it shall be getting well where it first began. This cannot be merely constitutional; for if it was, the parts already inflamed could not recover, if its increase in new parts arose from the constitution; but it gives the idea that when the parts have once gone through this action that they lose the disposition and become healthy. This property is not peculiar to this inflammation, the ringworm has this peculiarity, as also many cutaneous ulcers*.

This inflammation is more common in the summer than in the winter, more especially in hospitals; and I think takes place oftener after wounds on the head than any other. I have often seen it begin round a wound, on the scalp, extending itself over the whole head and face; the eyelids

* There appear to me two ways of accounting for this: one is, that the whole skin is very susceptible of such action, and readily goes on with it by continued sympathy, and the part having gone through the action, like the smallpox, &c., loses the disposition, and the action ceases. The other is, that the inflammation is such as to contaminate while it spreads, but when it has once acted it is cured as above observed. If this last be a true solution, then the right practice would be to stop its progress by destroying the parts beyond it.

being very much swelled, the ears thickened, and it has advanced to the neck, shoulders, and body, creeping along both arms, and terminating at the fingers' ends; that which attacks the body often goes along the body to both thighs, down the legs, and terminates at the ends of the toes; and while this is going on, it is as expeditiously cured behind, and the skin peels off the cured parts. However, this is not always the case; it often stops, and where it proceeds so far, it is commonly becoming milder. This inflammation, when it runs along the skin, has a determined edge, not losing itself gradually and insensibly in the skin beyond, as in the true adhesive, and indeed most of the inflammations; the skin feels as if only a little thickened, and not so pliable; for by passing the finger along the sound skin to the inflamed we feel an evident difference. The colour of the skin is of a darkish red. When it goes deeper than the skin into the cellular membrane it often suppurates; but then I suspect it is not the true erysipelatous, for in such cases it commonly produces mortification in the cells, by which air is let loose: this gives a strange feel, neither of fluctuation nor crepitation, and as there are no adhesions the matter finds an easy passage into the common cellular membrane, increasing the same kind of suppuration wherever it comes; and as mortification is a consequence of these inflammations, putrefaction ensues, and the discharge becomes very offensive. Whether this difference in the effect of the inflammation arises from the nature of the parts, I will not pretend to say. This effect takes place about the buttocks and side of the anus oftener than anywhere else, as indeed does common inflammation and suppuration.

This inflammation commonly begins with fever, lowness of spirits, prostration of strength, loss of appetite, &c.; but it commonly does not last long, and the inflammation shall spread even when the fever is gone off, but then it is not so violent. When it produces suppuration in the cellular membrane it is often dangerous, both from the disease itself and the consequences of the matter diffusing itself much further. This effect frequently takes place when this inflammation attacks the buttocks or parts near the anus, and often proves fatal. In such cases, as the sores seldom ulcerate, they should be opened early, for the matter either gets into the cellular membrane from the want of adhesions, or it separates parts that are only attached, as the periosteum from the bone, muscles from muscles, &c., whereas the true suppurative ulcerates briskly, which therefore should not be opened early, but allowed to burst.

Many inflammations on the skin which come to suppuration have something of the erysipelatous disposition, for we see them increasing the circle of inflammation, the cuticle separating, matter forming underneath from the cutis, and the sore healing in the centre; they perhaps begin like a pimple, but spread in that way to the breadth of a sixpence, shilling, or crown-piece; such often take place on the fingers.

[3.] The inflammation that produces the carbuncle is of a different nature from any of the former; it is stationary with respect to place, and is pretty much circumscribed, even forming a broad flat firm tumour; it begins in the skin almost like a pimple, and goes deeper and deeper, spreading with a broad base under the skin in the cellular membrane; and although considerably tumefied, yet this does not arise from the extravasation of coagulating lymph producing adhesions which are to retain life, for the very cells into which it is extravasated become dead. It produces a suppuration, but not an abscess, somewhat similar to the erysipelatous when the inflammation passes into the cellular membrane, for as there are no adhesions the matter lies in the cells where it was formed, almost like water in an anasarca; but still it is not diffused through the uninflamed cellular membrane, as in the erysipelatous, for it appears to extend no further than the inflammation: one would almost imagine that there was a limitation to the extent, beyond which this species of inflammation could not go, and at these limits the adhesive inflammation took place to confine the matter within the bounds of the carbuncle. A diffused ulceration on the inside for the exit of the matter takes place, making a number of openings through the skin.

There are generally more carbuncles than one at the same time, a great number succeeding each other, which would almost seem to produce each other in this succession; they are commonly more on the trunk of the body than anywhere else. However, I have seen them on the head, and sometimes on the extremities, although but seldom. They are more commonly on the posterior part of the body than the anterior. This inflammation attacks more beyond the middle age than at it, and very few under it. It is most common in those that have lived well. I never saw but one patient of this kind in an hospital. It appears to have some affinity to the boil; but the boil differs in this respect, that it has more of the true inflammation, therefore spreads less, and is more peculiar to the young than the old, which may be the reason why it partakes more of the true inflammation.

As death is produced in a great deal of the cellular membrane, and I believe in it only, except the skin giving way, which I believe is by ulceration principally, it becomes a question whether this mortification arises from the nature of the inflammation, or rather from the matter being confined in the cells of the cellular membrane. I rather suspect the latter; for I find that if this matter escapes from these cells and comes into uninflamed cells, it produces mortification there. This is like the urine, for whenever the urine escapes into the cellular membrane it there produces mortification; the colour of the skin is at first more vivid than afterwards, for it becomes of a purple colour[a].

[4.] Inflammation often produces mortification or death in the part inflamed. This commonly takes place in old people that are become very much debilitated, and chiefly in the lower extremities. I suspect it to be somewhat similar to the carbuncle, viz. principally in those who have lived well, although not so much confined to them as the carbuncle; however, it takes place in the young, where great debility has been produced from disease, especially those diseases that have debility as a principle, such as what are commonly called putrid fevers; but the situation of these is not so determined, and in such inflammation hardly takes place without an immediate exciting cause, as the application of blisters, &c. Death in a part sometimes takes place almost immediately without inflammation; but this is not to the present purpose. Where mortification succeeds inflammation in the extremities, especially in elderly persons, there is often an early separation of the cuticle which forms a blister, filled with a bloody serum; and we shall observe dark brownish spots, which consist of extravasated blood in the true cutis, and which shall at last blister, and then the cutis forms a slough.

Such inflammations have little of the adhesive tumefaction in them, but more of the œdematous; are not clear or transparent, but rather of a dusky red. As the colour of the inflamed parts shows something of its nature, it is to be observed that it is different in all these inflammations from that of the true adhesive; and as we have reason to believe that the circulation is quicker in the adhesive inflammation than is natural, and that the colour arises from this cause, we may suppose that the motion of the blood in these is languid, and that it assumes the venal appearance even in the arteries.

In most of these four inflammations there is an appearance that often arises, which is a reddish streak commonly passing from the inflamed parts towards the source of the circulation, but not always in this direction, sometimes just the contrary; and this is more certain when it happens to take place in an extremity, because there we know the course of all the vessels better; but it does not always arise from the part inflamed. I have seen this last species of inflammation attack the toes,

---

[a] [Probably the scarlet colour may in some measure arise from the salts of the urine. Afterwards, as the urine putrefies, ammonia is evolved, which changes the natural colour of the blood to a deep black.]

[b] [See *Leçons Orales de Clinique Chirurgicale*, par M. Dupuytren. According to this gentleman, the spontaneous, dry, or senile gangrene (which is here principally referred to) is generally the consequence of spontaneous arteritis and obliteration of the principal vessels. According to Cruveilhier, the same effect may be produced by arterial inflammation induced by direct experiment on living animals.]

and red streaks run up the foot, terminating about the ankle, while there were several arising on the fore part of the leg just below the knee. They often make a network on the leg, and are frequently a forerunner and an attendant on mortification. They seldom go further than a blush in the skin, seldom thicken, but are more of the œdematous kind; however, we sometimes find hard cords running from sores and inflammations, but these are commonly deeper-seated, and I have suspected them to be veins. As a proof of this, I have seen the superficial veins of the leg have the skin red over them, similar to those above described, and the veins have felt hard under the finger.

These reddish streaks are supposed to be absorbents, becoming inflamed by their carrying a stimulating fluid. I am apt to suppose them to be absorbents, but I do not conceive that this effect arises from absorption. If it arose from such a cause it should be uniform; the cause should always exist when the effect takes place. It is first to be observed that it only takes place in certain constitutions, in which absorption one way or other explains nothing; and I find, upon observation, that this effect shall be coeval with the inflammation where no suppuration has taken place. I have even seen it arise from accident, prior to the possibility of inflammation taking place, viz. in the time of the pain arising from the immediate effects of the accident: this was in the finger, from the prick of a clean needle, which had been for some time piercing new buckskin leather; the glands in the armpit were sore; sickness, attended with its usual symptoms, such as oppression, was nearly as immediate. Its direction from the source of the circulation is another strong proof of its not arising from absorption, and its taking place at some distance is also a corroboration of the same opinion. Another strong circumstance in favour of this opinion is that the morbid poisons do not produce this effect, where we know absorption has taken place. Thus the venereal seldom if ever produces it. The hard cord passing from the prepuce along the upper part of the penis I do not conceive to be of this kind. In the smallpox after inoculation it has been observed, but I imagine it was only in the above-mentioned constitutions. I could conceive it to arise in the plague, if there was any local disease. I am therefore rather apt to attribute this appearance to the irritation running along the lymphatics, more especially in such constitutions; and as we do not allow the veins to be absorbents, their being affected must be supposed to arise from the same cause[a]. Whenever we see this effect we may, in some degree, form an opinion of the kind of inflammation, and that it is not the most favourable.

---

[a] [See paper *On Absorption by Veins* in Vol. IV., and *On Inflammation of the Veins* at

CHAPTER III.

THE ADHESIVE INFLAMMATION.

I SHALL begin by treating of the nature and effects of what I have called the adhesive inflammation, as well as giving a proper idea of it. I shall also open the way to a clear understanding of the many phenomena which attend the suppurative inflammation. But as inflammation does not produce one effect only, but several, and as most of them take place about the same time, it is difficult to determine in the mind which to describe first.

Inflammation in most cases appears to begin at a point: for at the very first commencement all the local symptoms are within a very small compass; and they afterwards spread according to the violence of the cause, the disposition in the parts for inflammation, and the nature of the surrounding parts themselves, which susceptibility in the surrounding parts may be either constitutional or local. This is so much the case that inflammation shall come on at once in a fixed point, giving great pain, and which shall be soon followed by tumefaction. This is also the case with those inflammations which arise from accident, for all accidents are confined to fixed and determined limits; but the inflammation which follows is not; it spreads over a large extent; yet the inflammation is always the greater the nearer it is to the first fixed point, and gradually becomes less and less in the surrounding parts, till at last it is insensibly lost in them.

This spreading of the inflammation is owing to continued sympathy, the surrounding parts sympathizing with the point of irritation; and in proportion to the health of the surrounding parts and constitution this

---

the end of this volume. The symptoms and phenomena of inflammation of the absorbents and inflammation of the veins are analogous in many respects, and very often occur together, particularly after parturition. The particular conditions which dispose to these inflammations are very imperfectly understood, but in general they undoubtedly point to a broken down and highly irritable state of the constitution. Inflammation of the absorbents is the most frequent of the two, and very often is the first symptom of an attack of erysipelas, the inflammation passing outwards, as it were, with great facility, and extensively spreading on the skin. It is probably from the interposition of the lymphatic glands preventing the circulation of pus, that inflammation of the absorbents is so much less fatal than that of the veins.]

sympathy is less; for we find in many states of parts, and many constitutions, that there is a disposition to this sympathy, and in such the inflammation spreads in proportion[a].

§. 1. *Action of the Vessels in Inflammation.*

The act of inflammation would appear to be an increased action of the vessels*; but whatever action it is, it takes place most probably in the smaller vessels, for it may be confined almost to a point where nothing but the smallest vessels exist. The larger vessels may be considered as only the conveyers of the materials, for the smaller to act upon and dispose of according to the different intentions; however, inflammation in a part is not only an action of the smaller vessels in the part itself, but in the larger vessels leading to it. This is proved by a whitlow taking place on the end of a finger; for although the inflammation itself shall be confined to the end of a finger, and the inflammatory sensation or throbbing be situated in this part, yet we can feel by our hands, when we grasp the finger, a strong pulsation in the two arteries leading to the inflamed part, while no such pulsation can be felt in the other fingers; and if the inflammation is very considerable, the artery, as high as the wrist, will be sensibly affected, which proves that the arterial system is at that time dilating itself, and allowing a much larger quantity of blood to pass than is usual. This is probably by continued sympathy.

Where the inflammation affects the constitution, the vessels of the system rather contract, and keep as it were stationary, which stationary contraction is more or less according to the state of the constitution. In strong healthy constitutions, whose powers are equal to the necessary actions, or in parts that affect the constitution less, this contraction is less and less stationary.

The very first act of the vessels when the stimulus which excites in-

* It may be here remarked, that the action of vessels is commonly supposed to be contraction, either by their elastic or muscular coats; but I have shown that their elastic power also dilated them, and I have reason to believe their muscular power has a similar effect.

---

[a] [The disposition to spread may depend on many causes, as the nature of the part affected, the quality of the exciting cause, or the state of the constitution at the time. Where it depends on the constitution, it may be affirmed almost certainly that the nervous system is much debilitated and that locally there is a defective power of effusing coagulable lymph; a circumstance of which Mr. James has ingeniously availed himself to form the basis of his classification of inflammations.]

flammation is applied, is, I believe, exactly similar to a blush. It is, I believe, simply an increase or distension beyond their natural size. This effect we see takes place upon many occasions: gentle friction on the skin produces it, gently stimulating medicines have the same effect; a warm glow is the consequence, similar to that of the cheek in a blush; and if either of these be increased or continued, real inflammation will be the consequence, as well as excoriation, suppuration, and ulceration. This effect we often see, even where considerable mischief has been done; and I believe it is what always terminates the boundaries of the true inflammation. A musket-ball shall pass a considerable way under the skin, perhaps half-way round the body, which shall be discovered and traced by a red band in the skin, not in the least hard, only a little tender to the touch; and it shall subside without extending further. This appearance I shall term a blush; for although this may be reckoned the first act of inflammation, yet I would not call it inflammation, having produced a lasting effect. I should rather say that inflammation sets out from this point, and that afterwards a new action begins, which is probably first a separation of the coagulating lymph, and the throwing it out of the vessels.

The parts inflamed appear to become more vascular; but how far they are really so I am not certain; for this appearance does (at least in part) arise from the dilatation of the vessels, which allows the red part of the blood to go into vessels where only serum and coagulating lymph could pass when they were in a natural state; and till the newly-extravasated substances become vascular, the effect is most probably owing wholly to the above cause.

This incipient enlargement of the vessels upon the first excitement of inflammation is satisfactorily seen in the following manner. Make an incision through the skin on the inside of the upper part of a dog's thigh, three inches long. By pulling the cut edges asunder, and observing the exposed surface, we shall see the blush or ash-coloured cellular membrane covering the different parts underneath, with a few arteries passing through it to the neighbouring parts. But in a little time we shall see these vessels increasing in size, and also smaller vessels going off from them that were not before observable, as if newly formed or forming; the number and size shall increase till the whole surface shall become extremely vascular, and at last the red blood shall be thrown out in small dots on the exposed surface, probably through the cut ends of the arteries that only carried the lymph before. This surface will become in time more opake and less ductile. Parts inflamed, when compared with similar parts not inflamed, show a considerable difference in the size of the vessels, and probably from this cause bring an increased number to view. I froze the ear of a rabbit and thawed it again: this excited a considerable inflammation, an increased heat, and a considerable thickening of the part. This rabbit was killed when the ear was in the height of inflammation, and the head being injected, the two ears were removed and dried [see Pl. XX.]. The uninflamed ear dried clear and transparent, the vessels were distinctly seen ramifying through the substance; but the inflamed ear dried thicker and more opake, and its arteries were considerably larger.

In inflammation of the eye, which is commonly of the tunica conjunctiva, the progress of inflammation may in part be accurately observed, although not so progressively as in a wound. The contrast between the red vessel and the white of the eye, under this coat, is very conspicuous; and although we do not see the vessels enlarging in this coat, yet we see the progress they have made: the white appears as if it was becoming more vascular, and these vessels larger, till at last the whole tunica conjunctiva shall appear as one mass of blood, looking more like extravasated blood than a congeries of vessels, although I believe it is commonly the last.

From these circumstances it must appear that a much larger quantity of blood passes through parts when inflamed than when in a natural state[a], which is according to the common rules of the animal œconomy; for, whenever a part has more to do than simply to support itself, the blood is there collected in larger quantity. This we find to take place universally in those parts whose powers are called up to action by some necessary operation to be performed, whether natural or diseased.

As the vessels become larger, and the part becomes more of the colour of the blood, it is to be supposed there is more blood in the part; and as the true inflammatory colour is scarlet, or that colour which the blood has when in the arteries, one would from hence conclude either that the arteries were principally dilated, or at least, if the veins are equally distended, that the blood undergoes no change in such inflammation in its passage from the arteries into the veins, which I think is most probably the case; and this may arise from the quickness of its passage through those vessels.

When inflammation takes place in parts that have a degree of transparency, that transparency is lessened. This is, probably, best seen in membranes, such as those membranes which line cavities, or cover bodies in those cavities, such as the pia mater, where, in a natural state, we may observe the blood-vessels to be very distinct. But when we see

[a] [Recent microscopical investigations have demonstrated the error of this opinion, as will be shown more fully presently.]

the blood-vessels fuller than common, yet distinct in such membranes, we are not to call that inflammation, although it may be the first step, as we find to be the case in the first action of the vessels in consequence of such irritation as will end in inflammation. As it may not, however, be the first step, there must be other attending circumstances to determine it to be the very first action of the vessels in inflammation, for as that appearance may either belong to a briskness in the circulation in the part at the time, or be the very first step in inflammation, their causes are to be discriminated by some other symptom. They are both a kind of blush, or an exertion of the action of the vessels; but when it is an effect of an inflammatory cause, it is then only that the inflammation has not yet produced any change in the natural structure of the parts, but which it will soon do*. What the action is, or in what it differs from the common action of the vessels, is not easily ascertained, since we are more able to judge of the effects than the immediate cause. However, it is probably an action of the vessels, which we can better observe than any diseased action in the body, for we can observe the state in which the arteries are, with their general effects; we feel also a different temperature respecting heat, yet the immediate cause may not be ascertainable.

The vessels, both arteries and veins, in the inflamed part are enlarged, and the part becomes visibly more vascular; from which we should suspect, that instead of an increased contraction, there was rather what would appear an increased relaxation of their muscular powers, being, as we might suppose, left to the elasticity entirely. This would be reducing them to a state of paralysis simply; but the power of muscular contraction would seem to give way in inflammation, for they certainly dilate more in inflammation than the extent of the elastic power would allow; and it must also be supposed that the elastic power of the artery must be dilated in the same proportion. The contents of the circulation being thrown out upon such occasions, would, from considering it in those lights, rather confirm us in that opinion; and when we consider the whole of this as a necessary operation of nature, we must suppose it something more than simply a common relaxation; we must suppose it an action in the parts to produce an increase of size to answer particular purposes; and this I should call the action of dilatation, as we see the uterus increase in size in the time of uterine-gestation, as

* When this appearance is seen anywhere after death it should not be called inflammation, even although we knew it was the first action of inflammation; for as we are then only looking out for the causes of death, or the symptoms prior to death, we are only to look out for such as can be a cause, and not lay hold of those that cannot possibly be a cause, which those first actions cannot be.

well as the os tincæ in the time of labour, the consequence of the preceding actions, and necessary for the completion of those which are to follow.

The force of the circulation would seem to have some share in this effect, but only as a secondary cause; for I could conceive a part to inflame, or be in a state of inflammation, although no blood were to pass. As a proof of this, we may observe, that by lessening either the action of the heart, or the column of blood, inflammation is lessened; and I may also observe, that we have an increased pain in the inflamed part in the diastole of the artery, and a part inflamed by being gently pressed is made easier. Thus a person with an inflammation in the finger will find relief by gently pressing it in the other hand. These are strong proofs that it is not a contractile action of the muscular coat of the vessel; for in such a sensible state of vessels, if they contracted by their muscular power, the pain would be in their systole; for we find in all muscles which are in a state of great sensibility, from whatever cause, that they cannot act without giving great pain. Thus an inflamed bladder becomes extremely painful when expelling its contents; an inflamed intestine in the same manner. I should say, therefore, that in inflammation the muscular coats of the arteries do not contract.

Whatever purpose this increase of the size of the vessels may answer, we must suppose it allows a greater quantity of blood to pass through the inflamed part than in the natural state, which supposition is supported by many other observations. The part inflamed, I have already observed, becomes to appearance more vascular than when in the natural state, and it is probable that it is really so, both from new vessels being set up in the inflamed part, as well as from the new and adventitious uniting substance becoming vascular. Besides, the vessels of the parts are enlarged, so that the red blood passes further than common, which increases those appearances. But the brain appears to be an exception to these general rules; for in all diseases of the brain, where the effects were such as are commonly the consequence of inflammation, such as suppuration from accidents, I never could find the above appearances; the brain may, perhaps, go directly into suppuration, as sometimes the peritonæum does; but its slowness of going into suppuration after the accident would make us suppose, *à priori*, that there was sufficient time for adhesions to form[a].

---

[a] [In an inquiry into the proximate cause of inflammation, two principal considerations occur: first, as to the state of the capillary circulation, and, secondly, as to the influence of the nervous system.

1. When the web of a frog's foot, or the transparent mesentery of a warm-blooded animal, are viewed in the field of a good microscope, and at the same time irritated,

§. 2. *Of the Colour, Swelling, and Pain of Inflamed Parts.*

[*Colour.*]—The colour of an inflamed part is visibly changed from the natural, whatever it was, to a red. This red is of various hues, accord-

---

effects very different are observed to ensue in different cases; but in all instances where inflammation is well established the vessels are observed to be increased in number as well as size, and the course of the blood to be much retarded. The evidence upon this point is so universal, precise, and satisfactory, as to render any detail on the subject quite unnecessary and any doubt upon the question a mere excess of scepticism. (See *Treatise on Inflammation, by Dr. C. Hastings*, p. 67. *Hist. des Inflam., par M. Gendrin*, ii. 475, (1453 et seq.) *Lectures on Inflam., by Dr. J. Thomson*, p. 61. *Treatise on Febrile Diseases, by Dr. W. Philip*, 3rd edit. ii. 17. *Kaltenbrunner*, op. cit. See ante, p. 142.) It would appear, however, that there is a great difference between actual inflammation and that precedent state of erubescence which is excited by slight stimulants, or which bounds the outer circumference of an inflamed part, a difference which has not always been attended to, and which in many instances has led to mistakes on this subject. At first the effect of stimulation is generally to contract the small vessels and to accelerate the circulation; but as soon as inflammation is unequivocally established, the circulation is invariably retarded. In severe cases indeed the retardation amounts to a complete *stasis*, although in the surrounding parts the blood is observed to flow with more rapidity than usual.

Arguing from these facts, Dr. Hastings and others have drawn the conclusion that debility of the capillaries is the cause of inflammation; or, in other words, that the increased action of the vessels, consequent on the application of stimuli, exhausts and impairs their irritability, and gives rise to their subsequent dilatation, followed on the other hand by an increased action of the larger vessels; so that, according to this gentleman, "Inflammation consists in a weakened action of the capillaries, by which the equilibrium between the larger and smaller vessels is destroyed, and the latter become distended;" while the restoration of an inflamed part is supposed to be effected by the capillary vessels being so excited, and the larger vessels so far weakened, by the preternatural action of the latter, that the two are again brought into correspondence and proportion to each other.

The objections to this theory are sufficiently obvious, as it not only places the two extremities of the vascular system in opposition to each other, without any apparent cause, but makes the recovery of inflammation to depend upon the reaction of the larger vessels, which, if we may judge from the effect of remedies, or from the common sense of the case, should appear to be one of the most certain means of increasing it. Besides, why the larger vessels should be excited by the debility of the smaller, or the latter recover themselves from their debilitated state by the excitement of the larger, is not pretended to be accounted for; not to mention that every physiological fact is strongly repugnant to the notion of an action, essentially reparative, like that of inflammation, being dependent on debility for its principle.

The other most prevailing opinion on this subject is that which was adopted by our author, viz. that inflammation is an increased action of the natural powers of a part attended with an accelerated circulation. The grounds for this opinion are as follow: 1. That when a part has more to do than simply to support its own life, an increased activity of the circulation becomes necessary; as, for instance, in the growth of the stag's horn, the enlargement of the vessels of the uterus during gestation, and the augmented supply of blood to secreting organs during the period of their activity. 2. That the

ing to the nature of the inflammation; if healthy, it is a pale red; if less healthy, the colour will be darker, more of a purple, and so on till it shall

---

arteries and capillaries visibly enlarge in size and increase in number in inflammation exactly as they are observed to do when the healthy functions of any part are unusually exerted. 3. That as, under ordinary circumstances, the heat and sensibility of parts are in proportion to the quantity of blood going to these parts, so it is reasonable to conclude that the same effects, observable in inflammation, are dependent on the same causes. 4. That inflamed parts bleed more copiously than those which are uninflamed, and that the redness returns more rapidly after pressure than is observed to happen in parts which have been stricken with cold, and are consequently congested. 5. That the returning veins from an inflamed part are more distended than naturally, which perfectly accords with the observation made by Mr. Lawrence that when venesection is simultaneously performed on both arms, one of which is inflamed, the blood which flows from the inflamed side, in a given time, is twice and sometimes three times as great as that which flows from the sound side. 6. That periodic determinations of blood consequent on increased activity of function are apt, when excessive either in degree or duration, to terminate in inflammation, in the same manner exactly as great or prolonged constitutional excitement from exercise or mental causes may terminate in fever. 7. That the arterial colour of the blood in inflamed parts depends (as Mr. Hunter supposed) on the rapidity of its transmission through the parts, which does not allow sufficient time for the usual changes to take place; an effect, however, which it seems more reasonable to refer to the perverted state of the vital functions. 8. That the pulsatory and throbbing pain of inflammation indicates an increased local activity, just as any sudden or great exertion of muscular power occasions throbbing of the whole system. The augmented volume and stroke of the pulse, and the increased impetus with which the blood is projected from an inflamed vessel when divided, are additional proofs of the same kind. 9. That as the application of stimuli, ex vi termini, excites an unusual activity of function in all the organs of the body, it seems unreasonable to assign a sedative effect to these agencies where they occasion inflammation. 10. That the causes of inflammation, immediate as well as predisponent, are of such a nature as to give increased vigour to most of the operations of the economy, as on the other hand the nature of the remedies employed is precisely of that kind which is known, from experience, to be best calculated to diminish strength as well as to reduce action. 11. That the ordinary functions of an inflamed part, and sometimes of the whole system, are suspended and as it were concentrated on the process of reparation, agreeably to what is observed to happen when other important operations are carried on in the animal body. These reasons seem sufficient to lead to the conclusion that inflammation is an act in which, if there is not increased power, there is at least increased action.

The capital objection to this theory is, that the circulation is demonstratively retarded, and sometimes completely arrested, in inflammation; an objection which is partly removed, however, by the consideration, that although retarded in the most inflamed parts, it is accelerated in the parts adjacent. The statement, however, is objectionable on other accounts. It makes increased action, in parts professedly contractile, to consist in dilatation, for which we have no authority, and which obviously confounds congestion with inflammation; besides, dilatation can only influence the circulation by giving increased effect to the heart's action; an effect, however, which by no means universally follows; and in regard to the larger arteries the same consequences must ensue, for it has been proved by Dr. Alison, that instead of their contractility being increased,

be a bluish purple, which I took notice of in the short sketch of the peculiar inflammations; but the parts inflamed will in every constitution be

as the hypothesis supposes, it is certainly impaired (4th and 5th Rep. of Br. Assoc.). In the sense, therefore, in which the author understood the term, increased action certainly does not take place, although in another sense it certainly must. Probably the effect of inflammation is to approximate the structure of an inflamed part to that of a gland, requiring, on the one hand, a slow circulation, in order that the important offices of reparation may be carried on; and on the other hand, an extensive supply of the vital fluid as aliment to this function. It is at least remarkable, that the whole internal arrangements of glands, as well indeed as of the whole capillary system, seem designed to retard the circulation, while the most prominent symptom of inflammation, and that which forms the only unequivocal proof of its presence, is the slowness of the circulation and the extraordinary quantity of effusion which is poured out.

Inflammation, however, is an act which involves all the functions of a part. The blood itself is affected. It loses its globular structure, and the globules are observed to lose their repulsive properties, and either to agglomerate together, or to adhere to the sides of the vessels. At first it is generally redder than usual, but afterwards it assumes various shades of brown or yellow, until at length, when suppuration is fairly established, it has the character of pus, which some have been able to trace, as it slowly moved along the vessels, until it finally exuded on the surface. (Gendrin, *op. cit.*, ii. 479. (1457, 1458.)) Along with these appearances are sometimes observed irregular flocculi, floating in a transparent fluid, which have the appearance of ragged portions of lymph, or decolorated and broken-down globules of blood. As soon as the inflammation begins to subside, the globules reappear, and the current of the circulation is slowly re-established; but should the inflammation increase still further in violence, the blood then entirely loses its red colour, complete stagnation of it takes place, and the part becomes gangrenous. More or fewer of these changes invariably attend inflammation, which cannot therefore be supposed to consist in a simple alteration of the circulation, but principally of those vital affinities subsisting between the vessels and their contents, which are the peculiar attributes of life.

As soon as inflammation is established, an increased secretion takes place from the cells of the cellular membrane, which at first is limpid and colourless, and contains little albumen, but becomes more yellow and more charged with albumen as the inflammation advances. Then it becomes semi-gelatinous, depending on a small admixture of fibrin with it. Bloody striæ and puncta now appear in it, the fibrin becomes more abundant, blood is poured out in a pure state, and finally pus is formed. These successive degenerations are fully exhibited in the section of an inflamed part, beginning from the circumference to the centre, and correspond precisely with the effusions which take place from the surfaces of inflamed membranes, being in fact so many degenerations of the natural secretions of the parts. From these facts, therefore, it is obvious that inflammation induces a new state of the secretory function, and that all the results of inflammation are the consequence of this modification, an inference which perfectly coincides with Mr. Hunter's views of suppuration, although it is opposed to those of M. Gendrin, who supposes that the various matters effused in inflammation are spontaneously convertible into pus, without the aid of the proper vessels. (*Op. cit.*, ii. 471. (1447, 1448.))

2. The facts which relate to the influence of the nervous system in the production of inflammation are neither numerous nor precise, which is probably the reason why this part of the subject has received less attention than the state of the capillaries. There

more of the healthy red when near to the source of the circulation, than when far from it. This increase of red appears to arise from two causes;

---

can be no doubt of the general analogy which exists between the reparation of the accidental lesions of the frame, and the ordinary nutrition of the body, and also that the functions of secretion, excretion, absorption, sensibility, and the due venalization of the blood, are all more or less modified and affected by the process of inflammation; so far, therefore, as these functions are dependent on or liable to be affected by the nervous system in a state of health, so far it seems reasonable to conclude that they are similarly affected in the process of inflammation. 1. The circulation and nutrition of parts are greatly impaired by a paralysis of the nerves, while, from the best observation of physiologists, it appears that deficiency or imperfect development of the normal organization is exactly correspondent to the deficiency or imperfect development of the corresponding portions of the spinal marrow. 2. The experiments of physiologists have demonstrated that the functions of secretion and excretion, and the general offices of a part, are greatly dependent on the integrity of the nervous system. The urine is not secreted after decapitation, nor the gastric juice after the division of the eighth pair of nerves. 3. The nutrition of the body is affected by various influences of the mind, which can only be supposed to operate through the medium of the nerves. 4. Intense pain often ushers in the inflammatory attack, and precedes every other apparent symptom. So also hysterical and sympathetic pains, obviously depending on some distant source, often excite inflammation, while the operation of cold can only be explained on the same principle. From facts of this kind some have inferred the invariable precedence of some disturbance of the nervous system. 5. Metastatic inflammations are plainly referrible to the same cause, unless they are to be explained on the humoral pathology. Thus also the appearances of local inflammation, especially of the exanthematous eruptions, are often preceded by constitutional rigors and fever, which plainly evince an antecedent disturbance of the nervous system. 6. Blushing, the contraction of the extreme capillaries from fear and other causes, and the effects produced by the sudden crushing of the nervous centres, are proofs of the influence which the nervous system has over the circulation. 7. Division of the fifth pair of nerves gives rise to inflammation and consequent destruction of the globe of the eye. Similar effects have been known to ensue from compression of the fifth pair within the cranium (Med. Gaz., i. 531.), or by division of the nerve of a horse's foot above the fetlock joint (*op. cit.*, xvi. 140.); and occasionally in the human subject, when the principal nerves of the limb have been divided by a gunshot wound, inflammation and mortification have taken place. The interesting facts communicated on this subject by Mr. Earle (Med. Chir. Tr., vii. 173.) render it probable that these effects depend on the impairment of vitality consequent on the deficient innervation, which renders parts incapable of supporting stimuli, which in a healthy state would not be injurious. The sloughing of the nates in injuries of the spinal marrow, and of frost-bitten parts when hastily restored to life, strongly corroborate this opinion. 8. Direct irritation of the adjacent nerves has sometimes been found to excite inflammation at their extremities. (Phil. Trans. 1814, p. 583; Med. Gaz., i. 531; Med. Chir. Trans., vii. 191.) 9. The generally acknowledged fact that the condition of the nervous system has great effect in determining the course of common inflammation. From these facts, therefore, it is clear that the nervous system exercises an important influence in inflammation, although from the illustrations which have been given, it is equally clear that this influence is rather of a negative than a positive kind. In fact the office of the nerves in inflammation appears to hold precisely the same relation to this action that it does to the other organic functions of the body. It is regulative, but not essential.]

the first is a dilatation of the vessels, whereby a greater quantity of blood is allowed to pass into those vessels which only admitted serum or lymph before*. The second is owing probably to new vessels being set up in the extravasated uniting coagulating lymph. This colour is gradually lost in the surrounding parts if the inflammation is of the healthy kind, but in many others it has a determined edge, as in the true erysipelatous, and in some specific diseases, as in the smallpox, where its quick termination is a sign of health.

[*Swelling.*]—From the account I have given of the immediate effects of inflammation of the cellular membrane (in which I include the larger cavities), the volume of the part inflamed must be increased. This, when a common consequence of inflammation, is not circumscribed, but rather diffused. As the inflammation, however, begins in a circumscribed part (which is at least the case with that arising from violence), the inflammation, as I just now observed, is always the greatest nearest to that point, and is gradually lost in the surrounding parts, the swelling of course being the greatest at or nearest to this point, and it is also lost in the surrounding sound parts. This takes place, more or less, according to the constitution, or the situation of the inflammation; for if the constitution be strong and healthy, the surrounding parts will sympathize less with the point of irritation, so that inflammation and its consequences, viz. extravasation, will be less diffused. There will be less of the serum, and of course a purer coagulating lymph, so that the swelled parts will be firmer; but in some specific diseases or dissimilar parts, as a gland, it has a more determined edge, the surrounding parts not so readily taking on specific diseased action as in other cases. In this both the colour and swelling correspond very much, since they both depend on the same principle.

This increase of volume is owing to the extravasation of the coagulating lymph and some serum. In proportion to the inflammation (the degree of which depends on the causes above mentioned,) this effect is more or less, and therefore is greatest at the point of inflammation, becoming less and less as it extends into the surrounding parts, till it is insensibly lost in them.

The extravasation of the serum along with the coagulating lymph is, probably, not a separation of itself, as in a dropsy, but a part of it being separated from the lymph in the coagulation of that fluid, is squeezed into the surrounding cellular membrane, where there is but little extra-

* The tunica conjunctiva of the eye when inflamed is a striking instance of this; but the visible progress of inflammation I have already described in the experiment on the dog, p. 279.

vasation, and where the cells are not united by it[a]. Thus the circumference of such swellings is a little œdematous; but the whole of the serum, if there be a depending part, will move thither, and distend it considerably, as in the foot in consequence of an inflammation in the leg. But in most cases there is a continued extravasation of serum, long after the extravasation of the coagulating lymph is at an end; so that depending parts will continue œdematous while the inflammation is resolving, or while suppuration, or even healing is going on. The whole swelling looks like a part of the body only a little changed, without any appearance of containing extraneous matter; and indeed it is simply formed by an extravasation of fluids without their having undergone any visible or material change, except coagulation.

[*Pain.*]—As few uncommon operations can go on in an animal body without affecting the sensations, and as the first principle of sensation arises from some uncommon action, or alteration being made in the natural position or arrangement of the parts, we should naturally suppose that the sensation would be in some degree according to those effects, and the sensibility of the parts. One can easily form an idea of an alteration in the structure of parts giving sensation which may even be carried to pain, but that the simple action of parts should produce sensations and even violent pain is but little known, or at least has been, I believe, but little attended to; all these effects, I think, may justly be included under the term spasm*; at least we are led by analogy to suppose that they belong to that class.

By spasm I should understand a contraction of a muscle without the leading and natural causes. Thus, the contraction of a muscle of the leg, called the cramp, gives considerable pain, often violent; as also the tetanus; and when in a less degree, as in the twinkling of the eyelid, it gives only sensation, whereas if the muscles were to act by the will no sensation would be produced.

We find that those sensations are more or less acute, according to the quickness or slowness of the progress of these causes; from whence we are naturally led to assign two causes, which must always attend one another; for when both do not take place at the same time, the mind

* How far a nerve from a part, or how far the materia vitæ of a part, can act so as to convey sensation I do not know; but we all know that an involuntary action of a voluntary muscle, or the spontaneous action of an involuntary muscle, will produce it.

---

[a] [This accords with the opinion of Dr. B. C. Babington, who has attempted to prove that the fibrin and serum are always effused in the same relative proportions to each other. Observation, however, and the account which has been formerly given (see *note*, p.328.) of the gradual transformation of the secretions of an inflamed part, are opposed to this notion.—Med. Chir. Trans., xvi. 311.]

then remains insensible to the alteration. This is its being produced in a given time, for the alteration in the position of the parts may be produced so slowly as not to keep pace with sensation, which is the case with many indolent tumours, ascites, etc.; on the other hand, this alteration in the natural position of parts may be so quick as to exceed sensation, and therefore there is a certain medium, which produces the greatest pain.

The actions I have been describing being pretty quick in their effects, we cannot fail to see why the pain from the inflammation must be considerable; however, the pain is not the same in all the different stages. In the adhesive state of the inflammation it is generally but very inconsiderable, especially if it is to go no further, and is perhaps more of a heavy than an acute pain; when it happens on the skin it often begins with an itching, but as the inflammation is passing from the adhesive to the suppurative, the parts then undergo a greater change than before, and the pain grows more and more acute, till it becomes very considerable. The nerves also acquire at that time a degree of sensibility, which renders them much more susceptible of impression than when they are in their natural state; thus, an inflamed part is not only painful in itself, but it communicates impressions to the mind independent of pain, which do not arise from a natural sound part. This pain increases every time the arteries are dilated, whence it would appear that the arteries do not contract by their muscular power in their systole, for if they did, we might expect a considerable pain in that action, which would be at the full of the pulse. Whether this pain arises from the distension of the artery by the force of the heart, or whether it arises from the action of distension from the force of the artery itself, is not easily determined. We know that diseased muscles give much pain in their contraction, perhaps more than they do when stretched*.

That the degree of inflammation which becomes the cause of adhesions gives but little pain, is proved from the dissections of dead bodies, for we seldom or never find a body in dissection which has not adhesions in some of the larger cavities; and yet it may reasonably be supposed that many of these persons never had any acute symptoms or

* This is very evident in the bladder of urine when inflamed, for in the contraction of that viscus to expel the urine there is more pain than in the dilatation; indeed the distension is gradual; and when the urine is wholly evacuated, the irritation produced by the contraction still continues, which produces a continuance of the straining[a].

---

[a] [It seems more reasonable to suppose that the pain in this instance is produced by the compression of the inflamed and highly sensible mucous membrane of the bladder against itself. The first efforts to evacuate the urine are not nearly so painful as those which follow.]

violent pain in those parts; indeed we find many strong adhesions upon the opening of dead bodies, in parts which the friends of these persons never heard mentioned, during life, as the subject of a single complaint.

That adhesions can be produced from very slight inflammation, is proved in ruptures in consequence of wearing a truss; for we find the slight pressure of a truss exciting such action as to thicken parts, by which means the two sides of the sac are united, though there be hardly any sensation in the part; we also see, in cases where this inflammation arises from violence, that it gives little or no pain. A man shall be shot through the cavity of the abdomen, and if none of the contained parts are materially hurt, the adhesive inflammation shall take place in all the internal parts contiguous to the wound made by the ball, and yet no great degree of pain shall be felt. This assertion is still proved by the little pain suffered after many bruises, where there is evident inflammation; and in simple fractures the pain from the inflammation is very trifling, whatever it may be from the laceration of the parts. But this will be according to the degree of inflammation, what stage it is in, and what parts are inflamed, as will be fully explained hereafter.

We find it a common principle in the animal machine, that every part increases in some degree according to the action required[a]. Thus we find muscles increase in size when much exercised; vessels become larger in proportion to the necessity of supply, as, for instance, in the gravid uterus: the external carotids in the stag, also, when his horns are growing, are much larger than at any other time; and I have observed, that in inflammation the vessels become larger, more blood passes, and there appear to be more actions taking place; but the nerves do not seem to undergo any change. The nerves of the gravid uterus are the same as when it is in the natural state; neither do the branches of the fifth and seventh pair of nerves in the stag become larger; and in inflammation of the nerves their blood-vessels are enlarged, and have coagulating lymph thrown into their interstices, but the nerve itself is not increased, so as to bring the part to the state of a natural part, fitted for acute sensation, which shows that the motions of the nerves have nothing to do with the œconomy of the part; they are only the messengers of intelligence and orders. It appears that only the action of the materia vitæ in the inflamed parts is increased, and this increase of action in the inflamed part is continued along the nerve which is not in-

---

[a] [This observation may be true of those parts which have naturally a fibrous texture, but certainly not of the internal viscera of the body and organs of the senses, the perfection of which is not observed to bear any proportion to their size. How far the brain is subject to this law it is for the cranioscopist to decide.]

flamed, to the mind, so that the impression on the sensorium is, probably, equal to the action of the inflamed materia vitæ.

The quantity of natural sensibility is, I believe, proportioned to the quantity of nerves, under any given circumstance; but I apprehend the diseased sensibility does not take place at all in this proportion, but in proportion to the diseased action of the materia vitæ. Thus a tendon has very little sensation when injured in a natural state; but let that tendon become inflamed, or otherwise diseased, and the sensation shall be very acute.

It may not be improper to observe, that many parts of the body in a natural state give peculiar sensations when impressed; and when those parts are injured they give likewise pain peculiar to themselves; it is this latter effect which I am to consider. I may also observe, that the same mode of impression shall give a peculiar sensation to one part, while it shall give pain to another. Thus, what will produce sickness in the stomach, will produce pain in the colon. When the sensation of pain is in a vital part it is somewhat different from most of those pains that are common. Thus, when the pain arises from an injury done to the head, the sensation is a heavy stupifying pain, rendering the person affected unfit to pay attention to other sensations, and is often attended with sickness, from the stomach sympathizing with it. When the pain is in the heart or lungs it is more acute, and is very much confined to the part diseased. When in the stomach and intestines, especially the upper part of them, it is a heavy oppressive sickly pain, but more or less attended with sickness according to its pressure or proximity to the stomach; for when situated in the colon it is more acute, and less attended with sickness.

We cannot give a better illustration of this than by taking notice of the effects of a purge. If we take such a purge as will produce both sickness and griping, we can easily trace the progress of the medicine in the canal; when in the stomach it makes us sick, but we soon find the sickness becoming more faint, by which we can judge that it has proceeded to the duodenum; and then a kind of uneasiness, approaching to pain, succeeds; when this is the case we may be certain that the medicine is passing along the jejunum; it then begins to give a sickish griping pain, which I conceive belongs to the ilium; and when in the colon it is a sharp pain, soon after which a motion takes place.

The liver, testicles, and uterus are subject nearly to the same kind of pain as the stomach. A tendon, ligament, and bone give something of the same kind of pain, though not so oppressive, namely, a dull and heavy pain, often attended with some little sickness, the stomach generally sympathizing in such cases. But the skin, muscles, and the cellular membrane, in common, give an acute pain, which rather rouses than oppresses, if not too great. All of this will be further mentioned when we treat of each part.

One cause of this variety of sensations, according as the parts inflamed are vital or not vital, seems to consist in the different systems of materia vitæ with which those parts are supplied, having, probably, nerves peculiarly constructed for this purpose; for all the parts which are supplied with branches from the par vagum and intercostals affect the patient with lowness of spirits from the very first attack of the inflammation: the actions of those parts are involuntary, and therefore are more immediately connected with the living principle, and consequently that principle is affected whenever anything affects these nerves. The other system of the materia vitæ, when affected by this inflammation, rather rouses at first the constitution, which shows signs of strength, unless the parts have rather weak powers of recovery, such as tendon, bone, etc., or are far from the heart, in which cases the signs of weakness sooner or later appear: hence it would seem that this difference in the constitution, arising from the difference in parts and their situation, arises from the constitution having a disease which it cannot so easily manage, as it can in those parts which are not vital, and in parts that are near to the heart; which circumstances alone become a cause of irritation in the constitution.

§. 3. *The Heat of Parts in Inflammation.*

When I was treating of the blood I observed that the heat of the animal was commonly considered as connected with that fluid; but as I had not made up my mind about the cause of the heat of animals, not being satisfied with the opinions hitherto given, I did not endeavour to offer any account of that property; but I shall now consider this power when the animal is under disease, where it would appear often to be diminished, and often increased, and of course the animal often becomes colder and hotter than its natural temperature.

There is an endeavour to bring the heat of a living body to the temperature of the surrounding medium, but in the more perfect animals this is prevented by the powers in the animal to support its own temperature, more especially in and near the vital parts[a]; therefore, in

[a] [This uniformity of temperature is not, however, by any means so universal, even in health and in the higher animals, as has often been supposed. De la Roche and Berger found that warm-blooded mammalia, exposed for long periods to a high tempe-

making experiments, to ascertain any variation, it is not necessary to ascertain at the same time the temperature of the atmosphere.

Heat, I imagine, is a sign of strength and power of constitution, although it may often arise from an increased action either of weak constitutions or of weakened parts.

Heat is a positive action, while cold is the reverse, therefore producing weakness, and often arising from a diminished action of strong parts[a].

It has not yet been considered whether an animal has the power of producing heat equally in every part of the body, although, from what is generally advanced on this subject, we are led to suppose that every part has this power, or whether it is carried from some one source of heat by the blood to every part; this may probably not be easily determined; but I am apt to suspect there is a principal source of heat, although it may not be in the blood itself, the blood being only affected by having its source near the source of heat.

That this principle resides in the stomach is probable, or at least I am certain that affections of the stomach will produce either heat or cold. There are affections of the stomach which produce the sensation of heat in it, and the air that arises in eructations feels hot to the mouth of the person; but whether these sensations arise from actual heat, or from sensation only, I have not been able to determine. Stimulating substances applied to the stomach will produce a glow. Affections of the mind produce the same effect, which last circumstance might seem to contradict the idea of its arising from the stomach; but I suspect that the stomach sympathizes with those actions of the brain which form the mind, and then produces heat, which will be better illustrated in treating of cold. I suspect that the cold bath produces heat in the

---

rature, experienced an elevation equal to 10°, and sometimes 13°. Dr. Edwards and M. Despretz found a difference of 6° in birds in the winter and summer months, being in the former 105° and in the latter 111°. Dr. Davy found that the standard heat of the Cingalese varied from 1° to 2° above the average in more temperate climates. Dr. Fordyce and his friends experienced an elevation of 2° or 3° in their experiments on heated air, and De la Roche an elevation of 5° after remaining seventeen minutes in a vapour bath at 120°. The singular power which the body possesses of accommodating itself to the extremes of external circumstances, is well exemplified by a fact recorded by Capt. Lyon in Capt. Parry's second voyage to the arctic regions, where the temperature of eleven out of sixteen foxes, killed in Winter Isle (lat. 66° 11′, temp. −3° to −32°) varied from 100° to 106¾° at their vital parts; as well as by the counter-fact that the temperature of persons exposed to very high degrees of natural heat, as at Sierra Leone, (100° to 103°), Senegal (108½° to 117½°), Oronoco (110° to 115°), &c., does not in general vary more than a few degrees from the standard heat. How this is accomplished has been fully shown by M. De la Rôche, *Journal de Physiologie*, lxiii., lxxi., and lxvii.]

[a] [See Note, §. i. 279.]

same way, from the sympathizing intercourse between the skin and the stomach.

That diseases augment or lessen this power in the animal is evident; for in many diseases the animal becomes much hotter, and in many others much colder than is usual to it. This fact was first discovered by simple sensation alone, both to the patients themselves and the practitioner, before the absolute measurement of the degrees of heat by instruments was known; but it was impossible that such knowledge of it could be accurate, for we find by experiment that the measurement of degrees of heat by sensation is very vague. This happens because the degree of heat in ourselves (which in such experiments is the instrument) is not of one standard, but must vary pretty much before we are made sensible of the difference, and therefore there can be only a relative knowledge respecting our own heat at the time. But now our measurement is more determined, and can be brought even nearer to the truth than is absolutely necessary to be known in disease.

The increase and decrease of the heat of an animal body may be divided into constitutional and local. The constitutional arises from a constitutional affection, and may arise primarily in the constitution itself; or it probably may arise secondarily, as from a local disease with which the constitution sympathizes; but of this I am not yet certain, for from several experiments made to ascertain this point, it seemed to appear that local inflammation had little power of increasing the heat of the body beyond the natural standard, although the body was under the influence of the inflammation by sympathy, called the symptomatic fever; but if the heat of the body is below the natural heat, or that heat where actions, whether natural or diseased, are called forth, then the heat of the body is raised to its natural standard*.

As it is the principle of increase of local heat in inflammation I am now to consider, it should be first ascertained how far such a principle exists in a part, and what that principle may be; the constitutional principle being in some measure not to the present purpose, although it may throw some light on the difference between the powers of the constitutional and those of the local principle. It is said that disease, as fever, has been known to raise the heat of the body to twelve degrees above the natural heat; and if so, then there is in such cases either an increased power or an increased exertion of that power; and to know whether this arises only from a constitutional affection at large, or whether it can take place in parts when the constitution is affected by those parts, is worthy of inquiry.

* Vide Animal Œconomy, iv. 131.

The principal instance of supposed increased local heat is in inflammation, and we find that external parts inflamed do actually become hotter; but let us see how far the increase goes. From all the observations and experiments I have made, I do not find that a local inflammation can increase the local heat above the natural heat of the animal; and when in parts whose natural heat is inferior to that which is at the source of the circulation, it does not rise so high: those animals, too, which appear to have no power, either of increase or decrease in health, naturally appear to be equally deficient in disease, as will be seen in the experiments.

I suspect that the blood has an ultimate standard heat in itself when in health, and that nothing can increase that heat but some universal or constitutional affection; and probably the sympathetic fever is such as has no power in this way, and that the whole power of local inflammation is only to increase it a little in the part, but that it cannot bring it above the standard heat at the source, nor even up to it in parts that naturally or commonly do not come up to it, as just above mentioned.

As inflammation is the principal instance capable of producing local increased heat, I have taken the opportunity of examining inflammations, both when spontaneous and in consequence of operations. I have also made several experiments for that purpose, which are similar to operations, and cannot say that I ever saw, from all these experiments and observations, a case where the heat was really so much increased as it appeared to be to the sensations.

Experiments on Internal Surfaces.

Experiment I. A man had the operation for the radical cure of the hydrocele performed at St. George's Hospital. When I opened the tunica vaginalis I immediately introduced the ball of the thermometer into it, and close by the side of the testicle. The mercury rose exactly to 92°. The cavity was filled with lint, dipped in salve, that it might be taken out at will; the next day, when inflammation was come on, the dressings were taken out, and the ball of the thermometer introduced as before, when it arose to 98¾° exactly.

Here was an increase of heat of 6¾°, but even this was not equal to that of the blood, probably, at the source of the circulation in the same man. This experiment I have repeated more than once, and with nearly the same event.

As the human subject cannot always furnish us with opportunities of ascertaining the fact, and it is often impossible to make experiments when proper cases occur, I was led to make such experiments on animals as appeared to me proper for determining the fact; but in none of them could I ever increase the inflammatory heat so as to make it equal to the natural heat of the blood at its source.

Experiment II. I made an incision into the thorax of a dog; the wound was made about the centre of the right side, and the thermometer pushed down, so as to come in contact, or nearly so, with the diaphragm. The degree of heat was 101°; a large dossil of lint was put into the wound to prevent its healing by the first intention, and covered over by a sticking-plaster. The dog was affected with a shivering. The day following the lint was extracted, and the thermometer again introduced; the degree of heat appeared exactly the same, viz. 101° This dog recovered.

Experiment III. An oblique incision was made about two inches deep into the gluteal muscles of an ass, and into this wound was introduced a tin canula about an inch and half long, so that half an inch of the bottom of the wound projected beyond the canula; into this canula was introduced a wooden plug, which projected half an inch beyond the canula, so as to fill up the bottom of the wound, and which kept that part of the wound from uniting. The whole was fastened into the wound by threads attached to the skin.

Immediately upon making the wound the ball of the thermometer was introduced into it to the bottom, and the mercury rose to 100° exactly, as it did also at the same time in the vagina. On the next morning the wooden plug was taken out, and the ball of the thermometer (being previously warmed to 99°,) was introduced down to the bottom of the wound, which projected beyond the canula, and the mercury rose to 100°. The wooden plug was returned and secured as before. In the evening the same experiment was repeated, and the mercury rose to 100°. Friday morning it rose only to 99°. Friday evening it rose to near 101½°. Saturday morning, 99°, and in the evening 100°. A similar experiment to this was made on a dog, and the heat was 101°. The day following the heat was the same, as also on the third day, when suppuration was taking place.

Experiment IV. Although in the experiment upon the dog, by making an opening into the thorax so as to excite an inflammation there, and to affect his constitution, the heat of the part was not increased; yet in order to be more clear with regard to the result of such an experiment, a wound was made into the abdomen of an ass, and a solution of common salt and water thrown in (about a handful to a pint of water), to excite a universal inflammation in the cavity of the abdomen. This produced great pain and uneasiness, so as to make the animal lie down and roll, becoming as restless as horses when griped. The next morning, Friday, the thermometer was introduced into the vagina, and the mercury stood at 99½°, nearly the same heat as before the experiment; in the evening, 101½°. Saturday morning, 100½°; evening, 100½°. The vagina, therefore, was not rendered hotter by an inflammation which produced what we may call the sympathetic fever. The animal was now killed, and on examining the abdomen, the side where the wound was made appeared much inflamed, as well as the intestine opposite to this part. All of them adhered together, and the intestines surrounding this part of the adhesions had their peritoneal coat become extremely vascular, and matter was formed in the abdomen.

But that the heat of a part can be increased above the common standard of a healthy person is certain, when it is such a part as is naturally of the standard heat, as, for instance, the abdomen. For in Lord Hertford's servant, who was tapped eight times, and seven of them in thirteen weeks, the seventh time I held the ball of a thermometer in the stream, as it flowed from the canula of the trocar, and it raised the mercury to 101° exactly, through the whole time. Twelve days after I tapped him the eighth time; the water was pretty clear; when I held the thermometer in the stream it rose to 104°. Now as the heat of the abdomen was 104°, we must, I think, suppose that the general heat of the man would also be 104°.

Experiments on Secreting Surfaces.

Experiment I. I took the degree of heat of a dog's rectum, by introducing the thermometer about three inches; and when it was ascertained, four grains of corrosive sublimate were dissolved in two ounces of water, and the solution thrown up the rectum. The day following the thermometer was again introduced, and then I found the heat somewhat increased, but not quite a degree. As far as one might judge from external appearances, the rectum was very much inflamed, as there was a considerable external swelling, forming a thick elevated ring round the anus.

Experiment II. I introduced into the rectum of an ass the thermometer, and the mercury rose to 98½° exactly: this was repeated several times with the same result. I then threw up the rectum an injection of flour of mustard and ginger, mixed in about a pint of water. About twelve hours after I introduced the thermometer, and it rose to 99½°. The injection was repeated several times, but the heat did not increase.

Experiment III. To irritate the rectum still more, I threw up a solution of corrosive sublimate, and about twelve hours after I introduced the thermometer, and found no increase of heat. Twenty hours after I introduced the thermometer, but the heat was the same. Sixty hours after the injection, the thermometer being introduced, the mercury rose to 100° exactly. This injection had irritated so much as to give a very severe tenesmus, and even blood passed.

Experiment IV. The natural heat of the vagina of a young ass was 100°. A solution of corrosive sublimate, as much as would dissolve in a teacup full of water, viz. about ten grains, was injected into the vagina. In about two hours after the mercury fell to 99°. Thursday morning, 99°; evening, 100°. Friday morning, 99°; evening, near to 101°. Saturday morning, 99°; evening, 100°. This experiment was repeated several times upon the same ass with the same result.

In these experiments it can hardly be said that the heat was increased. That the inflammation had been raised to a very considerable degree was plain, for it produced a discharge of matter which was often bloody, and upon killing the ass for another experiment, the following appearances were found in the uterus. The horns of the uterus were filled with serum, and the inflammation had run so high by the stimulating injections which were used for the experiments on the vagina, that the coagulating lymph had been thrown out so as almost to obliterate the vagina, uterus, etc. by those adhesions which are the ultimate effects of inflammation on secreting canals, while suppuration is the ultimate effect of inflammation on internal surfaces: there were no signs of inflammation on the external surface of the uterus, which is covered by the peritonæum.

It may just be remarked, that in most of those experiments the heat in the morning was a degree less than in the evening; and I may also remark, that this is commonly the case in the natural heat of the animal.

I wished to know whether such animals as have little or no power of varying their natural heat had a power of increasing their heat in consequence of injuries, for which purpose I opened into circumscribed cavities in frogs, toads, and snails, and at different periods, after the opening was made, the thermometer was introduced. As the heat of those animals is principally from the atmosphere, the external heat is to be connected with the experiments.

Experiments on cold-blooded Animals.

Nov. 27, 1788. A healthy toad and frog, after having the heat in the stomach ascertained, had openings made through the skin of the belly, large enough to admit a thermometer, and the orifice was kept open by a piece of sponge.

Atmosphere, 36°; stomach of both, 40°; underskin of the belly, 40°.

	Atm.	Frog. (Under the skin.)	Toad. (Under the skin.)	Stom.
Half an hour after the opening ..	35°	40°	40°	40°
Hour and a half	35	39	39	—
Two hours and a half	—	39	39	—

The abdomen was now opened, and a piece of sponge kept in the orifice.

	Atm.	Frog. (Abdomen.)	Toad. (Abdomen.)	Stom.
The heat	36°	40°	40°	40°
Hour and a half after opening	36	39	39	39
Four hours and a half	38	39	39	—

Part of the left oviduct protruded, of the natural colour and appearance.

	Atm.	Frog.	Toad.	Stom.
Nine hours after	38°	38°	38°	38°
Twenty-one hours and a half	35	35	35	35

The protruded oviduct was more vascular, and of a uniformly red appearance; it was returned into the belly and retained there.

	Atm.	Frog.	Toad.	Stom.
Twenty-four hours	32°	32°	32°	32°
Forty-six hours	34	34	34	34

The toad died, and the frog was become very weak and languid: part of the oviduct protruded, and had the small vessels loaded with blood. It lived one hundred and eighteen hours; that is, seventy-two longer than the toad, during which period its heat corresponded with the atmosphere. Upon examining the abdomen after death, there were no adhesions nor any appearances from inflammation, except on the protruded oviduct.

Some healthy shell-snails had openings made into the lungs, and their heat ascertained at the following times:

	Atm.	Snail.
The heat at the time	34°	38°
One hour and a half	32	32
Six hours and a half	32	35
Ten hours	31	36
Twenty-four hours	30	30

To ascertain the standard heat of a snail:

	Atm.	Snail.
A fresh lively snail had its heat in the lungs ..	30°	36°
Another	28	35
Another	30	37

Experiments to ascertain the heat of worms, leeches, and snails, when compared with the atmosphere, and the changes produced in their heat by inflammation.

Exp. I.	Heat of the air in the room	56°
	——— water in the room	57
	——— some earth-worms	58½
Exp. II.	Water as a standard	56¼
	Leeches in the same quantity	57
Exp. III.	Water as a standard	56
	Fresh egg	55
	Leeches alone	60
	Worms alone	57
	Air	54
	Worms .. } two hours after being wounded	58
	Leeches .. } two hours after being wounded	57
	Slugs .... } two hours after being wounded	58
	Air	55
	Worms .. } twenty-four hours after being wounded	55
	Leeches .. } twenty-four hours after being wounded	55
	Slugs .... } twenty-four hours after being wounded	55

They were all very weak and dying[a].

[a] [The production and phenomena of animal temperature have been referred to more specifically elsewhere. (I. 278, and IV. 131.) It only, therefore, becomes necessary to mention here the intimate association which exists in all instances between the calorific and respiratory functions, so that throughout the animal series the degree of temperature evolved is in accurate correspondence with the elaborateness of the respiratory apparatus and the perfection with which the chemical changes on the blood are accomplished, leaving no doubt in the mind as to the relation in which these functions stand to each other. If we adopt the view formerly suggested (see *note*, p. 94), of the absorption of oxygen into the blood, and its gradual conversion into carbonic acid in the course of the circulation, especially in the peripheral capillaries, it will not be difficult to explain the variations which sometimes occur in the local temperature, depending, as they would seem to do, on the varying afflux of blood to particular parts, or to the varying activity of the nutritive functions. That these circumstances, however, are greatly under the dominion of the nervous system, the observations and experiments of Brodie, Home, Earle, Wilson Philip, Mayo, Le Gallois, and others have incontestably proved (Phil. Trans., ci. 36, cii. 380, cxv. 7; Med. Chir. Trans., vii. 173; *Ann. de Chimie*, iv. (1817); and Wilson Philip, On the Vital Functions, 2nd edit., p. 168), although in no

§. 4. *Of the Production of Cold in Inflammation.*

The production of cold is certainly an operation which the more perfect animals are endowed with; and this power would appear to be both constitutional and local, similar to the power of producing heat. As the word inflammation implies heat, and has been used to express that action of the vessels where heat is commonly an effect, it may seem strange that we should treat of cold in the action of inflammation. But probably we have no action in the body that is not attended with an occasional production of cold. How far this takes place in parts I do not know; but that it takes place constitutionally, from almost every affection, is evident, whether it be inflammatory fever or local inflammation. As an animal has no standard of cold but at the source, which is also the standard of heat, it is perhaps impossible to ascertain with certainty the degree of cold produced either by disease or from the surrounding cold; but perhaps, by comparing the part suspected of being colder, than is natural, from disease, with a similar part under the same external influence of heat and cold, as, for instance, one limb with the other, or one hand with the other, a pretty fair inference may be made; and we often find that diseased parts shall become extremely cold, while from other circumstances than disease they should not be so.

I suspect that coldness in disease arises either from weakness, or a

---

other manner dependent than all the other functions of organic life. The observation of Hunter, that the generation of heat cannot essentially "depend upon the nervous system, for it is found in animals that have no brain or nerves," is still further corroborated by the fact that the same phenomenon is observed in vegetables, in which there is still less pretence or proof of a nervous system. Thus, during the germination of seeds, the temperature is elevated at least ten degrees. Hubert found that the thermometer was raised to 108° Fahrenheit when surrounded by the spadices of the *Arum cordifolium* during the process of fecundation, the temperature of the atmosphere being 70°; and Sennebier, that it was raised from 70° to 143° under the same circumstances. (Ellis on Respiration, p. 204.) The phenomena which appear most difficult to account for are the occasional exaltation of temperature in parts, beyond the standard heat of the body; especially where, as in fractures and injuries of the spine, the cause would appear not only inadequate to the effect, but to have a directly contrary tendency. In inflammation, on the contrary, the reparative and nutritive functions are in an undue state of activity, and therefore it is reasonable to suppose that the peculiar changes consequent on the circulation of the blood are carried on with greater vigour.

The author, it may be observed, accounts for the production of animal heat by referring to the vital principle, which, after all, throws no light upon the subject, nor gives any account of the immediate agency by which this is produced. That the stomach may often indirectly become the cause of the production of partial cold, is readily explained, when we consider the influence which it is admitted that the nervous system exercises over the function of calorification, and the power which the stomach has of affecting the former.]

feel or consciousness of weakness, in the whole constitution or a part, joined with a peculiar mode of action at the time. Thus we have many constitutional diseases beginning with absolute coldness, which seems afterwards to terminate in a sensitive coldness only, as the cold fit of an ague; for I apprehend that the sickness which generally precedes such complaints produces universal cold, and once having produced the action of the body arising from absolute cold, the action goes on for some time, although the cause no longer exists, which continues the sensation; and although the absolute coldness is gone, yet the action of the parts, which is a continuation of and therefore similar to the action of the absolute cold, is capable of destroying itself by producing the hot fit, if there be power or disposition.

That weakness, or a feel of weakness, produces cold is evident, and that universal or constitutional cold arises from the stomach is also evident; for whenever we are made sick an universal coldness takes place; and this is best proved by producing sickness on animals that we can kill, or that die while they are under these affections of the stomach. The experiments I made to ascertain this were not conducted with great accuracy, as I trusted in them entirely to my own sensations or feelings.

Experiment I. I threw three grains of tartar emetic into the veins of a healthy bitch, the quantity of water near an ounce. In about twenty minutes she had a stool and voided some single tape-worms. Some of the stools were extremely thin, and made up principally of bile. Some time after she had two more stools, which were thin and bilious. She continued pretty easy for about three hours, but became a little convulsed, which increased, and at last she became senseless, with little twitchings; hardly breathing, except with the diaphragm, and having a low slow pulse. She was very cold to our feel, when applying our hand on the skin of the body. In about ten or twelve hours after the injection she died.

Experiment II. I repeated the above experiment on another bitch, adding a full grain more to the medicine. She vomited in less than a minute after it was thrown in, and strained excessively hard, throwing up a great deal of froth, which was only the mucus of the stomach mixed up with the air in the act of retching. In less than three minutes she had a stool, which was pretty loose and partly of the natural appearance. She continued retching and purging for above an hour, and was extremely uneasy; at last she got into a dark corner and lay there, frothing at the mouth, was taken with convulsive twitchings like the former, and died in about five hours after the injection. I opened her body immediately after death, and found the intestines, liver, and heart not so warm as we usually find them.

I have known people who had affections of the stomach and bowels say that they had plainly the feeling of cold in their bellies. I knew a gentleman who told me that often when he threw the wind off his stomach it felt cold to his mouth and even to his hands, which was by much the best guide respecting sensation.

A lady, near seventy years of age, has a violent cough, which often makes her puke, and what comes off her stomach feels like ice to the mouth.

Affections of the mind also produce constitutional coldness; but they are such affections as the stomach sympathizes with, producing sickness, shuddering, &c. A disagreeable idea or sight will sometimes give a quick sensation of sickness, and the skin shall sympathize with the stomach. It shall appear to begin, as it were, in the mouth or throat, as if something there had a tendency to come up; the muscles of the neck shall become convulsed, and the head shall be violently shaken; from thence a disagreeable feeling shall spread over the whole body, passing directly down the back to the feet, commonly expressed by saying, "one's flesh creeps;" and hence the words shudder and horror express mental as well as bodily affections. Another action shall be joined with the cold, viz. the action of sweating, so that a cold sweat shall take place over the whole body. This cold shall be partial, for under many diseases a partial cold sweat will sometimes come on, while other parts remain tolerably temperate.

§. 5. *Of the time the Adhesive Inflammation commences after its cause; and in what cases and parts it is imperfect in its consequences.*

It will be often impossible to determine the distance of time between the impression which becomes the cause of inflammation and the action itself; which will depend upon two circumstances, viz. the nature of the exciting cause, and the susceptibility for such action in the parts.

In the exposure of internal surfaces, inflammation is perhaps sooner brought on than in most others; for the incitement is immediate, and there is no remission in the cause itself. In specific diseases the time is perhaps more regular, each having a determined interval between the application of the exciting cause and the appearance of the disease, although even in some of these there is a vast difference in the time after contamination; but in those arising spontaneously it must be uncertain. Yet in some cases it can be pretty well ascertained, supposing sensation the first effect of the inflammatory impression; and in such instances we often find it very rapid. They shall be attacked with a violent pain in the part, so much so as hardly to be able to bear it, which shall be immediately succeeded with a violent inflammation.

A lady was walking in her garden, and at once was attacked with a violent pain in the middle of the fore part of the thigh, which made her immediately lame. Soon after, the skin appeared discoloured, which spread nearly over one half of the thigh: this part became thick and swelled, which appeared to go as deep as the bone. It afterwards suppurated; all in a few days. This appeared to be a well-marked case.

The commencement of inflammation after accidents is more easily ascertained, for we must date it from the accident, and we find it is not immediate; for after a wound has been received, inflammation does not begin for twelve, eighteen, or twenty-four hours.

It sometimes happens, however, that the adhesive state cannot set bounds to itself, and therefore cannot set bounds to the suppurative. This may be owing to two causes: the one is the violence of the inflammation, and quickness of the attack of the suppurative spreading before parts have had a sufficient union, and even perhaps joined with a species of suppuration from the very first, so that union is prevented. Secondly, the inflammation may, I suspect, be of the erysipelatous kind, especially when there is a tendency, from the beginning, to mortification. This mixing of the suppurative with the adhesive, or the hurrying on of the suppurative, or this mixture of the erysipelatous with the others, I have frequently seen in the abdomen of women who have been attacked with the peritonæal inflammation after childbirth, and which from these circumstances became the cause of their death. In such cases we find matter mixed with coagulating lymph, as if formed with it; for without having been formed with it, it could not have mixed with it after coagulation. We find also coagulating lymph mixed with the matter, as it were, separated from the inflamed surface by the formation of the matter; and in those cases where there is a tendency to mortification from the beginning, as in strangulated ruptures, we often find the adhesive and suppurative inflammation going hand in hand. All of these causes and effects account for the violence of the symptoms, the quickness of the progress of the disease, and its fatal consequences, beyond such inflammations as have only the true adhesive progress, or where it takes place perfectly prior to suppuration.

It seems to appear, from observation, that some surfaces of the body do not so readily unite by the coagulating lymph as others, and therefore on such surfaces there is commonly a much larger quantity of this matter thrown out than probably would have been if union had readily taken place; for we may suppose that where once union has taken place extravasation is at an end. Thus we see in (what we may suppose) inflammation of the heart, that the coagulating lymph is thrown out on the exterior surface in vast quantities, while at the same time the heart shall not adhere to the pericardium. This is not only seen in the human subject, but in other animals: in an ox the heart was furred all over, and in some places the coagulating lymph was near an inch in thickness. The external surface of such hearts has an uncommon appearance: the outer surface of the coagulable lymph is extremely irregular, appearing very much like the external surface of a sponge, while the base or attachment to the heart is very solid and firm. However, in many instances we find the pericardium adhering to the heart, and generally in pretty close contact, which would make us suppose that the extent of motion of those two parts on one another is not great. These adhesions affect the pulse much, which is a good reason why nature avoids them as much as possible. On the other hand, it seems deducible from observation that neither the pia-mater nor dura-mater is apt to throw out much coagulating lymph, for here it would produce compression; and therefore we seldom find adhesions between them, in consequence of such accidents as produce suppuration between these two membranes: we seldom if ever find the surrounding parts adhering so as to confine the matter to the suppurating surface.

Inflammation of the skin, or such as approaches to the skin, produces in general a separation of the cuticle, often of the hair or the nails. These effects arise sooner or later, according to the nature and degree of the inflammation, but more particularly according to its nature; they take place the least and latest in the true adhesive inflammation, which is always attended with the greatest strength. In such cases the separation does not happen till the inflammation has subsided; and, as a proof of this, in the gout it is least and latest of all, for this is always a healthy inflammation, otherwise it would not take place; but in weak habits, at the early part of the disease, there are often vesications, which are filled with serum, sometimes with coagulating lymph, &c., both of which are sometimes tinged with red blood. When the inflammation is of a weak kind, tending to mortification, the cuticle commonly separates early during the time of inflammation, almost beginning with it, and of course the vesications will be filled with serum, and often with the red globules. We may observe in wounds of the skin which are not allowed to heal by the first intention, that a separation of the cuticle will take place at the edges of the wound, and this will extend according to the nature of the inflammation, which is according to the nature of the constitution. This will be attended with other concomitant appearances, such as flabby edges and thin matter. I conceive in the weak habit it depends on an action of the inflammation itself, but in the strong it depends on a state in which the parts are left to separate the cuticle.

This separation arises, I apprehend, from a degree of weakness approaching to a kind of death in the connexion between the cuticle and cutis, from life being in this part naturally very weak. In the beginning of mortification it is produced; in the œdematous and erysipelatous inflammations it is greatest, and in putrefaction of dead bodies it is the first operation. I suspect too that a blistering plaster, hot water, &c. only kill the uniting parts, by which means an irritation is produced in the cutis, and the extravasation is according to that irritation.

The connexion of the cuticle is more or less destroyed in every inflammation of the skin, for we seldom see an inflammation attack the skin but the cuticle comes off sooner or later. We generally observe it peeling off in flakes, after inflammation has subsided, and it begins nearest the point of inflammation*.

§. 6. *Of the Uniting Medium in Inflammations.*

Every new substance that is formed is either for a salutary purpose, or it is diseased. The first consists either of adhesions or granulations, whether with the first or second intention; and these may be considered as a revival of the natural principles, and powers of growth, whereas diseased substances are, as it were, monsters.

In the adhesive inflammation, the vessels being enlarged, as above described, similar to what they are in the young subject, begin to separate from the mass some portion of the coagulating lymph, with some serum, and also red globules, and throw it out on the internal surface, probably through the exhaling vessels, or perhaps open new ones, and cover the sides of those cells, which easily unite with the opposite, with which they are in contact, forming the first progress of adhesions. That this is really the case, and that this effect has taken place in consequence of inflammation, is evident from the following observations. In all large cavities where we can make our observations with certainty, when in the state of inflammation, we find diffused over the sides, or through

* It may be observed, that when an inflammation attacks the finger-ends or toes, so as to produce suppuration either in the substance of these parts, although not larger than a pimple, or only on the surface of the cutis, an extensive separation of the cuticle takes place, not entirely from the inflammation, but assisted by it. This is owing, principally, to the cuticle in such places not giving way, being there strong, so that a seeming abscess almost occupies the whole finger, &c. This should be opened early to prevent this separation as much as possible, or to prevent the separation from extending too far.

the cavity, a substance exactly similar to the coagulating lymph when separated from the serum and red blood, after common bleeding. That the blood, when thrown out of the circulation from an inflammatory state of the vessels, as well as the blood itself, unites parts together, is probably best seen in the inflammation of the larger cavities above mentioned. The following I shall give as an example, which I have often observed on the peritonæum of those who have died in consequence of inflammation of this membrane. The intestines are more or less united to one another, and, according to the stage of the inflammation, this union is stronger or weaker; in some it is so strong as to require some force to pull them asunder*; the smooth peritonæal coat is, as it were, lost, having become cellular, like cellular membrane. When the vessels of this part are injected, we shall find that in those parts where a separation has been made by laceration, previous to the injecting, the injection will appear on that surface like small spots or drops, which shows that the vessels had at least passed to the very surface of the intestines.

In parts where the union was preserved I have observed the three following facts. On separating the united parts I have observed in some places the vessels come to the surface of the intestines, and then terminate all at once. In other places I could observe the vessels passing from the intestine into the extravasated substance, and there ramifying, so that the vessel was plainly continued from the old into the new. In a vast number of instances I have observed, that in the substance of the extravasation there were a great number of spots of red blood in it, so that it looked mottled. The same appearance was very observable on the surface of separation, between the old substance and the new, a good deal like petechial spots. How this red blood got here is the thing to be considered, especially as a good deal was within the substance of the coagulum. Was it extravasated along with the coagulated lymph? In this case I should have rather supposed it would have been more diffused, and if not diffused, more attached to the intestine, and not in the centre of the coagulum; if it had been extravasation, one would have expected extravasation of injection, but we had none in any of these places; I have therefore suspected that parts have the power of making vessels and red blood independent of circulation. This appears to be evidently the case with the chick in the egg[a].

* Adhesions in consequence of inflammation become very soon strong, and are very soon elongated; probably as soon as they become organized they adapt themselves to their situation or the necessity. Thus the dog which had his belly opened to wound some lacteals, when killed on the ninth day, had his intestines connected by adhesion in several places, and those very firm and long.

[a] [See p. 67, and note, and also the note to the explanation of Plate XVI.]

I have observed, when I was treating of the blood, that it was capable of becoming vascular, when deposited either by accident, or for particular purposes; and I had reason to believe that a coagulum or coagulating lymph had a power of becoming vascular in itself when it could be supplied with blood, and mentioned the coagulum in a large artery as an instance. Likewise, when I was treating of union by the first intention, I explained the intercourse established by the uniting medium becoming vascular, and those vessels uniting across by a process called inosculation. The same reasoning is applicable to the union by means of the adhesive inflammation; for it is the blood in all cases that is to become vascular[a]; but this takes place sooner or latter, according to the apparent necessity. In some it becomes vascular immediately, in others very late, and indeed in some hardly ever, according to the degree of utility to arise from that change. Where it becomes vascular soonest, there the vessels are found also in greatest numbers, the two effects depending on the same principle.

Extravasation, whether of blood or only of lymph, becomes vascular almost immediately when thrown out into the cavity of the human uterus in the state of pregnancy. Here is an operation necessary to go on, which is more than the simple support of the extravasation itself; but when the extravasation is thrown out by accident, or for the purpose of producing adhesions, the immediate intent is answered without the vessels, and vascularity only becomes necessary afterwards; therefore vascularity in such cases is the second consideration, not the immediate one. But in the case of impregnation it must be immediate, for the simple extravasation would not answer the intention. This shows that this extravasation is very different from that of the menses.

The new vessels which are formed in the newly extravasated and uniting substance become of use, both during the state of adhesion and suppuration. In the first they serve to give powers of action to this new substance, which assists in preventing suppuration. In the second, where this cannot be done, they assist in forming a vascular basis for the granulations.

When we cut into inflamed parts after death we find them firm and solid, resembling the section of a lemon, or some œdematous tumour, where we know extravasation has taken place. This appearance arises from the cells in the cellular membrane, and other interstices of parts, being loaded with extravasated coagulating lymph; from this circumstance they are cemented together, and become impervious to air, not similar in these respects to common cellular membrane or natural parts.

---

[a] [See Note, p. 267.]

In many places where this extravasation has been in considerable quantities, it is formed in time into cellular membrane. I have observed that this mode of separation of the coagulating lymph is not peculiar to inflammation; it is separated in many diseases. It is thrown out to form tumours, etc. where inflammation does not seem to be a leading cause[a]; and we often find the adhesive stages, as it were, degenerate into, or terminate in the formation of a cyst, to contain the body that was the cause of the inflammation. Thus, a sac is formed for bullets, pieces of glass, etc.

It is unnecessary to instance every possible situation where adhesions could be produced; they can take place wherever there are two internal surfaces in contact, or that can be brought into contact. I cannot give a better instance of its utility in the animal œconomy than in the following experiment: I wished to know in wounds which penetrated into the chest (many of which I have seen in the army), where suppuration had come on the whole cavity of the chest, as well as on the surface of the lungs, and where the lungs collapsed, how parts were reinstated, or in what form they healed; whether the lungs, etc. lost their suppurating disposition, and dilated, so as to fill the chest again. To ascertain this as far as one well could, I made the following experiment on a dog.

October 1779 I made an opening between the ribs into the chest of a dog, and touched the edges of the wound all round with caustic, to prevent it from healing by the first intention, and then allowed the dog to do as he pleased. The air at first passed in and out of his chest by the wound. He ate, etc. for some days, but his appetite gradually began to fall off. He breathed with difficulty, which increased; he lay principally on that side which we find people do who have the lungs diseased on one side only or principally; and he died on the eleventh day after the opening. On opening the body I found the collapsed lungs passing directly across the chest, and attached to the inside of the wound all round, so that they excluded the cavity of the chest from all external communication. This circumstance, of the lungs falling across the chest, was owing to his having lain principally on that side, which I conceived to have been only accidental. The cavity of the chest all round was filled with air. That part of the external surface of the lungs which did not adhere, that is to say, the part opposite the upper surface of the diaphragm, and that part of the pleura which covered the ribs, were entirely free from inflammation or suppuration; this cavity, from these adhesions, being rendered a perfect cavity, shows that air, simply,

---

[a] [See I. 367, note.]

has no power to excite inflammation when the cavity is otherwise perfect, which the adhesions had effected; this shows also that adhesions of two surfaces round the exposed part exclude every part from the necessity of inflammation, as was explained when treating of inflammation.

From the connection between the living powers of the solids and the fluids, we can hardly suppose that such an uncommon action could take place in the vascular system without producing its effects upon the fluids; and therefore, from reasoning, we might suppose that the coagulating lymph undergoes some changes in its passage through the inflamed vessels, which obliges it to coagulate more immediately, or much sooner than it otherwise would*. For in those cases of inflamed arms, after bleeding, and in inflammations in consequence of other causes, we find that the cavities of the veins are in many places furred over, and in others [the sides] united by means of the coagulating lymph. Now if this coagulating lymph is similar in its production to that which we have been describing, it must have been thrown out from the vasa vasorum, these vessels having separated it and poured it into the cavity of the veins, and it must there have coagulated immediately; in this separation, therefore, from the blood, it must have undergone some change, arising from the actions of the vessels; for if this lymph was no more than the coagulating lymph with its common properties, or the properties common to that which is circulating in the same vein which receives it, it would in such cases only continue to throw in more coagulating lymph, in addition to what was circulating, and therefore, probably, it would be carried along with the blood to the heart, as a part of the common mass.

From this we should infer that this coagulating matter is not simply the coagulating lymph, such as it is when circulating, but somewhat different, from having undergone a change in its passage through the inflamed vessels, partaking of the disposition of those solids which are inflamed through which it passed. This process cannot therefore be supposed to be merely extravasation; for I conceive that an œdema would be a consequence of simple extravasation. But this may be taken up in another point of view, and upon the same principle. The inflamed vessels may give a disposition to the blood, as it is moving slowly along, to coagulate on its surface; and this is probably the more just idea of the two, as we find that the vessels, both veins and arteries, can give

* This is contrary to the disposition of inflammatory blood when taken out of the vessels and allowed to go through its spontaneous changes; from which it would appear that the general affection of the blood (which I would call sympathy of the coagulating lymph with the universal irritation,) is different from its affection or disposition when employed for the purposes of union.

this disposition, and to a very great extent[a]. We find in the beginning of mortification the blood coagulating in the vessels, so as to fill them up entirely; and this, preceding the mortification, seems to be for the purpose of securing the vessel before it is to give way. We therefore cannot doubt of a coagulating principle being given to the blood from the vessels; and, as a further proof of this, we may observe that the extravasated coagulating lymph, which produces either adhesions or forms tumours (which is often the case), is always of the nature of the diseased solids that produced it. If the case is venereal, the new substance is of the same nature: if cancerous, it is cancerous; for I find that it has, when absorbed, the power of contaminating, similar to matter or pus produced by the sores or ulcers of such diseases; the absorbent glands being often affected by the absorption of the coagulating matter of a scirrhous breast.

Whatever change the coagulating lymph has undergone in this operation of inflammation, it seems so far the same as to retain still the nature of the coagulating lymph, and to possess the living principle. This is most probably in a greater degree; and therefore the coagulating lymph is still better fitted to be formed into a part of the solids of the body, as will be taken notice of when we come to treat of the state of the blood in inflammation. But it is not absolutely necessary that the coagulating lymph should first undergo a change in the extravasated vessels before it can become a living solid, or unite living solids: for we find that common blood extravasated from a ruptured vessel is, perhaps, equally efficacious in this respect; therefore the red globules do not retard union, but they may promote it.

§. 7. *The state of the Blood and of the Pulse in Inflammation.*

From what has been said of the living power of the blood, I think we must allow that it will be commonly affected much in the same manner with the constitution, and that disease will have nearly the same effect upon it as it has on the body, because the same living principle runs through the whole. We find this to be nearly the case: for till a disease has affected the constitution, the blood continues the same as be-

[a] [We can have no difficulty in rejecting this opinion; especially as it is opposed to the author's own observations elsewhere (p. 254 *et passim*) as well as the whole analogies of the subject (p. 328 *note*). The reason for assigning a different cause for the obliteration of the cavities of blood-vessels, than that which is employed by Nature for the union of divided parts, derives no support from observation. The coagula which form in blood-vessels and aneurismal sacs is not found to form any vascular connexion with the containing parts.]

fore; but as the constitution becomes affected, the blood also becomes affected, and undergoes the same changes, which probably may be ascribed to contiguous sympathy between the vessels and the blood; and we shall find that the changes in the blood are often as much expressive of disease as any other part of the body. It is expressive of strong action as well as of weak action; but as it does not give sensation it cannot convey to the mind all the varieties of disease that may take place in it; yet I could conceive, if the blood was to be primarily affected, that an impression would be made upon the mind, from its affecting the vessels in which it moved. However, it is not always the case that the state of the blood and the other symptoms are expressive exactly of the same thing; the blood often expressing less, and often more. When the action of the solids is of the inflammatory kind, or, which perhaps is the same thing, when there is too great an action of the solids, the blood more readily admits of a separation of its visible parts, and the coagulating lymph coagulates more slowly, but becomes firmer when coagulated. This last circumstance, however, might be supposed not to be so clear, for its firmness may be owing to its want of the red particles, which certainly give the blood a brittleness in proportion to their quantity; but although this may have some effect, yet it is very little, for we find blood of loose texture in some inflammations when deprived of its red part. When blood has this disposition it is called sizy blood.

These changes in the nature of the blood depend so much upon the above-mentioned causes of inflammation, that it is impossible to say whether they do not constitute the first universal effect produced from the local inflammation, and whether the constitutional is an effect of this change in the blood. I knew a man who was stabbed in the loins, and, according to the consequent symptoms, was most probably wounded or hurt in some viscus within the abdomen. At first he had no symptoms, but simple pain in the part; I therefore only bled him, by way of precaution, and the blood was perfectly natural; in less than a quarter of an hour after, constitutional symptoms came on, such as rigor, sickness, &c., and on opening the same orifice, and taking away more blood, this second quantity had a very thick and strong buff upon it, having all the appearance of inflammatory blood. While this constitutional disposition lasted, which was some time, his blood continued the same, which was proved by the subsequent bleedings. The subsiding, however, of the red globules in the blood when in an inflamed state, although pretty frequent, is not always an attendant, or, in other words (and perhaps upon some other principle), the blood is not always attended with this appearance, when the visible symptoms are the same. A young woman was attacked with a violent cough, oppression in breathing, quick, full, and hard pulse. She was bled, which gave her ease; the blood was sizy; the symptoms again returned, and she was bled a second time, which also relieved her, and the blood was more sizy than before; so far all the symptoms agreed. The symptoms again recurred, and were more violent than before: she was bled a third time, and a third time relieved; but this blood was not in the least sizy, although it came from the vein very freely. Here then the blood, under the same disease, lost this disposition, although the symptoms remained the same.

As inflamed blood leaves a portion of the coagulating lymph free from the red globules at the top, and as that can be accounted for upon the principle of the coagulating lymph, in such cases, not coagulating so fast as when the blood has not this appearance, and as the coagulation hinders any comparative experiment respecting the weight of the red globules of each, I tried to see if they sunk in serum faster in the one kind of blood than in the other. I took the serum of inflammatory blood, with some of the red part, and also some serum of blood free from inflammation, with nearly the same quantity of the red part. They were put into phials of the same size; I shook them at the same time, then allowed them to stand quiet, and observed that the red globules subsided much faster in the inflammatory blood than in the other. To ascertain whether this arose from the red globules being heavier or the serum lighter, I poured off the serum from each, as free from red blood as possible; then put the red part of the one into the serum of the other, and shook them to mix them well; and, upon letting them stand quiet, the red globules appeared to fall equally fast. From these experiments it appears that the red part of inflammatory blood was heavier than that which was not so, and the serum was lighter, and the difference pretty nearly equal; for if we could suppose that the red globules were one tenth heavier, and the serum one tenth lighter, then the difference in the subsiding of the red globules of inflammatory blood in its own serum, to that which is not inflammatory, would be as one to five; and if they were to be changed, then they would be equal[a].

To see whether the blood from an inflamed part was different from that drawn from a part not inflamed, the following experiment was made:—A large leech was applied to an inflamed surface, and when it had sucked itself full, another leech was suffered to fill itself from the breast where no inflammation existed. They were both cut in two, and

[a] [This accords with the fact before mentioned of the proportion of fibrin in inflamed blood being increased at the expense of the albuminous parts of the serum. The results of ten experiments on inflamed blood gave the following average, viz. 4·2 fibrin, and 30·13 solid contents of the serum; the standard of health being respectively 2·8 and 42·2.—Thackrah, p. 212, and *notes* pp. 37, 39.]

the blood received into two teacups, kept moderately warm in a dish of warm water. Both of them coagulated without the serum separating; but the inflamed blood was evidently of a lighter colour than the blood from the uninflamed part, but neither had the appearance of a buffy coat.

Whether the disposition for inflammation, and the change produced in the blood, arise from a real increase of animal life, or whether it is only an increase of a disposition to act with the full powers which the machine is already in possession of, is not easily determined; but it appears to be certain that it is either the one or the other. There are some circumstances, however, that would incline us to suspect it to be the latter, because there is often inflammation when the powers of the machine are but weak, where it appears to be only an exertion of very weak powers, arising from some irritation produced; in such cases the blood will show signs of weakness although sizy. This appears to be equally the case in local inflammation, and inflammatory fevers, or in the symptomatic fever *. That it is an increase of the one or the other, and that the sensible effect produced arises from the action taking place, both in the solids and fluids, is proved by the method of treatment, which will be further illustrated in speaking of the mode of cure. On the other hand, where there is great debility in the solids, where the powers of preservation (the first animal powers) are weak, and therefore the action weak, and where of course the body must have a tendency to dissolution, there we find the very reverse of the former appearance in the blood: instead of separating distinctly, and coagulating firmly, we have the whole mass of blood keeping mixed, and hardly any coagulation, only becoming of a thicker consistence. This effect, or appearance, often takes place in those who die instantaneously. I suspect that in such cases the blood dies first, and also instantaneously.

In the commencement of most diseases, and even through the whole course of many, the situation of the blood appears to be an object with Nature. In some the blood forsakes the skin and extremities, and we

* On the other hand it would appear reasonable to suppose that there was really an increase of animal life, for women who are breeding, and are in perfect health, always have sizy blood; and this is most remarkably the case with all animals in similar situations. Now it would appear necessary for an animal, whenever put into a situation where greater powers are wanted, to have these powers increased. In a breeding woman there is a process going on, though natural yet uncommon, and which requires a greater exertion, or a greater quantity of powers than usual, and therefore we have them produced. This process of breeding, although in many of its symptoms it is similar to fever, is yet very different; for actual fever kept up for nine months would destroy the person, while, on the other hand, many are relieved by the process of breeding. If these observations are just, this blood should not be called inflammatory blood, but blood whose powers of life are increased.

may suppose the smaller vessels in general; for when we can observe internal parts, so we find it, such as the mouth in general, eyes, &c.; a general paleness takes place, which is best seen in the lips, and even a shrinking of the external visible parts takes place, especially the eyes, so that the person looks ill, and often looks as if dying. The pulse is at this time small, which shows that the whole arterial system is in action. This appears to arise from debility, or the want of powers in the constitution to be acted on by such a disposition at the time, so that the whole powers or materials of life are called into the vital parts or citadel, and the outworks are left to themselves. Such is the case with fainting, the cold fit of an ague, the cold fit or beginning of a fever, and the rigors or beginnings of exacerbations: it is also the case with the hectic.

In the commencement of diseases it does not appear to arise from real debility of constitution, but from the novelty of the action, and of course a debility in that action, and from that only; but in the hectic, where a real debility has taken place, those appearances are owing to that cause; however, even in the hectic, this debility is assisted by the unnaturalness of the action. In the first, where there are real powers, it would appear as if Nature was struggling with the new disposition, and it either becomes destroyed entirely or in part, and the blood is then determined to the skin, and we may suppose into the smaller vessels in general; then the pulse becomes full; the whole action now appears to be there [in the skin], and it becomes hot; when that action in the skin ceases a perspiration takes place, and nature seems in many cases to be at rest: in some disorders this cessation is perfect for a time, as in agues; sometimes wholly, as in slight colds; but often imperfectly, as in continued fevers, where the cessation appears only to arise from weariness, which prevents the continuance of the action, not from an alteration of the disposition. In other diseases the blood is thrown very early upon the exterior parts. The face shall look bloated, the eyes full, the skin red, dry, and hard to the touch. These symptoms, I suspect, belong more to fevers of the putrid kind, and have less connexion with surgery than the former.

The pulse is often as strong a sign of the state of the constitution as any other action that takes place in it, though it is not so always; but as the pulse has but one circumstance attending it that we can really measure, all the others being referable to the sensation or feeling of the person who is to judge of it, the true state of the pulse is not easily ascertained. The knowledge of the soft, the hard, and the thrilling, are such as can only be acquired with accuracy by the habit of feeling pulses in these different states, and by many is not to be attained, for simple sensation in the minds of any two men are seldom alike. Thus we find it happens with respect to music, for what would be disagreeable and not in harmony to one ear, which is nice and accustomed to the harmony of sounds, will not be so to another. The late Dr. Hunter was a striking instance of this, for though he was extremely accurate in most things, he could never feel that nice distinction in the pulse that many others did, and was ready to suspect more nicety of discrimination than can really be found. Frequency of pulsation in a given time is measurable by instruments; smartness or quickness in the stroke, with a pause, is measurable by the touch; but the nicer peculiarities in the pulse are only sensations in the mind. I think I have been certain of the pulse having a disagreeable jar in it when others did not perceive it, when they were only sensible of its frequency and strength; and it is perhaps this jar that is the specific distinction between constitutional disease, or irritation and health; frequency of pulsation may often arise from stimulus, but the stroke will then be soft; yet softness is not to be depended on as a mark of health; it is often a sign of dissolution; but then there must be other attending symptoms.

In the consideration of the peculiarities of the pulse it is always necessary to observe, that there are two powers acting to produce them, the heart and the arteries; that one part of the pulse belongs to the heart alone, another to the arteries alone, and the third is a compound of both; but the actions of the heart and arteries do not always correspond; the heart may be in a state of irritation, and act quickly in its systole, while the arteries may be acting slowly; for the heart is to be considered as a local part, while the vessels must be considered as universal, or even constitutional. The stroke (which is the pulse), with the number of them that are made in a given time, whence the pulse is commonly called quick or slow, their regularity and irregularity as to time, and the quickness of the stroke itself, belong to the heart. The quickness of the heart's action often takes place, although the pulsations are not frequent, which gives a kind of rest or halt to the artery or pulse, especially if the pulse be not frequent. The hardness, the vibratory thrill, the slowness of the systole, with the fulness and smallness of the pulse, belong to the arteries. As the pulse arises from the actions of the solids or machine, its state will be of course according to the nature of the machine at the time, and therefore is capable of being in one of these states,—natural or diseased.

In most diseases of the constitution, whether originating from it, or arising in consequence of diseases of parts, where the constitution becomes affected by sympathy, the pulse is altered from a natural to a diseased state, the degree of which will be regulated by those affections. This alteration is commonly so constant, and so regularly of the nature of the disease, that it is one of the first modes of intelligence we have recourse to in our inquiries into its nature; but alone it is not always a certain guide, for where there are peculiarities of constitution we find the pulse corresponding to those peculiarities, and perhaps in direct contradiction to the accustomed state of the local affection. The same parts, too, under disease, give very irregular or uncertain signs in the actions of the heart and vessels, such as diseases or injuries done to the brain.

The varieties which the pulse admits of are several. It is increased in its number of strokes, or it is diminished; it is regular or irregular, as to time, in its strokes; it is quick in its stroke or diastole, and slow in its systole; it is hard in its diastole, and it vibrates in its diastole. In most cases, probably, where the constitution is in a state of irritation, the pulse will be quick and frequent in its number of strokes in a given time, and the artery will become hard from a constant or spasmodic contraction of its muscular coats, so as to give the feel of hardness to the touch; besides which, the diastole of the artery is not regularly uniform and smooth, but proceeds by a vast number of stops or interruptions, which are so quick as to give the feel of a vibration, or what we would express by a thrill. The pulse, under such a disposition or mode of action, may be either full or small.

These two very opposite effects do not seem to arise from a difference in the quantity of blood, which might at first be supposed; I should rather suspect that they arise from a difference in the degrees of strength; which will be more or less, according to the nature of the parts inflamed, and the degree of irritability of the patient at the time. These give, more or less, an anti-diastolic disposition to the arteries; and while the arteries have the power of contraction, and are in a state of irritation, this effect will always take place. It is certain, at least, that the arteries do not commonly, in such a state of constitution, dilate so freely and so fully as at other times; and as this will vary very quickly (if the constitutional irritation varies quickly), it is more reasonable to suppose that it is an immediate effect of the arteries, than an increase and decrease of the quantity of blood.

If this be really the case, then we should naturally suppose that the motion of the blood in the arteries would be increased in proportion to their diminished size; except we should also suppose that the diastole, or the systole or contraction of the heart, is also diminished in the same proportion. The first of these, I think, may probably be the case, as we find that the blood forsakes the surface of the body in such a state of the constitution, as will hereafter be observed, and therefore must be collected in the larger veins about the heart. If the heart was to dilate [as usual] and throw out its whole contents at each systole, then the velocity of the blood in the arteries, under such a state of contraction of arteries, would be immense, and it might then be pushed into the smaller vessels on the surface of the body, which it certainly is not.

The quick, hard, and vibratory pulse is generally an attendant upon inflammations, and whether it be attended with fulness, or the contrary, depends a good deal upon the part that is inflamed, which either increases or decreases the irritability, which will be described in treating of the different parts inflamed.

In such a state of the constitution as produces such a pulse, the blood, which appears to be only a passive body, acted upon by the heart, so as to produce the diastole of the artery, and reacted on by the vessels, making the complete pulse, this blood, I say, is generally found in a different state from that where there are not these symptoms in the pulse; they, as it were, constantly attend each other, or are the reciprocal causes and effects of one another, as was taken notice of when I was speaking of the state of the blood in inflammation.

From the account I then gave of the state of the blood in inflammation, and have now given of the pulse, under the same action, it should naturally be expected that they should explain each other, which, for the most part, they certainly do; yet these appearances of the blood, and the kind of pulse, are every now and then appearing to be in opposition to each other in their common attending circumstances; but this cannot be known till the person is bled. When the pulse is quick and hard, with a kind of vibration in the action, we generally have sizy blood. This may arise from fever, or such inflammation, etc. as affects the constitution or vital parts, these being so diseased as to keep up a constitutional irritation, which will always be an attending symptom; but when we have neither a quick nor hard pulse, but both, perhaps, below par and rather small, with no visible fever nor inflammation, but probably some strong undetermined symptoms, such as pain, which is moveable, being sometimes in one place, sometimes in another, but at the same time seeming to impede no natural function, yet upon bleeding the blood shall be sizy, and the size shall have strong powers of contraction, so as to cup.

A gentleman was ill with a pain, chiefly in his right side, but upon the part being rubbed, or upon applications being made to it, the pain seemed to move to some other part, from which circumstance it was supposed to have connexion with the bowels: at other times he was tolerably well. His pulse was slow, small, and soft, and not at all, to the feel, like a pulse which required bleeding. He desired to be bled, and when bled the blood was extremely sizy, the size being strong, and contracting so much as to draw in the edges, forming the upper surface into a hollow or cup. His pulse became fuller, quicker, and harder; he was bled a second time; the blood was the same, and the above symptoms increased so much that I observed, immediately after the second bleeding, his pulse was quicker, harder, and fuller than it was just before the bleeding. That it might be quicker and fuller I could conceive, because I have often seen such effect from bleeding where there had been an oppressed and languid pulse; but I cannot say that I ever saw a case where the pulse became harder, and acquired the vibration, except when debility or languor was produced, and where the blood was weak in its powers of coagulation, being flat on the coagulated surface[a].

Another want of correspondence, or irregularity, takes place when a constitution sympathizes with a local inflammation. There are cases where the pulse becomes slow, and often irregular; such are mostly to be found in old people, when the constitution is affected either originally or sympathetically, and in such I suspect that a disposition for dissolution, and perhaps mortification, is much to be feared. A man, aged sixty-eight years, had an occasional inflammation in one of his legs, which often ulcerated, and which seemed to arise more from a defect in the constitution than to be simply local. In those indispositions his pulse seldom exceeded forty in the minute; and as he began to get better his pulse became more and more frequent.

The varieties of the pulse, arising from the seat of the inflammation and the nature of the part inflamed, will be explained when I treat on inflammations in different situations and parts.

§. 8. *The effects of Inflammation on the Constitution, according to the structure of parts, situation of similar structures, and whether vital or not vital.*

These circumstances make a very material difference in the effects on the constitution arising from local inflammation; for we shall find that the effects on the constitution are not simply as the quantity of inflammation, but according to the quantity and parts combined, (supposing constitutions to be equal,) which I shall now consider separately.

In common parts, as muscle, cellular membrane, skin, &c., the symptoms will be acute, the pulse strong and full, and the more so if it be felt near to the heart; but perhaps not so quick as when the part is far

---

[a] [See Vol. I. p. 537; and Dr. Marshall Hall, On the Effects of Loss of Blood, in Med.-Chir. Trans., vol. xvii.]

from it, since there will be less irritability. The stomach will sympathize less, and the blood will be pushed further into the smaller vessels. If the inflammation is in tendinous, ligamentous, or bony parts, the symptoms will be less acute, the stomach will sympathize more, the pulse will not be so full, but perhaps quicker, because there will be more irritability, and the blood will not be so much pushed into the smaller vessels, and therefore forsake the skin more.

It seems to be a material circumstance whether the inflammation is in the lower or upper extremity, that is, far from or near to the heart; for the symptoms are the more violent, the constitution is more affected, and the power of resolution seems to be less when the part inflamed is far from the source of the circulation than when near it, even when parts are similar both in texture and use. Whatever course the inflammation is to run, or in whatever way it is to terminate, it is done with more ease when near to the heart than when far off.

All the parts that may in one sense be called vital do not produce the same effects upon the constitution; and the difference seems to arise from the difference in their connexions with the stomach. It is to be observed that vital parts may be divided into two, one of which is in itself immediately connected with life, as the stomach; the other, where life only depends upon it in its action or use. The heart, lungs, and brain are only to be considered in this last light; and therefore they have a considerable sympathizing affection with the stomach: the symptoms are rather depressing, the pulse is quick and small, and the blood is not pushed into the smaller vessels.

If the heart or lungs are inflamed, either immediately, or affected secondarily as by sympathy, the disease has more violent effects upon the constitution than the same quantity of inflammation would have if it was not in a vital part, or was in one with which the vital parts did not sympathize; for if it is such as the vital parts sympathize with readily, then the sympathetic action of the vital parts will affect the constitution, as in an inflammation of the testicle.

In such cases the pulse is much quicker and smaller than when in a common part, as a muscle, cellular membrane, or skin; but not so much so as in the stomach, and the blood is more sizy. When the inflammation is in the heart only, its actions are extremely agitated and irregular. If in the lungs, singly, the heart in such cases would appear to sympathize, and not allow of a full or free diastole. The stomach does not in common sympathize in such cases, which is the reason perhaps of the inflammation not depressing; but it is to be observed that I make a material difference between the inflammation of the lungs, commonly called a pleurisy, and those diseases that begin slowly and spin out to great lengths, and which are truly scrofulous, producing the hectic, for in them we have the hectic pulse and not the inflammatory.

If the stomach is inflamed, the patient feels an oppression and dejection through all the stages of the inflammation; simple animal life seems to be hurt and lessened, just as sensation is lessened when the brain is injured; the pulse is generally low and quick, the pain is obtuse, strong, and oppressing, such as a patient can hardly bear[a].

If the intestines are much affected, the same symptoms take place, especially if the inflammation be in the upper part of the canal; but if it is the colon only which is affected the patient is more roused, and the pulse is fuller than when the stomach only is inflamed.

If it be the uterus, the pulse is extremely quick and low. If it be a testicle that is inflamed, the pain is depressing, the pulse is quick but not strong.

When the inflammation is either in the intestines, testicle, or uterus, the stomach generally sympathizes with them, which will produce or increase the symptoms peculiar to the stomach. In inflammation of the brain, I believe, the pulse varies more than in inflammations of any other part; and perhaps we are led to judge of inflammation there more from other symptoms than the pulse. I believe the pulse is sometimes quick, slow, depressed, full, &c., and which may accord with the other symptoms, such as delirium, stupor, &c.

It is to be observed, when the attack upon these organs (which are principally connected with life) proves fatal, that the effects of the inflammation upon the constitution run through all the stages with more rapidity than when it happens in other parts; so that at its very beginning it has the same effect upon the constitution which is only produced by the second stage of fatal inflammation in other parts. Debility begins very early, because the inflammation itself is interfering immediately with the actions of life; and also in such parts universal sympathy takes place more readily, because the connexion of these parts by sympathy is more immediate; and if the sympathy is similar to the action, then the whole is in some degree in the same action.

If the inflammation comes on in a part not very essential to life, and with such violence as to affect the actions of life or to produce universal sympathy, the pulse is fuller and stronger than common; the blood is pushed further into the extreme arteries than when the inflammation is in a vital part; the patient, after many occasional rigors, is at first rather roused, because the actions of the part are roused; and the effects

[a] [It may be asked, if inflammation consists of an increase of animal life, or of a disposition to act with all the powers of which the machine is possessed, how comes it to pass that inflammation of the stomach produces such depressing effects?]

in the constitution are such as do not impede any of the operations of the vital parts. It is allowed to proceed to greater lengths, or greater violence in itself, before the constitution becomes equally hurt by it; and the constitutional symptoms produced at last may be said to arise simply from the violence of the inflammation. But this will take place more or less according to circumstances: it will be according to the nature of the parts, whether active as muscles, or inactive as tendons; also according to the situation of the same kind of parts, as well as according to the nature of the constitution. If the constitution is strong and not irritable, the pulse will be as above; but if the constitution is extremely irritable and weak, as in many women who lead sedentary lives, the pulse may be quick, hard, and small at the commencement of the inflammation, similar to what happens in the inflammation of vital parts. The blood may be sizy, but will be loose and flat on the surface.

§. 9. *General Reflections on the Resolution of Inflammation.*

I now come to the most difficult part of the subject, for it is much more easy to describe actions than to assign motives[a]; and without being able to assign motives, it is impossible to know when or how we may or should check actions, or remove them. I have endeavoured to show that an animal body is susceptible of impression producing action; that the action, in quantity, is in the compound ratio of the impression, the susceptibility of the part, and the powers of action of the part or whole; and in quality that it is according to the nature of the impressing power and the parts affected. I have also endeavoured to show that impressions are capable of producing or increasing natural actions, and are then called stimuli; but that they are likewise capable of producing too much action, as well as depraved, unnatural, or what are commonly called diseased actions. The first of these I have mentioned by the general term, irritations; the depraved, &c. come in more properly in treating of peculiar or specific actions.

Since then an animal body can be made to increase its natural action, or to act improperly by impression, so we can see no reason, when it is acting too violently, why it should not be restrained by impression; or when acting improperly, in consequence of these impressions, why it should not be made to act properly again by the same mode, namely, by impressions.

---

[a] [By "motives" the author must here be understood to mean all the causes of inflammation, whether original or modifying.]

These modes of action we are first to understand, and then the power of correcting or counteracting those impressions, in order to diminish or prevent the action, so as to produce one that is healthy or natural. Besides, an injury which produces a new mode of action, and a disease, which is a new mode of action, often happen when the machine is in perfect health, and in such a state as is perfectly in harmony with that health; but which state is not suitable to disease. Therefore it is to be presumed the more perfect health the body enjoys the less it bears a change in its actions. Thus we know that strong health does not bear considerable injuries, such as accidents, operations, &c. A man in strong health, for instance, will not bear a compound fracture in the leg, or an amputation of the same, so well as a man accustomed to such diseases and reduced by them. We find, commonly, that our artificial mode of reduction is by far too quick, and is almost as much a violence on the constitution as the injury; when therefore considerable injuries or diseases commence, the constitution is to be brought to that state which accords best with that accident or disease [see p. 281.]. The knowledge of that state of the body at that time, as well as of the operations of the whole animal, or of its parts, when arising from a disturbed or deranged state, or a diseased disposition, are to be considered as the first steps towards a rational cure. But this alone is insufficient: the means of bringing the body to that state are also necessary, which will include the knowledge of certain causes and effects, acquired by experience, including the application of many substances, called medicines, which have the power of counteracting the action of disease; or of substances perfectly inefficient in themselves, but capable under certain circumstances of producing considerable effects, such as water when hot and cold, or a substance when it varies its form, as from fluidity to vapour. Of these virtues we know nothing definitely: all we know is, that some are capable of altering the mode of action, others of stimulating, many of counter-stimulating, some even of irritating, and others of quieting, so as to produce either a healthy disposition and action in a diseased part, or to change the disease to that action which accords with the medicine, or to quiet where there is too much action; and our reasoning goes no further than to make a proper application of those substances with these virtues.

The difficulty is to ascertain the connexion of substance and virtue, and to apply this in restraining or altering any diseased action; and as that cannot be demonstrated *à priori*, it reduces the practice of medicine to experiment, and this not built upon well-determined data, but upon experience, resulting from probable data.

This is not equally the case through the whole practice of medicine, for in many diseases we are much more certain of a cure than in others; but still, even in them, the certainty does not arise from reasoning upon any more fixed data than in others where the certainty of a cure is less, but it arises from a greater experience alone: it is still no more than inferring, that in what is now to be tried, there is a probable effect or good to arise in the experiment, from what has been found serviceable in similar cases. Diseases, however, of the same specific nature, not only vary in their visible symptoms or actions, but in many of those that are invisible, arising probably from peculiarities of constitution and causes, which will make the effects of applications vary probably almost in the same proportion; and as those varieties cannot be known, so as either to adapt the specific medicine to them, or to suit the disease to the medicine, it will then be only given upon a general principle, which of course may not correspond to the peculiarities. Even in well marked specific diseases, where there is a specific remedy, we find that there are often peculiarities which counteract the simple specific medicine. This we even see in poisons, which produce the simplest instances of specific disease, because the effects always depend on the same causes[a]. The peculiarities therefore in the disease must arise from a peculiarity in the constitution, and not from the cause of the disease.

The inflammation I have been treating of is the most simple of any, because it is the simple action of the parts unmixed with any specific quality, arising from causes of no specific kind, and attacking constitutions and parts not necessarily having any specific tendency. The cure therefore, or method of terminating the inflammation, which is called resolution, (in cases that will admit of it,) must also be very simple, if we knew it; and accordingly, when the cure of such is known, it lays the foundation of the general plan for the treatment of all inflammations of the same kind. But it very rarely happens that a constitution is perfectly free from a tendency to some disease*; we seldom therefore see simple salutary actions of parts tending to relieve themselves from a violence committed: some constitutions being so irritable that the inflammation has no disposition to terminate, and others so indolent that the inflammation passes into another species, as into scrofula; all of which will require very different treatment.

The same varieties take place in specific inflammations, as also in inflammations arising from poisons; for many will have the true inflammatory disposition joined with the specific. In such therefore the same

* Vide the varieties of the inflammation, in the Introduction.

---

[a] [The passage in the original text runs thus: "This we even see in poisons, the most simple specific of all, because its effect arises in all cases from one cause."]

plan is to be pursued, with the addition only of the specific treatment; but this must not be omitted, as the inflammation depends upon the specific disease. It is this critical knowledge which becomes the basis of practice, and it is this which requires the greatest sagacity; and I must own it requires more knowledge than comes to the share of most practitioners. As every inflammation has a cause, that cause should be removed before resolution can take place; for the animal œconomy having a disposition within itself to discontinue diseased action, that of course subsides upon the removal of the cause, and this disposition is so strong in some as to appear to act alone. That removing the cause is a mode of resolution is proved in the venereal bubo; for by taking off the venereal action with mercury, the inflammation subsides, if another mode of action does not arise*.

Inflammation, where it must suppurate, is most probably a restorative act, and cannot be resolved in those cases where restoration becomes necessary: as, for instance, in a wound that is kept exposed, the inflammatory act of restoration becomes or is rendered necessary, and it takes place; but bring those parts together, or let the blood coagulate and dry upon it, and it becomes unnecessary. I have already observed, when treating of the causes of inflammation, which might be called the spontaneous, that they probably arose from a state of parts in which they could not exist, similar to exposed surfaces, and therefore this act of restoration became necessary. If this be true, then probably by altering that state of parts, as we can [in the latter instances] by bringing the divided parts together, the inflammation would either not rise or immediately cease; but as we are not in all cases acquainted with the mode of restoring those natural actions, we are obliged to be restricted to those methods that render them easier under this state, and which are often capable of turning the balance in favour of resolution.

As inflamed parts are not always visible, it becomes necessary that we should have some rule to inform us whether the part is inflamed or not; to ascertain which we must have recourse to all the symptoms formerly mentioned, except the visible ones. We ought also to have a guide respecting the kind of inflammation, more especially as it is not sufficient, in many cases, to be guided entirely by its appearances, even where it is in sight. It is often therefore very necessary to inquire into the cause of the inflammation, the nature of the constitution, the effects that former inflammation has produced, and even into the temper and mind of the patient.

The cure of inflammation is resolution, and the attempt towards it is principally to be made when the inflammation is in the adhesive state; for we find that often it goes no further, but subsides, and this is reso-

* Vide Treatise on Venereal Disease, Vol. II.

lution. Probably the sooner [the attempt is made] after its commencement the better it is. The object of the attempt is to prevent suppuration taking place, although suppuration may be considered as a resolution; but it is the mode of resolution we commonly wish to avoid. Resolution is in general only to be attempted, with any probability of success, under the following circumstances, viz. first, when the inflammation is in consequence of the constitution, or a disease of the part; secondly, in cases of accident, where there is either no exposure, or where it has been removed in time, as, for example, by bringing the parts in contact; thirdly, where the life of the part has not been destroyed. In all such cases we find that resolution can take place; but in those cases arising from accident and a continuance of exposure joined, or where death of the parts is produced by the accident, it becomes impossible to hinder the suppuration from taking place.

I have already observed, that in many bruises, as well as simple fractures, where the cavities are not exposed, and where they are to heal by the first and second intention, the inflammation, in most of these cases, is capable of being resolved, although in some such cases the inflammation runs so high as to threaten suppuration. I have also already shown that, in parts which have been divided and exposed, the inflammation is, in a great measure, prevented by bringing them together; or, if it has taken place previous to the union, that the same operation of union is sufficient to produce resolution; and I have likewise shown, that where parts were not brought together, Nature attempted to prevent inflammation by covering the wound with blood and forming an eschar, which in many cases will either prevent or remove inflammation: all of which shows a power of resolution even in cases where the parts have been exposed.

As it is commonly supposed that there are a great many local diseases that should not be resolved, the first thing necessary to be considered is when the resolution should or should not be attempted. On the contrary, there are cases where inflammation is to be excited; but these arise commonly from disease, which is not to our present purpose. Yet it sometimes happens in accidents, where inflammation is necessary, that it is not sufficient for the reinstatement of the injured parts, as in some simple fractures, where the first bond of union, the extravasated blood, had not fulfilled its purpose, and had been absorbed, and where the inflammation was too slight to supply its place; so that the union of parts being prevented, another mode became necessary, not at all a consequence of inflammation, viz. by granulations without suppuration[a];

---

[a] [See Vol. I. p. 427.]

all of which retard still more the restoration of the parts. As this defect can only be known in bone, and in the soft union of the bone, which is similar to the union in the soft parts, it is reasonable to suppose it may also take place in the soft parts, more especially those which are tendinous or ligamentous, where we find recovery very slow, for the soft union in bones differs in nothing from that of the soft parts; it may therefore be a much more common defect than is generally imagined. In such cases, if it could be known, it would be proper to encourage or even excite inflammation. If we cannot probably in any case determine where it should be excited, nor even where it should be checked, yet we can say in many cases where it is unnecessary to check it.

Before we attempt to check inflammation, we should have reason to suppose it is going further than is necessary for the natural cure, and that it is therefore laying the foundation of work for the surgeon. It may be very difficult to say, in many cases, when it should be checked. The most simple reason will be to lessen pain, arising in a part not merely when moved or touched, but from the act of inflammation. Secondly, where it may be uniting parts, the union of which we wish to avoid; but this is an uncertain guide, even if we knew adhesions were taking place, for adhesions often prevent suppuration. Thirdly, to prevent the inflammation from suppurating; and in this last, although the most obvious, yet there is less certainty how far we may advise the attempt. It is also the most difficult to effect; for in many cases of spontaneous inflammation, if it arises from a state under which the parts cannot exist nor their functions go on, similar to an exposed breach in the solids, then resolution should not be attempted. It may be palliated when going beyond what is necessary for suppuration; but when this practice is carried further, it rather retards that salutary process. From the foregoing statement of particulars it must appear that in many cases it is unnecessary to check inflammation, in others it would be wrong, and in many very necessary; and probably the best guide is its going further than appears, from the [nature of the] cause, to be salutary. Yet in practice we find applications, and other modes of resolution, immediately had recourse to, which must be considered as opprobrious to surgery.

Inflammations, in consequence of accidents, ought in general to be resolved, if possible. It is perhaps impossible to produce a single instance where a contrary practice would be preferable, except as above related, where its consequence would be to answer some great purpose; and it is also conceivable that this local disease, produced by accident, might relieve the constitution from some prior disorders, similar to what is understood to be the effects of an issue. Mr. Foote was relieved of head-ache, of long standing, by the loss of a leg, which may be considered as a proof of this; but he afterwards died of a complaint in his head, very similar to an apoplexy. It might be supposed, on the other hand, that the temporary cure was the cause of the apoplexy.

Inflammation, in consequence only of a disease in a part, appears to be under the same circumstances with respect to resolution; but an inflammation arising from a preceding indisposition in the constitution (commonly called critical) has always been classed among those which should not be cured locally, and this has got the term of repulsion: it has been insisted on that the inflammation should rather be encouraged, and suppuration produced, if possible. If the inflammation is really a concentration of the constitutional complaint, and that by not allowing it to rest here, the same disposition is really diffused over the whole animal again, and at liberty to fix on some other part, it certainly would be better to encourage its stay; but in such cases it is always to be understood that the inflammation is in such parts as will readily admit of a cure when suppuration takes place; for if the disease be otherwise situated, then the cure of the constitution by suppuration will be a mode of cure which will reflect back another disease upon it, under which it will sink: resolution of inflammation, therefore, in the first of these situations, should if possible be brought about. For instance, many deep-seated inflammations, if allowed to suppurate, would of themselves most certainly kill. This might be illustrated by the gout, when either in the head or stomach, for when in such parts it had better be repelled, and left to find another part less connected with life, which, if in the feet, would be called repelling of it; but still it does not appear to me necessary that it should suppurate, for suppuration is only a consequence of the inflammation, and not an immediate consequence of the original or constitutional disease, but a secondary one*: as suppuration, therefore, is only a thing superadded, and as we shall find that inflammation generally subsides when suppuration comes on, I see no reason why inflammation, in the present case, should not as well subside by resolution as by suppuration: however, it may be supposed that although suppuration is not the natural or immediate effect of the disease, yet as it is a continued local action, and the thing sought for by the constitution,

* This is contrary to the common received opinion, but it is according to my idea of suppuration; for I have all along considered inflammation as the disease, and suppuration only as a consequence of that disease, and have supposed the disease to be gone when suppuration has taken place; but, according to the common opinion, suppuration was the thing to be wished for, because all diseases arose from humours; but as we have not once mentioned humours, and therefore made it no part of our system, we must also drop it at present.

and as inflammation must precede it, the parts must submit to those regular processes, for it must be supposed to be capable of diverting the disease to this part.

§. 10. *Of the Methods of Resolution by constitutional means.*

The first thing to be considered is the kind of inflammation, when visible, which will in some degree show the kind of constitution; the next is the nature of the part inflamed, and the stage of inflammation; for upon these depend in some measure the method of relief. In cases of exposed internal surfaces the inflammation cannot be resolved, because the cause still exists till inflammation has resolved itself; but it may be lessened, and this probably takes place by lessening everything which has a tendency to keep it up; and in all likelihood little more can be done in spontaneous inflammations; for as yet we know of no method which will entirely quiet or remove the inflammatory disposition or mode of action, as there is no inflammatory specific with which we are acquainted.

When I described inflammation I observed there was either an increase of life, or an increased disposition to use with more violence the life which the machine or the part was in possession of; and also there was an increased size of vessels, and of course an increased circulation in the part inflamed, and in the constitution in general. If this theory of the mode of action of the vessels in inflammation is just, then our practice is reducible to two principles, one consisting in removing the cause of that action, the other in counteracting the effect. As to the first, as we seldom know the cause, but only see the effect, except in some specific diseases, for which we have a specific remedy, we do not know with any degree of certainty how to act; but as to the second, that is, the effect, as it is more an object of our senses, we can apply with more certainty our reasoning upon it, for reasoning from analogy will assist us in our attempts. We find, from common observation, that many circumstances in life, as also many applications to parts, will call forth the contraction of the vessels; we are, therefore, from the above theory, to apply such means: and whatever will do this, without irritation, will so far counteract the effect*.

I have already observed, that wherever there has been a violence committed, or some violent action is going on, there is a greater influx

* As this is a new theory of the action of the vessels in inflammation, and the only one that can possibly direct to a method of cure, it is to be hoped that attention will be paid to it, and, if just, that more certain methods of resolution will be discovered.

of blood to that part. Lessening, therefore, that influx, becomes one mode of relief, for as the vessels dilate, they should not be encouraged in that action. Although the increased influx is to be considered chiefly as an effect, yet it is to be considered as a secondary cause[a]; and from our ignorance of the immediate cause, it is probably only through such secondary causes that we can produce any effect; and upon these principles most likely rests, in some measure, the method of resolution, for whatever will lessen the power and disposition will also lessen the effect, and possibly these will likewise lessen the force of the circulation.

If the inflammation is attended with considerable action and power, as it were, increasing itself, then the modes of resolution are to be put in practice; the one by producing a contraction of the vessels, the other by soothing or lessening irritability, or the action of dilatation[b].

The first, or contraction of the vessels, is produced in two ways; one by producing weakness, for weakness excites the action of contraction of the vessels; the other, by such applications as induce the vessels to contract.

1st. The means of producing absolute weakness are bleeding and purging; but the bleeding also produces irritability for a time, and is often attended by a temporary weakness of another kind, viz. sickness. The inconvenience, however, arising from this practice is, that the sound parts must nearly, in the same proportion, suffer with the inflamed, for by bringing the inflamed part upon a par with health, the sound parts must be brought much lower, so as to be too low. 2nd. The soothing may be produced by sedatives, relaxants, anti-stimulants, etc., such as many sudorifics, anodynes, etc.

The first method will have the greatest, the most permanent, and the most lasting effect, because, if it has any effect at all, the diseased action cannot be soon renewed. The second will act as an auxiliary, for so far as irritation is a cause this will also lessen it, and the two should go hand in hand; for wherever we lessen power, we should at the same time lessen the disposition for action, or else we may increase the disposition; but neither bleeding, purging, nor sickness can possibly lessen the original inflammatory disposition [Vol. I. 301.], for none of them

---

[a] [This is consistent with Mr. Hunter's language elsewhere, where he says that he "could conceive a part to inflame, or be in a state of inflammation, although no blood were to pass" (p. 325); but it is difficult to imagine the popriety of calling that a cause which is the essential part of the thing intended. Inflammation could not exist, or certainly could not be defined, without taking into account the augmented influx of blood.]

[b] [The reader will observe that an hypothesis is involved in this expression which does not appear to be supported by any substantial facts. That vessels presumed to be contractile should yet *actively* dilate under increased action, seems not only to imply a contradiction in terms, but to be wholly unsupported by any other consideration.]

will resolve a venereal inflammation when mercury will; nor will they resolve the erysipelatous inflammation, although that inflammation has the very action for which we should bleed in the common inflammation, viz. dilatation of vessels. However, these means may, in some sense, be reckoned direct, for whatever will produce the action of contraction in the vessels is counteracting the action of dilatation. Lessening the power of action belonging to any disposition can only lessen or protract the effects, which, however, will be of singular service, as less mischief will be done, and it will often give the disposition time to wear itself out. Means employed on this principle should be such as give the feel of weakness to the constitution, which will affect the part, and will make the vessels contract; but this practice should not be carried so far as to produce the sense of too much weakness, for then the heart acts with great force, and the arteries dilate.

Bleeding then, as a general principle, is to be put in practice, but this must be done with judgment, for I conceive the effects of bleeding to be very extensive. Besides, the loss of any quantity of blood being universally felt, in proportion to the quantity lost, a universal alarm is excited, and a greater contraction of the vessels ensues, than simply in proportion to this quantity, in consequence, as it would appear, of a sympathetic affection with the part bleeding[a].

Too much blood in an inflammation is a load upon the actions of the circulation. Too little produces debility and irritability, because there is a loss of powers, with an increased action to keep up, which is now not supported. It would seem that violent actions of a strong arterial system required less blood than even the natural actions, and even less still than a weak or irritable system; from whence we must see that bleeding can either relieve inflammatory action or increase it, and therefore is not to be used at random.

As many patients that seem to require bleeding have been already bled, it may not be improper to inquire how they bear, or are affected by bleeding, for certainly all constitutions (independently of every other circumstance,) do not bear this evacuation equally, and it is probable that its effects on inflammation may be nearly in the same proportion; if so, it becomes a very useful caution; for although the loss of blood may, as a general principle, be set down as a weakener, and probably

---

[a] [This effect is with more probability to be ascribed to the approach of the state of syncope, which state, it may be observed, is often signally beneficial in the incipient stages of inflammation; not merely by its tendency "to lessen and protract the effects," but by cutting short and at once removing the diseased action. The dangers or ill effects of blood-letting lie principally on the side of delay and too frequent repetition, and less in having vigorous recourse to this remedy in the first instance.]

the greatest, as we can kill by such means, yet the loss of certain quantities in many constitutions is necessary for health: this is either when there is a disposition to make too much blood, or a constitution that cannot bear the usual quantity; in such, when known, bleeding with freedom is certainly necessary. If the inflammation is known to be attended with real powers bleeding is absolutely necessary, in such quantity as to take off from the force of the circulation, which arises from too much blood; or if that is not sufficient, then as much as will cause a contraction of the vessels; but in cases of too great an action of weak parts, then the proper quantity to be taken is no more than may assist the dilatation of the vessels, which will lessen the violence of motion in the blood, or remove the sensation in the part inflamed, of having too much to do[a]: the quantity, therefore, must be regulated according to the symptoms and other circumstances; for instance, according to the visible indications.

We are to remark here, that every part of the body under inflammation will not bear bleeding alike. I believe that the constitution bears bleeding best when the inflammation is in parts not vital, and those near the source of the circulation: whatever disturbs some of the vital parts, depresses, but not equally in all; and in them it becomes more necessary to be particular; for in accidents of the brain, bleeding freely, even so as to produce sickness and fainting, is necessary. It is probable that the sickness attending such accidents is designed to lessen the influx to the head, and occasion the vessels of the brain to contract.

The indications for bleeding are, first, according to the violence of the inflammation, joined with the strength of the constitution, which will in general point out the kind of inflammation. Secondly, according to the disposition to form much blood; thirdly, according to the nature of the part, whether vital or not; fourthly, according to its situation, in point of distance from the heart; fifthly, according to the effect of the inflammation on the constitution[b]

With regard to this evacuation, it is worthy of particular consideration, whether or not, in all cases where it can be put in practice, bleeding in or near the part will answer better than taking the blood from the general habit, for certainly less may be removed in this way, so as to have equal effect upon the part inflamed (and probably upon every other disease that is relieved by bleeding), and yet affect the constitution less;

---

[a] [These modes of expression, which are evidently unphilosophical, have been already noticed. (See CONSCIOUSNESS in the Index.) For the word "assist" in this paragraph, I should apprehend we ought to read *relieve*.]

[b] [See Note, Vol. I. p. 402.]

for although in many cases the general habit may be relieved by bleeding, yet the part affected, where it can act, will in all cases require this evacuation most, and local bleeding will keep nearer these proportions; whereas taking blood from the general system is just the reverse. That local bleeding has very considerable effects on the inflamed part, is proved by the gout; for applying leeches to the part inflamed commonly relieves that part, and often almost immediately*. We find that bleeding by leeches alone will remove a tumour in the breast, having all the appearances of a scirrhus, which cannot be considered as inflammatory; its powers, therefore, extend beyond inflammation. We find relief by bleeding in the temporal artery or jugular vein, for complaints in the brain; or cupping and bleeding with leeches on or near the part, as applying leeches to the temples, in inflammations of the eye.

I have observed that there is something similar to sympathetic affection in bleeding. I conceive that all the sympathetic powers, the universal, continued, and contiguous, may be brought into action from the local influence of bleeding. Thus, bleeding in the part inflamed, I can conceive, does more than simply empty the vessels mechanically, for that would be soon restored from the general circulation; but it acts by continued sympathy, viz. the vessels of the part being opened, they contract for their own defence, and this is carried further along the vessels of the part; so that bleeding from the part acts in two ways, viz. mechanically, by relieving the vessels of some blood, so as to allow them to contract in proportion as the load is taken off; and also by exciting them to contraction, in order to prevent the effusion of blood. I suppose, likewise, that contiguous sympathy comes into action, for this would appear from practice and observation to be a principle in bleeding; therefore, in inflammation of contiguous parts, it is proper to bleed from the skin opposite to them, as from the skin of the abdomen in complaints of the liver, stomach, and bowels; and likewise from the loins in inflammatory affections of the kidneys. In affections of the lungs bleeding opposite to them is of service; but in such cases it is not clear where the inflammation is, for if in the pleura, then it does not act upon this principle, but by continued sympathy: bleeding on the scalp relieves head-aches; and the relief given to the testicle by bleeding from the scrotum, in inflammation of that body, proves the principle.

Where the first indication for bleeding takes place, viz. where there is violent inflammation, with strength of constitution, bleeding freely will be of singular service. The same mode of practice is also to be followed under the circumstance of strength, with respect to the second, third, fourth, and fifth; but each will not require the same quantity to

* It is not meant here to recommend bleeding in this disease.

be taken under equal strength of constitution, as will be taken notice of when treating of them separately. As it seldom happens that bleeding once will be sufficient in a considerable inflammation, the first, or preceding blood taken becomes a symptom of the disease. If the coagulating lymph is long in coagulating, so that the globules have time to subside, there will be what is called a thick buff; and if its surface is considerably cupped, then future bleedings may be used with less caution; because such appearance indicates strong powers of coagulation, which always shows strength in the solids; but if the blood is weak in its powers of coagulation, and lies flat in the dish, then we must be cautious in our future bleedings; or if it was strong at first in its powers of coagulation, and after repeated bleedings becomes weak, then we must not pursue this further; but in some cases it is proper to pursue it to this point, for we shall sometimes find that the inflammatory symptoms shall not cease after repeated bleedings, if the strength continues; but the moment a degree of looseness is produced in the blood, that moment will the inflammatory action cease. The following case is a strong instance of this:

A lady had a violent cough, tightness in respiration, loss of appetite, strong sizy blood, and the symptoms continued to the sixth bleeding, when the blood was not quite so sizy; but the most remarkable change was its remaining flat on the surface. Upon this bleeding all the symptoms disappeared; and here, although the blood became weak in its power of coagulation, yet it did not produce irritability in the constitution, the vessels of the inflamed parts having still had power to contract. On the other hand, there may be indications for bleeding sparingly; first, when there is too much action, with weakened powers; secondly, when there is a disposition to form but little blood; thirdly, when the part affected is far from the source of the circulation.

From the above three dispositions that require bleeding sparingly, or with caution, I may observe that it will most probably be proper in all such cases to bleed from, or as near the part affected as possible, in order to have the greatest effect, with the loss of the least quantity of blood; more so than when the constitution is strong; because the constitution in such cases should feel the loss of blood as little as possible. If from the part, leeches will answer best, because commonly little irritation follows the wound of a leech*: however, this can only be put in prac-

* However this is not always the case, for it sometimes happens that an unkindly inflammation attends the wound, though not extensive. It sometimes also happens that the lymphatic glands swell in consequence of their bite; but these so rarely occur, and are of such little consequence when they do, that they are not to be regarded. From hence it has been conceived that there is something poisonous in the bite of a leech,

tice in inflammations not very remote from the surface. But in many cases the blood cannot be taken away from the part itself, but only from some neighbouring part, so as to affect the part inflamed: thus, we bleed in the temporal artery for inflammation of the eyes; we bleed in the jugular veins for inflammation of the brain; and also in the temporal artery to lessen the column of blood going to the brain, by the internal carotids. But in many situations it will probably be impossible to do this with any hopes of success, and therefore we may have recourse to the sympathetic affections before described.

Too much action with small powers may often, if not always, be classed with the irritable constitution, and bleeding should then be performed with very great caution: one case out of many I shall relate as an instance of great action with debility.

A gentleman had one of the most violent inflammations I ever saw in one of his eyes, attended with violent pain in his head and the blood extremely sizy, all of which denotes great action of parts: yet the buff of the blood was so loose when coagulated that it could hardly bear its own weight, or make any resistance to the finger when pressed; and although he was bled pretty freely, yet he never found any relief from it. This blood becoming a symptom, both of the constitution and disease, manifestly showed weak powers from its looseness, and too great action from its slowness of coagulation, which was the cause of the buff. The following case is another strong instance of great action in a weak irritable habit.

A lady had a violent inflammation at the root of the tongue, so as to form a considerable suppuration, with a pulse of 120, 125, and often 130 in a minute. Her blood was extremely sizy, yet she received but little benefit from the first bleeding, although the blood coagulated pretty firmly, which indicated strength. She was of an irritable constitution, so as to receive less benefit from bleeding than another; and when bled three times, the blood became extremely loose in its texture, which bark removed, as well as the other symptoms. Upon leaving off the bark the symptoms all recurred, and when she was bled again for the second attack, which was the fourth time, the blood, although inflammatory, had recovered a good deal of its proper firmness; but in the second bleeding for this second attack it was less so; and in the third it was still less. Suspecting that bleeding in the present case would not produce resolution, I paid particular attention to the pulse at the time of bleed-

but I think there are no proofs of it: however, from another effect, I conceive there is a power or property applied to the wound, which hinders the irritation of contraction that naturally takes place in a wounded vessel, producing, probably, a paralysis for a time.

ing, and found that in this last bleeding the pulse increased in its frequency even in the time of bleeding; and within a few minutes after the bleeding was over, it had increased ten strokes in the minute*. These bleedings retarded suppuration, but by producing irritability they could not effect resolution.

Where there is a disposition to form but little blood (when known), bleeding should be performed with great caution.

When the inflammation is far from the source of the circulation the same precautions are necessary. In general it can be taken away from the part in such cases. But these are only so many facts, that require peculiar symptoms to ascertain them.

The common indications of bleeding, besides inflammation, are too often very little to be relied upon, and I shall consider them no further than as it concerns inflammation, which will indeed throw light on other cases. The pulse is the great indication in inflammation, but not always to be depended upon.

In inflammations that are visible a knowledge of the kind of inflammation is in some degree ascertained, as has been observed; we therefore go upon surer ground in our indications for bleeding. But all inflammations are not visible; and it is therefore necessary to have some other criterion. However, if we could ascertain the pulse peculiar to such and such appearances in visible inflammation, and that was universally the same in all such appearances, we might then suppose that we had got a true indicative criterion for our guide, and therefore apply it to invisible inflammations, so as to judge of the kind by the state of the pulse. But when we consider that the same kind of inflammation in every part of the body will not produce the same kind of pulse, but very different kinds, not according to the inflammation, but according to the nature of the parts inflamed, and those other parts also not visible, we lose at once the criterion of the pulse as a guide. When we consider also that there shall be every other sign or symptom of inflammation in some viscus, and from the symptoms the viscus shall be well ascertained, yet the pulse shall be soft and of the common frequency; and upon bleeding, in consequence of these inflammatory symptoms, the blood shall correspond exactly with all of them, except the pulse, it shall be sizy, firm, and cupped, as was the case in the lady, which has been before described, we shall be still further convinced that the pulse is a very inadequate criterion. If a pulse be hard, pretty full, and quick,

* This, of the pulse increasing upon bleeding, is not always to be set down as a sure sign of irritation being an effect; for in a sluggish pulse, arising from too much blood, the increase of stroke, and freedom given to the circulation is salutary; but when a pulse is already quick, an increase must arise from irritation.

bleeding appears to be the immediate remedy, for hardness rather shows strong contractile action of the vessels not in a state of inflammation, which also implies strong action of the blood, and from such a pulse a sizy blood will generally be found. But even a quick hard pulse and sizy blood are not always to be depended upon as sure indications of bleeding being the proper method of the resolution of inflammations: more must be taken into the account.

The kind of blood is of great consequence to be known; for although it should prove sizy, yet if it lies squat in the bason, and is not firm in texture, and if the symptoms at the same time are very violent, bleeding must be performed very sparingly, if at all; for I suspect that under such a state of blood, if the symptoms continue, bleeding is not the proper mode of treatment. The cases of this kind which have been related are strong proofs of this.

As the pulse, abstracted from all other considerations, is not an absolute criterion to go by, and as sizy blood and a strong coagulum are after-proofs, let us see if there are any collateral circumstances that can throw some light on this subject, so as to allow us to judge *à priori* whether it be right to bleed or not, where the pulse does not of itself indicate it. Let us remember that in treating of inflammation of different parts I took notice of the pulse peculiar to each part, which I may now be allowed to repeat. First, I observed that an inflammation in parts not vital, or such as the stomach did not sympathize with, if there were great powers and the constitution not very irritable, the pulse was full, frequent, and hard. Secondly, that on the contrary, in inflammations of the same parts, if the constitution was weak, irritable, &c., that then the pulse was small, frequent, and hard, although perhaps not so much so as when in vital parts. Thirdly, that when the inflammation was in a vital part, such as the stomach or intestines, or such as the stomach readily sympathizes with, then the pulse was quick, small, and hard, similar to the above. Now in the first stated positions we have some guide, for in the first of these, viz. where the pulse is strong, &c., there bleeding is most probably absolutely necessary, and the symptoms, with the state of blood joined, will determine better the future conduct; but in the second, where the pulse is small, very frequent, and hard, bleeding should be performed with great caution. Yet in inflammations of the second stated parts the constitution seems to be more irritable, giving more the signs of weakness, as if less in the power of the constitution to manage. Bleeding, restricted to two or three ounces, can do no harm by way of trial, and, as in the first case, the symptoms and blood are to determine the future repetition; but in the third, or vital parts, viz. either the stomach or such as the stomach sympathizes with, we are yet, I am afraid, left in the dark respecting the pulse. Perhaps, bleeding at first with caution, and judging from the blood and its effects upon the other symptoms, is the only criterion we can go by.

The kind of constitution will make a material difference, whether robust or delicate.

The mode of life will also make a material difference, whether [the patient is] accustomed to considerable exercise, and can bear it with ease. Constitutions so habituated will bear bleeding freely; but those with contrary habits will not. The sex will likewise make a difference, although the mode of life will increase that difference: therefore men will bear bleeding better than women. Even age makes a material difference, the young being able to lose more blood than the old, for the vessels of the old are not able to adapt themselves so readily to the decreased quantity; it even should not be taken away so quickly, and probably the constitution may in some degree have lost the habit of making blood, since it has lost the necessity.

The urine will throw some light on the disease. If high-coloured, and not much in quantity, it may be presumed, with the other symptoms, that bleeding will be of singular service; but if pale and a good deal of it, although the other indications are in favour of bleeding, yet it may be necessary to do it with caution.

However, bleeding should in all cases be performed with great caution, more particularly at first, and no more taken than appears to be really necessary. It should only be done to ease the constitution or the part, and rather lower it where the constitution can bear it; but if the constitution is already below or brought below a certain point, or gives the signs of it from the situation of the disease, then an irritable habit takes place, which is an increased disposition to act without the power to act with. This of itself becomes a cause of the continuance of the original disposition, and therefore will admit neither of resolution nor suppuration, but continue in a state of inflammation, which is a much worse disease than the former.

Upon any other principle than those above mentioned I cannot see why bleeding should have such effects in inflammation as it sometimes has. If considered in a mechanical light, as simply lessening the quantity of blood, it cannot account for it; because the removal of any natural mechanical power can never remove a cause which neither took its rise from, nor is supported by it. However, in this light it may be of some service; because all the actions relative to the blood's motion will be performed with more ease to the solids when the quantity is well proportioned.

It is probably from this connexion between the solids and fluids, that the constitution or a part is in a state of perfect quietude or health; in which [state] we find that the fluids are, and ought to be, in a large quantity; but in a state of inflammation, or increased powers and actions, those proportions do not correspond, at least in the parts inflamed; and by producing the equilibrium between the two, suitable to such a state, the body becomes, so far as this one circumstance can affect it, in a state of health, and this in many cases will cast the balance in favour of health. It is not, however, sufficient to produce this effect in all inflammations.

How far taking the blood from parts, peculiarly situated with respect to the parts inflamed, is more efficacious, I believe, is not yet determined, as bleeding in the left side for an inflammation in the right, upon the supposed principle of derivation, which might be classed with remote sympathy; but so far as the loss of the blood acts mechanically, viz. so far as it simply empties the vessels, it certainly can have no more effect than if taken in any other way; nor can it affect the living principle, either universally or locally, more in this mode than in any other. But how far it can affect the sympathizing principle I do not know.

Bleeding is often performed from no constitutional indication, but only as a preventive arising from experience, such as in consequence of considerable accidents, as blows on the head, fractured bones, &c.; but this is not to the present purpose.

§. 11. *The Use of Medicines internally, and of Local Applications in Inflammation.*

Everything given to the body, or applied to the part inflamed, that can abate inflammation, or its effects in the constitution, may be called medicine. Such, therefore, divide themselves into constitutional and local. The first will be internal, the second external; but whichsoever way they are applied, they that tend to lessen inflammation have their effects local: for mercury, although given internally for a venereal ulcer in the throat, yet acts locally on the disease; but those that tend to remove constitutional affections have their effects constitutional.

The internal medicines generally ordered for the resolution of inflammation are such as tend to have similar effects to that which is produced by bleeding, namely, lowering the constitution or the action of the parts, and this has usually been performed principally by purges; and the medicines that were given to remove or lessen the effects of inflammation on the constitution, have been such as generally tend to lessen fever, or the effects that the inflammation has upon the constitution.

Purges were generally given in cases of inflammation (probably at first from the idea of humours to be discharged), and such practice will answer best where bleeding succeeds, because it will lower the body to a more natural standard, and of course the inflamed part, as a part of that constitution; but here the same cautions are necessary that were given upon bleeding, because nothing debilitates so much as purging when carried beyond a certain point. One purging stool shall even kill, where the constitution is very much reduced, as in many dropsies; therefore, keeping the body simply open is all that should be done. However, although purging lowers considerably, yet its effect is not so permanent as that of bleeding. It rather lowers action, without diminishing strength; for if a person was to feel the loss of blood equal to a purge, that sensation would be more lasting.

Many constitutions rather acquire strength upon being gently purged, particularly such as have been living above par. But such strength as is acquired by putting the body in good order, I should suppose, is not inimical to inflammation.

In irritable habits, where the inflammation becomes more diffused, greater caution is necessary with regard to purging as well as bleeding; for I observed on the subject of bleeding, that in such constitutions no more blood should be taken than would relieve the constitution, as it were mechanically, but not such a quantity as to have a tendency towards lowering or weakening that constitution, for in such cases the action is greater than the strength; and whenever the disposition between these two, is of this kind, we cannot expect anything salutary from this mode of treatment, and therefore should not increase it. In such cases, the very reverse of the former method should often be practised: whatever has a tendency to raise the constitution above irritability should be given, such as bark, &c. The object of this last practice consists in bringing the strength of the constitution and part as near upon a par with the action as possible, by which means a kindly resolution or suppuration may take place, according as the parts inflamed are capable of acting.

Medicines which have the power of producing sickness lessen the action, and even the general powers of life, for a time, in consequence of every part of the body sympathizing with the stomach; and their effects are pretty quick.

Sickness lowers the pulse, makes the smaller vessels contract, and rather disposes the skin for perspiration, but not of the active or warm kind; but I believe it should proceed no further than sickness, for the act of vomiting is rather a counteraction to that effect, and produces its effects from another cause, and of course of another kind, which I believe rather rouse. It is probably an action arising from the feel of weakness, and intended to relieve the person from that weakness. It is similar to the hot fit of an ague, a counteraction to the cold one. There are few so weak but they will bear vomiting, but they cannot bear sickness long.

If we had medicines which, when given internally, could be taken into the constitution, and were endowed with a power of making the vessels contract, such I apprehend would be proper medicines. Bark has certainly this property, and is of singular service I believe in every inflammation attended with weakness, and therefore, I conceive, should be oftener given than is commonly done; but it is supposed to give strength, which would not accord with inflammations attended with too much strength and considerable irritation.

Preparations of lead, given in very small doses, might be given with success in cases attended with great strengtn.

Applications to the body to cure or resolve inflammations are, with regard to their mode of application, of two kinds: one is applied to the part inflamed, the other to some distant part. The first may be called local, or absolute respecting the part itself; the second relative. But even the first may be considered as having a relative effect in one of its modes of action, viz. that called repulsion, from which local applications have by some been objected to, and it is principally local applications that can repel, although not literally.

The first, or absolute effects of medicine, may be divided into two kinds, viz. one the simple cure of the part, the other producing an irritation of another kind in the part; both, however, act locally, and their ultimate effect is local. Local applications to a part, where those applications possess really the powers of resolution, must be much more efficacious than any of the other modes of resolution. For instance, mercury has much greater powers when applied immediately to the venereal complaint, than when applied to the nearest surface; where, however, we have not medicines that can resolve inflammation by application, then of course the other method is the most efficacious; but whether we have external or local applications which have really a tendency to lessen the inflammatory disposition is not well ascertained. I doubt our being in possession of many that can remove the immediate cause. Such would of course remove the action, or, if not wholly, would at least lessen it, and allow the inflammation to go off. But most of our powers in this way appear to be of the soothing kind, which therefore lessen the action (although the cause may still exist), and hence the effects are also lessened. This either produces a termination of the inflammation; or it is protracted, the cause lessens, and the inflammation wears itself out.

As inflammation has too much action, which action gives the idea of strength, such applications as weaken have been recommended, and cold is one of them. Cold, according to its degrees, produces two very different effects, one is the exciting of action without lessening the powers, the other is absolutely debilitating, while at the same time it excites action, if carried too far. In the first it becomes like suitable exercise to the vascular system, as bodily exercise is to the muscles, increasing strength; but when carried or continued beyond this point it lessens the powers, and becomes a weakener, calling up the action of resistance after the powers are lessened: therefore cold should not be indiscriminately used, and should be well proportioned to the powers.

Cold produces the action of contraction in the vessels, which is an action of weakness. A degree of cold suddenly applied, which hardly produces more than the sense of cold, excites action after the immediate effect is over, which is the action of dilatation, and which is the effect of the cold bath when it agrees; and as cold produces weakness in proportion to its degree, its application should not be carried too far, for then it produces a much worse disease, viz. irritability, or over-action in respect to the strength of the parts, and then indolence too often commences. Cold might be supposed to act on an inflamed part similarly to its action on a frozen part, restraining action, keeping it within the strength of the part in the one case, so as not to allow death to take place from over-action, and in the other keeping it within bounds*.

Lead is also supposed to have considerable effects in this way; but I believe much more is ascribed to it than it deserves. The property of lead appears to be that of lessening the powers and not the action; it therefore should never be used but when the powers are too strong, and acting with too much violence. However, lead certainly has the power of producing the contraction of the vessels; and therefore, where there is great strength, lead is certainly a powerful application.

Applications which can weaken should never be applied to an irritable inflammation, especially if the irritability arises from weakness. I am certain I have seen lead increase such inflammations, particularly in many inflammations of the eyes and eyelids, and I believe it is a bad

* As cold can be applied upon two very different principles, it is necessary to mention which is here meant. When cold is applied either within the powers of resistance of the part to excite heat, or only for so short a time as to give the stimulus of cold, then a reaction takes place, and warmth is the consequence; but if cold is applied beyond the powers of resistance, then a contraction of the vessels takes place, and that contraction is in some degree permanent. But this must be done with caution; for if continued too long it will produce debility, and action will be excited which will be irritable. In the present case the application of cold should only be sufficient to excite the contraction of the vessels, and that not continued too long, for reasons above assigned.

application in all scrofulous cases; in such cases the parts should be strengthened without producing action.

Warmth, more especially when joined with moisture, called fomentation, is commonly had recourse to, but I am certain that warmth, when as much as the sensitive principle can bear, excites action; but whether it is the action of inflammation, or the action of the contraction of the vessels, I cannot determine. We see that in many cases they cannot bear it, and therefore it might be supposed to increase the action of dilatation, and do hurt; but if that pain arises from the contraction of the inflamed vessels, then it is doing good; but this I doubt, because I rather conceive the action of contraction would give ease.

Acids have certainly a sedative power, as also alcohol, and I believe many of the neutral salts.

I believe it is not known that we have the power of adding strength to a part by local applications: that in general, I believe, must arise from the constitution; for although we have the power of giving action, yet this does not imply strength.

Many local applications are recommended to us, respecting many of which I have my doubts.

The mode of cure by an irritation different from the disease appears to increase the disease; but by destroying the first mode of action it produces another disease, viz. one according to the mode of irritation of the application, and which more easily admits of a cure than the first. I believe, however, that this takes place principally in specific diseases, and not so readily in common inflammation; for a common inflammation most probably would be increased by it. I have known specific inflammations much more easily cured by their specific medicine than the common inflammation of the same constitution, viz. I have seen a gonorrhœa and a chancre cured much more easily in some constitutions than an inflammation from an accident, and oftener than once or twice in the same person. However, this mode will not do in all specific diseases, for the scrofula will not change its nature by it, nor will the irritable, although specific. The venereal gonorrhœa (if parts are very irritable) is an instance of this, for irritating injections increase it; still we have many cutaneous inflammations cured in this way, for a pretty strong solution of corrosive sublimate will remove an inflammation of the skin. The *unguentum citrinum*, mixed with any common ointment, cures many inflammations of the eyelids; yet I believe that artificial irritations are similar to one another, and I do not know if there be any difference between them, although I can conceive one may agree better with some constitutions than others. However, these local or immediate applications can only be such as come in contact with the disease, which always must be some exposed surface, as when the skin of the eyelids, tonsils, &c. are inflamed; but even there some part must be affected by continued sympathy if they produce a cure, as the inflammation generally goes beyond the surface of immediate contact.

That inflammation which admits of repulsion, although by local means, might be considered here; but, from its effects and connexion with the constitution, it comes in more properly with the several relations under which I shall consider it[a].

---

[a] [The three great means of reducing inflammation must ever consist in the use of bloodletting, purging, and the adoption of an antiphlogistic regimen. In regard to which it may be observed, that the first should be had recourse to early in the disease, and be carried to such an extent as to produce an evident abatement of the symptoms: the second should be so contrived as to ensure a regular and continued action of the bowels during the whole course of the disease; and the third should not be relaxed in until all the symptoms of active inflammation have disappeared. To these all other measures must be regarded as subsidiary in cases of extensive inflammation affecting vital parts, although in cases of less severity it may happen that the auxiliary measures, or some particular methods of treatment adapted to the peculiar circumstances of the case, may claim the principal attention. Among the auxiliary measures brought forward since the author's death, two or three may here be briefly adverted to, for the purpose chiefly of pointing them out to the student's attention rather than of forming any exact appreciation of their value.

1. The efficacy of mercury in controlling the inflammatory action is in no instance so well exemplified as in inflammation of the iris; for, as the parts are here open to our view, we obtain demonstrative evidence of its power, not only in checking the morbid action but in occasioning the absorption of adventitious deposits. The efficacy of mercury, however, is limited to particular cases. It is greatest in iritis, laryngitis, hepatitis, and inflammation of the testicle; less in the mucous and serous membranes and the parenchymatous viscera; and still less in the common cellular membrane and other tissues. Its success is most marked in dispelling the remaining inflammation after the acute symptoms have been subdued, and therefore it should not be administered until a proper measure of bloodletting and purging have been previously adopted. Its administration should also be continuous, so as to keep the constitution under its influence, and if it excites either local or constitutional irritation its use should be immediately discontinued.

2. It has been proposed to accomplish all the beneficial objects of depletion by the administration of sedative medicines, such as digitalis and prussic acid, which by acting directly on the heart reduce the strength and frequency of the pulse; but experience has not confirmed these pretensions, nor was it indeed to be expected, since the same or very nearly the same effects are produced by many forms of visceral inflammation, which proceed nevertheless to a fatal termination, and that too with the greater certainty in proportion as these symptoms continue: neither have emetics, except in a few instances, any decided effect in checking inflammatory action, although the depression which they produce is very nearly analogous to that produced by the above-mentioned medicines. Excitability and stimulants are correlative terms, but very different effects are produced by the temporary reduction of the former and the actual reduction of the latter: by the latter the disease is removed, but by the former it is merely masked.

3. The effect of antimonial medicines is to lower the pulse and to restore the actions

§. 12. *General Observations on Repulsion, Sympathy, Derivation, Revulsion, and Translation.*

These terms are meant to be expressive of a change in the situation of diseased actions in the body, and they are so named according to the immediate cause, for any one disease may admit of any of these modes equally; that is, a disease which admits of being repelled may admit of being cured by sympathy, which probably includes derivation, repulsion, and translation. That such a principle or principles exist is, I think, evident, but the precise mode of action is, I believe, not known; that is, it is not known what part of the body more readily accepts of the action of another; if there are such parts, they might be called correspondent parts, whether the action changes its place from repulsion, sympathy, derivation, or translation. In derivation and repulsion, whether one mode of irritation is better than another, to invite or divert the action, and whether parts of a peculiar action do not require a peculiar irritation to divert them; to all this we are likewise totally strangers.

It is not to my present purpose to go into the different effects of this principle, although I must own it might be as useful a part of the healing art as any; and even more, for it is probably the least known, as being the least intelligible, and therefore the more use may be derived from its investigation.

The operations denominated by these terms, so far as they exist, ap-

---

of the skin; but it has been proposed by Tommasini and the Italian physicians to administer the antimonium tartarizatum in large doses of from ten to sixty or even ninety grains, two or three times a day, which in cases where it is likely to prove beneficial are said not to produce sickness and purging, except after the first dose, but to act specifically on the extreme vessels so as to correct the morbid action. The plan, however, has been tried in this country without success, and in those cases where it has appeared to be of service, the good effects have seemed to arise either from the evacuation of the stomach in the first instance by vomiting, or by keeping up a gentle action of the bowels by purging, or else by subduing to a certain extent the heart's action; effects which may clearly be attained with more safety and ease by other means.

4. The last measure which I shall mention is the adoption of incisions, for which we are chiefly indebted to Mr. Copland Hutchinson and Mr. Lawrence. This method is principally serviceable in erysipelas, or diffuse inflammation of the cellular membrane. In the former case it relieves the tension of the skin and effectually unloads the vessels, while in the latter it gives exit to sloughs or putrid matter, and excites the parts to a healthy action. The length and depth of the incisions may vary from mere superficial incisions of a half inch in length to deep incisures extending through the whole adipose structure and reaching to a foot in extent. This plan is often very successful where the patient has a robust constitution, and has besides the courage to submit to so severe a method of procedure; but in other cases, especially if the incisions are of great extent, the loss of blood may prove fatal, or at least so weaken the patient as considerably to protract the convalescence.]

pear all to belong to the same principle in the animal œconomy, for they all consist either in a change of the situation of a disease or its action; —a change of the situation, as in the gout; a change of the action, as a swelling of the testicles in the stopping of a gonorrhœa. This last is not properly a change of the situation of the disease, but only of the general inflammatory action without the specific action; these principles can only produce a change in the seat of action, not in any of the consequences of disease; they have in some instances a connexion with the natural operations of the body, as it were, interfering with them; and when that is the case they in general must produce disease of some kind. Thus the stopping of the menses, which is a local natural action arising from the constitution, may be effected by local applications called repelling, by a derangement of the constitution, and by many consequences which depend on a deranged constitution simply; or it may be drawn off by a derangement of the constitution, which is a kind of derivation or revulsion. We find that local applications derange also other parts, which have no visible effect upon the part of application as the above, nor any visible connexion with the parts which assume the action. Thus cold, especially if wet be applied to the feet, will bring on complaints in the stomach and bowels by sympathy; and the same mode of application of cold, if looal, will produce a local complaint, as cold air blowing on a part will bring on rheumatism.

These changes were all supposed formerly to be of more consequence than I apprehend they really are, for they are only the change of situation of disease. They were introduced into the œconomy of disease from the idea of humours. Repellents were such applications as drove the humours out of a part, which would fall on some other; sympathy consisted in another part taking them up; derivation was a drawing off, or inviting the humours; revulsion was the same; and translation was the moving of humours from one part to another. Thus we have those different terms applied to that connexion of parts, by which one part being affected, some other is affected or relieved; or, as in translation, some other part takes up the disease as it were voluntarily, as is often the case in the gout. All of these produce one of the symptoms of a disease, viz. sensation and inflammation, but I believe seldom if ever real diseased structures. This agrees with what was formerly observed, that local inflammations depending on the constitution seldom if ever suppurate[a].

[a] [The present state of our knowledge does not enable us to give a complete account of these varieties of action, viz. repulsion, derivation, and metastasis; but it seems probable that they are all ultimately to be referred to the same general principle. The

I believe that these powers have greater effects in diseases depending on or producing action and sensation, which are called nervous, than on those producing an alteration in the structure of parts. Thus we have the cramp in the leg cured by a gentle irritation round the lower part of the thigh, such as a garter, which may be said to arise from derivation or sympathy; and I have known, in a nervous girl, a pain in one arm cured by rubbing the other.

These cures by derivation, repulsion, translation, etc. do not deserve that name, although the patients are cured of the original disease, as in many cases there is as large a quantity somewhere else in the body uncured; for example, in those cases where the cure is from some local inflammation being produced, and perhaps more violent than the first; but in other cases, where the cure arises only from an action in a part without a diseased alteration of structure, then the cure in such cases is performed without any other disease having been produced, such as sickness or vomiting curing a disease of the testicles.

I have already observed that local applications were principally supposed to repel, by the first or second mode of action; yet internal medicines having a specific, or what might be called a local action, although given internally, may repel by stopping the diseased action in the part which it chiefly affects, such as mercury falling on the mouth, might repel a disease from the mouth. Hemlock might do the same with regard to the head, or turpentine with regard to the urethra. In the last we often find by taking balsams, that by stopping the discharge a swelling of the testicles comes on, or an irritable bladder. As repulsion in this way is not so evident, it is less noticed. The uncertainty in the power of medicines respecting repulsion, has led surgeons into more errors than any other principle in the animal œconomy, with regard to diseases.

---

primary laws which appear to govern these phenomena are, first, the tendency which there is in all animal bodies to preserve an equilibrium, in consequence of which it happens that when any one part of the frame is unusually excited, a corresponding diminution takes place in the functions of other parts, so that in disease, the lesser disease gives way to the greater; and secondly, the affinities of structure and function, and the mutual relations which subsist between different parts, in a state of health; for it accords with experience, and at the same time is most agreeable to reason, to find that those parts which have a similarity of structure, and consequently of vital endowments, should be affected more readily by the causes of disease than parts of a different construction; and also, that parts associated in health should likewise become associated in disease. The former law explains in some measure the general principle of metastasis; the latter, the particular cause which determines the disease to any one organ rather than to another. The author has expressed his opinion, that in these affections the inflammation, but not the disease, is translated (p. 325); but this is a refined distinction, in opposition to the general fact, that the liability to metastasis is almost exclusively confined to specific diseases.]

It has prevented their acting in many cases where they might have done it with safety and effect. A stronger instance cannot be given than in that species of the venereal disease called a gonorrhœa, which they did not venture to cure by local applications, for fear of driving it into the constitution, and producing a pox; but they did not consider that a gonorrhœa did not arise from the constitution, but may be said to arise from accident, or at least is entirely local, and therefore no repulsion could take place. The idea of repelling was first introduced when local diseases were supposed to arise from a deposit or derivation of humours to a part, and is still retained by those who cannot or will not allow themselves to think better; yet still the term might be applied to diseased action; for the removal of many diseased actions from a part which fall on some other part is certainly the repelling of that diseased action; but since it is not subdued, but on y driven from the part, as is often the case with the gout, no cure is performed by this means.

Both or either of the two local methods of removing disease, just now mentioned, viz. whether by simply curing the disease, or by destroying the diseased action, in consequence of exciting an action of another kind, may produce the effect called repulsion; but the former, I believe, can only take place in inflammations arising from the constitution, and which being prevented from settling in this part, return upon the constitution again, and often fall upon some other part, viz. one next in order of susceptibility for such inflammation, as is often the case in the gout, and in many other diseases besides inflammation, as in many nervous complaints. St. Vitus's dance is a remarkable instance of it; but in this case it is not to be considered as a cure of the disease, but only as a suspension of its action in this part.

I could conceive it possible that the second mode of local cure, which is by producing an irritation of another kind, might not repel, although it cured the first or local complaint, because there is in such modes of cure still a larger quantity of inflammation in the part than was produced by the disease (although of another kind); but as the idea of repelling is to have a disease somewhere, although not in the same place, keeping it in the present situation may be as proper, if not more so, than in any other it might go to. But if, on the other hand, the constitution requires to have a local complaint arising from itself, which, as it were, is drawing off or relieving this constitutional disposition, then curing the one already formed, by producing another in the same part, can be of no service; for if the artificial disease is not of the same nature with the constitutional one (which it cannot be if it destroys it), then it cannot act as a substitute for it. We may observe, that by producing an irritation of another kind in the gout, we may destroy the gouty inflammation in the part, but cannot always clear the constitution of it; there is therefore no benefit arising from such practice in these cases.

The repelling powers which act from applications being made to the parts immediately affected, or by the change of one disease into another, become the most difficult of any to be ascertained; because it must be very difficult to say what will merely repel and what will completely cure, or perfectly change the disease. Repulsion is certainly to be considered as a cure of the part, whatever may be the consequence; and a change in the disease is certainly a cure of the first, although a disease may still exist in the part.

That an artificial irritation made on one part does not (always at least) cure or remove a diseased irritation of a specific nature in another part, is, I think, evident in many cases, even although that specific [disease] should be an affection of the constitution. This at least was evident in a case of the gout, for when the gout was in some of the vital parts, and sinapisms were applied to the feet, they did not relieve those vital parts, although the inflammation in consequence of the sinapisms was considerable; but this inflammation brought on the gout in the feet, and as soon as this happened the vital parts were relieved, from which it would appear that a specific irritation required a specific derivator. It may be supposed that the inflammation, in consequence of the sinapisms, brought on or produced such a derangement in the feet as made them more susceptible of the gout, or that the inflammation became an immediate cause of the action of the gout taking place there.

It is plain, too, that where there is a gouty disposition, or a gouty action in the constitution, a derangement in a part may bring it on, for in the above person, who had still those internal spasms recurring upon the least exercise or anxiety of mind, but was in all other respects, and at all other times, well, by applying sinapisms a second time to his feet, till a considerable cutaneous inflammation came on, the gout attacked the ball of the great toe of the right foot, and the last joint of the great toe of the left, which lasted about two days. This attack of gout, however, did not relieve him of the remaining spasms, as the first did, and therefore was to be considered an additional gouty action. This could certainly not have taken place if the constitution had not been gouty.

In diseases where we have no specific application capable of acting immediately, the advantages gained by derivation, revulsion, or sympathy are much greater in many cases than by the effects of any local application at present known; and the medicines which are capable of producing this effect are often such as would either have no[a] effect if ap-

[a] ["*an* effect" in the original text.]

plied to the diseased part, or would increase it. This arises from the dissimilar actions of the two parts; that is, the diseased actions of the one being similar[a] to, or producing the actions of recovery in the other; nor is it difficult to conceive why it should be so; for since the medicines are not specifics, but only invite or remove the disease by that connexion which the living powers of the one part have with those of another, it is reasonable to suppose that this principle of action between the parts must be much stronger than the effects of many medicines which have only a tendency to cure, or perhaps no tendency that way at all. Thus we find that vomits will often cure inflammations of the testicles when all soothing applications prove ineffectual, and when the same emetic could not have the least effect on the part itself were it applied to it. Thus we also find that a caustic behind the ear will relieve inflammations of the eyes or eyelids, when every application to the parts affected has proved ineffectual, and when this caustic, if applied to the parts themselves only as a stimulant, would increase the disease.

Sympathy, perhaps, (except the continued) includes the mode of action in all of those which I have called relatives, viz. repulsion, derivation, revulsion, and translation; at least it is probably the same principle in the whole. What I would call a cure by sympathy, is producing a curative action in a sound part, that the diseased may take on the same mode of action from sympathy that it would take on if the curative was applied to it; so that sympathy might even be supposed to repel in cases which would admit of repelling, and fall on some other part, although not the part necessarily where the application was made. The difference between derivation or repulsion, and sympathy, consists in derivation producing a disease in a sound part to cure a disease in another part, as was observed; while sympathy is applying the cure to a sound part to cure the diseased; but in many cases it will be very difficult to distinguish the one from the other. Sympathy is very universal, or more general than any [of the] others; for there are few local diseases that do not extend beyond the surface of contact, which produces continued sympathy; and also, there are few parts that have not some connexion with some other part, which gives us remote sympathy.

It may be recollected, that when sympathy was treated of, it was divided into continued, contiguous, remote, similar, and dissimilar.

The cure by continued sympathy is that application which we have reason to suppose would cure if applied to the part itself, such as applying mercury to the skin over a venereal node. The node is cured by its sympathizing with the mercurial irritation of the skin; and the

---

[a] [The sense of the passage seems to require that we should read *dissimilar*.]

action of the sympathizer here is similar to the action of the part of application. Remote sympathy is seldom if ever produced by a similarity of action in similar parts, but most probably cures by dissimilar modes of action in the two parts, and therefore might be called dissimilar sympathy, viz. by stimulating the part of application in such a way that the sympathizer shall act in the same way as if the real application of cure was made to it, and yet the mode of action of the part of application shall not be at all similar to the sympathizer. I can even suppose a local disease cured by sympathy, and by that medicine which would increase it, if applied immediately to it. Let us suppose, for example, any diseased mode of action, and that this mode could be increased by some irritating medicine, if applied [directly] to it; but apply this irritator to some other part which this diseased part sympathizes with, and [suppose] that the sympathetic act in the diseased part shall be the same as if its [proper] curative medicine was applied to it,—similar [in short] to what would have taken place if its specific irritator was applied,—then, in such a case the medicine would cure by sympathy, although it would increase the disease if applied locally, or have no effect at all.

The contiguous sympathy is where it would appear to act from the approximation of dissimilar parts, and therefore is not continued sympathy; neither can it be called remote sympathy, as there appears to be no specific connexion, but to arise entirely from contiguity or approximation of parts. Of this kind are blisters on the head, curing headache; on the chest, curing pains in the chest; to the pit of the stomach, to cure irritations there; to the belly, to cure complaints of the bowels. The applications which act by contiguous sympathy are only those which can be applied to the nearest surface to that which is inflamed, when the inflamed part beyond this surface becomes affected in some degree similar to the part of application, such as the applications to the eyelids, when the inflammation is in the eye; to the scrotum, when it is in the testicle; to the abdomen, when some of the bowels are inflamed; to the thorax, in inflammations of the lungs, etc. These may be either of the specific, stimulating, or soothing kinds,—something which affects the parts in such a manner as that a remote diseased action ceases. It may be specific, as opium applied to the pit of the stomach curing an irritation of that viscus; stimulating, as blisters to cure inflammation in the subjacent viscera, as has been mentioned; soothing, as fomentations to the abdomen to relieve complaints in the bowels.

Derivation means a cessation of action in one part, in consequence of an action having taken place in another; and when this is a cessation of a diseased action, then a cure of that action in the original part may be said to be performed: this cure was brought into use from the idea of humours, that is, the drawing off of the humours from the seat where they had taken possession; but I believe much more has been ascribed to it than it deserves. How far it really takes place I have not been able fully to ascertain in all its parts; that is, how far the real disease is invited, and accepts of the invitation; but I have already observed, that there is such a principle of disease in the animal œconomy, although we must see from derivation that the same quantity, or perhaps more irritation, is retained in the constitution; yet the artificial irritation produced being either such as more readily admits of a cure than the disease in the part, or being in parts which are not so essential to life, an advantage by this means is gained; thus, burning the ear is practised as a cure for the tooth-ache, and the part which is burnt more readily admits of a cure than the tooth. We also find that blisters often cure or remove deep-seated pains, such as head-ache, and relieve the bladder when applied to the perinæum. Blisters and caustics behind the ear cure also inflammations of the eye.

Less may be said on revulsion, since we have explained derivation. To draw off a disease always implies safe ground, and can be applied with safety in any disease; revulsion can best be applied when the disease attacks essential parts, where the application cannot be so near as to imply derivation. Thus we find that vomits will cure an inflammation of the testicles, white swellings, and even venereal buboes; and sinapisms applied to the feet relieve the head.

Translation differs from derivation, revulsion, and repulsion, only as it proceeds from a natural or spontaneous cause, whereas these proceed from an artificial, accidental, or external cause, and the common principle of them all seems to be sympathy; for if not an act of its own [i. e. of the disease itself], then it must be either repelled, derived, or from sympathy. Very strange instances of translation are given us; it has been supposed that pus already formed has been translated to another part of the body, deposited there in form of an abscess, and then discharged. This is an operation absolutely impossible[a]. Matter absorbed may be carried off by some of the secretions, such as that by the kidneys, which have a power of removing more than they secrete; but the deposition of pus is the same with its formation. Both revulsion and repulsion may be reckoned a species of translation. The gout moving of its own accord from the stomach to the foot, or from one foot to the other, may be reckoned a translation of the gout.

---

[a] [This opinion is nevertheless entertained by several justly celebrated physiologists of the present day. See Vol. I., 352, *note*, and Andral, Anat. Pathol., i. 405.]

§. 13. *Of the different Forms in which Medicines are applied, and the subsiding of Inflammation.*

Fomentations or steams, washes, and poultices are the common applications to a part in the state of inflammation. The first and last are commonly applied to inflammation arising from external violence, and proceeding to suppuration; the second, commonly to internal surfaces, as the mouth, nose, urethra, vagina, rectum, etc. The aetion of the two first is but of very short duration.

Fomentations and steams are fluid bodies raised into vapour: they may be either simple or compound; simple, as steam, or vapour of water; compound, as steam of water impregnated with medicines.

This mode of applying heat and moisture appears, from experience, to be more efficacious than when these are applied in the form of a fluid; it often gives ease at the time of the application, while at other times it gives great pain; but if it does give ease, the symptoms generally return between the times of applying it, and with nearly the same violence. How far the application of a medicine for fifteen minutes out of twenty-four hours can do good, I am not certain; we find, however, that the application of a vapour of a specific medicine, though but for a few minutes in the day, will have very considerable effects: fumigations with cinnabar may serve as an instance[a]. The fomentations are commonly composed of the decoction of herbs; sometimes of the marsh-mallows, but oftener of the decoction of herbs possessing essential oil, which I believe are the best; because I suppose that whatever will excite contraction of the vessels, will in some degree counteract the dilating principle. Vinegar as well as spirits are put into them, but how far they stimulate to contraction I do not know, but rather believe they remove irritation, which must lessen the inflammatory action.

Washes are in general fluid applications, and are more commonly applied to inflammations of internal surfaces than of the common integuments: there are washes to the eye called collyria; washes to the mouth and throat, called gargles; washes to the urethra, called injections; and to the rectum, called clysters; but I am fearful that we are not yet acquainted with the true specific virtues of these washes, at least there is something very vague in their application. There are, for instanoe, astringent washes for the inflammation of the eye, such as white and blue vitriol, alum, etc.; stimulating warm gargles for inflammations of the throat, such as mustard, red port, claret with vinegar and honey; but

[a] [But in this instance the mercury is rapidly absorbed into the system.]

to moderate or resolve external inflammations, they do not apply substances with any such properties[a]. How absurd would it appear to surgeons in general, if any one made use of the same applications to an inflammation in any other part; yet I do not know if there is any difference between an inflammation of the eye or throat, and one in any other part, if the inflammations are of the same kind: mercury cures a venereal inflammation, either of the eye or throat, as easily as a venereal inflammation any where else, because it is an inflammation of the same kind.

These applications, like fomentations, are of short duration, for there is no possibility of applying these powers constantly, except in the form of a poultice, whose operation is somewhat similar; and, indeed, they are only substitutes for a poultice, where that mode of application cannot be made use of, as I observed with respect to internal surfaces.

Poultices are constant applications, and, like fomentations, may be of two kinds, either simply warm and wet, or medicated. The greatest effect that a poultice can produce must be immediate, but its power will extend beyond the surface of contact, although only in a secondary degree.

To the common inflammation the simplest poultices are supposed to be the best, and produce their effect, I believe, only by keeping the parts easier under the complaint; but I am of opinion that such do not affect the inflammation any other way. A common poultice is, perhaps, one of the best applications when we mean to do nothing but to allow nature to perform the cure with as much ease to herself as possible. Poultices may be medicated, so as to be adapted to the kind of inflammation, as with the solution of lead, opium, mercury, etc.; in short, they may be compounded with any kind of medicine.

Whatever the disposition is which produces inflammation, and whatever the actions are which produce the effects, that disposition, under certain circumstances, viz. when it arises either from the constitution or the parts, can be removed, and of course the actions excited by it. The disposition for inflammation shall have taken place, and the vessels which are the active parts shall have dilated, and allowed more blood to enter them, so that the part shall look red; but no hardness or fulness shall be observed, and the whole shall subside before adhesions

---

[a] [The reason of this is sufficiently obvious, for if the external integuments of the body are deprived of their defence of cuticle, and assimilated therefore in conditions to the mucous membranes, the same effects are produced in them; which effects it may be observed are more or less of a permanent nature. The consequences which ensue from the application of various metallic or saline solutions to the web of a frog's foot, leave no doubt as to the fact of the imbibition of foreign substances by the lining cuticle, and of their influence upon the subjacent vessels.]

have been formed; or if inflammation has gone so far as to produce swelling, which is the adhesive stage of the disease, it by certain methods can be frequently so assuaged as to prevent suppuration taking place, and then the parts will fall back into their natural state, which is called resolution, some adhesions being perhaps the only remaining consequences of the inflammation.

The same methods are likewise often used with considerable success in lessening inflammation arising from violence, so as to prevent suppuration entirely; but in many of these cases they are not sufficient, and in those where it cannot be prevented, yet it may be lessened by the same means.

As the first symptom of inflammation is commonly pain, so is the first symptom of resolution a cessation of that pain, as well as one of the symptoms of suppuration, which is a species of resolution. I have known the cessation of pain so quick as to appear like a charm, although no other visible alteration had taken place, the swelling and colour being the same.

Why inflammation of any kind should cease after it has once begun is very difficult to explain, or even to form an idea of, since as yet we have no mode of counteracting the first cause, or irritation. It may be supposed to arise from the principle, of parts adapting themselves in time to their present situation, which I call custom; and that therefore, in order to keep up the inflammation, it would be necessary for the cause to increase in proportion as the parts get reconciled to their present circumstances. But, allowing this to be the cause, it will not account for their returning back to their natural or original state, when this increase of irritation ceases, and only the last or original irritation remains; for upon this principle they only grow more easy under their present state, or perhaps, which is worse, acquire a habit of it, which may be the cause of many indolent specific diseases.

If we suppose the removal of the original cause to be sufficient to stop the progress of inflammation, and when this is stopped that the parts cannot easily remain in the same inflamed state, but by their own efforts begin to restore themselves to health, (which we can easily conceive to be the case in specific diseases, especially those arising from poisons of such kinds as are capable of a termination, as the smallpox, or where a cure can be administered for the effects of the poison, as in the lues venerea,) then we must conclude that the inflamed state is an uneasy state,—a force upon the organs which suffer it, like the bending of a spring, which is always endeavouring to restore itself, and the moment that the power is removed returns back to its natural state again; or it may be like the mind, forgetful of injuries.

§. 14. *Of the Use of the Adhesive Inflammation.*

This inflammation may be said in all cases to arise from a state of parts in which they cannot remain, and therefore an irritation of imperfection takes place. It may be looked upon as the effect of wise counsels, the constitution being so formed as to take spontaneously all the precautions necessary for its defence; for in most cases we shall evidently see that it answers wise purposes.

Its utility may be said to be both local and constitutional, but certainly most so with regard to the first. Its utility is most evident when it arises from a disease in a part, whether this proceeds from the constitution or otherwise; and when it does, it must be considered as arising from a state in which that part cannot exist,—as in exposure,—and therefore is the first step towards a cure. It is often of service in those cases which arise from violence, although not necessarily so, the injured parts not being always under the necessity of having recourse to it, as was shown in treating of union by the first intention.

When the adhesive inflammation arises from the constitution, it may depend on some disease of that constitution; and if so, it may be conceived to be of use to it, especially if it should be supposed to be the termination of a universal irritation in a local one, by that means relieving the constitution of the former, as in the gout; but when it is only the simple adhesive inflammation that takes place, I am rather apt to think that it is more a part of the disease than a termination of it, or an act of the constitution.

The adhesive inflammation serves as a check to the suppurative by making parts, which otherwise must infallibly fall into that state, previously unite, in order to prevent its access, as was described when speaking of the adhesive inflammation being limited; and where it cannot produce this effect, so as altogether to hinder the suppurative inflammation itself from taking place, it becomes in most cases a check upon the extent of it. This we see evidently to be the case in large cavities, as in the tunica vaginalis after the operation for the hydrocele; for after the water has made its escape, parts of the collapsed sac frequently unite to other parts of the same sac by this inflammation, and thereby preclude the suppurative from extending beyond these adhesions, which so far prevents the intention of the surgeon from having its full effect; and often, on the other hand, the adhesive state of the inflammation takes place universally in this bag, in consequence of the palliative cure, which produces the radical cure, and prevents a relapse. In the hernia it performs a cure by uniting the two sides of the sac together, by means of slight pressure, so that we should understand perfectly its mode of action, where it can prevent a cure, and where it can perform one. In still larger cavities, such as the abdomen, (where often only a partial inflammation takes place, as is frequently the case after childbearing and in wounds of this cavity,) we find this inflammation produced; which either prevents the suppurative altogether, or if it does not, it unites the parts surrounding the suppurative centre, and confines the suppuration to that point; and as the abscess increases in size, the adhesive inflammation spreads, uniting the parts as it spreads, so that the general cavity is excluded. Thus the suppuration is confined to the first point, and forms there a kind of circumscribed abscess, as will be more fully explained hereafter.

In inflammations of the pleura or surface of the lungs, the same thing happens, for the adhesive inflammation takes place, and the surfaces are united, which union going before the suppuration confines it to certain limits, so that distinct abscesses are formed by this union of the parts, and the whole cavity of the thorax is not involved in a general suppuration; such cases are called the spurious empyema.

The cellular membrane everywhere in the body is united exactly in the same manner; the sides of the cells throw out, or as it were sweat out, the uniting matter, which fills the cavities and unites the whole into one mass.

The adhesive inflammation often disposes the parts to form a cyst or bag; this is generally to cover some extraneous body that does not irritate so much as to produce suppuration, such as a sac formed to inclose a bullet, pieces of glass, &c.

With the same wise views it unites the parts or cellular membrane which lies between an abscess and the spot where that abscess has a tendency to open, as will be more fully explained hereafter, when I come to treat of ulceration.

The lungs are so circumstanced as to partake of the effects of two principles: the one, as an internal uniting surface; the other, as a secreting surface: the last of which constitutes the peculiar structure and use of this viscus; and the first is no more than the reticular or uniting substance of the air-cells. The internal or the uniting membrane of the lungs unites readily by the adhesive inflammation, as the cellular membrane through the body generally; but the air-cells, like the inner surface of the urethra, nose, intestines, &c., pass directly into the suppurative inflammation, and therefore do not admit of the adhesive, by which means the matter formed is obliged to be coughed up, which produces symptoms peculiar to the parts affected; and it is perhaps almost impossible to produce an inflammation on either of those two surfaces without affecting the other; which probably is one reason why the treatment of inflammation in those parts is attended with such bad success.

We cannot give a better illustration of the use of the adhesions produced in consequence of this inflammation, than to contrast it with the erysipelatous, of which I have already given an account. When the erysipelatous inflammation takes place, the matter gets very freely into the surrounding and sound cellular membrane, and then diffuses itself almost over the whole body; while, in another kind of constitution, the adhesive inflammation would have been produced, to have prevented its progress.

A man was attacked with a violent inflammation on each side of the anus, which I did not see till some days after it began. It had the appearance of the suppurative inflammation joined with the erysipelatous; for it was not so circumscribed as the suppurative, nor did it spread upon the skin like the true erysipelatous, and the skin had a shining œdematous appearance. The inflammation went deeper into the cellular membrane than the true erysipelatous. He was bled; the blood was extremely sizy. He took a purge, and was fomented. He had a difficulty in making water, most probably from the pressure of the swelling upon the urethra. The day following I observed that the scrotum of that side was very much swelled, which had extended up the right spermatic chord; and on examining this swelling, I plainly felt a fluid in it, with air, which sounded on being shaken. The case now plainly discovered itself. I immediately opened the suppuration on each side of the anus, which discharged a dusky coloured pus, very fœtid, with a good deal of air, and upon squeezing the swelling in the scrotum, &c. I could easily discharge the matter and air by these openings: I therefore made him lie principally upon his back, and squeeze these swellings often, with a view to discharge this matter by the openings. The matter at the part where it was formed was not contained in a bag or abscess, but formed in the cellular membrane, without previous adhesion.

The scrotum now inflamed, and seemed to have a tendency to open; at least it looked livid and spotted. I opened it at this part, and it discharged a good deal of matter and air. A general suppuration came upon the whole cellular membrane of those parts, and the matter passed up through the cellular membrane of the belly; and the cellular membrane of the loins was loaded with matter, from its sinking down from the cells of the abdomen. I made openings there, and could squeeze out a great deal of matter and air. A mortification came on just above the right groin, and when I removed the slough matter was discharged. I also made openings on the loins, on the side of the abdomen, &c. He lived but a few days in this way, during which time the cellular membrane was hanging out of the wounds like wet dirty tow.

The adhesive inflammation takes place in consequence of accidents, (when it is impossible it should ever produce the same good effects,) such as wounds which are not allowed to or cannot heal by the first intention; for instance, a stump after amputation, and many other wounds: but it is one of those fixed and invariable principles of the animal machine, which upon all such irritations uniformly produces the uniting process, though, like many other principles in the same machine, the effects [which it produces] are perhaps not so much required; so that although a wound is not allowed to heal, or cannot heal by means of the adhesive inflammation, yet the surrounding parts go through the common consequences of being wounded, and the surrounding cells are united; as was described when I treated of union by the first intention. It first throws out the blood, as if the intention was to unite the parts again; the newly-cut or torn ends of the vessels, however, soon contract and close up, and then the discharge is not blood, but a serum with the coagulating part of the blood, similar to that which is produced by the adhesive state of inflammation, so that they go through the two first processes of union; therefore the use of the adhesive inflammation does not appear so evidently in these cases as in spontaneous inflammations: however, in case of wounds which are allowed to suppurate, it answers the great purpose of uniting the cells at the cut surface, from their being simply in contact with each other, as has been described, which confines the inflammation to that part, without which the irritation arising from this state of imperfection might have been communicated from cell to cell, and proceed further than it commonly does. The cut vessels, by this means, are also united, which hinders the progress of inflammation from running along their cavities, as we find sometimes to be the case in the veins of a wounded surface, where this inflammation has not taken place. From everything which has been said it must appear that all surfaces, which are suppurating in consequence of this inflammation, have their basis in that state of the adhesive inflammation which very nearly approaches to suppuration; and this inflammation is less and less as it recedes further from the suppurating centre.

CHAPTER IV.

OF THE SUPPURATIVE INFLAMMATION.

When the adhesive inflammation is not capable of resolution, and has gone as far as possible to prevent the necessity of suppuration, especially in those cases that might have admitted of a resolution, as in spontaneous* inflammations in general, where there has neither been an exposed laceration of the solids, nor, as before mentioned, loss of substance, but where the natural functions of the part have only been so deranged that it was unable to fall back into a natural and sound state again; or, secondly, where it was a consequence of such accidents, as the effects of the adhesive could not in the least prevent, (as in wounds that were prevented from healing by the first or second intention,) then, under either of these two circumstances, suppuration takes place.

The immediate effect of suppuration is the production of pus from the inflamed surface, which appears in such cases, or under such circumstances, to be a leading step to the formation of a new substance, called granulations, which granulations are the third method in the first order of parts of restoring those parts to health; but upon all internal canals suppuration is certainly not a leading step to granulations, which will be explained hereafter.

The same theory of the adhesive inflammation respecting the vessels is, I believe, applicable to the suppurative; for when suppuration is the first, we have the vessels in the same state as in the adhesive when it happens, but their dispositions and actions must have altered, there being a great difference in their effects.

This is so much the case, that the true inflammatory disposition and action almost immediately ceases upon the commencement of suppuration; and although the vessels may be nearly in the same state, yet they are in a much more quiescent state than before, and have acquired a new mode of action.

I shall endeavour to establish as an invariable fact that no suppuration takes place which is not preceded by inflammation; that is, that no

* I have used this word to denote a case where no visible cause of inflammation exists; for strictly there can be no such thing in nature as spontaneous.

pus is formed but in consequence of it. That it is an effect of inflammation only is proved in abscesses from a breach in the solids, attended with exposure, and from extraneous matter of all kinds, whether introduced or formed there. In abscess, suppuration is an immediate consequence of inflammation: from the exposure of internal cavities no suppuration comes on till inflammation has formed the disposition and action; and although we find collections of extraneous matter, something like pus, in different parts of the body, yet such extraneous matter is not pus. However, towards the last, in such collections, pus is often formed; but then this is in consequence of inflammation having taken place towards the surface, and when such collections are opened they immediately inflame universally, similar to every other breach of the solids, and then the future discharge is pus, all of which I shall now treat.

The irritation, which is immediately the cause of suppuration, is the same, from whatever cause it may proceed, similar to that which produces the adhesive stage; it [suppuration] is a similar process going through the same stages, and attended with nearly the same circumstances, whether it takes its rise from external violence, the constitution, or a disposition in the part, if all other circumstances are equal. However, it is not so general in its causes as the adhesive, for the thickening process will take place in many diseases where true suppuration is not admitted, as in some scrofulous cases, some venereal, and also some cancers. Suppuration, therefore, depends more on the soundness of parts than the adhesive inflammation; and this is so much the case that we can, in some degree, judge of a sore simply by its discharge.

It appears very difficult to give a true and clear idea of the whole chain of causes leading to suppuration. The immediate state of parts, which may be called the immediate cause, I conceive to be such as cannot carry on its usual functions of life, and which state of parts I have called the state of imperfection, let the cause of that state be what it will[a]. We have shown that irritation simply is not always sufficient; it often only brings on the adhesive stage, which is in most cases intended to prevent the suppurative, as has been observed.

It is a curious fact to see the same mode of action producing two such contrary effects, and each tending to a cure: the first producing from necessity the second, and being also subservient to it. Violence done to parts is one of the great causes of suppuration; but we have already remarked that violence simply does not always produce this in-

[a] [To say that the causes of suppuration operate by inducing a "state of imperfection," is, after all, a mere figurative generalization, which does not advance us a single step nearer the solution of the difficulty.]

flammation, but that it must be a violence followed by a prevention of the parts performing their cure in a more simple way, viz. a restoration of the structure, so as [to be able] to carry on the animal functions of the part, or, in other words, a prevention of union by the first or second intention; or [a violence] attended with this circumstance, viz. that the parts are kept a sufficient time in that state into which they were put by the violence; or, what is something similar to this, a violence attended with death in a part, such as in many bruises, mortifications, sloughs in consequence of caustics, &c., which, when separated, have exposed internal surfaces*.

Various have been the opinions on this subject; and as every violence committed from without, under the circumstances before mentioned, is exposed more or less to the surrounding air, the applications of this matter to internal surfaces has generally been assigned as a cause of this inflammation; but air certainly has not the least effect upon those parts, for a stimulus would arise from a wound were it even contained in a vacuum[a]. Nor does the air get to the parts that form circumscribed abscesses so as to be a cause of their formation, and yet they as readily suppurate in consequence of inflammation as exposed surfaces.

Further, in many cases of the emphysema, where the air is diffused over the whole body, (and this air not the purest,) we have no such effect, excepting there is produced an exposure or imperfection of some internal surface for this air to make its escape by, and then this part inflames. Nay, as a stronger proof, and of the same kind with the former, that it is not the admission of air which makes parts fall into inflammation, we find that the cells in the soft parts of birds, and many of the cells and canals of the bones of the same tribe of animals, which communicate with the lungs†, and at all times have more or less air in them, never inflame; but if these cells are exposed in an unnatural way,

* But here we may just remark, that the first processes towards suppuration in cases of mortification, where a separation must take place prior to suppuration, are different from the foregoing, because the living surface is to separate from it the dead parts, and therefore another action of the living powers is required, which is what I call ulceration. And by the phenomena on this occasion, it would appear that Nature can carry on two processes at one and the same time; for while the separation is carried on by the absorbents, the arteries are forming themselves for suppuration: so that at the same time the part is going through these two very different species of inflammation.

† Vide Observations on certain Parts of the Animal Œconomy, Vol. IV. p. 176.

---

[a] [The admission of fresh air to recent wounds and exposed suppurating surfaces undoubtedly excites pain and eventually an accession of inflammation; which effects were found by Dr. Beddoes to be considerably increased by the use of pure oxygen, and proportionably diminished by the employment of the inert gases, nitrogen, carbonic acid gas, and hydrogen.]

by being wounded, &c., then the stimulus of imperfection is given, and the cells inflame, and unite if allowed; but if prevented, they then suppurate, granulate, &c.

The same observation is applicable to a wound made into the cavity of the abdomen of a fowl, for here the wound inflames and unites to the intestines to make it a perfect cavity again; but if this union is not allowed to take place, then more or less of the abdomen will inflame and suppurate.

If it was necessary that air should be admitted in order for suppuration to take place, we should not very readily account for suppuration taking place in the nose from a cold, as this part is not more under the influence of air at one time than at another; nor is the urethra in a gonorrhœa affected by the air more at that time than at any other. These parts being at all times under the same circumstances with respect to air, therefore there must be another cause.

The sympathetic fever has been supposed a cause, which will be considered when I treat of the formation of pus.

In cases of violence I have endeavoured to give a tolerably distinct idea of the steps leading to suppuration; but we are still at a loss with respect to the immediate cause of those suppurations which appear to arise spontaneously, for in these it is almost impossible to determine whether the inflammation itself be a real disease, viz. an original morbid affection, or whether it may not be (as is evidently the case when from external violence) a salutary process of nature to restore parts whose functions, and perhaps texture, has been destroyed by some previous and almost imperceptible disease or cause. Suppuration being, in cases of violence, a means of restoration, affords a presumption that it is a like instrument of nature in spontaneous cases. If it is the first, viz. a real disease, then two causes that are different in themselves can produce one effect, or one mode of action, for the result of both is the same; but if it is the last, then suppuration must be considered as depending on exactly the same stimulus being given, as in the above-mentioned instance of violence.

Suppuration does not arise from the violence of the action of the parts inflamed, for that circumstance simply rather tends to produce mortification; and we see that in the gout, which does not suppurate, there is often more violent inflammation than in many others that do. All internal canals likewise suppurate with very slight inflammation, when not in an irritable habit; but if of a very irritable disposition, the action will almost exceed suppuration, and by its becoming milder, suppuration will come on.

But if we suppose the cause of inflammation to be a disposition in the parts for such actions, without the parts themselves being either diseased or in such a state as to be similar to the destruction or alteration of their texture, this inflammation then may arise from a vast variety of causes with which we are at present totally unacquainted; nay, which we do not perhaps even suspect: and this last opinion, upon a slight view, would seem to be the most probable, because we can frequently put back these spontaneous inflammations, which would not be the case if they came on from the destruction of a part, or anything else, whose stimulus was similar to it, for no such thing can be done with wounds: if they are not soon united by the first intention, they must suppurate. However, this argument is not conclusive; for we can prevent suppuration in those arising from accident, by uniting them by the second intention, which prevents suppuration by acting as a kind of resolution.

Although suppuration is often produced without much visible violence of action in the part, yet when it is a consequence of a healthy inflammation, we find in general that the inflammation has been violent.

It [the suppurative inflammation] is always more violent than the preceding inflammation; and in such cases it would appear to be little more than an increased action, out of which is produced an entire new mode of action, and which of course destroys the first.

It is from this violence that inflammation produces its effects so quickly, for the inflammation which is capable of producing quickly so great a change in the operations of the parts, as suppuration, must be violent, because it is a violence committed upon the natural actions and structure of the parts.

This inflammation will also be more or less, according to the violence of the cause producing it, compared with the state of the constitution and parts affected.

The inflammation which precedes suppuration is much more violent in those cases where it appears to arise spontaneously, than when it arises from any injury done by violence. A suppuration equal in quantity to that from an amputation of the thigh, shall have been preceded by a much greater inflammation than that which is a consequence of the amputation.

This inflammation would seem to vary somewhat in its effects, according to the exertion of that power [viz. of the cause] during its progress; for in proportion to its rapidity [of action] the cause is certainly more simple, and its termination and effects more speedy and salutary; and this idea agrees perfectly with inflammation in consequence of accidents, for here it runs through its stages more rapidly, and with less inflammation; necessity appears to be the leading cause here.

This seems to be the case even in those parts which have a tendency to slow and specific diseases, as, for example, the breasts of women, or the testicles of men; for if these parts inflame quickly the effects will be more salutary than if they inflamed slowly. In other words, those parts are capable of being affected by the common suppurative inflammation, which in most cases terminates well. Perhaps the specific inflammation is slow in its progress and operation, and such slowness marks it to be an inflammation of some specific kind. In whatever light we view this fact it at least leads us with more certainty to what the effects of an inflammation will be, and thus often to form a just prognostic.

Suppuration takes place much more readily in internal canals than internal cavities.

Suppuration takes place more readily upon the surface of canals than in either the cellular or investing membrane. The same cause which would produce a suppuration in the first parts, would only produce the adhesive inflammation in the other; for instance, if a bougie is introduced into the urethra for a few hours, it will produce suppuration; while, if a bougie was introduced into either the tunica vaginalis testis, or the abdomen, but for a few hours, it would only give the disposition for adhesions, and even might not go the length of exciting this stage of inflammation in so short a time; but such surfaces often produce a greater variety of matter than a sore: it is not always pus: and this probably arises from the cause not being so easily got rid of. An irritation in the bladder, from stone, stricture in the urethra, or disease of the bladder itself, gives us a great variety of matter; pus, mucus, slime, are often all found; sometimes only one or two of them. I have some idea that the mucus is easiest of production; but I am certain that for the formation of slime the greatest irritation is required.

§. 1. *The Symptoms of the Suppurative Inflammation.*

This inflammation has symptoms common to inflammation in general, but it has these in a greater degree than the inflammation leading to it, and has also some symptoms peculiar to itself; it therefore becomes necessary to be particular in our description of these peculiarities.

The sensations arising from a disease generally convey some idea of its nature; the suppurative inflammation gives us as much as possible the idea of simple pain, without having a relation to any other mode of sensation: we cannot annex an epithet to it, but it will vary in some degree according to the nature of the parts going into suppuration; and what was remarked, when treating of the adhesive state, is in some degree applicable here. This pain is increased at the time of the dilating of the arteries, which gives the sensation called throbbing, in which every one can count his own pulse, from paying attention merely to the inflamed part; and perhaps this last symptom is one of the best characteristics of this species of inflammation. When the inflammation is moving from the adhesive state to the suppurative, the pain is considerably increased, which would seem to be the extent of this operation in the part; but when suppuration has taken place the pain in some degree subsides; however, as ulceration begins, it in some degree keeps up the pain, and this is more or less, according to the quickness of ulceration; but the sensation attending ulceration gives more the idea of soreness.

The redness that took place in the adhesive stage is now increased, and is of a pale scarlet. This is the true arterial colour, and is to be accounted a constant symptom, as we find it in all internal inflammations when at any time exposed, as well as in those that are external. Besides, I observed in the introduction to Inflammation, and when treating of the adhesive state, that the old vessels were dilated, and new ones were formed; these effects, therefore, are here carried still further in the surrounding parts which do not suppurate, and constitute two other causes of this redness being increased, by the vessels becoming still more numerous, and the red part of the blood being pushed more forward into many vessels, where only the serum and coagulating lymph went before.

The part which was firm, hard, and swelled while in the first stages, or the adhesive state, now becomes still more swelled by the greater dilatation of the vessels, and greater quantity of extravasated coagulating lymph thrown out in order to secure the adhesions. The œdematous swelling surrounding the adhesive gradually spreads into the neighbouring parts.

In spontaneous suppurations, one, two, three, or more parts of the inflammation lose the power of resolution, and assume exactly the same disposition with those of an exposed surface, or a surface in contact with an extraneous body. If it is in the cellular membrane that this disposition takes place, or in the investing membranes of circumscribed cavities, their vessels now begin to alter their disposition and mode of action, and continue changing till they gradually form themselves to that state which fits them to form pus; so that the effect or discharge is gradually changing from coagulating lymph to pus; hence we commonly find in abscesses both coagulating lymph and pus, and the earlier they are opened the greater is the proportion of the former. This gave rise to the common idea and expression, "That the matter is not concocted"; or "The abscess is not yet ripe ; the real meaning of which is, the abscess is not yet arrived at the true suppurative state.

From hence it must appear that suppuration takes place upon those surfaces without a breach of the solids or a dissolution of the parts, a circumstance not commonly allowed*[a]; and when got beyond the adhesive state they become similar in their suppuration to the inner surfaces of internal canals.

There is a certain period in the inflammation when the suppurative disposition takes place, which is discovered by new symptoms taking place in the constitution, viz. the shivering.

Although the sudden effects produced in the constitution would show that this change of disposition is pretty quick, yet its effects in the parts must be far from immediate, for some time is required for the vessels to be formed by it, so as to produce all the consequences intended by nature; and, indeed, we find it is some time before suppuration completely takes place, and that it is sooner or later, according as the inflamed state is backward in going off; for while the inflammation lasts, the part, as it were, hangs between inflammation and suppuration.

The effect of inflammation appears to be the producing of the suppurative disposition, or that state of a part which disposes it to form pus; in doing this the inflammation seems first to be carried to such a height as to destroy that state of the parts on which itself depends, the consequence of which is, that they lose the inflammatory disposition, and come into that which fits them for forming pus.

It seems to be a fixed and most useful law in the animal œconomy, that in spontaneous inflammation, when it has either destroyed the natural functions of parts, so much as to prevent their returning by a retrograde motion, as it were, to the state from whence they set out, or

* The knowledge of this fact in some of the larger cavities is not quite new, for I remember, about the year 1749 or 1750, that a young subject came under our inspection, and on opening the thorax it was found on the left side to contain a considerable quantity of pus. Upon examining the pleura and surface of the lungs, they were found to be perfectly entire. This was taken notice of by Dr. Hunter as a new fact, that suppuration could take place without a breach of surface, and he sent to Mr. Samuel Sharp to see it. It was also new to him, and he published it in his Critical Inquiry. Since that period it has been often observed in the peritonæal inflammation.

---

[a] [According to Dr. Thomson (Lectures on Inflammation, p. 316,) this doctrine was first distinctly suggested by Dr. Simpson of St. Andrew's, in his *Dissertationes de Re Medicâ*, published in the year 1722. De Haen, in 1756, adopted the same view, and Dr. Morgan more fully in 1763. Still, however, the prevailing opinion may have been different, and Mr. Hunter must certainly be supposed to have known what that was.]

where the first cause was a destruction of the natural functions, as an exposure of internal surfaces, that they form a disposition to the second method of cure. That the disposition for suppuration is very different from the actual state of inflammation, though produced by it, is proved by a variety of observations, for no perfect suppuration takes place till the inflammation is gone off; and as the inflammation ceases the disposition to suppuration gradually comes on. If, too, by any peculiarity in the constitution, or inflammation by which it is continued, or if by any accident an inflammation is brought on a healthy sore, the discharge and other appearances become the same as they were when the part from whence they arose was first in an inflamed state, very different from those observed when it was arrived at the state of a kind of suppuration.

§. 2. *Of the Treatment necessary in Inflammation when Suppuration must take place.*

In cases of inflammation arising from accident, but so circumstanced that we know suppuration cannot be prevented, the practice will be to moderate the inflammation if necessary, but not with a view to prevent suppuration; for if the powers are very great, and the violence committed very considerable, the inflammation will probably be very violent; and if it should have equal effects on the constitution, which will be in proportion to the quantity of surface inflamed, then certain constitutional means of relief will be necessary, such as bleeding, purging, regimen, and perhaps producing sickness; because, while that inflammation, continues to have effects upon the constitution, the suppuration which takes place will not be so kindly as it would otherwise be; but if the constitution is of the irritable kind, which will be generally known by the inflammation, the same practice as mentioned above is necessary; in short, whatever is to be the consequence, whether resolution or suppuration, the irritability and the too great action of the vessels, whether arising from too great powers, or too great action with small powers, are to be corrected or removed, as they in all cases counteract salutary operations.

In cases where the constitution has sympathized much with the inflamed part, such medicines as produce a slight perspiration much relieve the patient, such as antimonials, Dover's powder, saline draughts, spirits of mindererus, etc., because they endeavour to keep up a universal harmony, by putting the skin in good humour (which quiets every sympathizing part), and by counteracting the effects of the irritability.

Opium often lessens actions, although it seldom alters them, when only given as an opiate, and may be of a temporary service : however, this is not always a consequence of opium, as there are constitutions where it increases irritation, and of course diseased action.

Fresh wounds, considered simply as wounds, are all of the same nature, and require one uniform treatment, the intention being to put them into that situation in which they can suppurate with most ease to themselves ; and the first dressings commonly remain till suppuration comes on, unless some peculiarity from the situation of parts, or other collateral circumstances, should make it necessary to remove the dressings or vary the treatment.

The difference between one wound and another, with respect to the nature of the part wounded, will vary very much ; some will have small vessels wounded that cannot be conveniently got at, in order to tie them up, yet should be stopt from bleeding, which can be done by the mode of dressing, and therefore require dressing suitable to this circumstance alone.

Wounds opening into cavities, where peculiarities of the contained parts are joined with the injury done to them by the accident, will require a suitable mode of dressing ; the influence, too, that a simple wound in the containing parts may have upon those in the cavity, as a wound into the belly, thorax, joints, skull, etc., will oblige the surgeon to vary the mode of dressing from that of a simple wound ; while many wounds will require being kept open for fear of uniting again, in order to answer some future purpose, as the wound made into the tunica vaginalis testis, for the radical cure of the hydrocele; others may require attention being paid to them before suppuration comes on, and therefore should be so dressed as to admit of being soon and easily removed, to examine the parts occasionally as the symptoms arise. This ought to be the case in wounds of the head, attended or not attended with fracture of the skull. But whatever mode of application may be thought necessary to answer the various attending circumstances, yet as they are all wounds which are to come to suppuration, one general method is to be followed respecting them all, as far as those peculiarities will allow.

The application which has been made to wounds for some years past in this country has been in general dry lint. What brought this application into common practice most probably was, its assisting to stop the hemorrhage; and as most wounds are attended with bleeding, it became universal; but as it became universal, the first intention was lost sight of, and it became simply a first dressing.

I need hardly remark here, that all wounds that are to suppurate are first attended with inflammation, and therefore are so far similar to spontaneous inflammations which are to suppurate. If this observation is just, how contradictory must this mode of treatment be to common practice, when spontaneous inflammation has already taken place; for let me ask, where is the difference between an inflammation with a wound, and one without? And also, what should be the difference in the application to a part that is to inflame (while that application is made to the part), and one applied to an inflammation which has already taken place? The answer I should make to such a question is, there is no difference.

Wounds that are to suppurate, I have already observed, are first to go through the adhesive and suppurative inflammation. These inflammations in a wound are exactly similar to those spontaneous inflammations which suppurate and form an abscess, or those inflammations which ulcerate on the surface, and form a sore.

The applications to these which are now in practice, I have formerly observed, are poultices and fomentations; these, however, appear to be applied without much critical exactness or discrimination, for they are applied before suppuration has taken place, and where it is not intended it should take place; they are applied to inflammations where it is wished they should suppurate, and applied after suppuration has taken place. Now, with respect to suppuration itself, abstracted from all other considerations, the indication cannot be the same in all of those states; but if poultices and fomentations are found to be of real service in those two stages of the disease, then there must be something common to both, for which they are of service, abstracted from simple suppuration. I also formerly observed, that poultices were of service when the inflammation had attacked the skin, either of itself, or when an abscess had approached so near that the skin had become inflamed, and that this service consisted in keeping the skin soft and moist. This appears to me to be the use of a poultice in an inflammation, either before suppuration or after, as inflammation still exists, till it is opened; for inflammation is necessary in an abscess while it is making its approaches to the skin, which I have called the ulcerative; and then, and only then, it begins to subside; it is therefore still proper, inasmuch as it is of service to inflammation: so far, therefore, their practice is right and consistent, as the first reason exists through the whole; but when applied to inflamed parts, which are meant not to suppurate, their reasoning or principles upon which they applied it must fail them, although the application is still very proper.

If my first proposition is just, viz. that wounds which are allowed to suppurate are similar to inflammations that are also to suppurate, then let us see how far the two practices agree with this proposition. Lint,

I have observed, is applied to a fresh wound, which is to inflame; and the same lint is continued through the whole of the inflammation till suppuration comes on, because it cannot be removed. Lint, considered simply as an application to fresh wounds which are to inflame, is a very bad one, for it more or less adheres to the surface of the wound, by means of the extravasated blood; hence it becomes difficult of removal, and often shall remain in sores for months, being interwoven with the granulations, especially when applied to the surface of circumscribed cavities, such as the tunica vaginalis testis, after the operation for the hydrocele; however, this is not always the greatest inconvenience; the circumstance of its being loaded or soaked with blood, subjects it to become extremely hard when it dries, which it always does before the separation takes place, which separation is only effected by the suppuration. In this way it becomes the worst dressing possible for wounds.

As poultices are allowed by most to be the best application to an inflamed part, not attended by, or a consequence of, a wound, but considering it simply as an inflammation, I do conceive that the same application is the best for every inflammation, let it be from whatever cause; for the idea I have of the best dressing to a wound, simply as a wound, which is to inflame, is something that keeps soft and moist, and has no continuity of parts, so that it is easily separated. The only application of this kind is a poultice, which, from these qualities, is the very best application to a fresh wound. It keeps it soft and moist, and is at all times easily removed, either in part or the whole. The same medical advantage is gained here, as when it is applied to an inflamed part; but although it had not these advantages, yet the circumstance of being easily removed is much in its favour, especially when compared to dry lint.

But a poultice, from other circumstances, cannot at all times and in all places be conveniently applied. To preserve the above properties, it is necessary there should be a mass, much too large for many purposes; but when they can be used with tolerable convenience, they are the best applications. When they cannot be applied with ease, I should still object to dry lint, and would therefore recommend the lint to be covered with some oily substance, so that the blood shall not entangle itself with the lint, but may lie soft, and come easily off.

This mode of dressing should be continued for several days, or at least till fair suppuration comes on, and when that has taken place, then dry lint may be with great propriety used, except the sore is of some specific kind, which is seldom the case in fresh wounds; for accidental wounds seldom happen to specific diseases; and a wound in consequence of an operation should not be specific, because the specific affection (if there is any) should have been removed by the operation; and should therefore be a wound in the sound part, as after an amputation of a scrofulous joint, or the extirpation of a cancerous breast. Or if they take on some specific disposition afterwards, then they must be dressed accordingly, as will be explained hereafter.

Poultices are commonly made too thin, by which means the least pressure, or their own gravity, removes them from the wound; they should be thick enough to support a certain form when applied. They are generally made of stale bread and milk; this composition, in general, makes a too brittle application; it breaks easily into different portions from the least motion, and often leaves some part of the wound uncovered, which is frustrating the first intention. The poultice which makes the best application, and continues most nearly the same between each dressing, is that formed of the meal of linseed; it is made at once*, and when applied it keeps always in one mass. Fomentations are generally applied at this stage of the wound, and they generally give ease at the time of application, which has (joined with custom) been always a sufficient inducement to continue them. As soon as suppuration is well established, the part may then be dressed according to the appearances of the sore itself.

The kind of wound to which the above application is best adapted, is a wound made in a sound part which we intend shall heal by granulation. The same application is equally proper where parts are deprived of life, and consequently will slough. It is therefore the very best dressing for a gunshot wound, and probably for most lacerated wounds. For lint applied to a part that is to throw off a slough will often be retained till that slough is separated, which will be for eight, ten, or more days.

In the treatment of wounds that are to suppurate, it is in one view of the subject right to allow the parts to take their natural and spontaneous bent. From the natural elasticity of the skin, and the contraction of muscles, the parts wounded are generally exposed, and from the consequent inflammation they generally become more so. This is commonly more the case in wounds produced by accident; for [in operations,] as a small wound and much old skin are always desirable, surgeons very wisely are anxious to wish for both. In many operations they are desirous of preserving the skin, viz. where they are removing parts. as a limb, dissecting out tumours, or opening an abscess; all of which is extremely proper, and they continue to practice upon this principle immediately upon the receiving the wound, and in performing

* Take boiling water q. s. and stir in the linseed till it becomes of a sufficient thickness. and then add a small quantity of some sweet oil.

any of the above-mentioned operations; for the skin, after amputation, is drawn down and bound down, and the wounds are pressed together by bandages. In one point of view this is beginning too early; it is beginning it when Nature has the very opposite principle in view: inflammation the parts must submit to, and as inflammation by its effects will generally have a tendency to make them recede more, in this light it is proper not to check the effects of inflammation; therefore let them take their own way till inflammation subsides and granulations are formed, which granulations, I have already observed, by their power of contraction, will do what we wanted to have done; and if, from some of the first circumstances not being properly attended to, the contraction of the granulations is not sufficient, then is the time to assist, and not before. However, if we take up this in another point of view, we shall see a considerable utility arising from bringing the skin as much as possible over the wound, and keeping it there; for in the time of inflammation the parts will adhere or unite in this situation, by which means the sore will be less than it otherwise would; and I conceive that this practice, when begun, should be for some time continued, for fear the adhesions may not be sufficient to stand their ground till the granulations can assist.

It often happens in many wounds, both from accident and operations, that part of the wound may with great propriety be healed by the first intention; such as in many accidents on the head, when a part of the scalp has been torn off, on the face, &c., as also after many operations, especially where the skin is loose, as in the scrotum; or where the skin has been attended to in the time of the operation, as in some methods of amputation, extirpation of breasts, &c., a part of the saved skin, &c. may be made to unite to the parts underneath by the first intention, and therefore only part of the wound be allowed to suppurate. In all such cases a proper contracting or sustaining bandage may be applied with great advantage; even stitches may be used with great propriety, as was recommended in the healing of wounds by the first intention.

§. 3. *The Treatment of the Inflammation when Suppuration has taken place.*

In spontaneous inflammations, whether from a constitutional or local affection, when suppuration has taken place, it is most probable that another mode of practice must be followed than that which was pursued to prevent it; but even now, if a stop could be put to the further formation of matter, after it has begun, it would in many cases be very proper, and still prevent a great deal of mischief. Suppuration does certainly sometimes stop, after having begun, which shows that there is a principle in the animal œconomy[a] by which the machine is capable of producing this effect*.

I have seen buboes cured by vomits, after suppuration has been considerably advanced, and it is a very common termination of scrofulous abscesses; but in scrofulous abscesses we very seldom find inflammation This process appears to be a leading circumstance in ulceration, which is the very reverse of union[b] even in superficial sores, which are the most likely to continue suppuration if excited, we find by allowing them to scab, when they will admit of it, that the act which admits of scabbing is the reverse of suppuration, and it ceases; however, it is a process which the animal œconomy does not readily accept of, and our powers in producing this effect are but very small. If these powers could be increased by any means it would be a salutary discovery, be-

* I have formerly observed, that the inflammation often goes off without producing suppuration; and I have also mentioned instances of suppuration going off without the parts having produced granulations, and then the parts fall back into the adhesive state, and the matter being absorbed, they are left in nearly the same state as before the inflammation came on: as a presumptive proof of this, in many of the large cavities which have been allowed to inflame and suppurate (by having been opened) we find them often doing well, without ever forming granulations, and that suppuration generally goes off; and I do not believe that they ever fall back into the adhesive state, so as to unite the parts, but the parts resume their original and natural state or disposition, and no adhesions are formed. This appears sometimes to happen in cases of the empyema after the operation has been performed[c]. I have seen cases where wounds had been made into the cavity of the thorax, where there was every reason to suppose the whole cavity was in a state of suppuration, and yet those patients got well. I can hardly suppose that in these cases the parts had granulated and united in the cure, as the cellular membrane does, because I have seen many similar cases where the patients have died and no granulations have been found; and I have seen cases of the hydrocele attempted to be cured radically by the caustic, in which, when the slough came out, suppuration came on, but the orifice healing too soon, suppuration has ceased, and the cure was thought to be completed; but a return of the disease has led to another attempt, and, by laying open the whole sac, it has been found that the tunica vaginalis was perfectly entire: in such the fluids were a mothery serum. I have seen abscesses go back in the same manner; but I believe that this process is more common to scrofulous suppurations than any other, and I believe to the erysipelatous. I have seen joints heal after having suppurated and been opened, without having produced granulations, leaving a kind of joint, even when the cartilages have exfoliated from the ends of the bones, which was known by the grating of the two ends of the bones on one another.

[a] [" Animal œconomy of diseases" in the text.]

[b] [The meaning of the author I apprehend to be, that even in ulceration, which is an act directly opposed to reunion, the cessation or diminution of discharge is a leading circumstance towards the cure.]

[c] [See Vol. I., p. 443, *note.*]

cause suppuration itself in many cases proves fatal: for instance, suppuration of the brain and its membranes, of the thorax and its contents, as well as of the abdomen and its contents, in short, suppuration of any of the vital parts, often kills of itself, simply from the matter being produced. But this practice will by most be forbidden in many cases of suppuration, for it is supposed this very suppuration is a deposit of matter or humours already formed in the constitution; but it is to be hoped that time and experience will get rid of such prejudices.

When suppuration cannot be stopped or resolved, then in most cases it is to be hurried on, which generally is the first step taken by surgeons.

How far suppuration can be increased by medicine or applications I do not know; but attempts are generally made, and thence we have suppurating cataplasms, plasters, &c. recommended to us, which are composed of the warmer gums, seeds, &c., but I doubt very much if they have considerable effect in this way: for if the same applications were made to a sore they would hardly increase the discharge of that sore, but probably rather decrease it. However, in many cases, where the parts are indolent and hardly admit of true inflammation, in consequence of which a perfect suppuration cannot take place, by stimulating the skin a more salutary inflammation may be produced, and of course a quicker suppuration; but in the true suppuration, where inflammation has preceded it, I believe it is hardly necessary to do anything with respect to suppuration itself: however, from experience, I believe these applications have been found to bring the matter faster to the skin, even in the most rapid suppurations, which was supposed to be an increased formation of matter; but it can only be in those cases where the inner surface of the abscess is within the influence of the skin. This effect arises from another cause or mode of action being produced than that of quickening suppuration, which is the hastening on of ulceration. I have mentioned that ulceration was an effect of, or at least attended by, inflammation; and therefore whatever increases that inflammation will also increase the ulceration, which will bring the matter sooner to the skin, without an increased formation of matter.

Poultices of bread and milk are commonly used to inflamed parts when suppuration is known to have taken place. These applications can have no effect upon suppuration, excepting by lessening inflammation, or rather making the skin easy under them, for we observed that true suppuration did not begin till inflammation was abated; but the inflammation must have reached the skin before poultices can have much effect, for they can only affect that part.

It may be thought necessary that the ease of the patient should be considered, and we find that fomentations and poultices often produce that effect; we find too, that by keeping the cuticle moist and warm the sensitive operations of the nerves of the parts are soothed or lulled to rest; while, on the contrary, if the inflamed skin is allowed to dry, the inflammation is increased; and as probably suppuration is not checked by such treatment, it ought to be put into practice: as warmth excites action, it is probable the warmer the fomentation so much the better; and in many cases the action is increased so that they can hardly bear it.

§. 4. *Collections of Matter without Inflammation.*

I have hitherto been describing true suppuration, which I have said, "I believe is a consequence only of inflammation," a process generally allowed. Also in treating on the cause of suppuration, viz. inflammation, I hinted that there were often swellings, or thickening of parts, without the visible or common symptoms of inflammation, viz. without pain, change of colour, &c.; and I also hinted, in treating of suppuration, that there were collections of matter, somewhat similar to suppuration, which did not arise in consequence of the common inflammation: these I shall now consider. I conceive all such collections of matter to be of a scrofulous nature: they are most common in the young subject, and seldom found in the full-grown or old: they are commonly called matter or pus, and therefore I choose to contrast true suppuration with them. Although I have termed this suppuration, yet it has none of its true characters, any more than the swellings, which are the forerunners of it, have the true characters of inflammation; and as I did not call them inflammatory, strictly speaking I should not call this suppuration; but I have no other term expressive of it.

Many indolent tumours, slow swellings in the joints, swellings of the lymphatic glands, tubercles in the lungs, and swellings in many parts of the body, are diseased thickenings, without visible inflammation; and the contents of some kinds of encysted tumours; the matter of many scrofulous suppurations, as in the lymphatic glands; the suppuration of many joints, viz. those scrofulous suppurations in the joints of the foot and hand; in the knee, called white swellings; the joint of the thigh, commonly called hip-cases; the loins, called lumbar abscesses; the discharge of the above-mentioned tubercles in the lungs, as well as in many other parts of the body, are all instances of matter being formed without any previous visible inflammation, and are therefore in this one respect all very similar to one another. They come on insensibly, the first symptom being commonly the swellings, in consequence of the thickening;

which is not the case with inflammation, for there the sensation is the first symptom.

These formations of matter, although they do approach the skin, yet do not do it in the same manner as collections of pus. They do not produce readily either the elongating or the ulcerative process, and as the matter was not preceded by the adhesive inflammation, these collections are more easily moved from their original seat into some other part by any slight pressure, such as the weight of their own matter; from which I have called them abscesses in a part, in opposition to abscesses of a part: when the matter does approach the skin, it is commonly by merely a distension of the part, coming by a broad surface, not attended with any marks of pointing. Their surrounding parts or boundaries are soft, not being attended with thickening; more especially those in a part.

Such collections of matter are always larger than they would have been, if they had been either a consequence of inflammation or attended by it: this is owing to their indolence, allowing of great distention beyond the extent of the first disease, and even of their moving into other parts; whereas an abscess in consequence of inflammation is confined to the extent of inflammation that takes on suppuration, and its rapid progress towards the skin prevents distention, and of course extension of the disease.

All those formations of matter not preceded by inflammation, nor a consequence of it, are I believe similar to each other, having in this respect one common principle, very different from inflammation. The cancer, although it produces a secretion, yet does not produce pus till exposed; it is therefore one of those diseases, like the scrofula, which does not suppurate till inflammation comes on, and even seldom then; for true suppuration arises from inflammation, terminating in a disposition to heal, which is not the case with cancer. In the scrofulous suppuration there is often a like reluctance to heal.

The kind of matter is another distinguishing mark between that produced in consequence of inflammation and what is formed without it, the last being generally composed of a curdly substance mixed with a flaky matter. The curdly substance is, we may suppose, the coagulating lymph deprived of its serum*, and the other or flaky is probably the same, only in smaller parts; it looks like the precipitate of animal matter from an acid or an alkali.

So far these productions of matter in their remote and immediate

* I may observe here that the coagulating lymph of long standing is not similar to the recent. This is similar to blood in general, for we find that the blood in aneurisms, which was first coagulated, is very different from that which has only coagulated lately.

causes are not in the least similar to that arising from common inflammation; nor is the effect, viz. the matter, similar; and to show still further that suppuration is always preceded by inflammation, the very surfaces which form the above matter immediately produce true matter when the inflammation comes on, which it always does whenever opened; which I shall now consider.

Since they are not similar in their causes or modes of production, let us next examine how far they are similar in their first steps towards a cure.

All parts which form matter of any kind, viz. whether in consequence of inflammation or otherwise, must go through similar processes to produce the ultimate effect or cure. The first step in either is the evacuation of this matter, for till this is effected, Nature cannot pursue the proper means towards a cure; and if opened, the second step is granulation, and the third cicatrization. To accomplish the evacuation of the matter there are two modes: one is the absorption of the matter, which is very common in the scrofula, or those productions of matter not preceded by inflammation: this produces no alteration in the part, except that it gradually creeps into a sound state, the parts uniting again that had been separated by the accumulation of the matter; it produces also no alteration in the constitution: absorption, however, seldom takes place in suppuration which is the consequence of inflammation. The other mode of discharging this matter is either by opening the abscess, in order to allow it to pass out, or by allowing ulceration to take place from the inside to produce its escape; and this process, in the present case, having peculiarities different from those arising from inflammation, it is necessary they should be understood. Ulceration in consequence of suppuration arising from inflammation is very rapid, especially if the suppuration is so likewise; but ulceration in consequence of matter being formed which is not the effect of inflammation is extremely slow: it will remain months, even years, before the parts have completely given way; they commonly come to the skin by a broad surface, and not pointing like a circumscribed abscess in consequence of inflammation; so far are these two different[a].

---

[a] [That Mr. Hunter should have overlooked the analogies which connect the class of facts, referred to in this section, with ordinary suppuration, and insisted only on their dissimilarities, might justly excite our surprise, if we did not reflect that his argument is ultimately based on the assumption that inflammation is a salutary process, and not a diseased action; a doctrine which it is evident could derive no support from the phenomena of chronic abscesses. In this mode of argumentation, however, the same fallacy is involved as in the author's speculations on the venereal disease, in which, having laid down the proposition that mercury is essential to its cure, he afterwards argues on this fact, adopting it as the only unequivocal test of the existence of the dis-

§. 5. *Of the effects such Formations of Matter have on the Constitution.*

Whatever may be the extent of such collections of matter, they seldom if ever affect the constitution, unless they are seated in a vital part, or so connected with it as to disturb its functions. This is an effect of indolence in any disease. A young person shall have a lumbar abscess, for instance, for years, without a single constitutional symptom. It shall appear to be making its way through a number of parts, such as the loins behind, the buttocks, the lower part of the abdomen before, and through the upper part of the thigh; and in each part shall show large collections of matter. All these shall even attend the same person, and yet not any bad symptoms nor any shiverings shall accompany this suppuration*. In some there is not even the least degree of lameness, but this is often the first symptom of the disease in the lumbar abscess.

Let us next consider and compare the consequences attending these two collections of matter when opened. When an abscess, in consequence of inflammation, is opened, it immediately proceeds towards a cure, and

* I have heard surgeons ask such patients if they had rigors, even alluding to the time of increase; this was applying the idea of the symptom of one disease to another, and also the first stage of a disease to the second.

---

ease; just as in the present case, having determined that "true suppuration arises from inflammation, terminating in a disposition to heal," the cases which do not correspond with this condition are considered as non-inflammatory. Undoubtedly the symptoms which mark the presence of inflammation in many chronic suppurations are often obscurely developed, but so are those which characterize the adhesive inflammation which precedes the approach of aneurisms and foreign bodies to the surface, or the formation of internal cysts, or the ulceration of the bones of the spine. Such indolent swellings, however, and chronic collections of matter, as are referred to by the author, almost always exhibit indications of increased heat, vascularity, and sensibility when near the surface of the body, while the causes to which they may in most cases be referred, the products in which they commonly result, and the adhesions which invariably accompany their progress, so closely resemble those belonging to genuine inflammation that it is impossible to distinguish them. Whatever differences therefore may exist must be regarded as differences of degree. Still, however, the question cannot be considered as decided whether suppuration may not take place independently of inflammation; for large collections of matter are sometimes found to occur simultaneously in various parts of the body without any well-defined marks of inflammation before or after death, or even the existence of mischief having been suspected until it has been fully revealed by dissection. Such purulent collections are most commonly found to occur in certain forms of constitutional irritation, of which that attending phlebitis may be regarded as the type, and often present the appearance of purulent metastases. I should conceive, however, that even these cases depend on inflammation, as it often happens that coagulable lymph, either alone or in conjunction with pus, is poured out under such circumstances.]

perhaps it may have gone some steps towards a cure before opening; the inflammation still lessens, the suppuration becomes more perfect, granulations begin to form, and all of these steps naturally take place, because inflammation had been the cause; but when a collection of matter not preceded by inflammation is opened, a very different process is first to take place, viz. inflammation is now excited over the whole cavity of the abscess, which afterwards produces a perfect matter, similar to that produced in consequence of inflammation, when it is the original disease, and which now produces its constitutional affection, if it is such as to have connexion with the constitution; but this will depend on the size of the abscess, the situation and the nature of the parts, &c. However, it sometimes happens that they inflame before they are opened; but this is in consequence of the matter distending the cavity, and thereby acting as an extraneous body. I have seen white swellings in the knee inflame before they were opened, then ulceration take place, and the pus brought soon to the skin, even after it had been confined for months, without producing the least tendency to ulceration, because there had been none to inflammation; but the confinement of the matter becomes a cause of the inflammation, and then ulceration takes place.

The inflammation and new suppuration taking place in consequence of opening into these abscesses is exactly similar to those arising in consequence of wounds or openings made into natural cavities; it was still, therefore, necessary that they should go through all the common steps towards restoration; but unfortunately such inflammations have begun at the wrong end; they have also set down upon a specific disease, which they can seldom alter to their own nature. The inflammation is in such cases extended over a much larger surface than the original; which is not the case in abscess in consequence of inflammation, for there the inflammation was the cause and confined to the point. In some cases, as in lumbar abscess, the extent of surface to inflame is immense in comparison to the extent of the original disease; and of course, when such abscesses inflame, the symptoms in the constitution are in the same proportion.

How different is this from the opening of the abscess in consequence of inflammation! There we have no inflammation following, except what arises in consequence of the wound made in the solids in the operation of opening; but when it is allowed to open of itself there is no consequent inflammation, but suppuration goes on. But it would appear that when those collections of matter are allowed to open of themselves, that the succeeding inflammation does not so readily take place as when opened by art. I have seen large lumbar abscesses open of themselves on the lower part of the loins, which have discharged a large quantity of matter, then closed up, then broke out anew, and so on for months, without giving any other disturbance[a]; but when opened, so as to give a free discharge to the matter, inflammation has immediately succeeded, fever has come on, and, from the situation of the parts inflamed, as well as their extent, death in a very days after has been the consequence: it therefore often becomes a question whether we should enlarge the first opening or not. We may observe in general that in cases of this kind, where they are to terminate ill, that is, where they cannot be cured, and are such as to affect the constitution, the consequent inflammation upon opening them, which produces the sympathetic fever, has that fever commonly terminating in the hectic, or continued into the hectic, before any recess takes place, so that the one is continued into the other without any intermission; however, this is not always the case, and those variations will depend on the state of the sore, the state of the constitution, &c.

§. 6. *The Effects of the Suppurative Inflammation on the Constitution.*

It is to be observed, that every local complaint of any consequence, or which has considerable and quick action within itself, although not of considerable magnitude, affects more or less the constitution, and gives rise to what has been commonly called the symptomatic fever. These symptoms are the sympathies of the constitution with a local disease or injury, and will vary according to a vast variety of circumstances. They will vary according to the nature of the constitution, which admits of great differences, and which will include different ages; they will vary according to the nature of the part in a state of disease, which also admits of great differences; they will vary according to the quantity of mischief done, as well as the manner of its being done; that is, whether so as to call forth immediate inflammation, as a wound; or not so immediate, as from having only killed a part: they will vary according to the situation of similar parts in the body; and they will vary according to the stage of the disease. This last variation may be divided into two

---

[a] [It was in imitation of this method of Nature that the late Mr. Abernethy suggested the propriety of opening large abscesses by a small valvular aperture, discharging part of the contents, and then healing up the opening. (See his Works, vol. ii.) There is reason to believe that the inflammation which frequently succeeds the discharge of large abscesses in the common way is due to the admission of air, which acting on the effused blood, or perhaps on the matter itself, occasions decomposition. In this manner the sac is directly irritated, and the constitution greatly disturbed by the absorption of putrid matter.]

kinds, the one which begins slowly and increases progressively, as in the venereal disease, and the sympathetic affections of course come on gradually; the other, where it begins at once with violence, and afterwards diminishes. The first of this last division we have nothing to do with at present; it is, therefore, the kind of constitution, the kind of parts, the diseases which commence with so much violence as to affect the constitution at once, with the constitutional effects arising from the local disease being incurable, that form our present subject.

I shall observe here, that every disease, whether local or constitutional, that has the power of termination in itself, commonly has its regular progress and stated times of action; in some, however, there are no changes in the modes of action, the disease coming on and dying away; but in others there are; and in those where changes take place there are stated periods for those changes, so as to render them regular. As regularity in the modes of action in disease is conducive to the termination of that disease, it is a thing very much to be desired, for these changes are a cessation of the action, either temporary or permanent.

As the constitution sympathizes with a local irritation, and as that sympathy is according to the constitution, to the violence of the irritation, and to the nature of the parts irritated; and as the symptoms of that sympathy must be similar to constitutional complaints that are commonly taking place; if the local complaint should not be known, then they will be taken for constitutional complaints wholly, and treated as such: but often, from their continuance, some local affection is suspected: local complaints, however, are commonly preceded or attended with some local symptom, either directly or indirectly, or with some collateral symptom or symptoms, so as to direct us to the cause.

Local complaints attended with inflammations, the objects of surgery, are often attended with, or rather consequent upon, violence of some kind, such as the loss of a part, either fluid or solid, which the constitution feels, and which loss or violence adds to the constitutional affection. This will be according to the quantity of injury or loss of living matter, whether blood or some solid, the time in the operation, the state of the parts operated upon, and the nature of the part removed. I have seen a man die almost immediately upon the loss of a testicle: I have seen convulsions immediately attend the operation for the hydrocele, so that I have almost despaired of recovery: I have seen a most violent sympathetic fever, delirium, and death follow, in consequence of dividing parts in the leg, and searching after a bleeding artery. The loss of a limb above the knee is more than many can bear: the cutting for the stone, where it breaks, and may be an hour in extracting, is also more than many can bear; the parts being in such a diseased state as not to be relieved, have continued the symptoms of the disease: and the loss of a testicle, although of so small a size, when compared with many other parts which we can lose with impunity, yet from its vital connexion is more serious. We cannot bear to lose much brain.

The loss of too much blood is often an attendant on, or a consequence of operations, but sometimes takes place without much violence. This produces very considerable constitutional effects; bringing on weakness, and many complaints, depending, as it were, upon debility, which are what are commonly called nervous. I have seen a locked-jaw come on in consequence of the loss of a considerable quantity of blood, the cause of the loss being but trifling, and giving no symptoms whatever.

The nature of the cause of inflammation produces, I believe, but little variation in the constitution, for of whatever kind it is, the symptoms in the constitution will be in all cases nearly the same, proportioned only to the violence and rapidity of its progress; and as this [viz. the suppurative] inflammation is pretty violent, more especially if it produces healthy suppuration, it generally produces more violent effects upon the constitution than any other; this, however, will be in some degree according to the susceptibility of the constitution for inflammation; and if any difference takes place in the inflammation in one constitution from that of another, it will arise from the nature of the constitution, and the nature of parts and their situation, and not from the nature of the cause.

The sympathy of the constitution with a local disease is what I have called universal sympathy, and is, perhaps, the most simple act of a constitution; it is the sympathy with a simple violence, as a cold, etc., but still it will vary in different constitutions, because all constitutions will not act alike under the influence of a local disease, although it will vary according to the stages of inflammation, according to the natural disposition of the parts inflamed, and according to the situation of those parts in the body; yet it may be the most simple act of that constitution at the time, for although it would appear at the time to be an increase of the disease by its becoming universal, yet as it is a natural consequence it is a much better sign of health than if no fever had occurred in consequence of considerable injuries, for if there was no inflammation, there would probably be little or no fever. Nature requires to feel the injury; for where, after a considerable operation, there is rather a weak quiet pulse, often with a nervous oppression, with a seeming difficulty of breathing and a loathing of food, the patient is in a dangerous way. Fever shows powers of resistance; the other symptoms show weakness and sinking under the injury. This is like the effects of the cold bath; yet we see it calling forth, or rousing up to action, some peculiarity in the constitution, or a part, which may be continued after the sympathetic action is lost, and which may again reflect back upon the part its reluctance to heal. This may be exemplified by the affections of scrofula, and even cancer, arising in consequence of injury*[a].

Rigors are commonly the first symptom of a constitutional affection; but a rigor is productive of other effects or symptoms, as it were naturally arising out of the rigor; and these are according to the nature of the constitution. In a strong constitution a hot period succeeds, as if the constitution was roused to action to resist debility, which terminates the rigor; and this hot fit terminates in perspiration, which is the complete action of the disease, restoring tranquillity, which is the cure, and the best termination that can happen where a rigor takes place, for it shows that the constitution has the power of terminating the effects of the cause. I believe, however, that in most cases it shows a degree of weakness, especially if easily excited, or a peculiarity of constitution. But as the cause is still continuing in cases of rigor arising from local irritation, these rigors may recur; and if they recur, it shows a constitution ready to be affected; however, if they do recur at stated periods, it still shows the constitution to be able to resist the effects of the disease. Further, if the constitution is weak a rigor comes on, and no hot fit succeeds, but it runs directly into the sweat, which will probably be cold and clammy. If it is a constitution of another kind the hot fit will continue, having only a kind of abatement; but no sweat or perfect intermission will take place, and therefore the whole action has not taken place.

Rigors from local irritation, attended with the full action, and at re-

* I believe that local specific irritations do not produce much variety in the constitution; for I am persuaded that specific local irritations are not capable of altering that constitution, similar to the plague and other contagious diseases. I believe that morbid poisons do not act by any peculiar mode of action in the part, so as to affect the constitution in any peculiar way, if we except such as are capable of continuing so long as to weaken that constitution, as, for instance, the lues, when of long standing; but even this will be similar to every other lasting disease, for at first it certainly does not affect the constitution so as to alter the disposition of a wound made upon another part. I am not so certain respecting natural poisons. The ticunas, poisoned arrow, [*Upas tieuté*,] etc. would seem to produce a peculiar constitutional affection from a local cause, for we can hardly suppose absorption to have taken place in so short a time[b].

---

[a] ["This may be exemplified by affection or injury, scrofula, even cancer, &c."—*Original text.*]

[b] [This question, which has been made the subject of a great deal of interesting discussion and experiment of late years, must still be considered as undecided, although, upon the whole, the balance still inclines to the doctrine as here laid down by the author. The late ingenious researches by Mr. Morgan and Dr. Addison on this subject strongly confirm this view.]

gular stated times, have all the characters of an intermittent fever; but it may be observed that, in common, rigors preceding suppuration are not followed by so much heat and sweating as those in an intermittent.

In spontaneous inflammations it is not so easy to ascertain whether the constitution or the part is first affected; and if we always could, it would be the best guide to know whether the inflammation was local entirely, or an effect of a constitutional affection: nothing but the priority of the symptoms can in some degree fix this; but the constitutional symptoms are often so slight, at least at first, as not to be taken notice of. However, we know that indispositions of the constitution are productive of local complaints, which are often attended with inflammation, but which is often according to the nature of the parts*, the constitution being first diseased; and we know that in many fevers there is suppuration in some part of the body, and often in particular parts, such as the parotid glands, probably according to the nature of the fever; such inflammations will, according to their violence, add to the constitutional affection. Constitutional affection arising from inflammations will be almost coeval with the inflammations, or at least will very soon follow; however, that will be according to the circumstance before related, for inflammation is an act of the part, attended with a degree of violence, and the constitution will feel it sooner or later, according to circumstances: we see in cases of inflammation of the testicles from a gonorrhœa (which must be considered as entirely local), that the constitution is soon affected by it. But constitutional symptoms arise from external violence alone, and more especially when attended with loss of substance; and they will be sooner or later, according to the degree of the violence, and the importance of the parts lost, agreeably to what has been said; but simple violence, even with the loss of a part, I have already observed, is not of such consequence as we should at first imagine, for in consequence of the loss of a limb, if the parts are allowed to heal by the first intention, the constitution is but little affected; it is, therefore, violence with loss of substance, and which is to produce inflammation and suppuration, that gives rise to the constitutional symptoms; and when these commence, or more probably when the part sets about these operations, the constitution becomes affected. It is more the new disposition in the parts, than the quantity of inflammatory action in them, by which the constitution is affected, for we shall see that upon

* Local inflammations arising from derangement of the constitution I think are most commonly of the scrofulous kind, more especially when in parts of a particular nature, such as lymphatic glands and ligamentous or tendinous parts, which, when in particular situations, are often supposed to be venereal. Vide Treatise on Venereal Disease, Vol. II.

the simple commencement of the suppurative disposition, before it has taken place, rigors, etc. come on.

The constitutional effects arising upon the commencement of inflammation, independent of situation, of vital parts, nerves, &c., are greater or less according to the nature of the disease. When the adhesive stage commences it has but very little effect upon the whole system; there is sometimes, however, a rigor, although not always; this is more in common spontaneous inflammations than in those arising from an injury done to a part, but such are seldom or ever alarming. When the suppurative disposition takes place, new effects upon the constitution arise, which are very considerable and varying in themselves. The cold fits or rigors are more frequently felt at the commencement of the suppurative than at the beginning of the adhesive inflammation, more especially too if it is what we commonly call spontaneous inflammations, which advance to suppuration; for in those inflammations occasioned by an accident or an operation, which must suppurate, they [the inflammations] appear to set out at the very first with a kind of suppurative disposition. Those arising in consequence of spontaneous inflammation, or from an injury, are not lasting, are often succeeded by hot fits, and if they terminate in perspiration then the patient is relieved; and are more or less so according to the greatness of the present inflammation, and the suppuration that is likely to follow, joined to the nature of the parts and their situation: if in vital parts they will be most violent, and, next to these, in parts far from the heart. This cold fit is indeed a constant symptom in most local diseases which affect the constitution, and in this case plainly shows that the constitution is so affected, or sympathizes with the part. It is thus also that fevers usually commence, and upon the absorption of any poisonous matter the same symptoms appear. I have seen them arise from a simple prick in the end of a finger, made with a clean sewing needle*, exactly similar to those arising from the absorption of poison. Disagreeable applications to the stomach produce them, and also disagreeable affections of the mind; but rigors are not confined to the commencement of disease, for they occur in its progress and sometimes at its termination, as will be mentioned.

It is probable that the stomach is the cause of those rigors by its taking part in the diseased action of the constitution; for as the stomach is the seat of simple animal life, and thereby the organ of universal sympathy of the materia vitæ or the living principle, it is of course more or less affected upon all these occasions; so that an affection of any part of the body and of the mind can produce very nearly

* Hence it would seem as if simple irritation in a part was capable of affecting the whole nervous system.

the same effect as that which arises from disagreeable applications to the stomach itself; which accounts for that viscus taking part in all constitutional affections. I am inclined to believe that sympathy of the stomach which occasions sickness arises from causes producing weakness or debility. It takes place from injuries or disorders of the brain, which occasion universal debility; it arises from loss of blood, and also from epileptic fits. How far the sickness is to be considered as an effect which is to produce action, viz. vomiting, and which action is to reflect strength back upon the constitution, I do not know; but it is certain that people who are sick and going to faint are prevented by the action of vomiting; the act of vomiting, therefore, appears often to be a cause of the prevention of the fits coming on, by rousing up the actions of life. The rigors I should be apt to suspect arise from weakness at the time. A sudden alteration, a sudden call, or a sudden and universal irritation upon the constitution will, I imagine, produce immediate weakness; for every new action in a constitution must produce or tend to produce a weakness in that function, the effects of which will vary according to the necessity and state of the constitution. In some cases where the constitution is strong, and as it were equal of itself to the task, it will call up the animal powers to action, and produce the hot fit of a fever; but in weak constitutions, or in such as threaten dissolution, as in many diseases, especially towards the close, it loses by every rigor, and is seldom capable of producing a hot fit, but only occasions a cold clammy sweat; hence cold sweats, when a person is in extremities, is a common symptom. That rigors are an effect of every sudden change in the constitution, and are not peculiar to the commencement of disease, is evident from the following cases; which also prove that even the change to health shall produce the same effect, so that not only in its commencement and in its different stages a disease shall produce rigors, but in its termination or crisis.

A boy about eleven months [years?] old was taken ill with a complaint, which could not be well understood from the symptoms, and which came on insensibly; his pulse was quick and full, for which he was bled three times, and the blood was rather sizy; the tongue was white; he was not very hot, but uneasy and restless, with loss of appetite. His stools were upon the whole pretty natural; he was observed to be every other day rather worse, although there never was a perfect intermission, but only a kind of remission. After having been ill for about a fortnight in this way, he was taken with a cold shivering fit, succeeded by a hot fit, and then a sweat. My opinion was that the disease was now formed, and that he would have more at the intermitting times; but he had no more after. In short, the disease formed itself into that which has but one fit, and in this formation he had those symptoms. I have seen the same symptoms in many diseases, especially those occasioned by an operation, which in general alarm, but which should not if they go through their stages.

A patient of mine, at St. George's Hospital, was cut for the stone; he had no uncommon symptoms for several weeks, when he was taken with a cold fit, which was succeeded by a hot one, and then by a profuse sweat. The young gentlemen of the hospital were rather alarmed, conceiving them to be the signs of dissolution; but I told them that this was of no consequence, as the disease had completed its full action; that it was either a regular ague, or arose from the irritation of the wound; and if the first, he would have more of them at stated periods, which the bark would probably cure; but if the second, it might not return, for since the constitution was in possession of the complete action, that when the parts got better he would be well. He had no more, and went on doing as well as if no such fit had ever taken place. This is not the only instance of this nature.

Here it is to be considered that those affections of the constitution are effects of the local action of the solids, either when produced by spontaneous causes or by accident; but there are sometimes constitutional symptoms or universal sympathies, which arise immediately out of the act of violence itself, and which are often dangerous. Loss of blood may be reckoned one cause, which will bring on all kinds of constitutional complaints, in consequence of weakness being produced; either immediate, as fainting, or secondary, as dropsies, as well as nervous affections, the locked jaw, for instance; or violence alone, without the loss of blood, may often produce immediate fatal effects.

I have seen a man thrown into such convulsions from the operation of the hydrocele being performed upon him, that I began to despair of his recovery. I have known a man die immediately of castration. These symptoms are somewhat similar to the second, or nervous, but are still very different; for in the present the persons are as it were lost to themselves, being rendered senseless, therefore it is probably more an affection of the brain than the nerves.

Another symptom attending inflammation, when it has affected the constitution, is frequent exacerbations, or periods in which the inflammation appears to be increased. They have great affinity to the rigors we have been mentioning. Exacerbations are common to all constitutional diseases, and would often appear to belong to many local complaints. They are commonly regular if the constitution is strong, having their stated times, and in proportion as they are so the disease is less dangerous. They are a repetition of the first attack, but seldom so strong, except where there is a perfect cessation in the disease between the fits. This is an attribute belonging to life, and shows that life cannot go on the same continually in any state, but must have its hours of rest and hours of action.

In this, as in almost every other symptom of disease, the effect has been considered as a cause; for exacerbations have always been considered as owing to the disease having its time of subsiding or lessening and its time of increase. This idea might pass as just in fevers, where causes are not known; but where the causes continue the same, as in local diseases, we *à priori* should not expect it; yet we find in such cases periods of increase and decrease of the symptoms in the constitution, and therefore we must search after some principle belonging to animal life as a cause of this.

We shall find that an animal is so constituted as to be incapable of existing for any continuance of time in any one state whatever. The actions of the sensitive principle, when in perfect health, have their regular exacerbations, viz. watching and sleep: it is disease that interrupts this regularity of the actions of health, therefore we find that the actions of disease cannot always go on in the same way; Nature rests insensible of the disease [as in ague], while the disease exists at all times alike. Since this is the case where we see evidently a continuance of the remote cause, and that the constitution is only capable of being affected by this cause at stated times, according to the species of irritation given and the constitution at the time, may we not reasonably suppose this to be the case where the cause is invisible, as in fevers?

Whether these exacerbations are an effect of an occasional increase of the inflammation, or whether the inflammation is increased by the paroxysm of the fever, is not easy to determine; but they attend each other.

An ague is a disease which exists in the constitution between the fits as much as at the time of the fit; but the constitution becomes insensible of it, and the action can only last a stated time.

The process of ulceration seldom appears to affect the whole system; it is hardly known to exist, but in the appearance of the parts, viz. when the part which contains the matter gets softer to the touch, or when an ulcer becomes larger. But that rigors take place upon the commencement of ulceration I think is evident, although it cannot well be known in all cases; for ulceration will be so close upon suppuration in most cases that it will be difficult to distinguish which was the cause of the rigor; but where suppuration has taken place, and the abscess is opened, so that the first act of suppuration is finished, yet if it is not opened, so as to allow of a ready outlet to the matter, for instance, if it is not opened at a depending part, the pressure of the matter against the most depending part of the abscess will produce ulceration there, and rigors will take place. Those rigors, however, will not commence for some time after the first opening, because the first opening will for some time remove the disposition for ulceration all over the surface of the abscess; but when it finds that this opening is not sufficient to take off the pressure, then it sets about forming another opening, and when it does so the rigors will recur, and with as much severity as before. This is supposed by some to be new matter forming from fresh inflammation, and by others to be the absorption of matter already formed. Although ulceration does not affect the constitution equal to the mischief it is doing, yet its operations are often much affected by indispositions of the constitution; in some indispositions its progress is increased; in others it is even brought on, as in many old sores, especially of the lower extremities; and in some indispositions its progress is lessened or stopped.

The constitutional symptoms arising from a local complaint may be divided into three as to time, the immediate, indefinite, and remote. Of the first, or immediate, there appears to be but one; of the second, there is probably a great variety, at least [a great many] appearing in very different forms and at very different periods, in respect of the original cause. Of the remote there is probably only one. The immediate I shall reckon that which is called the symptomatic fever, and what I shall reckon the second are, nervous affections, as spasms, both temporary and permanent, and delirium. Whether the symptomatic fever, the spasms, or the delirium, come first, is not certain, for often all concur or occur at the same time; but as the sympathetic fever is most constant, and is more an universal principle, it is to be reckoned the first, And the third, which I have called remote, is what is understood by the hectic, to which may be added the symptoms of dissolution, which is the last stage of all, and may be a consequence of either the above or any other disease.

The first of the constitutional affections is commonly called the symptomatic fever, but which I choose to call the sympathetic inflammatory fever. This is immediate, or nearly so, and is the sympathy of the constitution, with the first stages of a local disease, which excites an alarm in the constitution, thereby rousing up its powers to produce succeeding actions. This would appear to show very much the nature of the constitution at the time; for not being of any specific nature, both inflammation and fever are led of course into the nature of the constitution by the natural tendency of the constitution itself, and therefore partake of it, and only become more or less of a specific, in proportion as the constitution has more or less of a specific susceptibility or disposition.

I have already observed, that affections of the constitution often commence with rigor. However, the commencement of the sympathetic fever is not always attended with that effect, and I believe it is the best constitution where it is not; and in that case it changes into a regular fever of the inflammatory kind. If the constitution has powers, heat comes on, attended with dry skin, frequent, and commonly a full pulse, having at the same time a degree of hardness in the stroke; watchfulness, high-coloured urine, loss of appetite for solids, and thirst; all these will vary according to various visible circumstances, as well as according to many invisible ones, some one symptom being more in one constitution, and less in another.

It is in many instances difficult to determine what is cause and what is effect. It has been commonly supposed that this fever was necessary for the operation of suppuration, and therefore the fever did not arise from the sympathy of the constitution with a local injury, but as a necessary effect to become a cause of suppuration. If this was the case, we could have no suppuration which had not been preceded by fever; and the fever must have been equal in all cases in the same constitution, let the quantity of injury be what it will. For if a pimple, or the suppuration of a scratch, depended upon fever, they would require as much fever for their production of inflammation and suppuration as the largest abscess, or largest wound; for a point that inflames and suppurates is under the same predicament with respect to the whole that a thousand are; and a large abscess is to be considered as only made up of a thousand points. One venereal sore requires as much mercury to cure it as a thousand. One plant requires as much wet weather and sunshine as a million. A principle that affects universally can only affect a part in proportion to the quantity of the universal affection there is in the part: each part has just its portion of general influence.

Now, according to this proposition, which is undeniable, a scratch requires the same quantity of fever that an amputation of the thigh does. Let us see how this accords with common experience; we find that inflammations and suppurations of sores shall take place without any fever; that the fever, in consequence of an injury, is not in all cases in the least proportioned to the quantity of injury, inflammation, and suppuration, which it always should be if the last was an effect of it; and we know if an increase of fever comes on, superadded to the sympathetic, that suppuration is retarded or stopped altogether instead of being quickened[a].

---

[a] [The former and latter parts of this paragraph are plainly contradictory; for if, upon the supposition, a scratch and an amputation require the same quantity of fever, then the degree of fever should not be in proportion to the suppuration, which, however, it is asserted it should be in the latter part of this paragraph.]

From the same mode of reasoning it should be exactly the same, whether the fever produce suppuration in a vital part or in one that is not vital. It is much more easy to conceive that an injury done to a vital part shall be the cause of universal sympathy, than that a vital part should require more fever to make it inflame and suppurate than a part does which is not vital. This theory would at once overset our observation that the constitution is affected or sympathizes more readily with some parts than with others. In many cases of spontaneous inflammations and suppurations it was natural to suppose that the fever was the cause of the suppuration; but if persons who thought so had observed accurately, they would have divided spontaneous suppurations into two kinds; one, whose remote and immediate cause was local, and therefore in such the fever followed the local action, as [happens] in injuries; the other, where the remote cause was fever, which produced the injury, and the injury, whatever it was, produced the inflammation and suppuration; so that here fever preceded, and was necessary for the remote cause, but not as the immediate; and indeed, as a proof of this, suppuration hardly takes place till the fever is gone[a]. The smallpox is of this last kind, as probably many other contagious diseases.

Those symptoms continue, more or less, according to the degree of injury, the nature and situation of parts, and the constitution; but as they arise from a local cause, which subsides, they of course subside also; however, as the constitution has often an inflammatory tendency, or a tendency to some other disease, besides the action arising from the violence singly, the parts often run into it, and this is reflected upon the constitution, which passes into that action to which it has a tendency, by which fever is kept up, and thereby inflammation.

The subsiding of these symptoms is the cure; and where they are simply the effects of the violence, the fever cures itself; therefore the only thing necessary is to lessen its violence; but if the injury is of any specific kind, that specific quality must be corrected, if possible, and then the cure will take place.

As the motion of the blood in the whole system is increased, and as we have reason to suppose it is locally increased, then what will diminish the motion of the blood will relieve in this respect. There are two methods of doing this. The first is by taking off its force, and this will be effected by bleeding. This, if it does not lessen its motion, or take

[a] [That is, if I rightly apprehend the passage, the fever is supposed to induce a condition of parts similar to a breach of surface, which state of parts again is supposed to induce a condition of imperfection, which is the immediate cause of the inflammation and suppuration: however, it is difficult to conceive any possible cause of suppuration to which the same mode of reasoning would not be applicable.]

off from the sympathy of the constitution with the local disease, yet it lessens the momentum in the whole and in the part, which is taking off the effect of the excess of motion in the blood. The second is by diminishing the action of the parts by affecting the constitution, which may be done by purging; in this light bleeding may also be in some degree considered. It becomes in such cases very necessary to relieve the constitution by lessening the action of that constitution; for although what has been advised was to lessen the inflammation itself, and thereby lessen its effects on the constitution, yet as that seldom is done sufficiently to remove any affection of the constitution, we must therefore pay attention to that constitution; the two remedies will in some degree go hand in hand, one assisting the other; for instance, in a strong healthy constitution, where the symptomatic fever runs high, bleeding and purging will have their double effects; but still the constitution may require its peculiar medicines, which will in a secondary way relieve the inflammation.

The secondary constitutional symptoms are not so determined as to time; I have called them nervous, although not strictly so in every case, because more variety of affections are produced than from any cause I know; yet these affections seem all to have more connexion with the nervous than the vascular system, and are severally excited by the particular tendency or susceptibility of different constitutions. Many of them, I believe, are more common to the young than the old, which come under the doctrine of universal nervous sympathy with a local complaint; of this kind are universal convulsions from teething or worms, local convulsions, as St. Vitus's dance, and probably many others not so well marked, as those which worms and teething often produce. I have seen hiccup come on early in consequence of an operation; but in this stage of the nervous affection little was to be apprehended, although it certainly showed a peculiarity of constitution, and such as should be attended to; but when hiccup occurs towards the last stages, it shows strong signs of dissolution.

Many full-grown persons are also subject to very severe affections of the nervous kind, especially those people who are called nervous; and more particularly still those who have had affections in consequence of complaints of the stomach. In such constitutions there is observed great dejection, sinking, cold sweats, hardly any pulse, loss of appetite, no sleep, etc., seeming to threaten dissolution; and those symptoms are worse by fits. Delirium appears to arise from nervous affection of the brain, or sensorium, producing a sympathy of the action of the brain with the materia vitæ of the parts; not sensation as a head-ache, but action producing ideas without the exciting impression, and therefore delusive. This symptom is common to them all [viz. all the constitutional affections]; it is frequently a consequence of their being violent, or carried to considerable length in their several kinds; often arising in consequence of compound fractures, amputation of the lower extremities, injuries done to joints, brain, etc., but not so often attending the hectic, although it is often a symptom of dissolution. We have agues also from many diseases of parts, more especially of the liver, as also of the spleen, and from induration of the mesenteric glands[a].

The following cases are remarkable instances of well-marked constitutional diseases from local irritation, where the constitution took on a particular action, to which it had a strong tendency. A gentleman had a very bad fistula in perinæo from a stricture, and when the water did not come freely an inflammation in the part and scrotum was produced, and then he had an ague, which was relieved for a time by the bark. Two children had an ague from worms, which was not in the least relieved by the bark, but by destroying the worms they were cured.

As these diseases which I have brought into this class are of such various kinds, each must be taken up apart, and treated accordingly; but they are such as yield very little to medicine, for in some the constitutional disease is formed, and does not require the presence of the local disease to keep it up, as in the tetanus; and in others, the local disease being still in force, it is not to be expected that the constitutional affection is to be entirely relieved, although in some degree it may. In those which form a regular constitutional disease, such as an ague, although the local diseases may still exist in full force, yet some relief may be expected; the bark is to be administered, although not with a view to cure, as the immediate cause still exists; but bark will in some lessen that susceptibility in the constitution, and may cure, at least for a time, as I have seen in agues arising from the fistula in perinæo. But the susceptibility in the two children cited above was so strong for such a disease, that the bark was not sufficient; and therefore, when the local cause is not known, and when the common remedies for such effects do not cure them, some local disease should be suspected. We see often such symptoms arising from diseases of the liver, and the bark curing this symptom, yet the liver shall go on with its disease, and probably faster, as I believe bark is not a proper medicine for diseases of this viscus; such complaints of the liver have been too often attributed to the curing of the ague improperly by bark. St. Vitus's dance and many other involuntary actions have arisen from the same cause; such

---

[a] [These conditions of the liver and spleen are rather to be regarded as effects than as causes of the ague.]

constitutions required only an immediate cause to produce the effects. It is possible, however, that no other mode of local irritation would have produced the same effect, every constitution having a part that is capable of affecting it most. We find also local effects in consequence of local injuries, as the locked jaw, &c., which are remote sympathies with the part affected, which may become pretty universal, and which cannot be called immediate effects as to time, as they are often forming after the sympathetic fever has taken place, especially the locked jaw, which appears in many cases to be formed in the time of the preceding disease, and not appearing till it has subsided. There are certain intermediate steps between the inflammatory and the hectic state; but neither cure nor dissolution takes place in this period.

The following case illustrates the effects of inflammation on the constitution:

A lady, of what is called a nervous constitution, arising in some degree from an irritable stomach, often troubled with flatulencies and what are called nervous head-aches, with pale urine at those times, uncomfortable feelings, and often sinkings, had a tumour removed from the breast, and likewise from near the armpit; nothing appeared uncommon for a few days, when very considerable disorders came on. She was attacked with a shivering or cold fit, attended with the feel of dying, and followed with cold sweat. It being supposed that she was dying, brandy was thrown in, which soon brought on a warmth, and she was relieved; the fits came on frequently for several days, which were always relieved by brandy; and she took, in one of the most violent of them, about half a pint of brandy.

While under these affections she took the bark as a strengthener; the musk, occasionally, as a sedative in pretty large quantities; camphorated julep frequently, as an antispasmodic; and towards the last she took the valerian in large quantities; but whatever effect these might have in lessening the disease on the whole, they were certainly not equal to it without the brandy. Brandy removed those dying fits, and I thought they became less violent after taking the valerian.

A question naturally occurs, Would the brandy alone, if it had been continued as a medicine, have cured her, without the aid of the other medicines? The other medicines, I think, certainly could not have done it; nor do I believe that the brandy could have been continued in such quantity as to have prevented their returns; if so, then the two modes were happily united, the one gradually to prevent, the other to remove immediately the fits when they came on. This case, from the general tenour of the constitution, was running with great facility into the hectic.

CHAPTER V.

OF PUS.

HITHERTO I have been treating of the operations of parts preparatory to the formation of pus; I am now come to the formation of that fluid, its nature and supposed uses.

The immediate effect of the mode of action above described is the formation of a fluid, commonly termed pus; this is very different from what was discharged in the time of the adhesive stage of the inflammation, when either formed in the cellular membrane or circumscribed cavities; it is also very different from the natural secretion of internal canals, though it is probably formed in both by the same vessels, but under very different modes of action.

The cellular membrane, or circumscribed cavities, have their vessels but little changed from the adhesive state at the commencement of the suppurative disposition, so that they still retain much of the form they had acquired by the first state, the discharge being at the beginning little more than coagulating lymph mixed with some serum. This is scarcely different from the adhesive stage of the inflammation; but as the inflammatory disposition subsides, the new disposition is every instant of time altering those vessels to their suppurative state; the discharge is also varying and changing from a species of extravasation to a new-formed matter peculiar to suppuration; this matter is a remove further from the nature of the blood, and becomes more and more of the nature of the pus; it becomes whiter and whiter, losing more and more of the yellow and green, which it is apt to give the linen that is stained with it in its first stages, and in consistence more and more viscid or creamy.

By the formation of this new substance, the coagulating lymph, which was extravasated in the adhesive state of the inflammation, and adhered to the sides of the cells, either in cut surfaces as in wounds, in abscesses, or circumscribed cavities, is pushed off from these surfaces; and if it is the inner surface of a cavity, it is pushed into it, so that the cavity contains both coagulating lymph and pus; or if it is a cut surface, the coagulating lymph is separated from it by the suppuration taking place, and is thrown off; but as such surfaces are generally dressed immediately after the operation, while the wound is bleeding, this blood unites the dressings to the sore, which is assisted afterwards by the coagulating lymph thrown out in the adhesive stage; the whole, viz. dressings, blood, and coagulating lymph, are generally thrown off together, when suppuration commences on these surfaces. This is the process which takes place in the first formation of an abscess, and the first process towards suppuration in a fresh wound.

Upon the internal surfaces of the canals the parts do not go through all those steps; they would appear to run into suppuration almost instantaneously; however, inflammation even here is a kind of forerunner of suppuration. This discharge from internal canals has never been reckoned true matter; it has been called mucus, etc., but it has all the characters of true pus which I am yet acquainted with.

Pus is not to be found in the blood similar to that [viz. the coagulable lymph] which was produced in the first stage, but is formed from some change, decomposition, or separation of the blood which that undergoes in its passage out of the vessels, and for effecting which the vessels of the parts have been formed, which produces a subsiding of the inflammation from which it took its disposition; hence it must appear that the formation of pus consists of something more than a straining of juices from the blood. Many substances indeed which are to be considered as extraneous bodies in the blood, being only mixed with, and not making an essential part of that fluid, and perhaps even [some that are] necessary to it, may pass off with the pus, as with every other secretion, yet the pus is not to be considered on that account as simply parts of the blood unchanged; but we must look upon it as a new combination of the blood itself, and must be convinced that in order to carry on the decompositions and combinations necessary for producing this effect, either a new or peculiar structure of vessels must be formed, or a new disposition, and of course a new mode of action of the old must take place. This new structure or disposition of vessels I shall call glandular, and the effect, or pus, a secretion.

§. 1. *Of the general Opinion of the Formation of Pus.*

The dissolution of the living solids of an animal body into pus, and that the pus already formed has the power of continuing the dissolution, is an old opinion, and is still the opinion of many, for their language is "Pus corrodes, it is acrid, etc." If this idea of theirs was just, no sore which discharges matter could be exempted from a continual dissolution; and I think it must appear inconsistent, that the matter which was probably intended for salutary purposes should be a means of destroying the very parts which produced it, and which it is meant to heal. Probably they took their idea from finding that an abscess was a hollow cavity in the solids, and supposing the whole of the original substance of this cavity was now the matter which was found in it. This was a very natural way of accounting for the formation of pus by one entirely ignorant of the moving juices, the powers of the arteries, and the operation of an abscess after it was opened; for the knowledge of these three, abstracted from the knowledge of the abscess before opening, should have naturally led them to account for the formation of pus from the blood by the powers of the arteries alone, for upon their principle these abscesses should continue to increase after opening as fast as before. Upon this principle being established in their minds, viz. that solids were dissolved down into pus, they built a practice which was to bring all indurated parts to suppuration if possible, and not to open the suppuration in such parts early; this was done with a view to give such solids time to melt down into pus, which was the expression; but according to their own theory, they seemed to forget that abscesses formed matter after opening, and therefore the parts stood the same chance of dissolution into pus as before. Also, from being possessed of this idea, that solids went into the composition of pus, they never saw pus flowing from any internal canal, as in a gonorrhœa, etc., but they concluded that there was an ulcer; we would forgive such opinions before the knowledge that such surfaces could and generally did form pus without a breach of the solids; but that such an opinion should exist afterwards, is not mere ignorance, but stupidity; and the very circumstance of internal circumscribed cavities, as the abdomen, thorax, etc., forming pus, where they might often have seen pints of matter, and yet no breach in the solids to have produced it, which is a proof beyond controversy, should have taught them better; such ideas discover defect of knowledge and incapacity for observation.

The moderns have been still more ridiculous; for knowing that it was denied that solids were ever dissolved into pus, and also knowing that there was not a single proof of it, they have been busy in producing what to them seemed proof. They have been putting dead animal matter into abscesses, and finding that it was either wholly or in part dissolved, they therefore attributed the loss to its being formed into pus; but this was putting living and dead animal matter upon the same footing, which is a contradiction in itself: for if the result of this experiment was really according to their idea of it, the idea of living parts being dissolved into pus must fall to the ground, because living animal matter and dead animal matter can never stand upon the same ground.

Common observation in their profession should have taught them that even extraneous animal matter would lie in abscesses for a considerable time before it was even dissolved. They might have observed in abscesses arising either from violence or from a species of erysipelatous inflammation, that there were often sloughs of the cellular membrane, and that those sloughs would come away like wet tow, and therefore were not dissolved into pus. They might also have observed in abscesses of tendinous parts, as about the ancle, &c., that often a tendon became dead and sloughed away, and that these sores do not heal till such parts have sloughed, and this is often not accomplished for months, and yet all this time those sloughs are not formed into pus. They might have also known or observed that pieces of dead bone shall lie soaking in matter for many months, and yet not dissolve into pus; and although bones in such situations shall lose considerably of their substance (which might by the ignorant be supposed to have been dissolved into pus) yet that waste can be accounted for and proved on the principle of absorption; for they always lose on that surface where the continuity is broken off, and which is only a continuation of the separating process*.

To see how far the idea was just that dead animal matter was dissolved by pus, I put it to the trial of experiment, because I could put a piece of dead animal matter of a given weight into an abscess, and which could at stated times be weighed. To make it still more satisfactory, a similar piece was put into water, kept to nearly the same heat: they both lost in weight, but that in the abscess most, and there was also a difference in the manner, for that in the water became soonest putrid. But these experiments having been made as far back as the year 1757, I shall not rely on their accuracy, but state them as made by my brother-in-law Mr. Home, and as given in his Dissertation on the Properties of Pus, p. 32, under the idea that pus had a corroding quality.

"As pus has been supposed to have a corroding quality," I may add even upon the living solids, "I made the following experiments to ascertain the truth or fallacy of such an assertion, and found it to be void of foundation, and to have arisen from the inaccuracy of observers having prevented them from seeing the distinctions between pus in a pure state, and when mixed with other substances.

"I made a comparative trial upon matter contained in an abscess, and on pus and animal jelly out of the body. The matter and jelly were in equal quantities, and contained in glass vessels, kept nearly in the temperature of the human body. To make the comparative trials as fair as possible a portion of muscle, weighing exactly one drachm, was immersed

* It may be supposed that bones are not capable of being dissolved into pus; but we know that bone has animal substance in it, and we also know that this animal substance is capable of being dissolved into chyle.

in the matter of a compound fracture in the arm of a living man, and a similar portion into some of the same matter out of the body; also a third portion into fluid calf's foot jelly, in which the animal substance was pure, having neither wine nor vegetables mixed with it. These three portions of muscle were taken out once every twenty-four hours, washed in water, weighed and returned again. The results were as follows:

"In 24 hours the portion of muscle in the abscess weighed sixty grains, was pulpy and soft, but quite free from putrefaction: that portion immersed in the pus weighed forty-six grains, was pulpy, soft, and had a slightly putrid smell: the portion in the jelly weighed thirty-eight grains, was smaller and firmer in its texture. In 48 hours the portion of muscle in the abscess weighed thirty-eight grains, and had undergone no change; that in the matter weighed thirty-six grains, was softer and more putrid; that in the jelly thirty-six grains and smaller. In 72 hours the portion of muscle in the abscess weighed twenty-seven grains, was drier and firmer; that in the matter eighteen grains, and was rendered fibrous and thready; that in the jelly unaltered. In 96 hours the portion of muscle in the abscess weighed twenty-five grains; that in the matter was dissolved; that in the jelly weighed thirty-six grains*; In 120 hours the portion of muscle in the abscess weighed twenty-two grains, not at all putrid; that in the jelly thirty-four grains, not at all putrid. In 144 hours the portion of muscle in the abscess weighed twenty-two grains, and was free from putrefaction; that in the jelly thirty-four grains."

The supposed facts of the solids dissolving being established in the mind as so many data to reason from, they had now no difficulty to account for the formation of pus from both the solids and the fluids. Fermentation started up in the mind immediately as a cause; but there must be a cause for fermentation, and according to this idea there are facts which go against it. First, let us consider internal canals, where only mucus is naturally formed, taking on the formation of pus without the loss of substance or any previous ferment, and leaving it off.

Now if a fermentation of the solids and fluids was the immediate cause, I should beg leave to ask what solids were destroyed in order to enter into the composition of the pus discharged, for the whole penis could

* One reason, probably, for the piece of meat so soon becoming putrid and dissolving in the pus was its being kept in the same pus the whole time, therefore its dissolution was owing more to putrefaction than a dissolving quality in the pus; whereas the piece in the abscess had its matter continually changing, which is the common result in a sore, and if it had a corroding quality independent of the putrefaction, it ought to have been dissolved first; but we may observe that the piece of muscle in the abscess and the piece in the jelly were nearly upon a par.

not afford matter enough to form the pus which is discharged in a common gonorrhœa. I should also beg leave to be informed how that fermentation of the fluids ever ceased; for there is the same surface secreting its mucus whenever the formation of pus ceases. Besides, if dissolved solids enter necessarily into the composition of pus by the power of some ferment, it may be asked, by what power is the first particle of this fluid in an abscess or sore formed, before there is any particle existing which is capable of dissolving the solids? An abscess shall form, and, suppuration ceasing, it shall become stationary, perhaps for months, and at last be absorbed, and the whole shall heal; what becomes of the ferment the whole time it is stationary?

It has been supposed that blood when extravasated becomes of itself pus; but we find blood, when extravasated either from violence or a rupture of a vessel, as in an aneurism, never of itself becomes pus, nor was pus ever formed in such cavities till inflammation had taken place in them, and then in such cavities there was to be found both the blood and the matter: if the blood had coagulated (as it seldom does in those cases of violence) it would be found still coagulated, and if it had not coagulated the pus would be bloody.

True pus has certain properties, which when taken singly may belong to other secretions, but when all joined, form the peculiar character of pus, viz. globules swimming in a fluid, which is coagulable by a solution of sal ammoniac (which no other animal secretion that I know is); and at the same time a consequence of inflammation: these circumstances taken together may be said to constitute pus.

As inflammation does not produce at first true pus, I made the following experiments to ascertain its progress or formation. To do this it was only necessary to keep up an irritation on some living part a sufficient time to oblige it to set about the natural consequent actions, and the smooth coat of an internal cavity appeared to me to be well calculated for such an experiment, where nothing could interfere with the actions of the parts or their result; and it would also show its progress on internal surfaces, which shows its progress in wounds and abscesses.

§. 2. *Experiments to ascertain the Progress of Suppuration.*

Experiment I. The tunica vaginalis of a young ram was opened and the testicle exposed. The surface of the testicle was wiped clean, and a piece of talc was laid upon it. The surface almost immediately became more vascular; five minutes after, the talc was removed and examined in a microscope, but no globules could be observed, only a moisture, which appeared to be serum. Ten minutes after, there were irregular masses formed on the talc, some transparent, with determined edges, but no globules: fifteen minutes after, nearly the same. At twenty minutes there was an appearance of globules. At twenty-five minutes, there were globules in clusters; but I could not say exactly what those globules were. At thirty-five minutes, the globules more distinct, more diffused, and numerous. At fifty-five minutes, the globules still more perfect and distinct. At seventy, the globules more irregular, and of course less distinct. At eighty-five, the globules more distinct and numerous. At one hundred, more irregular and less distinct, forming little masses. At two hours, the masses more transparent, and the globules fewer. At two hours and a half, the masses transparent, and no distinct globules. At four hours, some transparent masses appearing to contain globules. At seven hours, distinct globules and numerous. At eight hours, the globules more distinct and somewhat larger. At nine hours, less appearance of globules. At twenty-one hours, the testicle was covered with lint, and the skin brought over and kept together with a ligature, and allowed to remain for twelve hours (which, from the first, was thirty-three hours); when it was opened it was wiped dry, and a piece of talc applied for five minutes; the quantity of fluid was very small, but containing globules small and numerous.

N.B. In this time, during which the testicle was covered, strong adhesions took place between the testicles and tunica vaginalis, which shows that probably the inflammation moved back to the adhesive stage whenever two similar surfaces were opposed.

Forty hours, the above repeated and the globules a little more distinct. Forty-four hours, the appearance of globules very distinct, and the pus looked like common matter diluted.

Experiment II. An opening was made through the linea alba below the navel, several inches long, into the cavity of the belly of a dog, care being taken that no blood should pass into that cavity; a piece of talc was applied to the peritonæum so as to be covered with the fluid which lubricates that surface; to do which it was found necessary to draw it over some considerable surface. This fluid was examined in the field of the microscope, and appeared to contain small semitransparent globules, few in number, swimming in a fluid.

The lubricating fluid in the cavity of the abdomen appears, from repeated experiments on healthy dogs, to be so small in quantity as only to give a polish to the different surfaces, but not sufficient to have a drop collected.

After five minutes, the surfaces had more moisture upon them, which being examined as before, the globular appearance was more distinct. In fifteen minutes the surfaces were more vascular; a portion of intestine was wiped dry, and a piece of talc applied to it; the fluid collected on it had a great number of globules, which were smaller than those at first observed. In an hour, this portion of intestine had its blood-vessels considerably increased in number, the whole surface appearing of a uniformly red colour: this was wiped dry, and a piece of talc laid upon it; the fluid collected did not appear to be made up of globules, but of very small parts, which had some transparency, but not exactly regular in their figure, which became still more evident on drying, when they lost the transparency altogether; these were most probably coagulating lymph. This was repeated upon the surface of the spleen, which had its surface excessively red, from the increased number of small vessels carrying red blood, and the result was exactly similar.

From these experiments the fluid which lubricates the peritonæum seems to undergo changes, in consequence of exposure, and at last, when inflammation takes place, to have coagulating blood substituted for it.

Although the lubricating fluid of the peritonæum is so small in quantity in a natural state, yet before that cavity has been exposed for half an hour the quantity is much increased, and has a mottled appearance of oil and water; but from the appearance in the microscope, it is only an increase of the original fluid with some coagulating lymph, although mistaken by some anatomists for an oily lubricating liquor.

Experiment III. At half-past seven o'clock in the morning, an incision was made with a lancet into the upper fleshy part of a young ram's thigh, into which was introduced a silver canula, about a quarter of an inch in diameter and three quarters long, with a great number of small holes in the sides and open at the bottom; it was fastened by means of ligatures to the skin, and a small cork adapted to it. The blood was sponged out several times, and the cork kept in during the intervals. At half-past nine the cork was withdrawn, and the canula was found to contain a fluid; a piece of talc was dipped in it, and the appearance was evidently globular, exactly like the red globules without the colour. At eleven, the quantity of fluid much increased, and the same appearance. At one, the quantity half filling the pipe, of a reddish brown colour; the globules more numerous, without colour when diluted with water. At three, the quantity considerable, the globules smaller, freer from colour. At half-past five, the same.

Experiment IV. In the same manner the canula was introduced into the fleshy part of an ass's thigh, at nine in the morning; and at one o'clock, as also at two, there was a fluid tinged with red globules. At four, there were no diffused globules, but there appeared to be small flakes in a transparent fluid; however, they proved to be clusters of globules. At seven, next morning, which was twenty-two hours, there was found in the canula common pus.

From the experiments on internal surfaces, it would appear that pus was formed coeval with its secretion; but from Mr. Home's experiments (*op. cit.*, p. 51,) it would rather appear that the globules were not formed till some time after secretion, and this sooner or later, according to circumstances, which we probably do not know.

So far these experiments explain the progress of suppuration on internal surfaces, and I shall now give its progress on the cutis, when deprived of its cuticle, from Mr. Home's Dissertation on that subject, before mentioned.

"I applied a blistering plaster of the size of a half-crown piece to the pit of the stomach of a healthy young man. In eight hours a blister arose, which was opened, and the contents removed; they were fluid, transparent, and coagulated by heat; had no appearance of globules when examined by the microscope, and in every respect resembled the serum of blood. The cuticle was not removed, but allowed to collapse, and the fluid which was formed upon the surface of the cutis was examined from time to time by a microscope, to determine as accurately as possible the changes which took place.

"The better to do this, as the quantity in the intervals stated below must be exceedingly small, a piece of talc, very thin and transparent, was applied to the whole surface, and covered with an adhesive plaster; and the surface of the talc applied to the skin was removed and examined by the microscope, applying a fresh piece of talc after every examination, to prevent any mistake which might have arisen from the surface not being quite clean.

"The fluid was examined by the microscope, to ascertain its appearance; but as the aqueous part in which the globules of pus swim is found by experiment to coagulate by adding to it a saturated solution of sal ammoniac, which is not the case with the serum of the blood nor the transparent part of the milk, I considered this as a property peculiar to pus; and consequently that it would be a very good test by which to ascertain the presence of true pus.

"In eight hours from the time the blister was applied the fluid discharged was perfectly transparent, and did not coagulate with the solution of sal ammoniac. Nine hours: The discharge was less transparent, but free from the appearance of globules. Ten hours: The discharge contained globules, which were very small, and few in number. Eleven hours: The globules were numerous, but still the fluid did not coagulate with the solution of sal ammoniac. Twelve hours: The appearance much the same as before. Fourteen hours: The globules a little larger, and the fluid appeared to be thickened by a solution of sal ammoniac Sixteen hours: The globules seemed to form themselves into masses, but were transparent. Twenty hours: The globules were double the size of those first observed at ten hours, and gave the appearance of true pus, in a diluted state; the fluid was coagulated by a solution of sal ammoniac, the globules at the same time remaining perfectly distinct, so that I should consider this as true pus. Twenty-two hours: No change appeared to have taken place. Thirty-two hours: The fluid was considerably thicker in consistence, the number of globules being very much increased; but in no other respect, that I could observe, did it differ from that formed twenty hours after the application of the blister."

To ascertain the progress of suppuration on canals or secreting surfaces, I have often examined the matter on a bougie that had been introduced into the urethra, and found it to be formed earlier than either of the times before mentioned: Mr. Home's experiment makes it five hours; but we often find a gonorrhœa coming on at once, not having in the least been preceded by a leading discharge.

Since that period experiments have been made on pus from different kinds of sores, with an intention to ascertain the nature of the sore by the result of such analysis. That sores give very different kinds of pus is evident to the naked eye; and that the different parts of which the blood is composed will come away in different proportions, we can make no doubt; and we find that whatever is in solution in the blood comes away more in one kind of pus than another, which are all so many deviations from true pus; we may also observe, that such kinds of pus change, after being secreted, much sooner than true pus, which will be observed by and by. From all this I should be apt to conceive that such experiments will throw little light on the specific nature of the disease, which is the thing wanted. From such experiments we may find out that pus from a venereal bubo in its height of malady, or that from a cancer, is bad matter, but cannot ascertain the difference between those two matters and all others, nor the specific difference between the two. The smallpox, although as malignant a disease as any, and one which produces a pus as replete with poisonous particles as any, yet gives a true pus, when not of the confluent kind, which disposition is not smallpox. The reason why it is good pus is because its inflammation is of the true suppurative kind; and the reason why it is of the true suppurative kind is because the parts have the power of curing themselves, just as much as in any accident which happens to such a constitution; but this is not the case with either the venereal disease or the cancer; from the moment these set out, their dispositions tend to become worse and worse; but the venereal bubo, if mercury is given so as to affect it, soon gives us another kind of pus, although this has the poison equally in it; therefore it is not the circumstance of containing a poison which makes it what is called a bad pus, but its being formed from a sore that has no disposition to heal: as we cannot give healing action to a cancer, so we never can have a good pus. The observation respecting the smallpox is applicable to the venereal gonorrhœa, for this complaint having the power of curing itself, its pus is good in proportion to that power; but as the periods of cure are not so determined as in the smallpox, neither is its time in producing good pus so determined; but, like the smallpox, as well as the venereal disease, when it is healing we have good pus, although it contains the poison.

From the above experiments it must appear unnecessary to give the chemical analyses of what is commonly called pus, for whatever comes from a sore has that name, although very different in many cases from what I should call true pus; and we shall find in those sores that have some specific quality which hinders them from healing, that the discharge is not pus. Probably the chemical properties may be nearly the same in them all.

§. 3. *Of the Properties of Pus.*

Pus, in the most perfect state, has at the first view certain peculiar qualities. These are principally colour and consistence; but it appears that the colour takes its rise from the largest portion of the whole mass being composed of very small round bodies, very much like those small round globules which, swimming in a fluid, make cream: I should suppose those round globules to be white in themselves, as cream would appear to be, although it is not necessary that the substance of matter which reflects a white should be itself white, for a vast number of transparent bodies being brought together will produce a white, such as broken glass, broken ice, water covering globules of air, making froth, &c.

These globules swim in a fluid, which we should at first suppose to be the serum of the blood, for it coagulates with heat like serum, and most probably is mixed with a small quantity of coagulating lymph; for pus in part coagulates, after having been discharged from the secreting vessels, as mucus is observed to do. But although it is thus far similar to serum, yet it has properties that serum has not. Observing there was a similarity between pus and milk, I tried if the fluid part of pus could be coagulated with the juice of the stomach of other animals, but found it could not. I then tried it with several mixtures, principally with the neutral salts, and found that a solution of sal ammoniac coagulated this fluid: not finding that a solution of this salt coagulated any other of our natural juices, I concluded that globules swimming in a fluid that was coagulable by this salt was to be considered as pus, and would be always formed in sores that had no peculiar backwardness to heal.

The proportion that these white globules in the pus bears to the other parts, depends on the health of the parts which formed it; for when they are in a large proportion the matter is thicker and whiter, and is called good matter; the meaning of which is that the solids which produced it are in good health, for these appearances in the matter are no more than the result of certain salutary processes going on in the solids, the effect of which processes is to produce the disposition on which both suppuration and granulation depend. All this is a good deal similar to the formation of milk; for in the commencement of the secretion of this fluid it is at first principally serum, and as the animal advances towards delivery the globules are forming and become more in quantity, and the animal that has them in largest quantity has the richest milk; likewise when they are naturally leaving off secreting milk, it again takes an exact retrograde motion; and we may also observe, that if any local affection attacks this gland, such as inflammation, the milk falls back to the state I have been now describing; or if any constitutional affection takes place, such as fever, &c., then this gland suffers in the same manner.

Pus is specifically heavier than water; it is probably nearly of the same weight with blood or any other animal substance rendered fluid.

Pus, besides the above-mentioned properties, has a sweetish and mawkish taste, probably from having sugar in it, which is very different from most other secretions, and the same taste takes place whether it is pus from a sore, viz. an ulcer, or an irritated inflamed surface. Thus, if any have an ulcer in their nose, mouth, throat, lungs, or parts adjacent, so that the matter shall come into the mouth unaltered by putrefaction, they will be able to taste it from its having this property; whereas the mucus and saliva of those parts are tasteless. The same thing happens when an irritation to inflammation takes place on the surface of those parts without ulceration.

If the internal surface of the nose is inflamed, so that when we blow it on a white handkerchief we see the substance discharged of a yellow colour, we also find that when we draw up the same substance into the mouth that it has a sweetish mawkish taste. If it is the surface of the mouth or throat that discharges this matter, the same taste is observable; and if it is brought up from the trachea and lungs, in consequence of the common effects of a cold on those parts, the same taste is also to be observed: so that pus, from whatever surface, whether an irritated natural surface or the surface of a common sore, has this property.

Pus has a smell in some degree peculiar to itself; but this differs. Some diseases, such for instance as the venereal gonorrhœa, it is pretended may be known by the smell.

To ascertain the properties of pus, or to distinguish it from mucus, it has, with mucus, been put to the test of chemistry. Solution in mentrua, and precipitation, were thought to be a test of their distinction.

This principle in its very first appearance is unphilosophical, and was at the very first treated by me as absurd. I conceived that all animal substance whatever, when in solution, either in acids or alkalis, would then be in the same state, and therefore that the precipitation would be the same in all. Calcareous earth, when dissolved in an acid, (for instance, the muriatic,) is in that acid in the same state, whether it has been dissolved from chalk, limestone, marble, or calcareous spar; and the precipitations from all are the same.

However, whatever my opinion might be, yet bold assertions, the result of described experiments, made me avoid falling into the same error, of describing what I never had seen. I made, therefore, some experiments on this subject; and, in consequence of having previously formed the above-mentioned opinion, I was more general in my experiments. I made them on organic animal matter as well as on inorganic, and the result was the same in all.

As organic animal matter, I took muscle, tendon, cartilage, gland, viz. liver and brain: as inorganic animal matter, I took pus and the white of an egg, and dissolved each in the vitriolic acid, and then precipitated the solution with vegetable alkali. Each precipitation I examined with such magnifiers as plainly showed the forms of the precipitate, all of which appeared to be flaky substances. The precipitate by the volatile alkali appeared exactly the same.

To carry those experiments a little further, I dissolved the same substance in the vegetable caustic alkali, and precipitated the solution with the muriatic acid, and examined each precipitate with the microscope, and the appearance was the same, viz. a flaky substance, without any regular form.

To see how far the nature of sores might be ascertained from the nature of their discharge, matter from a cancerous sore has been analysed, and the result has been that such matter differs from the true pus; but this explains nothing more than what the naked eye can perceive, that it is not pus, but it will not show the specific difference between the matter from a cancer and matter from a venereal bubo, where mercury has not been given, nor will it tell that one is cancer and the other is venereal. We might as well analyse the urine at different times, in order to ascertain the nature of kidneys at those times.

The quality of pus is always according to the nature of the parts which produce it, and whatever specific qualities the parts may have besides, the pus has also this specific quality; hence we have venereal matter from venereal sores, smallpox matter from smallpox sores, cancerous matter from cancerous sores, &c. It is not in the least affected by the constitution, except the parts which produce it are also affected by the constitution.

Pus is so far of the same specific nature with the part which produces it, that it does not become an irritator to that part; it is perfectly in harmony with it; the part is not in the least sensible of it: therefore the pus of a suppurating surface is not an irritator to the same surface, but may be an irritator to any other not of the same kind. Hence no suppurating surface of any specific kind can be kept up by its own matter; for if this had not been the case, no sore of any specific quality, or producing matter of an irritating quality, could ever have been healed. This is similar to every other secretion of stimulating fluids, as the bile, tears, &c., for those do not stimulate their own glands or ducts, but are capable of stimulating any other part of the body. The venereal gonorrhœa, smallpox, &c. healing or recovering of themselves, are striking instances of this. However, we find matter under certain circumstances stimulating its own sore, and also secretions stimulating their own canals, as the secretions of the intestines stimulating themselves; but how far this may not arise from one part of the intestines being so diseased as to secrete a stimulating fluid, and coming to a sound part stimulates that only, I will not determine. This I am certain happens to the rectum and anus; for it very often happens in purging that the watery stools shall irritate those parts so much as to make them feel as if they were scalded. This idea seems reasonable on another principle; for when we consider matter in the gross, we shall find that it is often mixed with extraneous substances which make no part of it, being probably strained from the blood, and also probably undergoing a change afterwards from its not being pure pus; nor do these always arise entirely from the nature of the sore, for they are produced by sores of very different specific qualities, it being the species of matter itself which arises from the nature of the sore; however, the kind of sore will often produce more or less of this extraneous matter, and this additional substance may act as a stimulus on every kind of sore.

What I have considered thus far is the natural process of a sound constitution and sound parts; since a sore that is going through all the natural stages to a cure is not to be called a disease.

A proof of this is, that whenever a real disease attacks either the suppurating surface, or the constitution, these processes of nature are destroyed, and the very reverse take place, the production of true pus ceases, and the fluid becomes changed in some measure in proportion to these morbid alterations; in general it becomes thinner and more transparent, as if the part was returning back to the adhesive state, it partakes more of the nature of the blood, as is the case in most other secretions under similar circumstances. This in common language is not called pus, but sanies.

Pus arising from such state of sores has more of the serum and frequently of the coagulating lymph in it, and less of the combination that renders it coagulable with a solution of sal ammoniac. It has a greater proportion also of the extraneous parts of the blood that are soluble in water, such as salts, and becomes sooner putrid. The two last species of matter not being of the same specific nature with the sore, they have the power of stimulating even their own sore.

On this last account too pus becomes more irritating to the adjoining parts with which it comes in contact, producing excoriation of the skin and the ulcerative inflammation, as the tears, when they run out, excoriate the skin of the cheek from the quantity of salts which they contain. From this effect the matter has been called corrosive, a quality which it has not; the only quality which it possesses being that of irritating the parts with which it comes in contact in such a manner that they are removed out of the way by the absorbents, as will be described when treating on ulceration.

In these instances of the change in the pus, we may say that the change is effected by the decomposition and new combination not being carried on so perfectly. This may probably depend on the secreting vessels having lost their due structure and action, and this appears to be so much the case that they not only fail in this operation, but the other offices of those vessels, viz. the production of granulations is also checked; for the vessels forming themselves into a certain structure which fits them for secreting pus, it is so ordered that the same structure also fits them for producing granulations; and thus those two processes are concomitant effects of the same cause, which cause is a peculiar organization superadded to the vessels of the part.

What organization this may be is not in the least known; nor must we wonder at this, for it is exactly the same with every other organ of secretion, about all which we are equally ignorant. Indeed, some of the differences between one gland and another are made out, and also something of their general structure, but not in such a way as can lead us to the actions and operations of the several parts upon which the nature of the different secretions depend, so as to enable us to conclude *à priori* that this or that gland must secrete this or that peculiar juice.

Pus, from several circumstances often attending it, would appear in general to have a greater tendency to putrefaction than the natural juices have; but I very much suspect that this is not really the case with pure pus, for when it is first discharged from an abscess it is in general perfectly sweet. There are, however, some exceptions to this, but these depend on circumstances entirely foreign to the nature of pus itself. Thus, if the abscess had any communication with the air while the matter was confined in it, (as is frequently the case with those in the neighbourhood of the lungs,) or if it has been so near the colon or rectum as to have been infected by the fæces, under such circumstances we cannot wonder that it becomes putrid. Matter formed early in the state of suppuration, either in abscesses, or more especially in consequence of any external violence committed on the solids, has always in it a portion of blood; or if some parts of the solids mortify and slough, these will mix with the matter. The same thing happens when the inflammation has something of the erysipelatous disposition, so as to have produced a mortification in the seat of the abscess: in all such circumstances we find the pus has a greater tendency to putrefy than the pure or true pus which comes to be discharged afterwards in sound abscesses or healing sores, and accordingly the matter from recent sores becomes very putrid between every dressing; whereas when the same sores are further advanced it is perfectly sweet at the same periods. But although the imperfect or heterogeneous matter that is formed at first is liable to putrefy when exposed, yet if it is perfectly confined in an abscess it will remain a considerable time without putrefaction. The suppuration, however, in consequence of the erysipelatous inflammation, which is often attended with suppuration produced by internal mortification, is, as we have observed, an exception to this rule; for although confined from external air, yet the matter becomes soon putrid, and this most probably arises from the solids themselves first becoming putrid.

A similar observation may be made with respect to sores which have been in the habit of discharging good pus; for if by any accident an extravasation of blood is produced in these parts, or a disposition is brought on to throw out blood, which mixes with the pus, the discharge changes from its former sweetness, and becomes much more putrid and offensive. It appears that pure matter, although easily rendered susceptible of change by extraneous additions, is in its own nature pretty uniform and immutable: it appears so unchangeable, that we find it retained in an abscess for weeks without having undergone any change; but these qualities belong only to perfect pus; for if a sore from a sound state changes its disposition and becomes inflamed, the matter now produced from it, though there be no extravasated blood or dead solids, becomes much sooner putrid than that which was discharged before this alteration of disposition, and will become much more irritating, as has already been observed.

From the above-mentioned considerations we can explain why the discharge in many specific diseases, although not in all, is so much more offensive than in common sores; for in these cases it is commonly not true pus, and is generally mixed with blood.

In the same manner, likewise, where there are diseased bones, or other extraneous bodies which excite irritation, sometimes even to so great a degree as to cause the vessels to bleed, and often wounding the vessels of the part, the matter is always found to be very offensive, one mark (although not commonly accounted for) of a diseased bone.

Our silver probes are rendered almost black when introduced into the discharge of an unhealthy sore; preparations of lead are the same, when applied to such matter: it even dissolves animal substance. If, for instance, a fresh wound has its lips brought together and held there with sticking-plaster spread upon leather, we shall find, if the wound suppurates, that the parts of the strips of leather going over the wound will be between the first and second dressing quite dissolved, dividing the strips into their two ends; and the plaster, which commonly has lead in it, shall become black where it has come in contact with this matter. This change in the colour of metals is also produced by eggs when not perfectly fresh, although not become putrid, and probably this property is assisted by the boiling or roasting. Dr. Crawford, in his experiments on the matter of cancers and animal hepatic air [sulphuretted hydrogen], attributes the dissolution of the metals to that air*.

§. 4. *Of the Use of Pus.*

The final intention of this secretion of matter is, I believe, not yet understood, although almost every one thinks himself able to assign one; and various are the uses attributed to it. It is by some supposed to carry off humours from the constitution. It is sometimes supposed to be a constitutional disease changed into a local one, and so discharged or thrown out of the body, either in form of, or with the pus, as in those cases to be called critical abscesses; but even those who see this final intention are very ready to overturn it, by supposing that this matter is

* Philos. Transact., vol. lxxx. year 1790, part 2nd, p. 385.

capable of being taken back again into the constitution by absorption, and producing much worse evils than those it was meant to relieve. I believe that the supposed cases of absorption are more numerous than those where it is supposed to relieve; if so, then by their own account nothing is gained. Or it is presumed to carry off local complaints from other parts of the body by way of derivation or revulsion; for this reason sores, as issues, are made in sound parts, to allow other sores to be dried up, or even with a view to oblige parts to dissolve themselves into pus, as indurated swellings; but we have endeavoured to show that the solids make no part of pus.

A secretion of pus is also looked upon as a general prevention of many or of all the causes of disease; issues, therefore, are made to keep off both universal disease as well as local. But I am apt to believe that we are not yet well or perhaps at all acquainted with its use, for it is common to all sores, takes place in the most perfect degree in those sores which may be said to be the most healthy, and especially in those where the constitution is most healthy. We find also that very large discharges, when proceeding from a part which is not essential to life, produces very little change in the constitution, and as little upon being healed up, whatever some people may suppose to the contrary.

One might naturally imagine that it was of service to the sore which formed it to keep it moist, &c., for all internal surfaces have their peculiar moisture; but as a sore is to heal, and if allowed to dry so as to form a scab, then a sore is disposed to form no more pus and heal faster, it is the mode of dressing external sores that keeps up this secretion, which in this respect maintains the sore in the state of an internal one. But this will not account for the formation of an abscess, which is the formation of pus we can best account for, since it produces the exposure of internal surfaces: in many cases it is of singular service to procure the second mode of cure, and open a communication between the disease and the external surface of the body. It also forms a passage for the exit of extraneous bodies: but all these are only secondary uses[a].

---

[a] [The chemical qualities of pus have not yet been accurately investigated, nor do we as yet possess any accurate test for distinguishing mucus from the purulent secretion. Dr. George Pearson, in his observations on this fluid in the Philosophical Transactions, 1810, p. 294, has distinguished four leading varieties, to which all the others may be referred, viz. 1. the healthy, or creamlike and equally consistent; 2. the curdy and unequally consistent; 3. the serous and thin; and 4. the viscid and slimy. As these, however, under the microscope all exhibit the same intimate structure, consisting of minute particles suspended in a transparent fluid, it is reasonable to infer that whatever differences exist depend on the relative proportions of their constituent parts, or the different degrees of aggregation in which their particles are united.

The globular structure of the pus, as first pointed out by Senac, has recently been called in question by the microscopical observations of Messieurs Hodgkin and Lister, who found that the particles above mentioned possessed the utmost variety in size as well as in external configuration.

According to Schwilgue pus consists of albumen in a particular state, extractive matter which appears to have no analogue in the healthy state, fatty matter, soda, muriate of soda, phosphate of lime, and other salts. According to some the particles of pus are merely the globules of the blood modified in size and colour, (Gendrin, ii. 479; Andral, Anat. Path., i. 389,) while by others they are regarded as the coagulable lymph existing in a very minute state of division and suspended in the serum of the blood, (Babington, Med.-Chir. Tr., xvi. p. 305,) an idea which agrees pretty nearly with that of Mr. Hunter, who says that "this matter (i. e. the matter which accompanies and precedes the suppurative stage) is a remove further from the nature of the blood, and becomes more and more of the nature of the pus." Pus from mucous membranes is said to contain a greater quantity of albumen than usual; from bone a greater quantity of the phosphates and muriates of lime; from the inflammation of gout a larger proportion of the carbonates and phosphates, and perhaps of the urate of lime; and from scrofulous abscesses a greater relative proportion of soda and the muriate of soda: but, as Mr. Hunter has justly remarked, such facts, even if well established, are of little real value.

The formation of pus was first philosophically classed by Mr. Hunter with the other secretions, and shown to be liable to all those modifications to which the secretions in general are subject from constitutional and local causes. M. Gendrin, in his elaborate work on inflammation, has admitted in general terms the correctness of this doctrine, and yet, inconsistently enough, has attempted to establish, not only the identity of the pus and blood globules, and their gradual metamorphosis *intra et extra vascula* into pus, but also the transformation of the coagulable products of inflammation after their effusion, so as to revive in almost direct terms the ancient doctrine on this subject, of the gradual melting down of the textures. If we examine, he says, a portion of cellular tissue under the microscope, infiltrated with a mixture of bloody serum and pus, we shal observe at the point furthest from the seat of suppuration a simple clear fluid, entirely devoid of globules; a little nearer and we shall perceive globules exactly resembling those of the blood; these, as we approach the seat of suppuration, lose a little of their transparency and deprive themselves of their external envelopes, which hang in striæ on their surfaces; still nearer they have a semi-opaque character and become yellowish; and finally they assume the genuine characters of pus. He has been able, he says, to trace these progressive mutations not only in the proper vessels, until it finally exuded on the surface, but also in all the coagulable fluids effused in inflammation, and cites several experiments to this purpose. (*Op. cit.* ii. 471 *et seq.* (1447.))

It does not appear to me, however, that the experiments which he has detailed at all warrant the conclusion which he has drawn from them, especially when we take into our consideration the following circumstances: 1. that the pus globules are nearly twice as large as those of the blood, and very irregular in size as well as figure; 2. that they display no organizable faculty; 3. that the theory assigns two causes, one chemical and the other vital, for the formation of pus (1461.), as well as two substances, one globular and the other not so, from which it is formed; and 4. that it is not supported by any analogy in regard to the secretions generally, nor account for the influence which the constitution exercises in modifying the time and mode of suppuration, or the superaddition of specific qualities to the pus.

The occurrence of purulent deposits, &c. in vascular coagula, unconnected with the surrounding solids, has been already adverted to (p. 269, *note*), and has been attempted to be explained by M. Andral by comparing them to the lowest order of animated beings, which, antecedent to any traceable organization, are capable of vital acts and of developing an organization by their own innate forces, similar to embryonic germs. Nay, he does not hesitate to ascribe the origin of parasitic acephalocysts and entozoa to this source (*op. cit.* p. 377 *et seq.*). These speculations, however, are scarcely admissible in the present state of science. The only thing which we are able to say with any certainty on this subject is, that these depositions are usually found to coexist with suppurations in other parts of the system, and therefore may with more probability be ascribed to the resorption of matter.]

CHAPTER VI.

THE ULCERATIVE INFLAMMATION.

IN considering the origin and course of the blood, it would have been most natural to have considered absorption, or the absorbing vessels; for in one point of view they may be considered as the animal consisting of so many mouths, everything else depending upon them or belonging to them, for in tracing these dependencies we find that there exists ultimately little else but absorbents. The stomach and the organs connected with it in such animals as have a stomach, are to be considered as subservient to this system; and many an animal is to be considered as consisting of a number of stomachs[a]. A piece of coral, for instance, appears to be no more than a thousand stomachs, all taking in food for digestion and absorption, for increase and support of the whole; for each stomach does not increase as the piece of coral increases, but they multiply in number, and of course the whole piece of coral increases; for although each appears to be a distinct animal yet it is not so. But as this is too general a view of this system for our present purpose, I shall leave it, and confine myself principally to the uses of the absorbents in the diseases of which I am going to treat; and as one of their uses in diseases, and indeed the principal one, has not been described, nor indeed in the least conjectured, that it may be clearly understood or distinguished from the other known uses, I shall relate first the more common uses which have been formerly assigned to this system.

First, the absorbents take up extraneous matter, in which is included nourishment.

Secondly, superfluous and extravasated matter, whether natural or diseased.

Thirdly, the fat.

Fourthly, they produce a waste of parts, in consequence of which muscles become smaller, bones become lighter, etc. Although these two last effects were perhaps not expressly said to be carried on by absorption, either by veins or any other system of vessels, yet we must suppose they were understood: so far the absorbents have in general been considered as active parts in the animal œconomy; but from a

---

[a] [See *note*, p. 116].

further knowledge of these vessels we shall find that they are of much more consequence in the body than has been imagined, and that they are often taking down what the arteries had formerly built up; removing whole organs; becoming modellers of the form of the body while growing; also removing many diseased and dead parts, which were beyond the power of cure; of all which I shall now take particular notice.

As these vessels are productive of a vast variety of effects in the animal œconomy, which are very dissimilar in the intention and effect, they may be viewed in a variety of lights, and admit of a variety of divisions[a]. I shall consider them in two views: first, as they absorb matter, which is not any part of the machine; secondly, as they absorb the machine itself.

The first of these is the well-known use, the absorption of matter, which is no part of the machine. This is of two kinds, one exterior matter, in which may be ranked everything applied to the skin, as also the chyle; and the other interior, such as many of the secreted juices, the fat, and the earth of bones, etc.*. These are principally with a view

* It may be necessary to remark here, that I do not consider either the fat, or the earth of bones, as a part of the animal; they are not animal matter; they have no action within themselves. They have not the principle of life.

---

[a] [The following tabular statement of Mr. Hunter's classification of absorption is introduced for the convenience of reference.

- Absorption connected with growth.
  - Absorption for nourishment.
    - Extraneous matter to become useful, as chyle, fat, &c.
    - Interstitial absorption of parts of the body itself, as cellular membrane, muscles, &c.
  - Absorption of useless, inconvenient, or hurtful parts.
    - Extraneous, that have been useful, as synovia and other secretions, become useless.
    - Parts of the body itself.
      - Producing wasting of a part, as a leg, an arm, &c.; or wasting of the whole body.
      - Absorption of the whole parts.
        - As modellers in the time of growth.
        - In consequence of weakness, as in the removal of calluses.
        - From parts becoming wholly useless, as the alveoli.
- Absorption in consequence of disease.
  - Interstitial absorption.
    - Partial wasting
      - of a leg, an arm, &c.; or of the whole body, as in atrophy.
      - of a callus, of a testicle.
    - Total wasting of calluses, alveoli, testicles, &c.
  - Progressive absorption.
    - Attended with suppuration.
      - As when pus or any extraneous body is brought to the skin,
      - In the process of exfoliation of bones,
      - In the process of sloughing,
      - In the formation of ulcers,
    - Without suppuration.
      - In the removal of the fangs of the teeth.
  - Mixed.
    - As in the progress of pus, tumours, &c. to the skin.]

to its nourishment, and also answer many other purposes; so that the action of absorbing foreign matter is extremely extensive, for besides its salutary effects, it is often the cause of a thousand diseases, especially from poisons, none of which are to my present purpose.

In the second of these views we are to consider them as removing parts of the body itself, in which they may be viewed in two lights. The first is, where only a wasting is produced in the whole machine or part, such as in the wasting of the whole body from an atrophy; or of a part, as in the wasting of the muscles of the leg, etc. from some injury done to some nerve, tendinous part, or joint, all of which I call interstitial absorption, because it is removing parts of the body out of the interstices of that part which remains, leaving the part still as a perfect whole*. But this mode is often carried further than simply wasting of the part; it is often continued till not a vestige is left, such as the total decay of a testicle, so that the interstitial absorption might be understood in two senses.

The second is, where they are removing whole parts of the body. This may be divided into the natural and the diseased†. In the natural they are to be considered as the modellers of the original construction of the body; and if we were to consider them fully in this view we should find that no alteration can take place in the original formation of many of the parts, either in the natural growth, or that formation arising from disease, in which the absorbents are not in action, and take not a considerable part: this absorption I shall call modelling absorption. If I were to consider their powers in this light, it would lead me into a vast variety of effects, as extensive as any principle in the animal œconomy, for a bone cannot be formed without it, nor probably many other parts. A part which was of use in one stage of life, but which becomes entirely useless in another, is thus removed. This is evident in many animals; the thymus gland is removed; the ductus arteriosus, and the membrana pupillaris are removed. This process is, perhaps, more remarkable in the changes of the insect than in any other known animal.

Absorption in consequence of disease is the power of removing complete parts of the body, and is in its operation somewhat similar to the first of this division, or modelling process, but very different in the intention, and therefore in its ultimate effects. This process of removing whole parts in consequence of disease in some cases produces effects which are not similar to one another; one of these is a sore or ulcer, and

* This mode of absorption has always been allowed or supposed, whether performed by the lymphatic veins or lymphatics.

† These uses I claim as my own discovery. I have taught them publicly ever since the year 1772.

I therefore call it ulcerative. In other cases no ulcer is produced, although whole parts are removed, and for this I have not been able to find a term; but both may be denominated progressive absorption.

This process of the removal of a whole solid part of the body, or that power which the animal œconomy has of taking part of itself into the circulation by means of the absorbing vessels whenever it is necessary, is a fact that has not in the least been attended to, nor was it even supposed, and having now been noticed, I mean to give a general idea of it. I may just be allowed once more to observe, that the oil or fat of animals, and the earth of bones, have always been considered as subject to absorption; and some other parts of the body being liable to wasting, have been supposed to suffer this by absorption; but that any solid part should totally be absorbed is a new doctrine. This use of the absorbents I have long been able to demonstrate, and the first hints I received of it were in the waste of the sockets of the teeth, as also in the fangs of the shedding teeth.

It may be difficult at first to conceive how a part of the body can be removed by itself, but it is just as difficult to conceive how a body can form itself, which we see daily taking place; they are both equally facts, and the knowledge of their mode of action would answer perhaps very little purpose; but this I may assert, that whenever any solid part of our bodies undergoes a diminution, or is broken in upon, in consequence of any disease, it is the absorbing system which does it.

When it becomes necessary that some whole living part should be removed, it is evident that nature, in order to effect this, must not only confer a new activity on the absorbents, but must throw the part to be absorbed into such a state as to yield to this operation.

This is the only animal power capable of producing such effects, and like all other operations of the machine, arises from a stimulus or an irritation, all other methods of destruction being either mechanical or chemical. The first by cutting instruments, as knives, saws, etc.; the second by caustics, metallic salts, etc.

The process of ulceration is of the same general nature in all cases, but some of the causes and effects are very different from one another.

The knowledge of the use of this system is but of late date, and the knowledge of its different modes of action is still later. Physiologists have laboured to account for its modes of action, and the principle of capillary tubes was at first the most general idea, because it was a familiar one. But this is too confined a principle of an animal machine; nor will it account for every kind of absorption. Capillary tubes can only attract fluids; but as these inquirers found that solids were often absorbed, such as scirrhous tumours, coagulated blood, the earth of bones, etc., they were driven to the necessity of supposing a solvent: this may or may not be true; it is one of those hypotheses that can never be proved or disproved, and may for ever rest upon opinion. But my conception of this matter is, that Nature leaves as little as possible to chance, and that the whole operation of absorption is performed by an action in the mouths of the absorbents: but even under the idea of capillary tubes, physiologists were still obliged to have recourse to the action of those vessels to carry it along after it was absorbed, and might therefore as well have carried this action to the mouths of these vessels.

As we know nothing of the mode of action of the mouths of these vessels, it is impossible we can form any opinion that can be relied upon; but as they are capable of absorbing substances in two different states, that of solidity and fluidity, it is reasonable to suppose that they have different modes of action; for although any construction of parts that is capable of absorbing a solid may also be such as is capable of absorbing a fluid, yet I can suppose a construction only capable of absorbing a fluid, and not at all fitted for absorbing a solid, though this is not likely; and to see the propriety of this remark more forcibly, let us only consider the mouths of different animals, and I will venture to say that the mouths of all the different animals have not a greater variety of substances to work upon than the absorbents have; and we may observe, that with all the variety of mouths in different animals, this variety is only for the purpose of adapting them to absorb solids, which admit of great variety in form, texture, etc., every one being capable of absorbing fluid matter, which admits of no variety.

This process of the removal of parts of the body, either by interstitial or progressive absorption, answers very material purposes in the machine, without which many local diseases could not be removed, and which, if allowed to remain, would destroy the person. It may be called in such cases the natural surgeon.

It is by the progressive absorption that matter or pus, and extraneous bodies of all kinds, whether in consequence of or producing inflammation and suppuration, are brought to the external surface; it is by means of this that bones exfoliate; it is this operation which separates sloughs; it is the absorbents which are removing whole bones while the arteries are supplying new ones; and although in these last cases of bones it arises from disease, yet it is somewhat similar to the modelling process of this system in the natural formation of bone; it is this operation that removes useless parts, as the alveolar processes when the teeth drop out, or when they are removed by art; as also the fangs of the shedding teeth, which allows them to drop off; and it is by these means ulcers are formed

It becomes a substitute in many cases for mortification, which is another mode of the loss of substance; and in such cases it seems to owe its taking place of mortification to a degree of strength or vigour superior to that where mortification takes place; for although it arises often from weakness, yet it is an action, while mortification is the loss of all action. In many cases it finishes what mortification had begun, by separating the mortified part.

These two modes of absorption, the interstitial and the progressive, are often wisely united, or perform their purposes often in the same part which is to be removed; and this may be called the mixed, which I believe takes place in most cases, as in that of extraneous bodies of all kinds coming to the skin; also in abscesses when in soft parts. It is the second kind of interstitial absorption, the progressive and the mixed, that becomes mostly the object of surgery, although the first of the interstitial sometimes takes place, so as to be worthy of attention.

This operation of the absorption of whole parts, like many other processes in the animal œconomy arising from disease, would often appear to be doing mischief, by destroying parts which are of service, and where no visible good appears to arise from it; for it is this process which forms a sore called an ulcer, such as in those cases where the solids are destroyed upon the external surface, as in old sores of the leg breaking out anew or increasing; but in all cases it must still be referred to some necessary purpose; for we may depend upon it that those parts have not the power of maintaining their ground, and it becomes a substitute for mortification; and indeed in many ulcers we shall see both ulceration and mortification going on, ulceration removing those parts that have power to resist death.

§. 1. *Of the remote Cause of the Absorption of the Animal itself.*

The remote cause of the removal of parts of the animal appears to be of various kinds, and whatever will produce the following effects will be a cause.

The most simple intention or object of nature seems to be the removal of a useless part, as the thymus gland, membrana pupillaris, ductus arteriosus, the alveoli when the teeth drop, or the crystalline humour after couching, and probably the wasting of the body from fever, either acute or hectic. These parts are removed by the absorbents, either as useless parts, or [in the latter case] in consequence of strength being unnecessary while under disease, or such as not to accord with disease*.

* It might be asked as a question, whether the waste of the constitution in disease

Another cause is a weakness, or the want of power in the part to support itself under certain irritations, which may be considered as the basis of every cause of removal of whole parts, as the absorption of calluses, cicatrices, the gums in salivation; also that arising from pressure or irritating applications, under which may be included the attachment of dead parts to a living one, all of which may be accounted for upon the same principle of parts or organs not being able to support themselves under the present evil.

From the above account of the final cause of the absorption of whole parts from disease, it would appear that they are capable of being absorbed from five causes. First, from parts being pressed; secondly, from parts being considerably irritated by irritating substances; thirdly, from parts being weakened; fourthly, from parts being rendered useless; fifthly, from parts becoming dead. The two first, for instance, parts being pressed and parts being irritated, appear to me to produce the same irritation; the third, or weakness, an irritation of its own kind; and the fourth, or parts being rendered useless, and the fifth, or parts becoming dead, may be somewhat similar.

It is probable that every cause above enumerated is capable of producing every mode, or rather effect, of absorption, whether interstitial or progressive; but pressure attended with suppuration always produces the progressive, whether applied externally or internally, as in the case of abscesses.

§. 2. *Of the Disposition of living Parts to absorb and to be absorbed.*

The dispositions of the two parts of the living body, which absorb and are absorbed, must be of two kinds respecting the parts, one passive and the other active. The first of these is an irritated state of the part to be absorbed, which renders it unfit to remain under such circumstances, the action excited by this irritation being incompatible with the natural actions and the existence of the parts, whatever these are, which therefore become ready for removal, or yield to it with ease. The second is the absorbents being stimulated to action by such a state of parts, so that both conspire to the same end.

When the part to be absorbed is a dead part, as nourishment or extraneous matter of all kinds, then the whole disposition is in the absorbents.

arises from the body becoming useless when under such diseases, as may be observed of muscles when their joint, tendon, &c. is diseased, or whether it accords better with the diseased state, and may even tend to a natural cure?

When the immediate causes arise in consequence of pressure, it would appear that absorption takes place more readily under certain circumtances than others, although the remote causes of them appear to be the same, and therefore there is something more than simple pressure. For we find that pressure from within produces ulceration or absorption much more readily than from without, for if it was pressure only, absorption then would be according to the quantity of pressure; but we find very different effects from the same quantity of pressure under the above-mentioned circumstances: for when from without, pressure rather stimulates than irritates, it shall give signs of strength, and produce an increase of thickening; but when from within, the same quantity of pressure will produce waste, for the first effect of the pressure from without is the disposition to thicken, which is rather an operation of strength; but if it exceeds the stimulus of thickening then the pressure becomes an irritator, and the power appears to give way to it, and absorption of the parts pressed takes place, so that Nature very readily takes on those steps which are to get rid of an extraneous body, but appears not only not ready to let extraneous bodies enter the body, but endeavours to exclude them, by increasing the thickness of the parts.

Many parts of our solids are more susceptible of being absorbed, especially by ulceration, than others, even under the same or similar circumstances, while the same part shall vary its susceptibility according to circumstances.

The cellular and adipose membranes are very particularly susceptible of being absorbed, which is proved by muscles, tendons, ligaments, nerves, and blood-vessels being found frequently deprived of their connecting membrane and fat, especially in abscesses, so that ulceration often takes a roundabout course to get to the skin, following the track of the cellular membrane; and the skin itself, when the pressure is from within, is much less susceptible of ulceration than the cellular and adipose membrane, which retards the progress of abscesses when they are so far advanced, and also becomes the cause of the skin's hanging over spreading ulcers, which are spreading from the same cause, more especially too if the part ulcerating is an original part. Ulceration never takes place on investing membranes of circumscribed cavities, excepting suppuration has taken place; and indeed ulceration in such parts would be a sure forerunner of suppuration.

New-formed parts, or such as cannot be said to constitute part of the original animal, as healed sores, calluses of bones, especially those in consequence of compound fractures, admit more readily of absorption, especially the progressive, than those parts which were originally formed.

This arises probably from the principle of weakness, and it is from this too that all adventitious new matter, as tumours, are more readily absorbed than even that which is a substitute for the old. Thus we have tumours more readily absorbed than a callus of a bone, union of a tendon, &c., because they have still less powers than those which are substitutes for parts originally formed.

Ulceration in consequence of death in an external part takes place soonest on the external edge between the dead and the living. This is visible in the sloughing of parts; for we may observe that sloughs from caustics, bruises, mortifications, &c. always begin at the external edge.

An internal pressure produced by an extraneous body acts equally on every side of the surrounding parts, and therefore every part being pressed alike ought, from this cause alone, to produce absorption of the surrounding parts equally on all sides, supposing the parts themselves similar in structure, or, which is the same, equally susceptible of being absorbed; but we find that one side only of the surrounding living parts is susceptible of this irritation, therefore one side only is absorbed; and this is always the side which is next to the external surface of the body. We therefore have always extraneous bodies of every kind determined to the skin, and on that side to which the extraneous body is nearest, without having any effect, or producing the least destruction of any of the other surrounding parts. From this cause we find abscesses, &c., whose seat is in or near the centre of a part, readily determined to the surface on the one side and not on the other; and whenever the lead is once taken, it immediately goes on. But as some parts from their structure are more susceptible of this irritation than others, we find that those parts composed of such structure are often absorbed, although they are not in the shortest road to the skin: this structure is the cellular membrane, as will be taken notice of hereafter

We find the same principle in the progress of tumours; for although every part surrounding a tumour is equally pressed, yet the interstitial absorption only takes place on that side next the external surface, by which means the tumour is, as it were, led to the skin. From hence we find that absorption of whole parts more readily takes place to allow an extraneous substance to pass out of the body than it will to allow one to pass in.

Thus we see that the slight pressure produced by matter on the inside of an abscess has a great effect, and the matter is brought much faster to the skin (although very deep) than it would by the same quantity of pressure applied from without; and indeed so slight a pressure from without would rather tend to have an opposite effect, namely, that of thickening.

The reasons of this are evident: one is, a readiness in the parts to be freed from a disease already existing; the other is, a backwardness in the parts to admit a disease. This principle therefore in the animal œconomy produces one of the most curious phenomena in the whole process of ulceration, viz. the susceptibility which the parts lying between an extraneous body and the skin have to ulcerate, while all the other sides of the abscess are not irritated to ulceration; and the necessity there is that it should be so must be very striking; for if ulceration went on equally on all sides of an abscess, it must increase to a most enormous size, and too great a quantity of our solids must necessarily be destroyed.

Bones, we have observed, are also subject to similar circumstances of ulceration; for whenever an abscess forms in the centre of a bone, or an internal exfoliation has taken place, the extraneous body acts upon the internal surface of the cavity, and produces ulceration.

If the matter or dead piece of bone is nearer one side than the other, ulceration takes place on that side only; and here too the provision of Nature in abscesses comes in, for the adhesive inflammation extends itself on the outside in proportion as ulceration extends itself on the inside of the cavity, and as ulceration approaches to the surface of the bone the adhesive disposition is given to the periosteum, then to the cellular membrane, &c. And what is very curious, this adhesive inflammation assumes the ossifying disposition, which I have called the ossific inflammation, and appears as a spreading ossification, in the same manner as in the callus of a simple fracture.

The consequence of these two processes taking place together in bones is very singular, for the ulcerative process destroying the inside of a bone while the ossifying makes addition to its outside, the bone often increases to a prodigious size, as in cases of spina ventosa; but in the end the ulceration on the inside gets the better, and the matter makes its escape.

Nature has not only made what might be called an instinctive provision in the parts to remove themselves, so as to bring extraneous bodies to the skin for their exit, and thereby from this principle has guarded the deeper-seated parts, but has also guarded all passages or outlets where, from reasoning, we might suppose no great mischief could arise from bringing extraneous bodies thither; and in many cases a seeming advantage would be gained, such passages appearing to be more convenient for the exit of such matter, and likely to produce less visible mischief in procuring them.

Thus a tumour in the cheek, close on the internal membrane of the mouth and some way from the skin, shall in its growth push externally, especially if there is matter in it, and in time come in contact with the skin and adhere to it, while it shall have made no closer connexion with the skin of the mouth. If it should suppurate, and more especially if it be of a scrofulous kind, which is slow in its progress, it will break externally; we even see abscesses in the gums opening externally, where the matter has been obliged to go a considerable way to get to the skin.

The same guard is set over the cavity of the nose: if an abscess forms in the antrum, frontal sinus, or saccus lachrymalis, all of which are nearer to the cavity of the nose than the external surface of the body, ulceration does not follow this shortest way, which would be directly into the nose, but leads the matter to the nearest external surface.

I have seen an abscess in the frontal sinus first attended with great pain in the part, then with inflammation on the whole forehead, at last matter has been felt under the skin, and on being opened it has led into one or both sinuses, and almost the whole bone has exfoliated. For such an abscess the nearest passage would have been directly into the nose. Abscess in the lachrymal sac, forming what is called the fistula lachrymalis, arises also from the same cause. A curious circumstance takes place here; but whether peculiar to this part or not, I do not yet know: besides the disposition for ulceration externally at the inner corner of the eye, there is a defence set up upon the inside, so that the membrane of the nose thickens very considerably. How far a thickening takes place on the inside of the nose, opposite to the antrum, in abscesses of that cavity, or how far it is a universal principle in other passages, I have not been able to learn, but I am inclined to believe it is not universal. From this principle we can see why openings made into these passages to make the matter come that way are more unsuccessful than reasoning (without the knowledge of this principle) would lead us to believe; the opening, therefore, should not be made on the inside, (even where we can do it,) excepting the matter is very near, or else the opening should be made very large; and probably in such cases it may be necessary to take out a piece, so as to prevent the uniting process, which is here very strong.

Illustrations will be given in other passages, when treating of ulceration in general tending to the external surface.

§. 3. *Of Interstitial Absorption.*

Interstitial absorption, I observed, was of two kinds with respect to effect, or rather had two stages. The first was where it took place only in a part, as in the wasting of a limb in consequence of its being rendered useless, whether from disease in a joint, a broken tendon, or the dividing of a nerve, whereby its influence is cut off; or where it takes place in the whole body in consequence of some disease, as in acute fever, hectic fever, diabetes, atrophy, or the like. The second is the absorption of a whole part, where not a vestige is left. This [latter] would seem to be of two kinds: one where it is only in consequence of another disease, and is a necessary and useful effect of that disease, as assisting in bringing parts to the surface; but the other appears to arise from a disease in the part itself, as the total decay of the alveoli, without any disease in the teeth or gums, which however in the end suffer, as also the total wasting of a testicle, the absorption of a callus, &c. It is the first of these two kinds which is most to my present purpose, and deserves our particular attention. It takes place in a thousand instances; we find it gradually taking place in the part of the body which happens to lie between encysted tumours and the external surface, when they are making their way to the skin. This absorption is commonly slow in its progress, so much so as even to make the ultimate effect, although considerable, not sensible till a certain length of time has elapsed.

This mode of removing parts appears to arise from pressure, as in the former; but here some principles are reversed. The contents of an encysted tumour do not give the stimulus of removal to that side of the cyst nearest to the external surface, as happens in an abscess, so as to produce a removal of the surface pressed by its contents, which would be the progressive ulceration, as in our first division; but the tumour gives the stimulus to the sound parts, between it and the skin, and an absorption of those parts takes place, similar to that which I suppose takes place in the removal of calluses of bones from weakness. We find whenever an encysted tumour is formed in the cellular membrane, it in time makes its approaches towards the skin, by the cellular membrane and other parts between it and the skin being absorbed, so that the whole substance between the cyst and skin becomes thinner and thinner, till the cyst and the external skin meet or come in contact, and then inflammation begins to take place; for as the parts are now soon to be exposed, inflammation takes place to produce a quicker absorption, which borders often upon ulceration. The mode of action in this last case may be, in one respect, very similar to the foregoing solid tumour, for besides the interstitial absorption, the cyst may be looked upon as a tumour acting upon or stimulating the parts between it and the skin; therefore the tumour causes absorption of the contiguous cellular membrane upon which it presses. This process of interstitial absorption of parts is very evident, even in common abscess; and where a progressive absorption is going on, it is assisted by this.

I have already observed that the interstitial absorption is not attended with, nor does it produce, suppuration.

§. 4. *Of the Progressive Absorption.*

The first or principal mode of this action is the removing of those surfaces that are immediately contiguous to the irritating causes, which is an absorption of necessity. These causes, I have observed, are of three kinds: one, pressure; another, irritating substances; and the third, considerable inflammation in a weak part, especially those new-formed parts that become a substitute for the old. Absorption from pressure is the removal of the part pressed, which may arise from a number of causes. There are tumours which, by pressing upon neighbouring parts, produce it; the pressure of the blood in aneurisms produces it, etc.; also that surface of an abscess, or any other extraneous body which is nearest the external surface[a]; or the ulceration of that part of the surface of the body which is in contact with a body pressing, as the buttocks or hips of those who lie long upon their backs; the heels of many people who lie long in the same position, as is the case with those who are under the cure of a fracture of the leg, in which case it seems to be a substitute for mortification, and is rather a proof of the strength of the patient; for if very weak constitutionally, the same parts certainly mortify; as also the constant pressure of chains on the legs of prisoners, and harness on the breasts of horses.

The second of these causes of absorption is the action of irritating substances, such as the tears passing constantly over the cheeks; as also many irritating medicines, producing too much action, and probably at the same time weakening the parts. The third is the formation of an ulcer or sore on a surface, in consequence of some disease, which has been the cause of inflammation. Bones are subject to the same effect from pressure as the soft parts, as in consequence of aneurisms; as also from the pressure from tumours: likewise in cases of the spina ventosa, where in some there is nothing to be found in the cavity of the swelling but blood coagulated, in others a grumous or curdly substance. This blood or curdly substance increasing, continues the pressure, and the inside of the bone is in time absorbed.

I have already observed that the progressive absorption is divisible into two kinds; one without suppuration, the other with. I shall now

---

[a] ["also that surface of an abscess which is in contact with the pus, or any other extraneous body."—*Original text.*]

observe that the absorption which does not produce suppuration may take place either from pressure made by sound parts upon diseased parts, or by diseased upon sound parts; as the effect that the pressure of the coagulated blood has in aneurisms, the moving blood in the same, which is a sound part, contained in diseased arteries not capable of supporting the pressure of the moving blood; as also many tumours, which are diseased parts, pressing upon natural sound parts; and these diseased parts are simply endowed with life, which I apprehend makes some difference in the effects respecting the formation of pus; also uncommon pressure made by such substances as are not endowed with any irritating quality sufficient to produce the suppurative inflammation, as a piece of glass, a lead bullet, etc., all of which I shall now more fully explain.

Of this first division, viz. from pressure without suppuration, we have several instances, as in aneurisms, especially when they are in the aorta, and principally at the curve; and when arrived at a considerable size, so as to press against the surrounding parts, particularly against the backbone, as also against the sternum; all of which will be according to the situation of the aneurism: we find in such cases, that from the dilatation of the artery (which arises from the force of the heart) the artery is pressed against those bones, and that the substance of the artery at the part pressed is taken into the constitution. This absorption begins at the external surface of the artery, where it comes in contact with the bone, and continues there till the whole artery is absorbed; then the bone itself comes in contact with the circulating blood, and not being naturally intended to be washed by moving blood, the bone or bones are also absorbed from this pressure and motion of the blood against them. The adhesive or strengthening disposition takes place in the surrounding parts, and is of great service here, as it unites the circumference of the unabsorbed part of the artery to the surrounding parts; as also the cellular membrane beyond the surface of absorption (when in soft parts), similar to the preceding adhesive inflammation going before ulceration in an abscess; but it is here much stronger, for strength is wanted as well as adhesion while it is dilating; so that a cavity of some strength for the moving blood is always kept entire, and no extravasation can take place, nor can the parts readily give way.

Another instance of this absorption occurs in those cases where living tumours make their way to the skin without the formation of an abscess. I once saw a remarkable instance of this in a Highland soldier in the Dutch service, who had a solid tumour formed, either in the substance of the brain, or, what is more probable, upon it, viz. in the pia-mater, for it seemed to be covered by that membrane: the tumour was oblong, above an inch thick, and two or more inches long; it was sunk near its whole length into the brain, seemingly by the simple effects of pressure; but the outer end of it, by pressing against the dura mater, had produced the absorbing disposition in that membrane, so that this membrane was entirely gone at that part. The same irritation from pressure had been given to the skull, which also was absorbed at this part; after which the same disposition was continued on to the scalp. As these respective parts gave way, the tumour was pushed further and further out, so that its outer end came to be in this new passage the absorbents were making for it in the scalp, by which it probably would have been discharged in time if the man had lived; but it was so connected with the vital parts that the man died before the parts could relieve themselves. While all these exterior parts were in a state of absorption, the internal parts which pressed upon the inner end of the tumour, and which pressure was sufficient to push it out, did not in the least ulcerate; nor did the tumour itself, which was pressed upon all sides, in the least give way in its substance. No matter was to be observed here from either the dura mater, the unconnected edge of the bones of the skull, nor from that part of the scalp which had given way; and perhaps the reason was, the tumour being a living part, and not an extraneous one. The general effect was, however, similar to the progress of an abscess, insomuch that it was on that side nearest to the external surface of the body that the irritation for absorption took place.

This first species of the absorption of whole parts is seldom or never attended with pain. Its progress is so very slow as to keep pace with our sensations, and in many cases it is not even attended with inflammation.

I believe that this absorption seldom if ever affects the constitution, although in some cases it takes its rise from affections of the constitution, as in the cases of the absorption of callus.

§. 5. *Of Absorption attended with Suppuration, which I have called Ulceration.*

I shall now give an account of that part of the actions of the absorbing system which I call ulceration, and which is the second of our first division respecting the formation of pus, viz. that which is connected with the formation of that fluid, being either a consequence of it, or producing it, and is that which in all cases constitutes an ulcer. It is this which principally constitutes the progressive absorption*.

* I have given it the term ulceration, because ulcer is a word in use to express a sore, and it is by this process that many ulcers are formed. The operations produced

This differs from the foregoing in some circumstances of its operations. It either takes place in consequence of suppuration already begun, and then the pus acts as an extraneous body, capable of producing pressure; or absorption attacks external surfaces from particular irritations or weakness, in which case suppuration, forming an ulcer, must follow, let the cause of that breach or loss of substance be what it may.

In order to produce ulceration from pressure, I may again take notice that it requires a much greater pressure from without than from within; and when it is from within, the ulceration is quicker when near to the skin than when deep or far from it; the nearer it is to the skin the more readily inflammation takes place; and I have also observed that inflammation, although it takes place in deep-seated parts, yet it seldom or never extends deeper, but approaches towards the external surface; and as inflammation seems to precede, and is essential to this process, we see the reason why it should take place sooner if near to the skin, and go on faster the nearer it comes to it.

The process of ulceration which brings matter to the external surface is not wholly the absorption of the inner surface of the abscess, for there is an interior or insterstitial absorption of the parts lying between the inner surface of the abscess and the skin, similar to the approach of encysted tumours, as has been described. And besides this assistance, I have already observed, there is a relaxing and elongating process carried on between the abscess and the skin, and at those parts only where the matter appears to point.

This process of ulceration, or absorption with suppuration, is almost constantly attended by inflammation; but it cannot be called an original inflammation, but a consequent, which gave rise to the term ulcerative inflammation. It is always preceded by the adhesive inflammation, and perhaps it is simply this inflammation which attends it. We find the adhesions produced answering very wise purposes; for although the adhesive inflammation has preceded the suppurative, and of course all the parts surrounding the abscess are united, yet if this union of the parts has not extended to the skin, where the abscess or matter is to be discharged, in such a case, wherever the ulceration has proceeded beyond the adhesions, there the matter will come into unadhering parts; the consequence of which will be that the fluid or matter will diffuse itself into the cellular membrane of the part, and from thence over the whole

in ulceration have not hitherto been in the least understood, therefore a very erroneous cause of these operations has been always supposed. It has always been supposed that those solids which were visibly gone were dissolved into pus; from whence arose the idea of matter being composed of solids and fluids, which we have endeavoured to refute.

body, as in the erysipelatous suppuration; but to prevent this effect, the adhesive inflammation takes the lead of ulceration. There are many other causes of ulceration, which operate on surfaces, where we do not see the same necessity for it, when the matter formed can be and is discharged without it; such parts are many old sores, the inside of the stomach and intestines, and indeed all the surfaces above mentioned; which do not admit readily of the adhesive inflammation, under some circumstances admit of the ulcerative. This effect would appear to arise from the violence of the inflammation, the parts being so weakened, either by it, or some former disease, that they can hardly support themselves; for we find in salivations, where the whole force of the mercury has been determined to the mouth, they have become weakened by long and violent action; the gums and inside of the mouth will ulcerate; also, from the same weakening disposition the gums will ulcerate in bad scurvies; therefore weakness joined with inflammation, or violence of action, appears to be the immediate cause in such cases.

The effect then of irritation, as above described, is to produce first the adhesive inflammation in such parts as will readily admit of it, and if that has not the intended effect, the suppurative takes place, and then the ulceration comes on to lead the matter already formed to the skin, if it is confined.

The natural consequence of suppuration in such parts is the growth of new flesh, called granulations, which are to repair the loss the parts have sustained by the injury done; but in all outlets, where the adhesive would be hurtful, the irritation first only produces the suppurative inflammation; but if carried further, the adhesive will take place, as has been described; and as in such parts the matter formed has an outlet, ulceration is also avoided; and as in such cases no parts are destroyed, granulations are also excluded.

There appears to be a curious circumstance attending ulceration, which is the readiness with which it seems to absorb every other substance applied to it, as well as the body itself; at least this appears to be the case with the smallpox after inoculation, as also the venereal chancre, whether arising from the absorbents at the time being in the act of absorbing, or whether they promiscuously absorb what is applied along with the parts themselves. In such cases it might be a question also whether the parts of the body which they do absorb have the same disposition with the pus of that part, as in the cancer, and therefore contaminate the constitution, as in the smallpox and venereal disease, as readily as if it was the pus.

From what has been observed, it must appear that any irritation which is so great as to destroy suddenly the natural operations of any one part, and the effect of which is so long continued as to oblige the parts to act for their own relief, produces in some parts, first the adhesive inflammation; and if the cause be increased, or continue still longer, the suppurative state takes place, and all the other consequences, as ulceration; or if in the other parts, as secreting surfaces, then the suppurative takes place immediately, and if too violent, the adhesive will succeed; or if parts are very much weakened the ulcerative will immediately succeed the adhesive, and then suppuration will be the consequence.

This species of ulceration in general gives considerable pain, which pain is commonly distinguished by the name of soreness; this is the sensation arising from cutting with an instrument, which operation is very similar to ulceration; but this pain does not attend all ulcerations, for there are some of a specific kind which give little or no pain, such as the scrofula; but even in this disease, when the ulceration proceeds pretty fast, it gives often considerable pain; therefore the pain may be in some degree proportioned to the quickness of its operation.

The greatest pain which in general attends this operation arises from those ulcerations which are formed for the purpose of bringing the matter of an abscess to the skin; as also where ulceration begins upon a surface, or is increasing a sore. Whether the increase of pain arises from the ulcerative inflammation singly, or from the adhesive and ulcerative going on together in the same point, is not easily determined; but in some cases these three are pretty rapid in their progress, and it is more than probable that the pain arises from all these causes.

In those cases where ulceration is employed in separating a dead part, such as sloughing, exfoliation, etc., it is seldom attended with pain; perhaps it may not be easy to assign a cause for this.

The effects that ulceration has upon the constitution I have mentioned, with the effects that other local complaints have upon it.

It is easy to distinguish between a sore that is ulcerating, and one which is standing still, or granulating. The ulcerating sore is made up of little cavities or hollows, and the edge of the skin is scolloped or notched, is thin, turned a little out, and overhangs more or less the sore. The sore is always foul, being probably composed of parts not completely absorbed, and discharges a thin matter. But when the ulceration stops, the edge of the skin becomes regular, smooth, a little rounded or turned in, and of a purple colour, covered with a semi-transparent white.

§. 6. *Of the Relaxing Process.*

Besides these two modes of removing whole parts, acting singly or together, there is an operation totally distinct from either, and this is a relaxing and elongating process carried on between the abscess and the skin, and at those parts only where the matter appears to point. It is possible that this relaxing, elongating, or weakening process may arise in some degree from the absorption of the interior parts; but there is certainly something more, for the skin that covers an abscess is always looser than a part that gives way from mere mechanical distention, excepting the increase of the abscess is very rapid.

That parts relax or elongate without mechanical force, but from particular stimuli, is evident in the female parts of generation just before the birth of the fœtus: they become relaxed prior to any pressure. The old women in the country can tell when a hen is going to lay, from the parts becoming loose about the anus.

That this relaxing process takes place between an abscess and the skin is evident in all cases, but was more demonstratively so in the following case than commonly can be observed, where an increase of surface takes place without the visible loss of substance, for here both could be exactly ascertained; and, indeed, no abscess could swell outwards, excepting by distention, without it. In the following case this process was particularly evident.

A lad about thirteen years of age was attacked with a violent inflammation in his belly, without any apparent cause. The usual means were used, but without effect. His belly began to swell in a few days after the attack, and his skin became cold and clammy, especially his feet and hands. Once when he made water it was transparent like spring water, with a little cloud of mucus. In several places of the belly there appeared a pointing, as if from matter; one of those, which was just below the sternum, became pretty large, and discoloured with a red tint. Although there was not any undulation or perfect fluctuation (there not being fluid enough for such a feel) yet it was plain there was a fluid, and most probably from the pointings, it was matter in consequence of inflammation, and was producing ulceration on the inside of the abdomen for its exit; therefore it was thought advisable, as early as possible, to open the belly at one of those parts. I made a small opening into the pointing part, just below the sternum, hardly an inch long: when I was performing the operation, I saw plainly the head of the rectus muscle, which I cut through in the direction of its fibres. There was immediately discharged by this wound about two or three quarts of a thin bloody matter. The swelling of the abdomen subsided of course; his pulse began to rise and become more full and soft; and his extremities became warmer; he was ordered bark, etc. but he lived only about sixty hours after the operation.

On opening his abdomen after death we found little or no matter lying loose; all had made its escape through the wound. The whole intestines, stomach, and liver were united by a very thick covering of the coagulating lymph, which also passed into all the interstices between them, by which means they were all united into one mass: the liver also adhered to the diaphragm, but none of the viscera adhered to the inside of the belly on its fore part, for there the matter had given the stimulus for ulceration, which prevents all adhesions. The process of ulceration had gone on so far as to have destroyed the whole of the peritonæum on the fore part of the abdomen, and the transversales and recti muscles were cleanly dissected on their inside. The tendons of the lateral muscles that pass behind the heads of the recti were in rags, partly gone, and partly in the form of a slough.

From this view of the case we must see how Nature had guarded all the most essential parts. In the time of the adhesive stage she had covered all the intestines with a coat of coagulating lymph, so as to guard them; and this probably upon two principles, one from their being canals, and therefore loth to admit of penetration in that way; the other from their being more internal than the parietes of the abdomen; one side is therefore thickened for their defence, while the other is thinned for the relief of the part.

Here the cavity of the abdomen had assumed all the properties of an abscess, but it was so connected with the vital parts, which also suffered much in the inflammation, that the patient could not support the necessary processes towards what would be called a radical cure in many other parts; and indeed, considering the mischief done to the abdomen and its viscera, it is astonishing he lived so long.

The most curious circumstance that happened was the appearance of pointing in several places; for why one part of the abdomen should have pointed more than another is not easily accounted for, since every part of the anterior portion was nearly equally thin, each part was equally involved in the abscess, and the ulceration had not yet begun with any of the muscles. To account for this, let us suppose that one, two, or three parts (by some accident) were more susceptible of the ulcerative stimulus than the others, and that the parts were ready to give way; but although these parts which were pointing were the places where ulceration would have gone on brisker, yet it had not proceeded further here than in any other part, it had only gone through the peritonæum and the tendons of the broad muscles, and the recti muscles were sound and perfect at the place where I made the opening, which was the most protuberant of any; therefore this pointing did not appear to arise from weakness or thinness of this part; and even supposing that the pointing was an effect of weakness, it would imply a great deal of pressure on the inside, (which at least was not the case here,) and simple pressure, although a hundred times greater, which we often see take place in dropsies, would not produce a pointing if not attended with some specific power[a].

If pressure then was not sufficient to produce this effect in the present case, and if the parts which pointed were as mechanically firm as at any other, to what other cause can we attribute the distention of this part, but to the weakening, elongating, and relaxing process which I have already described?

This observation of the relaxing process going on in the substance of the parts where it points is verified in a thousand instances. Suppose a large abscess in the thigh, only covered by the skin and adipose membrane, which shall go on for months without producing ulceration, and of course not point anywhere, but shall be a smooth, even, and uniform surface; let it receive the stimulus of ulceration in any one part, that

[a] [Having previously expressed my doubts as to the existence of any special law determining the course of foreign bodies to the surface (p. 300, *note*), I may here be permitted to express the same doubts respecting abscesses. "An internal pressure," Mr. Hunter observes, p. 467, "produced by an extraneous body, acts equally on every side of the surrounding parts, and therefore every part being pressed alike, ought, from this cause alone, to produce absorption of the surrounding parts equally on all sides," &c. A fallacy, however, is involved in this statement, arising from the omission of an important fact, viz. the resiliency or natural tonicity of the skin, which, being put still further on the stretch by the intrusion of a foreign body, reacts, so as to give a determinate direction to the force. In most cases this direction will be outwardly and inwardly, but inwardly the parts are not disposed to yield, and therefore in the same proportion as the external parts are more yielding than the internal, will there be an additional cause to determine the absorption in that direction; for I suppose it will not be doubted that extension and pressure are both powerful determining causes of inflammation and ulceration.

With regard to abscesses, other mechanical causes of a tendency to the surface will come into operation besides the greater extensibility of parts in that direction. For by the bulging thus originally produced, the area of the upper surface of the cavity will be greater, even from the first, than that of the base: and as fluids under pressure act equally on equal areas, the whole amount of pressure outwards will be increased in proportion to the local augmentation of area. This preponderance of pressure must produce a greater degree of stretching and a more active ulcerative absorption here than elsewhere; and the cause in question will grow more and more effective as the prominence which it contributes to produce is augmented,—so that the *pointing* of the abscess will proceed with a constantly accelerated rapidity.

These combined causes will manifestly be all in the fullest operation at the middle point of the outer surface of the cavity; here the cavities will be most stretched, because the least supported; here the vital processes which produce attenuation will be

part will immediately begin to point, although it may be thicker there than at some other parts of the same abscess.

The pressure necessary to allow extraneous matter to make its escape

---

most active because most stimulated; and it is in this situation that, *cæteris paribus*, the prominence is always observed to be most considerable, and that the abscess naturally bursts.

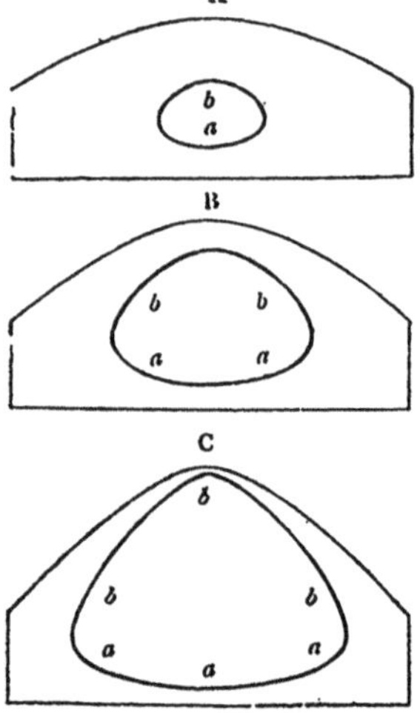

The annexed diagrams are intended to represent sections of an abscess in three several degrees of its progress towards the surface; and will serve to illustrate the suggestions that have been thrown out as to the causes of the outward tendency of the contained fluid. It will be seen that the surface of the cavity towards the skin (*b*, *b b*, *b b b*), progressively increases in area at a quicker rate than the *base* (*a*, *a a*, *a a a*).

This view I think is confirmed by the erratic course of internal abscesses, which only burrow in those directions in which the extensibility is greatest, as well as by the case of peritoneal abscess cited in the text, and that of chronic abscesses generally; for as the superficies of an abscess becomes more extended, and as the disposition to absorption becomes less active, so of course will the disposition to acumination become less evident. In dropsies both these causes combine to prevent pointing; for here there is no disposition to progressive absorption arising from inflammation, and no disposition to concentrate the acting force arising from inequality of extension.

The discovery of final causes appears to have been a principal object in all Mr. Hunter's investigations, and it must be confessed that few have ever been equally successful in this branch of inquiry. It was, however, the weakness as well as the strength of Hunter's physiology, as it often led him to substitute the final for the efficient causes of phenomena, of which, if I am not mistaken, several examples might be adduced from the present chapter.

As the above explanation is opposed to the received opinions of the profession, I offer it with much diffidence. As an instance of intelligent design, extending even to a provision for the accidental lesions of the frame, few examples are more beautiful than that of the adhesive inflammation, and especially of the approach of foreign bodies to the surface by progressive absorption; but nothing is detracted from the value of these facts by showing that mechanical causes are concerned in their operation.]

need not be great; for in many abscesses which have been opened, or have opened of themselves, but not at the most depending part, so that the matter is allowed to stagnate at the lower part of the cavity, making a very slight pressure, we find that this alone is sufficient to produce ulceration in that part, and of course a fresh opening is produced, more especially if near the skin. This we see often take place in abscesses of milk breasts, when the opening is not at a depending part, and appears to be common in the fistula in ano; for it frequently happens that the ulceration goes on at first towards the gut; but before this has taken place, ulceration has gone on some way by the side of it, to bring the matter externally, which weight of matter is alone sufficient to continue the same process.

§. 7. *Of the Intention of Absorption of the Body in Disease.*

This, like everything else in Nature, involves in it two consequences, the one beneficial, the other hurtful, both of which this has in a considerable degree; however, if we understood thoroughly all the remote causes, we should probably see its utility in every case, and that these effects, however bad in appearance, yet are necessary, and of course in the end salutary. The use arising from what may be called the natural absorption of parts, such as the forming or modelling process, as also the absorption of parts which have become unfit for the new mode of life, as the absorption of the thymus gland, &c., is involved in its necessity, and belongs to the natural history of the animal; but that arising from disease is directly to the present purpose. In the history I have just given, its use must, I apprehend, be evident; for we plainly see, in each mode of absorption, it often produces very salutary effects; and we may say that, although it often arises from disease, yet its operations and effects are often not at all a disease; and probably in those cases where we cannot assign a cause, as in wasting of parts, atrophy, &c., yet it is most probable that its use is considerable. It is likely that under such a disease, or state of body or parts, it would be hurtful to have them full and strong; where it produces a total waste of a part its utility is probably not so evident; but in the progressive absorption, where it is leading bodies externally, or in consequence of suppuration, where it is bringing matter externally, its use is plain; or even in the formation of an ulcer, or the spreading of an ulcer, its use may be considerable. I have formerly called it the natural surgeon; and where it can do its business it is in most cases preferable to art: this is so evident in many cases that it has been a constant practice to attempt to promote it in bringing abscesses to the surface, in the exfoliation of bone, &c., and although not accounted for upon the principle of absorption, yet the effect was visible, and its use allowed.

§. 8. *The Modes of promoting Absorption.*

The history that was given of the causes of absorption in some degree explains the modes of promoting it; but as there were some natural causes which we cannot imitate, it is principally those that can be rendered useful that we are to take notice of in this place.

To promote absorption of the body itself is no difficult operation: it is only to lessen the supply and increase the waste, which last is often done by medicine, or to take such things as will render the supply less efficacious, as vinegar or soap; but probably these act principally on the fat. To promote absorption of diseased parts, or parts increased, or parts newly formed is not so easy a task, although the latter may be the most easy of the whole, for I have asserted that newly formed parts are weaker in their living powers than the originally formed parts. This in some degree gives us a hint; for if we have a mode of producing a waste of the whole original body, under this general waste, new-formed parts must suffer in a degree proportional to their weakness, and therefore will suffer a diminution in the same proportion; but this is too often not sufficient, or at least what would be sufficient for the disease would be too great for the constitution to bear; however, we find in particular cases that this practice has some effect. Probably the best debilitating medicine is mercury, and it probably may act in more ways than one. It may promote absorption from a peculiar stimulus, producing necessity, or a state under which the parts cannot exist. Electricity and most other stimulants probably act in the same manner, for we find that violent inflammation is often a cause. Death in a part is sure to promote absorption, in order to produce a separation of the dead parts; and we even find that a part being diseased gives a tendency to separation, and only requires a considerable inflammation to promote it, such as warts coming away in consequence of inflammation. A diseased part has such power of giving the proper stimulus to the adjacent sound part, that if injured, or rendered dead in part by the application of a caustic for instance, the sound part underneath will begin to relax, and show more distinctly the limits or boundaries of the disease; so that a separation of the diseased parts begins to take place, although the caustic has not reached nearly so far, and may give us an intimation of the extent of the disease which we could not get before. It is in some measure upon this principle that arsenic removes tumours, which extend beyond the immediate effect of the medicine[a].

Pressure is one of the causes of absorption in general, particularly the progressive, which in the resolution of parts is not the mode wanted; but it also assists in producing the interstitial; and if it could be made to produce the second of the interstitial, viz. absorption of the whole, as in the total decay of the thymus gland, then it would be sufficient in those cases where it could be applied. But the pressure must be applied with great care, for too much will either thicken or ulcerate, which last may be a mode of absorption we do not want. However, these effects will happen according to circumstances; for I have an idea that entirely new-formed parts, as tumours, will not be made to thicken by pressure, and therefore may be pressed with all the force the natural surrounding parts will allow. On the other hand there are many cases where we would wish to prevent absorption; but when this is the case we should be certain that the part which was to have been absorbed is such as can be rendered useful afterwards, of which I have my doubts in many cases.

§. 9. *Illustrations of Ulceration.*

Now that I have been endeavouring to give ideas of these effects of inflammation, viz. adhesion, suppuration, and ulceration, let me next mention some cases which frequently occur, as illustrations, which will give a perfect idea of these three inflammations; and, for the clearer understanding them, I shall illustrate them upon the inflammation, suppuration, and ulceration of the large circumscribed cavities. For instance, an inflammation attacks the external coat of an intestine: the first stage of this inflammation produces adhesions between it and the peritonæum lining the abdominal muscles; if the inflammation does not stop at this stage, an abscess is formed in the middle of these adhesions, and the matter acts as an extraneous body; the abscess increasing in size from the accumulation of matter, a mechanical pressure is kept up, which irritates, and the side next the skin is only susceptible of the irritation: this irritation not destroying the disposition to form matter, suppuration is still continued, and the ulcerative inflammation takes place.

If suppuration began in more parts of the adhesions than one, they are commonly united into one abscess; an absorption of the parts be-

[a] [Yet as the irritation cannot fail but extend beyond the immediate effect, it is probable that these adventitious parts are thrown off in consequence of their not being able to support life under the inflammation which succeeds.]

tween the abscess and the skin takes place, and the matter is led on to the external surface of the body, where it is at last discharged.

If the disposition for ulceration was equal on every side of the abscess, it must open into the intestine, which is seldom the case, although it sometimes does; for the same precautions are not taken here as in many other situations; for in some others, as in the nose, in the case of an abscess of the lachrymal sac, the passage is thickened towards the nose. In the case above described, however, the abdominal muscles, fat, and skin are removed, rather than the coats of the intestine. Cases of this kind have come under my own observation.

In these cases if adhesions had not preceded ulceration, the matter must have been diffused over the whole cavity of the belly; if the adhesive inflammation had not likewise gone before the ulceration in the abdominal muscles, etc., the matter would have found a free passage from the abscess into the cellular membrane of the abdomen, as soon as the ulceration had got through the first adhesions, as is often the case in erysipelatous suppurations.

Abscesses between the lungs and the pleura, in the liver, gall-bladder, etc. rise to the surface from the same cause; also in lumbar abscesses, where one would at first imagine the readiest place of opening would be the cavity of the abdomen, or gut; the parts nearest to the skin are removed, and the matter passes out that way: however, in abscesses so very deep, it does not always happen that one side only is susceptible of the irritation, and we shall find that the matter is taking different courses.

Abscesses in the substance of the lungs sometimes differ from the above described, for they sometimes open into the air-cells: this occurs because the adhesive inflammation finds it difficult to unite the air-cells, and branches of the trachea, (as was described in treating of that inflammation,) and also because in the substance of the lungs, it may be difficult to say where it can take a lead externally, from which, probably, the air-cells become similar to an external surface, and then ulceration takes place on that side of the abscess which is nearest to the cells; therefore we find that the matter gets very readily into the air-cells, and from thence into the trachea.

That the air-cells do not take on the adhesive state is evident in most abscesses in this part; for we find in most of these cases that the air-cells are exposed, as also the branches of the trachea; and the parts of the lungs which compose this abscess have not the firmness and solidity which the adhesive inflammation generally produces in those parts where it takes place.

Thus too we find it going on in large abscesses, even after they have been opened, but are so situated or circumstanced as to have some part of the abscess on that side immediately under the skin pressed by some other part of the body which lies underneath. For instance, when a large abscess forms on the outer and upper part of the thigh, opposite the great trochanter, which is a very common complaint, and an opening is made into it, or it bursts below or on the side of that bone, but not directly opposite to the trochanter itself, in such cases it frequently happens that the pressure of the trochanter on the inside of the abscess, viz. the cellular and adipose membrane and the skin covering the trochanter, that this pressure produces ulceration of these parts; which process is continued on through the skin, and makes a second opening directly upon the trochanter.

It is curious to remark how these processes of nature fulfil their appointed purposes, and go on no further; for any young flesh, or granulations, which may have formed upon the trochanter, which very often happens before this ulceration is completed, yet these do not ulcerate, although the pressure was as great or greater upon them than it was upon the parts which gave way.

This is upon the principle that pressure from without has not the same effect as from within. The fistula lachrymalis is another strong proof of ulceration only taking place towards the external surface, and securing the deeper-seated parts; as also the ulceration in consequence of matter in the frontal sinuses.

An effect of the same kind we have observed in milk-breasts. In these cases the suppuration commonly begins in many distinct portions of the inflamed parts, so that it is not one large circumscribed abscess, but many separate sinuses are formed, all of which generally communicate: now it usually happens, that only one of these points externally; which being either opened or allowed to break, the whole of the matter is to be discharged this way; but it frequently happens that the matter does not find a ready outlet by this opening, and then one or more of these different sinuses make distinct openings for themselves; which shows how very easily the slight pressure of such a trifling confinement of matter can produce the ulcerative inflammation. Ulceration is therefore no more than an operation of nature to remove parts out of the way of all such pressure as the parts cannot support; and accordingly it begins where the greatest pressure is felt, joined with the nature of the parts and its vicinity to the skin.

It is curious to observe that the ulcerative process has no power over the cuticle, so that when the matter has got to that part it stops, and cannot make its way through till the cuticle bursts by distention; but in general the cuticle is so thin as to give but very little trouble*: however, in many places it is so thick as to be the cause of very troublesome consequences.

Thus far I have considered ulceration as arising from visible irritations, joined with a susceptibility of the parts for such particular irritation; but besides those above described, we often have instances of ulceration taking place from a disposition in a part, and where perhaps no reason can be assigned but weakness in the part. I observed before, that some parts of the body were more susceptible of ulceration than others. I then spoke of original parts; but I now remark that newly-formed parts are much more susceptible of ulceration than the original; such as cicatrices, granulations, calluses, etc., for we find this disposition often taking place in old cicatrices from very slight causes, such as irregularity in the way of life or violent exercise, which is seen every day in our hospitals, where the parts seem incapable of supporting them-

* This is the reason why many abscesses in the palms of the hands, soles of the feet, fore part of the fingers, and about the nails, commonly called whitloes, &c., more especially in working people, give so much pain in the time of inflammation, and are so long in breaking, even after the matter has got through the cutis to the cuticle; the thickness of the cuticle, as also the rigidity of the nail, acting in those cases like a tight bandage, which does not allow them to swell or give way to the extravasation; for in the cuticle there is not the relaxing power, which adds considerably to the pain arising from the inflammation; but when the abscess has reached to this thick cuticle it has no power of irritation, and therefore acts only by distention; and this is in most cases so considerable, as to produce a separation of the cuticle from the cutis for a considerable way round the abscess; for I observed, when on inflammation, that it commonly produced a separation of the cuticle; all of which circumstances taken together, make these complaints much more painful than a similar-sized abscess in any other soft part. The application of poultices in these cases is of more benefit than in any other, because here they can act mechanically, viz. the moisture being imbibed by the cuticle, as in a sponge, and thereby softening the cuticle, by which means it becomes larger in its dimensions and less durable in its texture. These cases should be opened as soon as possible, to avoid the pain arising from distention and the separation of the cuticle; when it is conceived it means to point at any one part, paring off the thick cuticle near the cutis, allows the matter to make its escape more readily, when it has got through the cutis. There is a circumstance which almost always attends the opening such an abscess, viz. the soft parts underneath push out through the opening in the cuticle, like a fungus. which when irritated from any accident, gives a greater idea of soreness perhaps than any other morbid part of the machine ever does: this is owing to the surrounding belts of cuticle not having given way to the increase of the parts underneath, by which means they are squeezed out of this small opening, like paint out of a bladder. It is a common practice to eat this down by escharotics, as if it was a diseased fungus; but this additional pain is very unnecessary, as the destroying a part which has only escaped from pressure, cannot in the least affect that which is within; and by simply poulticing till the inflammation, and of course the tumefaction, subside, these protruded parts are gradually drawn into their original situations.

selves. Remarkable instances of this are recorded in Anson's Voyages, where the habit was so much debilitated as to allow all the old sores to ulcerate, or break out anew: the calluses were absorbed and taken into the circulation; and we also find that all these parts perform the operation of sloughing when dead, much sooner than original parts.

Now it is evident, in those cases mentioned in Anson's Voyages, that the whole frame of body was weakened by the hardships suffered in this expedition; and that the young or new-formed substances would suffer in a greater degree, arising from their being less firm and fixed than that which had been an original formation, and subsisted from the first; and as no repaired parts are endowed with the powers of action or resistance equal to an original part, it is no wonder that this new flesh, sharing in the general debility, became incapable of supporting its texture: perhaps a very sense of this debility proved an irritation, or the cause of that irritation which produced the absorption of parts; however that may be, it is a general fact that parts which are not originally formed, commonly give way soonest in depravations of the habit: in like circumstances also old sores that are healing, will break out, spread, and undo, in twenty-four hours, as much of the parts as had been healing in so many weeks. All these observations tend to prove that new-formed parts are not able to resist the power of many diseases, and to support themselves under so many shocks, as parts originally formed; which will be still further illustrated in treating of the power of absorption.

I observed that, although a part is losing ground or ulcerating, yet it continues suppurating; for while a matter-forming surface is ulcerating, (whether an original-formed part of the body, such as most abscesses, or a new-formed substance, such as granulations,) we find that it still secretes pus. In such cases the adhesive inflammation proceeds very rapidly, and would seem to prepare the parts as it goes for immediate suppuration, the moment they are exposed.

CHAPTER VII.

GRANULATIONS.

WE come now to trace the operations of Nature in bringing parts whose disposition, action, and structure had been preternaturally altered, either by accident or diseased dispositions, as nearly as possible to their original state. In doing this we are to consider the constitution and the parts as free from disease, because all actions which tend to the restoration of parts are salutary, the animal powers being entirely employed in repairing the loss and the injury sustained both from the cause, and arising from the course of the immediate effects, viz. inflammation, suppuration, and ulceration: now such operations cannot certainly be looked upon as morbid.

Nature having carried these operations for reparation so far as the formation of pus, she, in such cases, endeavours immediately to set about the next order of actions, which is the formation of new matter, upon such suppurating surfaces as naturally admit of it, viz. where there has been a breach of solids; so that we find following and going hand in hand with suppuration, the formation of new solids, which constitute the common surfaces of a sore. This process is called granulating, or incarnation; and the substance formed is called granulation.

Granulations have, I believe, been generally supposed to be a consequence of, or always an attendant on, suppuration; but the formation of granulations is not confined to a breach of solids where the parts have been allowed to suppurate, either from accident or a breach of the solids in consequence of an abscess; but it takes place under other circumstances; for instance, when the first and second bond of union has failed, as in simple fractures, which will be noticed hereafter.

Suppuration, I observed, arose in consequence of an injury having been done to the solids, so as to prevent them for some time from carrying on their natural functions; and I also observed that it was immaterial whether this injury had exposed their surfaces, as in cases of accidents and wounds, or whether the surfaces were not exposed, as in cases of abscesses in general; for in either of them suppuration would equally take place: I likewise observed that it was not necessary that there should be a breach in the continuity of parts for suppuration to take place in many cases, because all secreting surfaces were capable of suppuration; but this last seems not to be so commonly the case with granulations. I believe that no internal canal will granulate, in consequence of suppuration, except there has been a breach of surface, and then it is not the natural surface which granulates, but the cellular membrane, etc., as in other parts.

Wounds that are kept exposed do not granulate till inflammation is over, and suppuration has fully taken place[a]; for as the suppurative inflammation constantly follows, when wounds come to be under such circumstances, it would seem to be in such cases a leading and necessary process for disposing the vessels to granulation.

Setting out then with the supposition that this inflammation is in general necessary, under the above circumstances, for disposing the vessels to form granulations, we shall at once see how it may operate in the same manner, whether it arises spontaneously from a wound, the laceration of parts, mortification, bruise, caustic, or in short any other power which destroys or exposes the innumerable internal cells or surfaces, so as to prevent their carrying on their natural functions.

Few surfaces in consequence of abscesses granulate till they are exposed, so that few or no abscesses granulate till they are opened, either of themselves or by art; and therefore in an abscess, even of very long standing, we seldom if ever find granulations. In abscesses, after they have been opened, there is generally one surface that is more disposed to granulate than the others, which is the surface next to the centre of the body in which the suppuration took place. The surface next to the skin hardly ever has the disposition to granulate: indeed, before opening, its action was that of ulceration, the very reverse of the other; but even after opening, that side under the skin hardly granulates, or at least not readily. I may further observe, that exposure is so necessary to granulation, even on such surfaces as arise from a broken continuity of parts, that if the abscess is very deep-seated they will not granulate kindly without being freely exposed, which alone often becomes a cause why deep-seated abscesses do not heal so readily, and often become fistulous.

Upon the same principle of granulations forming more readily upon that surface which is next to the centre, or opposite to the surface of the body, is to be considered their tendency to the skin. Granulations always tend to the skin, which is exactly similar to vegetation, for plants always grow from the centre of the earth towards the surface[b]; and this

---

[a] [It is a singular circumstance that although exposure seems to be a necessary condition for granulations to take place, yet subsequent seclusion seems to be equally necessary for their continuance, to effect which is one of the principal objects of all dressings.]

[b] [See *note*, p. 287.]

principle was taken notice of when we were treating of abscesses coming towards the skin.

§. 1. *Of Granulations independent of Suppuration.*

The formation of granulations, I have observed, is not wholly confined to a breach made in the solids, either by external violence and exposure, or in consequence of a breach in the solids, which had been produced by suppuration and ulceration, and afterwards exposed; for parts are capable of forming granulations, or what I suppose to be the same thing, new animal matter, where a breach has been made internally, and where it ought to have healed by the first intention; but the parts being baulked in that operation, often do not reach so far as suppuration, so as to produce the most common cause of granulation. The first instance of the kind that gave me this idea was in a man who died in St. George's Hospital.

January, 1777. A man about fifty years of age fell and broke his thigh-bone nearly across, and about six inches above the lower end. He was taken into St. George's Hospital; the thigh was bound up, and put into splints, etc. The union between the two bones did not seem to take place in the usual time. He was taken ill with a complaint in his chest, which he had been subject to before, and died between three and four weeks after the accident.

On examining the parts after death there were found little or no effects of inflammation in the soft parts surrounding the broken bones, except close to the bones where the adhesive inflammation had taken place only in a small degree. The bones were found to ride considerably, viz. near three inches. The cavity made in the soft parts, in consequence of the laceration made by the riding of the bones, had its parietes thickened and pretty solid, by means of the adhesive inflammation, although not so much as would have been the case if the parts had been better disposed for inflammation; and some parts had become bony. There hardly was found within this cavity any extravasated blood or coagulating lymph, except a few pretty loose fibres like strings, which were visibly the remains of the extravasated blood. From these appearances this cavity had evidently lost its first bond of union, viz. the extravasated blood, which took place from the ruptured vessels; and probably the second had never taken place, viz. the coagulating lymph, in consequence of the adhesive inflammation: however, there was an attempt towards a union, for the surrounding soft parts, we have observed, had taken on the adhesive and ossific inflammation, so that in time there might have been formed in the surrounding soft parts a bony case, which would have united the two bones; but the parts being deprived of the two common modes of union, they were led to a third.

From the ends of the bones, and some parts of their surface, as well as from the inner surface of the soft parts, there was formed new flesh, similar to granulations. The hollow ends of the bones were filled with this matter, which was rising beyond the common surface of the bone, and in some places adhesion had taken place between it and the surrounding parts, with which it had come in contact. The same appearance which this new flesh had in this case I have several times seen in joints, both on the ends of the bones and on the inside of the capsular ligament, but never before understood how it was formed; hence we find that granulations can and do arise in parts that are not exposed. This is what I have long suspected to be the case in the union of the fractured patella, and this fact confirms me more in that opinion[a].

Here then we are shown that the cause of granulation, or the forming of new flesh for union (independently of extravasation, or the adhesive inflammation), is more extensive in its effects than we were formerly acquainted with, and that granulations, or new flesh, arise in all cases from the first and second bond of union being lost in the part (which indeed seldom happens, except from exposure); it therefore makes no difference whether the first and second bond of union escape through an opening made in the skin, as in a compound fracture, or it loses its living powers, as in the present case, and as I suppose to be the case in a fracture of the patella, which obliges the absorbents to take it up as an extraneous body.

§. 2. *The Nature and Properties of Granulations.*

Granulations and this new-formed substance are an accretion of animal matter upon the wounded or exposed surface: they are formed by an exudation of the coagulating lymph from the vessels, into which new substance both the old vessels very probably extend, and also entirely new ones form, so that the granulations come to be very vascular, and indeed they are more so than almost any other animal substance. That this is the case is seen in sores every day. I have often been able to trace the growth and vascularity of this new substance. I have seen upon a sore a white substance, exactly similar in every visible respect

[a] [This opinion has not been confirmed by any subsequent and more unequivocal proofs, and therefore it is now generally considered to be erroneous.]

to coagulating lymph. I have not attempted to wipe it off, and the next day of dressing I have found this very substance vascular, for by wiping or touching it with a probe it has bled freely. I have observed the same appearance on the surface of a bone that has been laid bare. I once scraped off some of the external surface of a bone of the foot, to see if the surface would granulate. I remarked the following day that the surface of the bone was covered with a whitish substance, having a tinge of blue; when I passed my probe into it I did not feel the bone bare, but only its resistance. I conceived this substance to be coagulating lymph, thrown out from inflammation, and that it would be forced off when suppuration came on; but on the succeeding day I found it vascular, and appearing like healthy granulations.

The vessels of granulations pass from the original parts, whatever these are, to the basis of the granulations; from thence towards their external surface, in pretty regular parallel lines, and would almost appear to terminate there.

The surface of this new substance, or granulations, continues to have the same disposition for the secretion of pus as the parts from which they were produced; it is therefore reasonable to suppose that the nature of the vessels does not alter by forming the granulations, but that they were completely changed for the purpose before the granulations began to form, and that these granulations are a consequence of a change then produced upon them.

Their surfaces are very convex, the reverse of ulceration, having a great many points or small eminences, so as to appear rough; and the smaller these points are, the more healthy we find the granulations.

The colour of healthy granulations is a deep florid red, which would make us suspect that the colour was principally owing to the arterial blood*, but it only shows a brisk circulation in them, the blood not having time to become dark.

When naturally of a livid red they are commonly unhealthy, and show a languid circulation, which appearance often comes on in granulations of the limbs from the position of the body, as is evident from the following case.

A stout healthy young man had his leg considerably torn, and it formed a broad sore; when healing, it was some days of a florid red, and on others of a purple hue: wondering what this could be owing to, he told me when he stood for a few minutes it always changed from the scarlet to the modena. I made him stand up, and found it soon changed;

* I once began to suspect that the air might have some influence upon the blood when circulating in the vessels, but from its losing that florid colour in sores of the legs by standing erect, I gave up that idea.

this plainly showed that these new-formed vessels were not able to support the increased column of blood, and to act upon it, which proves that a stagnation of blood was produced sufficient to allow of the change in the colour, and most probably both in the arteries and veins.

These sores never heal so fast as the others, whether it is occasioned by the position of the body or the nature of the sore itself; but most frequently so in cases of the last-mentioned kind. As the position of the body is capable of producing such an effect, it shows us the reason why sore legs are so backward in healing when the person is allowed to stand or walk.

Granulations when healthy, and on an exposed or flat surface, rise nearly even with the surface of the surrounding skin, and often a little higher, and in this state they are always of a florid red: but when they exceed this, and take on a growing disposition, they are then unhealthy, become soft and spongy, and without any disposition to skin. Granulations are always of the same disposition with the parts upon which they are formed, and take on the same mode of action: if it is a diseased part, they are diseased; and if the disease is of any specific kind, they are also of the same kind, and of course produce matter of the same kind, which I observed when on pus.

Granulations have the disposition to unite with one another when sound or healthy; the great intention of which is to produce the union of parts, somewhat similar to that by the first intention, or the adhesive inflammation, although possibly not by the same means. The granulations having a disposition to unite with each other upon coming into contact, without the appearance of any intermediate animal substance, perhaps is in the following manner. When two sound granulations approach together, the mouths of the secreting vessels of the one coming to oppose the mouths of similar vessels of the other, they are stimulated into action, which is mutual; so that a kind of sympathetic attraction takes place, and, as they are solids, the attraction of cohesion is established between them: this has been termed inosculation. The vessels thus joined are altered from secreting to circulating; or it may be in this way, viz. the circulatory vessels come to open upon the surface, and there unite with one another, and the two become one substance; or it may be asked, do they throw out coagulating lymph when they come into contact and have a disposition to heal? and does this become vascular, in which the vessels may inosculate, similar to union by the first or second intention? [a].

---

[a] [This seems to be the most probable as well as most prevailing opinion at the present day.]

I have seen two granulations on the head, viz. one from the dura-mater after trepanning and the other from the scalp, unite over the bare bone which was between them so strongly, in twenty-four hours, that they required some force to separate them, and when separated, they bled.

The inner surface of the cutis in an abscess or sore does not only not readily granulate, as has been mentioned, but it does not readily unite with the granulations underneath. The final intention of both seems to be that the mouth of a sore, which is seldom so much in a diseased state, should have a natural principle which attends disease, to put it upon a footing with the disease which is underneath[a]; therefore when abscesses are allowed to become as thin as possible before they are opened, this proportion between the sound skin and the disease is better preserved, and the parts are not so apt to turn fistulous.

When the parts are unsound, and of course the granulations formed upon them unsound, we have not this disposition for union, but a smooth surface is formed, somewhat similar to many natural internal surfaces of the body, and such as have no tendency to granulate, which continues to secrete a matter expressive of the sore which it lubricates, and in some measure prevents the union of the granulations. I imagine, for instance, that the internal surface of a fistulous ulcer is in some degree similar to the inner surface of the urethra, when it is forming the discharge commonly called a gleet. Such sores have therefore no disposition in their granulations to unite, and nothing can produce a union between them but altering the disposition of these granulations by exciting a considerable inflammation, and probably ulceration, so as to form new granulations, and by these means give them a chance of falling into a sound state.

Granulations are not endowed with the same powers as parts originally formed. In this respect they are similar to all new-formed parts, and it is from this cause that changes for the worse are so easily effected: they more readily fall into ulceration and mortification than originally-formed parts, and from their readiness to ulcerate they separate sloughs more quickly.

The granulations not only show the state of the part in which they are formed, or the state in which they are themselves, but they show how far the constitution is affected by many diseases. The chief of those habits which affect the granulations in consequence of the constitution are, I believe, the indolent and irritable habits, but principally fevers;

[a] [As the aperture of an abscess is frequently observed to extend, by a continuance of the ulcerative action, at the same time that the bottom of the abscess is filling up with new granulations, the final intention would rather seem to be to preserve a free exit for the matter; but this meaning is probably included in the language of the author.]

and these must be such as produce universal irritation in the constitution. The unsound appearances of the granulations show to what a stand the animal powers are put on such occasions, which does not appear so visibly in the originally-formed parts; it is therefore evident that the powers of the granulations are much weaker than those of the original parts.

§. 3. *Longevity of Granulations.*

Granulations are not only weaker in performing the natural or common functions of the parts to which they belong, but they would appear often to be formed with only stated periods of life, and those much shorter than the life of the part on which they are formed. This is most remarkable in the extremities; but where they are capable of going through all their operations, as cicatrization, their life then seems to be not so limited, they are probably then acquiring new life, or longevity, every day. But while in a state of granulation we find them often dying without any visible cause. Thus a person shall have a sore upon the leg which shall granulate readily; the granulations shall appear healthy, the skin shall be forming round the edges, and all shall be promising well, when all at once the granulations shall become livid, lose their life, and immediately slough off; or, in some cases, ulceration shall in part take place, and both together shall destroy the granulations; and probably where ulceration wholly takes place it may be owing to the same cause. New granulations shall immediately rise as before, and go through the same process; this shall happen three or four times in the same person, and probably for ever, if some alteration in the nature of the parts be not produced. This circumstance of the difference in longevity of granulations in different people, is somewhat similar to the difference in longevity of different animals.

In cases of short-lived granulations I have tried various modes of treatment, both local and constitutional, to render the life of these granulations longer, but without success.

It would appear from what has been said of suppuration and granulation, that it is absolutely necessary they should take place in wounds which are not allowed to unite by the first intention, before union and cicatrization can take place. Although this in general is the case, yet in small wounds, such as considerable scratches, or where there is a piece of skin rubbed off, we find that by the blood being suffered to coagulate upon the sore and form a scab, which is allowed to remain, the sore will only be attended by the adhesive inflammation, and will skin over without ever suppurating. Where a small caustic has been applied we find also, by allowing the slough to dry or scab, that when this is completed the scab will drop off and the parts shall be skinned; but if the blood has not been allowed to coagulate and dry, or the slough has been kept moist, the sore will suppurate and granulate. We even see in small sores[a], which are perfectly healthy and suppurating, that if the matter be allowed to dry upon them, the suppuration will stop, and the skin form under the scab: the smallpox is a striking proof of this, which was fully treated of in a former part of the work.

A blister whose cuticle is not removed is similar to a scab, it does not allow of suppuration. If a separation takes place between the cutis and cuticle, and the cuticle be not removed, nothing will be collected through the whole course, and a new cuticle will be formed; but if the cuticle be removed, a greater degree of inflammation will come on, and suppuration will certainly take place.

§. 4. *Of the Contraction of Granulations.*

Immediately upon the formation of the granulations, cicatrization would appear to be in view. The parts which had receded, in consequence of a breach being made in them, by their natural elasticity and probably by muscular contraction, now begin to be brought together by this new substance; and it being endowed with such properties, they soon begin to contract, which is a sign that cicatrization is to follow. The contraction takes place in every point, but principally from edge to edge, which brings the circumference of the sore towards the centre; so that the sore becomes smaller and smaller, although there is little or no new skin formed.

The contracting tendency is in some degree proportioned to the general healing disposition of the sore, and the looseness of the parts on which it is formed; for when it has not a tendency to skin, the granulations do not so readily contract, and therefore contracting and skinning are probably effects of one cause. The granulations too, being formed upon a pretty fixed surface, which is a consequence of [the induration arising from] inflammation, are in some degree retarded in their contraction from this cause; but probably this does not act so much upon a mechanical principle as we at first might imagine, for such a state of parts in some degree lessens the disposition for this process; but this state is every day altering in proportion as the tumefaction subsides. Granulations are also retarded in their contraction from a me-

[a] [See p. 263, *note*.]

chanical cause, when they are formed on parts naturally fixed, such as bone; for instance, the skull, the bone of the shin, &c., for there the granulations cannot greatly contract*.

In cases where there has been a loss of substance, making a hollow sore, and the contraction has begun and advanced pretty far before the granulations have had time to rise as high as the skin, in such cases the edges of the skin are generally drawn down and tucked in by it, in the hollow direction of the surface of the sore.

If it is a cavity or abscess which is granulating, with only a small opening, as in many that have not been freely opened, the whole circumference contracts, like the bladder of urine, till little or no cavity is left; and if any cavity is remaining when they cannot contract any further, they unite with the opposite granulations in the manner above described.

This contraction in the granulations continues till the whole is healed, or skinned over; but their greatest power is at the beginning, at least their greatest effect is at the beginning, one cause of which is that the resistance to their contraction in the surrounding parts is then least.

The contractile power can be assisted by art, which is a further proof that there is a resistance to be overcome. The art generally made use of is that of bandages, which tend to push, draw, or keep the skin near to the sore which is healing; but this assistance need not be given, or is at least not so necessary, till the granulations are formed, and the contractile power has taken place: however, it may not be amiss to practice it from the very beginning, as by bringing the parts near to their natural position the adhesive inflammation will fix them there; they will therefore not recede so much afterwards, and there will be less necessity for the contractile powers of the granulations.

Besides the contractile powers of the granulations, there is also a similar power in the surrounding edge of the cicatrizing skin, which assists the contraction of the granulations, and is generally more considerable than that of the granulations themselves, drawing the mouth of the wound together like a purse; this is frequently so great as to occasion the skin to grasp the granulations which rise above the surface, and is very visible in sugar-loaf stumps, where the projection of the sore is to be considered as above the level of the skin. This contractile power of the skin is confined principally to the very edge where it is cicatrizing, and I believe is in those very granulations which have already cicatrized; for the natural or original skin surrounding this edge does not

* This observation should direct us, in operations on those parts, to save as much skin as possible.

contract, or at least not nearly so much, as appears by its being thrown into folds and plaits, while the new skin is smooth and shining. This circumstance of the original surrounding skin not having the power of contraction, makes round wounds longer in healing than long ones, for it is much easier for the granulations and the edge of the skin to bring the sides of an oblong cavity together, than the sides of a circle, the circumference of a circle not being so capable of being brought to a point.

Whether this contraction of the granulations is owing to an approximation of all the parts by their muscular contraction, like that of a worm, while they lose in substance as they contract, or whether they lose without any muscular contraction, by the particles being absorbed, so as to form interstices (which I have called interstitial absorption), and the sides afterwards fall together, is not exactly determined, and perhaps both take place.

The uses arising from the contraction of the granulations are various. It facilitates the healing of a sore, as there are two operations going on at the same time, viz. contraction and skinning. It avoids the formation of much new skin, an effect very evident in all sores which are healed, especially in sound parts. In amputation of a thick thigh (which is naturally seven, eight, or more inches in diameter before the operation,) the surface of the sore is of the same diameter, for the receding of the skin here does not increase its surface, as it does in a cut on a plane; yet in this case the cicatrix shall be no broader than a crown piece. This can be effected by the contractile power of the granulations, for it is bringing the skin within its natural bounds. The advantage arising from this is very evident, for it is with the skin as it is with all other parts of the body, viz. that those parts which were originally formed are much fitter for the purposes of life than those that are newly formed, and not nearly so liable to ulceration.

After the whole is skinned we find that the substance, which is the remains of the granulations on which the new skin is formed, still continues to contract, till hardly anything more is left than what the new skin stands upon. This is a very small part in comparison with the first-formed granulations, and it in time loses most of its apparent vessels, becomes white, and ligamentous. For we may observe that all new-healed sores are redder than the common skin, but in time they become much whiter.

As the granulations contract the surrounding old skin is stretched, to cover the part which had been deprived of skin, and this is at first little more than bringing the skin to its old position, which had receded when the breach was first made; but afterwards it becomes considerably more, so as to stretch, or oblige the old skin to elongate, from which we might ask the following question: Does the surrounding skin in the healing of a sore lengthen by growth, or does it lengthen by stretching only? I think that the former is most probable; and if this is the case I should call this process interstitial growth, similar to the growth of the ears of the people in the Eastern islands, particularly as it is an opposite effect to interstitial absorption.

Granulations appear to have other powers of action besides simply their œconomy tending to a cure. They have power of action in the whole, so as to produce other operations, and even to affect other matter. I conceive that a deep wound, such as a gun-shot wound, advanced to suppuration and granulation, and also a fistula, become in some degree similar to an excretory duct, having the powers of a peristaltic motion from the bottom towards the opening externally. Thus we find that whatever extraneous body is situated at the bottom of the sore, is by degrees conducted to the skin, although the bottom of the sore or fistula is of the same depth. This effect in such sores does not arise from the granulations forming at the bottom, and gradually raising the extraneous body as they form (which is commonly the case with exfoliations and sloughs), but we find extraneous bodies come to the skin when the bottom of the wound is not granulating[a].

[This effect is rather to be attributed to the gradual contraction of the fistula from the bottom, which may therefore be represented by an inverted cone. The ascent of fluids against the force of gravity, as of the semen along the Fallopian tubes, the secretion of the lungs along the surface of the trachea, &c., is probably referrible in many instances to the actions of vibratory cilia, with which, according to recent discovery, the mucous membranes are found to be abundantly provided.]

CHAPTER VIII.

OF SKINNING.

WHEN a sore begins to heal we find that the surrounding old skin close to the granulations (which had been in a state of inflammation, having probably a red shining surface, as if excoriated, and rather ragged,) now becomes smooth and rounded, with a whitish cast, as if covered with something white, and the nearer to the cicatrizing edge the more white it is. This is, I believe, a beginning cuticle, and this appearance is probably as early a symptom of healing, and as much to be depended upon, as any; so that the disposition in the granulations for healing is manifested in the surrounding skin; and while the sore retains its red edge all round, for perhaps a quarter or half of an inch in breadth, we may be certain it is not a healing sore, and is what may be called an irritable sore.

Skin is a very different substance, with respect to texture, from the granulations upon which it is formed, but whether it is an addition of new matter, viz. a new-formed substance upon the granulations, being produced by them, or a change in the surface of the granulations themselves, is not easily determined. In either case, however, a change must take place in the disposition of the vessels, either to alter the structure of the granulations, or to form new parts upon them. One would at first be inclined to the former of these opinions, as we have a clearer idea of the formation of a new substance than such an alteration in the old.

We find the new skin most commonly taking its rise from the surrounding old skin, as if elongated from it, but this is not always the case. In very large sores, but principally old ulcers, where the edges of the surrounding skin have but little tendency to contract, or the cellular membrane underneath to yield, as well as the old skin having but little disposition to skinning in itself, a cicatrizing disposition cannot be communicated from it to the nearest granulations by continued sympathy. In such cases new skin forms in different parts of the ulcer, standing on the surface of the granulations like little islands. This, I believe, never takes place in parts the first time of their being sore, nor in sores which have a strong propensity to skin. Skinning is somewhat like crystallization, it requires a surface to shoot from, and the edge of the skin all round would appear to be this surface.

Whatever change the granulations undergo to form skin, they may in general be said to be guided to it by the surrounding skin, which gives this disposition to the surface of the adjoining granulations, as adjacent bones give an ossifying disposition to the granulations that are formed upon them. This may arise from sympathy; and if it does I should call it continued sympathy. But when the old skin is unsound, and not able to communicate this disposition, then the granulations sometimes of themselves acquire it, and new skin begins to form where that disposition is strongest in them, so that the granulations may be ready to form new skin, if the surrounding skin be not in a condition to give the disposition. It would appear, however, that the circumference of the sore generally has the strongest disposition to skin, even although the surrounding skin does not assist, for in many old sores no new skin shall shoot from the surrounding skin, or be continued, as it were, from the old, and yet a circle of new skin shall form, making a circle within the old, and, as it were, detached from it.

Skinning is a process in which Nature is always a great œconomist, without a single exception; this, however, may probably arise from the granulations being always of the nature of the parts on which they are formed, and from seldom being formed on parts that are the least of the nature of the skin; they have therefore no strong disposition to form skin. What would seem to make this observation more probable is, that if the cutis is only in part destroyed, as by a hurt or caustic which has not gone quite through the cutis to the cellular membrane underneath, a new cutis will form immediately on the granulations, and in many cases it will form as fast as the slough will separate; the reason is, because the cutis has a stronger tendency to form cutis than any other part, and in many cases it may be said to form it from almost every point.

We never find that the new-formed skin is so large as the sore was on which it is formed: this, I have already observed, is brought about by the contraction of the granulations, which in some measure is in proportion to the quantity of surrounding old skin, attended with the least resistance. If the sore is in a part where the surrounding skin is loose, as in the scrotum, then the contractile power of the granulations being not at all prevented, but allowed full scope, a very little new skin is formed; whereas if the sore is on any other part where the skin is not loose, such as the scalp, shin-bone, &c., in that case the new skin is nearly as large as the sore. This we find to be the case also in parts which are so swelled as to render the skin tight, such as the scrotum, when under the distention of a hydrocele, and which sometimes happens where a caustic has proved ineffectual: we then find the new skin as extensive as in any other parts equally distended. The same thing takes place in white swellings of the joint of the knee; for if a sore is made upon such a part, as is frequently done by the application of caustics, we find that the new skin is nearly of the same size as the original sore. The general principle is also very observable after amputations of the limbs: for if much old skin has been saved, we find the cicatrix small; while, on the other hand, if such care has not been taken, the cicatrix is proportionably large.

The new skin is at first commonly on the same level with the old, and if there has not been much loss of substance, or the disease is not very deep-seated, it continues its position; but this does not appear to be the case with scalds and burns, for they frequently heal with a cicatrix higher than the skin, although the granulations have been kept even with the skin. It would appear in these cases that a tumefaction of the parts, which were the granulations, takes place after cicatrization.

Sometimes granulations cicatrize while higher than the common surrounding skin, but then they are such as have been long in that position, as is the case in some issues. I have seen the granulations surrounding a pea rise considerably above the skin, near half-a-crown in breadth, and skin over, all but the hole in which the pea lay, the whole looking like a tumour.

§. 1. *The Nature of the new Cutis.*

The new-formed cutis is neither so yielding nor so elastic as the original is, and is also less moveable upon the part to which it is attached, or upon which it is formed. This last circumstance is owing to its basis being granulations, which are in some degree fixed upon parts united by the adhesive inflammation; and more particularly so when the granulations arise from a fixed part, such as a bone, the new skin formed upon them being also fixed in proportion. It is, however, constantly becoming more and more flexible in itself, and likewise more loosely attached, owing to the mechanical motion to which the parts are subject afterwards. The more flexible and loose the parts become, it is so much the better, as flexibility, or the yielding of the parts, preserves it from the effects of many accidents.

Parts which have been thickened in consequence of inflammation, such as the surrounding parts of new skin, have always a less internal power of action in them than parts which have never been inflamed. This arises from the adventitious substance thrown out in the time of inflammation being a clog upon the operations of the original; and the new matter not being endowed with the same powers, the part affected, taken as a whole, is by these means considerably weakened.

Motion given to the part so affected must be mechanical; but that motion becomes a stimulant to the parts moved, that they cannot exist under such motion without adapting the structure of the parts to it, and this sets the absorbents to work, or they receive the stimulus of necessity, and absorb all the adventitious or rather superfluous substance; by which means the parts are as much as possible reduced to their original texture.

Medicines have not the powers we could wish in many such cases: mercury, however, appears to have the power of producing a stimulus similar to motion, and should be made use of where a mechanical stimulus cannot be applied; and I believe, when joined with camphor, its powers of producing absorption are increased: when both medical and mechanical means can be used, so much the more benefit will ensue. When everything else fails, electricity might be tried. It has been the cause of absorption of tumours. It has reduced the swellings of many joints in consequence of sprains, and thereby allowed of the freedom of motion.

The new-formed cutis is at first very thin and extremely tender, but afterwards becomes firmer and thicker: it is a smooth continued skin, not formed with those insensible indentations which are observed in the natural or original skin, and by which the original admits of any distention the cellular membrane will allow of, as is experienced in many dropsies, white swellings in the joints, &c. This is proved by steeping a piece of dead skin, with a cicatrix in it, in water, to make the cuticle separate from the cutis; there we find that the new-formed cuticle becomes but little larger by such a process, which plainly shows that the new-formed cutis upon which this cuticle was formed, has a pretty smooth continued surface, and not that soft unequal surface which distinguishes the original cutis.

This new cutis, and indeed all the substance which had been formerly granulations, is not nearly so strong, nor endowed with such lasting and proper actions, as the originally-formed parts. The living principle itself is also not nearly so active; for when an old sore once breaks out, it continues to yield till almost the whole of the new-formed matter has been absorbed or mortified, as has been already explained.

The young cutis is extremely full of vessels, which afterwards, in a great measure, either become lymphatic or impervious, or are taken into the constitution, so that the skin and granulations underneath are at last free from visible vessels, and become white.

The surrounding original cutis, being drawn towards a centre by the contraction of granulations, to avoid as much as possible the formation of new skin, is thrown into loose folds, while the new looks like a piece of skin upon the stretch, and the whole appears as if a piece of skin had been sewed into a hole by much too large for it; and therefore it had been necessary to throw the surrounding old skin into folds, or gather the surrounding skin, in order to bring it in contact with the new. The new cutis of a sore, I believe, never acquires a muscular structure; nor does it grow larger than the sore which it covers, so as to be thrown into wrinkles similar to the old, and therefore has always that stretched, shining appearance.

§. 2. *Of the new Cuticle.*

It does not appear to be so difficult a process for the cutis to form cuticle as it is for the granulations to form cutis; for we find in general, that wherever there is a new cutis formed, it is covered with a cuticle: and in cases of blisters, or any other cause which may have deprived the cutis of its cuticle, we find that the cuticle is soon restored. We are to observe, however, that in such cases it is a sound original cutis, forming its own cuticle, and having the whole power of forming the cuticle, the surrounding cuticle itself having no power of action of this kind: every point of cutis is forming cuticle, so that it is forming equally everywhere at once; whereas I observed that the formation of the cutis was principally progressive from the surrounding cutis.

It is at first very thin, and partakes more of a pulpy than a horny substance; as it gets stronger, it becomes smooth and shining, and is much more transparent than original cuticle, which shows more the colour of the rete mucosum. This account relates to the cuticle of sound parts which had gone through all the operations of health; but where there is a retardation in the healing we find that the cuticle is in some cases backward in forming, and in others it shall be formed very thick, so as to make it necessary to be removed, it appearing to be a clog upon the cutis, retarding the progress of its formation.

§. 3. *Of the Rete Mucosum.*

The rete mucosum is later in forming than the cuticle, and in some cases never forms at all: this is best known in blacks who have been either wounded or blistered, for the cicatrix in the black is a considerable time before it becomes dark; and in one black who came under my observation, a sore which had been upon his leg when young, remained white when he was old. After blisters, too, the part blistered remains white for some time after the cuticle is completely formed: however, in many cicatrices of blacks we find them even darker than any other part of the skin.

CHAPTER IX.

EFFECTS OF INFLAMMATION, AND ITS CONSEQUENCES ON THE CONSTITUTION.

THE constitutional affections arising from inflammation are immediate and remote.

The immediate affections have been already considered, viz. the sympathetic fever, and also the nervous. I shall now treat of the remote, viz. the hectic, and dissolution, which arise from the state of the local affection at the time; the inflammation not being able to go through all the salutary steps that have been described. We have diseases, however, sometimes accompanying those salutary processes; although we should naturally conclude from the foregoing account, that the suppurative inflammation, and suppuration itself, should produce no change in the constitution but what was attendant upon the inflammation, and might be supposed perhaps somewhat necessary to it; and that when inflammation had subsided, and a kind suppuration come on, the constitution should be left in a sound state, because it would now appear that all the future processes were settled; and [therefore that] a constitution that was capable of doing this, was also capable of going through all the succeeding operations, as they are only actions of restoration; but we find sometimes the contrary, and the condition in which the constitution is either left, or which it afterwards takes on, proves often much more hurtful than the inflammation itself.

It appears in many cases that the inflammation, the attendant fever, the going off of these, and the commencement and continuance of the suppuration produce in many persons a change in the constitution, giving a disposition to symptoms which are called nervous. The locked jaw is often the effect of this leading cause, as well as hysterics, spasms upon the muscles of respiration, and great restlessness, which often prove fatal to the patient; there are likewise signs of great and universal debility or signs of dissolution in the patient, all of which appear to be increased by a continuance of the suppuration. Each of these diseases is well marked; and it would appear that the locked jaw, hysterics, spasms, and great restlessness are of the nervous kind, and do not appear to arise from such a constitution as is not equal to overcome the cause, for the cause which produced them being removed, the effects are going on towards health now as well as before; and if the patient dies of any of those diseases, it is not from the cause, nor from the immediate effect, viz. the local disease, but from the effect which the preceding operations, joined with the healing, have on some constitutions. They all seem to derive their origin from the same root, viz. from all the foregoing processes, which we have been describing; but they are altogether too extensive for our present subject.

§. 1. *Of the Hectic.*

I have now described the injuries of which inflammation is a consequence; the progress of that action in different parts; its effects on the constitution; together with the mode of treatment of both, and have carried it through its various steps to a perfect restoration. I have also already mentioned that the act of absorption affects some constitutions; but I shall now take notice that nature is not always equal to those salutary processes, and hence the constitution sometimes becomes particularly affected, producing symptoms different from those formerly described, and which have been called the hectic.

This disease is one of our remote constitutional sympathetic affections, and appears to arise from a very different origin from the other sympathizing effects before mentioned. When it is a consequence of a local disease, it has commonly been preceded by the first process of the former, viz. inflammation and suppuration, but has not been able to accomplish granulation and cicatrization, so as to complete the cure. It may be said to be a constitution now become affected with a local disease or irritation, which the constitution is conscious of, and of which it cannot relieve itself, and cannot cure; for while the inflammation lasts, which is only preparatory, and an immediate effect of most injuries, and in parts which can only affect the constitution, so as to call up its powers, there can be no hectic.

We should distinguish well between a hectic arising from a local complaint entirely, where the constitution is good, but only disturbed by too great an irritation; and a hectic arising principally from the badness of the constitution, which does not dispose the parts for a healing state; for in the first, it is only necessary to remove the part (if removable) and then all will do well; but in the other we gain nothing by a removal, except the wound made by the operation is much less, and much more easily put into a local method of cure; so that this bad constitution falls less under this (the operation taken into the account) than under the former state; but all this depends on nice discrimination.

The hectic comes on at very different periods after the inflammation, and commencement of suppuration, owing to a variety of circumstances. First, some constitutions much more easily fall into this state than others, having less powers of resistance. The quantity of incurable disease must be such as can affect the constitution, and in whatever situation or in whatever parts, it will be always as to the quantity of disease in those situations or parts in the constitution, which will make the time to vary very considerably. In many diseases it would appear that the manner of coming on retards the commencement of the hectic, such as lumbar abscesses. But when such abscesses are put into that state in which the constitution is to make its efforts towards a cure, but is not equal to the task, then the hectic commences.

It takes its rise from a variety of causes, but which I shall divide into two species, with regard to diseased parts, viz. the parts vital and the parts not vital. The only difference between these two is probably merely in time, with respect to its coming on, and its progress when come on: but what is very similar to the disease of a vital part, is quantity of incurable disease.

The causes of hectic, arising from diseases of the vital parts, may be many, of which a great proportion would not produce the hectic if they were in any other part of the body; such, for instance, as the formation of tumours, either in, or so as to press upon some vital part, or a part whose functions are immediately connected with life. Scirrhi in the stomach or mesenteric glands, which tumours anywhere else would not produce the hectic; many complaints too of vital parts, as diseased lungs, liver, etc., all of these produce the hectic, and much sooner than if the parts were not vital. In many cases where those causes of the hectic come on quickly, it frequently follows so quick upon the sympathetic fever that the one seems to run into the other: this I have often seen in the lumbar abscess. They also produce symptoms according to the nature of the part injured, as coughs, when in the lungs; sickness and vomiting, when in the stomach; and probably bring on many other complaints, as dropsies, jaundice, etc., but which are not peculiar to the hectic.

When the hectic arises from a disease in a part not vital, it sooner or later commences, according as it is in the power of the parts to heal, or continue the disease. If far from the source of the circulation, with the same quantity of disease, it will come on sooner. When in parts not vital, it is generally in those parts where so great a quantity of disease can take place (without the power of being diminished in size, as is the case with the diseases in most joints*,) as to affect the constitu-

* The cavity of a joint is such as not readily to become smaller under disease, as in the soft parts, which was described in the contraction of sores.

tion, and also in such parts as have naturally but little powers to heal: we must at the same time include parts that are well disposed to take on such specific diseases as are not readily cured in any situation; such parts are principally the larger joints, both of the trunk and extremities; but in the small joints of the toes and fingers, although the same local effects take place as in the larger, yet the constitution is not made sensible of it; we therefore find a scrofulous joint of a toe or finger going on for years without affecting the constitution. The ankle, wrist, elbow, and even the shoulder may be affected much longer than either the knee, hip-joint or loins, before the constitution sympathizes with their want of powers to heal.

Although the hectic commonly arises from some incurable local disease of a vital part, or of a common part when of some magnitude, yet it is possible for it to be an original disease in the constitution: the constitution may fall into the same mode of action, without any local cause whatever. at least that we know of.

Hectic may be said to be a slow mode of dissolution: the general symptoms are those of a low or slow fever, attended with weakness, but more with the action of weakness than real weakness; for upon the removal of the hectic cause, the action of strength is immediately produced, as well as every natural function, however much it was decreased before. The particular symptoms are debility; a small, quick, and sharp pulse; the blood forsaking the skin; loss of appetite; often rejection of all aliment by the stomach; wasting; a great readiness to be thrown into sweats; sweating spontaneously when in bed; frequently a constitutional purging; the water clear.

This disease has been and is still in general laid to the charge of the absorption of pus into the constitution from a sore; but I have long imagined that an absorption of pus has been too much blamed as the cause of many of the bad symptoms which frequently attack people who have sores. This symptom almost constantly attends suppuration when in particular parts, such as the vital parts, as well as many inflammations before actual suppuration has taken place, as in many of the larger joints, called white swellings; while the same kind and quantity of inflammation and suppuration in any of the fleshy parts, and especially such of them as are near the source of the circulation, have in general no such effect; in those cases, therefore, it is only an effect upon the constitution produced by a local complaint, having a peculiar property, which I shall now consider.

I observed, that with all diseases of vital parts, the constitution sympathized more readily than with diseases of any other parts; and also, that all diseases of vital parts are more difficult of cure in general than those which are not vital: I have observed, likewise, that all the diseases of bones, ligaments, and tendons affected the constitution more readily than those of muscles, skin, cellular membrane, etc., and we find that the same general principles are followed in the universal remote sympathy, produced by local diseases of those parts. When the disease is in vital parts, and is such as not to kill by its first constitutional effects, the constitution then becomes teazed with a complaint which is disturbing the necessary actions of health, the parts being vital; there is, besides, the universal sympathy, with a disease which gives the irritation of being incurable. In the large joints it continues to harass the constitution with a disease where the parts have no power, or what is more probable, have no disposition to produce a salutary inflammation and suppuration; the constitution, therefore, is also irritated with an incurable disease.

This is the theory of the cause of the hectic, which will be further illustrated; but now let us consider how far the idea of the absorption of matter may be a cause.

If the absorption of matter always produced such symptoms, I do not see how any patient who has a large sore could possibly escape this disease, because we have as yet no reason to suppose that any one sore has more power of absorption than another. If in those cases where there is a hectic constitution, the absorption is really greater than when the habit is healthy, it will be difficult to determine whether this increase of absorption is a cause or an effect. If it be a cause, it must arise from a particular disposition in the sore to absorb more at one time than common, even while it was in a healthy state; for the sore must be healthy, and then absorb, which hurts the constitution; moreover, as the sore is a part of that constitution, it must of course be affected in turn; and what reason we have to suppose that a healthy sore of a healthy constitution should begin to absorb more at one time than another I must own I cannot discover. If this increase of absorption does not depend upon the nature of the sore, it must then take its rise from the constitution; and if so, there is then a peculiarity in the constitution, so that the whole of the symptoms cannot arise entirely from the absorption of matter as a cause, but must depend on a peculiar constitution and absorption combined.

If absorption of matter produeed such violent effects as are commonly ascribed to it (which, indeed, are never of the inflammatory kind, but of the hectic), why does not the venereal matter do the same? We often know that absorption is going on by the progress of buboes, and I have known a large bubo, which was just ready to break, absorbed, from a few days' sickness at sea, while the person continued at sea for twenty-four days after; yet in such cases no symptoms appear till the matter begins to have its specific effects, and these very symptoms are not similar to those which are called hectic. From reasoning, we ought to expect that the venereal matter would act with greater violence than the common matter from a healthy sore. Although matter, too, is frequently formed on the inside of the veins in cases of inflammation of their cavities*, and this matter cannot fail of getting into the circulation, yet in these cases we have not the hectic disposition, but only the inflammatory, and sometimes death. We likewise find very large collections of matter, which have been produced without visible inflammation, such as many of the scrofulous kind, and which are wholly absorbed, even in a very short time, yet no bad symptoms follow†.

We may therefore from hence conclude, that the absorption of pus from a sore into the circulation cannot be a cause of so much mischief as is generally supposed; and if it was owing to matter in the constitution, I do not see how these symptoms could ever cease till suppuration ceased, which does not readily happen in such constitutions, their sores being tedious in healing. We find, however, that such patients often get well of the hectic before suppuration ceases, even when no medicine was given; and in the case of veins there is great reason to believe that after all the bad symptoms are removed, suppuration is still going on, as we find it so in a sore; pus may therefore still pass into the constitution from the veins, and yet the hectic may not be produced, which would certainly be the case if those bad symptoms were occasioned by the matter getting into the circulation. But I very much doubt the fact of absorption going on more in one sore than another; and if ever it does I think it is of no consequence; I am much more inclined to believe that this hectic disposition arises from the effect which irritation of a vital organ and some other parts, such as joints (being either incurable in themselves, or being so to the constitution for a time), have on the constitution.

We may remark, that in large abscesses which have not been preceded by inflammation, the hectic disposition seldom or never comes on till after they are opened (although they may have been forming matter for months); but in such cases the disposition often comes on soon after opening, and in others very late. Till the stimulus for restoring parts is given, no such effect can take place; and if the parts are well disposed

* Vide Paper entitled "Observations on the Internal Coats of Veins," at the end of this volume.

† It may, however, be objected to this, that this is not true matter or pus; but it may be necessary to show that the one affects the constitution upon absorption more than the other.

to heal, no hectic disposition comes on, neither is the constitution at all affected. In diseased joints also, which are attended with inflammation, if the parts were capable of taking on a salutary inflammation, we should have only the first sympathetic fever; but as they seldom are capable of doing this, the constitution becomes teased with a complaint, not taking on the immediate and salutary steps towards a cure. In the venereal disease, too, where we know that the venereal matter has got into the constitution, and that the matter is producing its specific effects, no hectic comes on, till the constitution is harassed with an incurable disease, and this not till long after all the parts are healed with regard to recent disease, and no matter is formed for further absorption. That absorption does take place in sores we have reason to believe, and upon this fact a mode of dressing sores has been advised. The following is a remarkable instance of it in a bubo.

A young man had a chancre and three buboes, one of which appeared when the other two were almost cured. This was very large, and at the bottom of the belly. When it had suppurated, and was pretty near breaking, it diminished very quickly, and in two or three days was entirely gone While this was going on he observed that his urine was wheyish and thick while making it, which went entirely off when the bubo had subsided. Before the bubo began to subside he was rather mending in his health, which continued to mend; nor did the diminution of the bubo alter the state of his health.

The hectic, from what has been said, appears in some measure to depend on the parts being stimulated to produce an effect which is beyond their powers; that this stimulus is sooner or later in taking place in different cases, and that the constitution becomes affected by it. The hectic disposition arises from diseased lungs, lumbar abscesses, white swellings, scrofulous joints, etc.

§. 2. *The Treatment of the Hectic.*

We have as yet, I am afraid, no cure for any of the consequences above related; I believe that depends on the cure of the cause, viz. the local complaint, or on its removal; the effects, I fear, are not to be cured. Strengtheners, and what are called antiseptics, are recommended. Strengtheners are proposed on account of the debility which has taken place. Antiseptics have been employed from an idea that pus, when absorbed, gives the blood a tendency to putrefaction. To prevent both of these effects from taking place the same medicines are however recommended. These are bark and wine. Bark will, in most cases, only assist in supporting a constitution. I should suppose it impossible to cure a disease of the constitution till the cause be removed; however, it may be supposed that these medicines may make the constitution less susceptible of the disease, and may also contribute to lessen the cause, by disposing the local complaints to heal; but where the hectic arises from specific disease, as, for instance, if a hectic disposition comes on from a venereal disposition, bark will enable the constitution to support it better than it otherwise could have done, but can never remove it. Wine, I am fearful, rather does harm if it increases the actions of the machine without giving strength, a thing carefully to be avoided: however, I have not yet made up my mind about wine.

When the hectic arises from local disease in such parts as the constitution can bear the removal of, then the diseased part should be removed, viz. when it arises from some incurable disease in an extremity; and although all the symptoms above described should have already taken place, we shall find that upon a removal of the limb the symptoms will abate almost immediately. I have known a hectic pulse at one hundred and twenty sink to ninety in a few hours upon the removal of the hectic cause. I have known persons sleep sound the first night without an opiate, who had not slept tolerably for weeks before. I have known cold sweats stop immediately, as well as those called colliquative. I have known a purging immediately stop upon the removal of the hectic cause, and the urine drop its sediment. It is possible, too, that the pain in the operation, and the sympathetic affection of the constitution may assist in these salutary effects. It is an action diametrically opposite to the hectic, and may be said to bring back the constitution to a natural state.

§. 3. *Of Dissolution.*

Dissolution is the last stage of all, and is common to, or an immediate consequence of, all diseases, whether local or constitutional. A man shall not recover of a fever, whether original or sympathetic, but shall move into the last stage, or dissolution. It shall take place in the second stage of a disease, where the state of constitution and parts appears to be formed out of the first; as, for instance, a man shall lose his leg, especially if above the knee, or have a very bad compound fracture in the leg; the first constitutional symptoms shall have been violent, but all shall appear to have been got the better of, and there shall be hopes of recovery, when suddenly he shall be attacked with a shivering fit, which shall not perform all its actions, viz. shall not produce the hot fit and sweat, but shall continue a kind of irregular hot fit, attended with loss of appetite, quick low pulse, and sunken eyes, and the person shall die in a few days. Or he shall go into the common diseased symptoms of the second stage, viz. the nervous, with many of its effects, as the tetanus, and dissolution shall also be a consequence. Or if the local disease does not or cannot heal, and is such as to affect the constitution, it then brings on the hectic, and sooner or later dissolution takes place: for the hectic is an action of disease, and of a particular kind; but dissolution is a giving way to disease of every kind, and therefore has no determined form arising from the nature of the preceding disease.

It has been supposed that this disease arises also from the absorption of matter. It appears to be in many cases an effect arising from violent and long-continued inflammations and suppurations, although not incurable in themselves, (therefore in those respects not similar to the hectic,) and which in many instances are known to produce the greatest changes in the constitution. Such often arise from very bad compound fractures, from amputations of the extremities, especially the lower, and more particularly the thigh, in which cases the sympathetic fever has run high, which would appear to be necessary or preparatory; but in the hectic it is not necessary that the constitution should have suffered at all in the first stages of the disease: dissolution seems to be more connected with what is past than with the present alone, which is the reverse of the hectic. We never find this disease take place in consequence of small wounds, or such wounds as have affected the constitution but little in its first stages, but which may affect the constitution much in its second, such as small wounds producing the lock-jaw. It would appear to take place in our hospitals more generally than in private houses, and more readily in large cities than in the country. We shall find that the hectic and dissolution are by no means the same disease, but differ exceedingly in their causes and in many of their effects; for in the case of compound fractures and amputations, we find the constitution often capable of going through the inflammatory and sympathetic fever, producing suppuration and granulation, as well as continuing the production of these for some time, and yet sinking under them at last, and often immediately, without a seeming cause. This effect will more readily take place if the person was in full health before the accident or operation than if he had been somewhat accustomed to the other, or true hectic; for the symptoms of dissolution seldom or never take place, if the violence committed has been to get rid of a hectic cause. It sometimes takes place early, in consequence of local injury, and would seem to be a continuation of the sympathetic fever; as if the constitution was not able to relieve itself of the general affection, or that the parts could not go into the true suppurative disposition. We see this frequently after removing a limb, especially the lower extremity, and after cutting for the stone in very fat men, above the middle age, and who have lived well.

The first symptoms are generally those of the stomach, which produce shivering; vomiting immediately follows, if not an immediate attendant; there is great oppression and anxiety, the persons conceiving they must die; there is a small quick pulse; perhaps bleeding from the whole surface of the sore; often mortification, with every sign of dissolution in the countenance; and, as it arises with the symptoms of death, its termination is pretty quick. Here is a very fatal disease taking place, in some almost immediately, when all appeared to be within the power of the machine, and therefore cannot immediately arise from the sore itself, for it is very common after such operations as usually do well; but the hectic always takes place in consequence of those sores which seldom or never get well in any case; yet the sore certainly assists in bringing on dissolution, because we never see the disease take place when the sore is healed, nor in those where the constitution seems not to be equal to the task, as is the cause of the hectic.

The hectic is much slower in its progress, and seems to be a simple and an immediate effect, arising from a continued cause which is local; by removing the cause therefore the effect ceases, and the havoc made upon the constitution is soon restored: persons therefore do much better in consequence of the hectic having in some degree taken place prior to the removal of the cause. But dissolution is a change of the constitution in consequence of causes which now do not wholly exist, and in many cases it does not take place till the constitution appears to be capable easily of performing all its functions, and a removal of the parts does not relieve, as in the hectic; for dissolution does not depend for its continuance upon the presence of the disease.

Death or dissolution appears not to be going on equally fast in every vital part; for we shall have many people very near their termination, yet some vital actions shall be good and tolerably strong; and if it is a visible action, and life depends much upon this action, the patients shall not appear to be so near their end as they really are. Thus I have seen dying people whose pulse was full and strong as usual on the day previous to their death, but it has sunk almost at once, and then become extremely quick, with a thrill. On such occasions it shall rise again, making a strong effort, and after a short time a moisture shall probably come on the skin, which shall in this state of pulse be warm, but upon the sinking of the pulse shall become cold and clammy; breathing shall become very imperfect, almost like short catchings, and the person shall soon die. It would appear in many cases that disease has produced such weakness at last as to destroy itself: we shall even see the symptoms or consequences of disease get well before death.

A gentlewoman, who was above seventy-five, was anasarcous all over; the abdomen was very full and large; she made but very little water; her breathing was so difficult as to make her purple in the face, so that most probably there was water in the chest; her pulse was extremely irregular, fluttering, trembling, intermitting, and small. Her legs were punctured with a lancet, and discharged very freely for more than three weeks, which emptied the cellular membrane of the body, as well as in some degree the abdomen; the breathing became free and easy, so that we supposed the water in the chest was absorbed; the pulse became regular, soft, and fuller, and the appetite in some degree mended; in which state she seemed free from disease, having only some of the consequences still remaining: the quantity of urine increased to the natural quantity; but, notwithstanding actual disease seemed to be gone, yet she became weaker and weaker, in which state she existed for near a month, and died. Some days prior to death a purple and then a livid appearance came upon the legs, with some spots of extravasated blood above where the punctures had been made, on which blisters arose, at first filled with serum, then with bloody serum, all of them threatening mortification.

Even when in the state of approaching death we often find a soft, quiet, and regular pulse, having not the least degree of irritability in it, and this when there is every other sign of approaching death, such as entire loss of appetite, no rest, hiccup, the feet cold, and partial cold, clammy sweats, &c.

A lady appeared to have lost all diseased action, only the consequences of disease remaining, viz. weakness, with swelled legs: she made little or no water; at length she became so weak as hardly to articulate; she lay in a kind of doze, was only roused to impression, and only took food by spoonfuls when desired; the pulse so small as hardly to be felt. Her extremities were cold, and she had all the signs of approaching dissolution, which took place; yet within thirty-six hours before she died, the whole water in her legs and thighs was taken up, her urine increased, and about ten hours previous to her death, the legs, &c. were as small as ever. As I consider the dropsy to be a disease, and not simply weakness, which this case would in some measure show from the result, I should wish to ask whether the absorption of water was not owing to the disease being gone? and whether the disease being gone, the absorbents did not set to work? If so, then dissolution may be a cessation of disease, and persons die of weakness simply; or simply either the want of powers to act, or the want of that stimulus of necessity to act, by which means a cessation of action takes place.

Since bodies of persons who die suddenly, and even by violent death, as well as those who die soon after a considerable operation, are not capable of being preserved so long as those who have been ill for some time; and as those who have a considerable operation performed upon them, as the amputation of a leg, do not so readily recover as those who have been long ill, may not the more ready production of death and the more ready production of putrefaction be owing to the same principle, one more readily running into the action of death as also more readily into the action of putrefaction? But it is very probable that the action producing quick putrefaction is an action prior to absolute death.

PART III.

CHAPTER I.

THE TREATMENT OF ABSCESSES.

I HAVE endeavoured to lay down the general principles of suppuration, which principles of themselves lead to a general method of cure; but as it is only the proper application of art to those principles which completes the surgeon, and since it is the most difficult part to apply our knowledge of first principles to practice with readiness, especially when there appear some peculiarities, it will be necessary to bring the beginner from first principles to the practical part.

Abscesses are in general consequences of spontaneous inflammation, but not always so; for they may be consequences of some violence, as strains or bruises from some external violence, which has hurt deeper-seated parts than the skin over them, which inflame and form an abscess, as was described in treating of accidents; as also from the introduction of extraneous bodies, over which the parts have healed. Even when they appear to be spontaneous, they arise from so many causes, and from thence have so many dispositions, or are of so many kinds, that in general they become one of the greatest objects in surgery; because, from these circumstances, they require a vast variety in the manner of treatment.

I do not mean at present to enter into a full discussion of the cause, effect, and cure of every abscess, because that would be treating of every disease which is capable of producing such complaints, many of which would come under the article of specific diseases, which must be treated of separately; yet I mean here to lay down such general surgical rules for their treatment and many of their consequences, as will include almost every kind of disease of this kind, considered as an abscess simply. So that the specific treatment of any specific abscess will be principally confined to the medicinal treatment of the part and the constitution; thereby the treatment of the local complaint so produced, abstracted from the specific disposition, will for the most part come under our general rules.

As most spontaneous suppurations, from whatever cause, are deeper-seated than the surface of the body, such of course must form what are called abscesses, or collections of pus; therefore we have abscesses of all depths, from the pimple in the skin to the boil, and from the boil to deep-seated abscesses among the muscles, or in any other deep-seated part.

Abscesses are commonly formed where matter is found, especially the more superficial ones, and such may be justly called abscesses of this part; but collections of matter are often found in parts where not formed, more especially in the deeper-seated ones; the matter moving from the seat where it was formed to some more depending part, or having met with some obstruction in its course, it takes another direction and therefore may be called an abscess in this part; and I shall call them so in my descriptions of them. I believe such abscesses do not arise from inflammation, but are of the scrofulous kind, and therefore not so much to our present purpose.

It will be difficult to divide abscesses into absolutely distinct classes; but, similarly to inflammation, they may be divided into two kinds, the sound and the unsound; for I imagine these two first principles might lead to the method of cure; but at present I only mean to lay down the principles of an abscess.

The appearances which distinguish the sound from the unsound abscess are several; although there are many abscesses of particular kinds that give little or no information. They often differ from one another in their first appearance from the kind of inflammation, as also in their course, but more particularly in their efforts toward a cure. Thus we judge of the consequences of the smallpox from the first appearance of the arm after inoculation; for if the beginning inflammation is small, pretty much circumscribed, and of the florid red with some rising, then we may in our own minds expect a good kind; the same upon the first appearance of the smallpox themselves; as also the first appearance of chancre, etc., or almost of any other disease, either beginning with or attended by inflammation; for it is by the kind of inflammation we are to judge of the future event.

It might be thought almost unnecessary here to treat of sound abscesses, because in such our first principles will readily take place, and often little or no assistance is required; but abscesses may be attended with circumstances which may retard the cure, and which have nothing to do with unsoundness, such as extraneous bodies in sound parts; and these will most probably come under our general principles of cure, that is, require something to be done, because they will in many cases relieve themselves of the extraneous matter, and then they require but little assistance.

§. 1. *The Progress of Abscesses to the Skin.*

What I mean by a sound abscess, is where there is a sound constitution, the parts affected having all the disposition and powers to heal, and those dispositions and powers allowed to take place, which will happen more readily if in structures of the body which have naturally a ready disposition to heal; so situated in the body as to be able to support its actions, and not of a specific kind, for which we have no cure; for any specific disease, for which we have a cure, will come within our first division*.

The inflammation in a sound and active part, and of a sound constitution, in general is pretty violent, attended from the very beginning with a considerable deal of pain†; suppuration takes place quickly; the parts between the abscess and the skin are readily affected, and ulceration goes on fast; the skin becomes of the florid red; the matter comes soon to it, especially at a point‡, and it bursts; all this is done with great rapidity. The symptoms show such a degree of health in the constitution and the parts, that little is necessary for the surgeon to do in the first stages of the disease.

Poultices are recommended in such cases to assist that disposition which the parts have to give way between the skin and the abscess; but I have already observed, that they certainly can have no effect of this kind; however, they have their uses when the inflammation has reached the skin, for they keep it soft, allow the cuticle to distend, and give way to the swelling underneath, which eases the patient. Warmth and moisture act in many cases as sedatives to our sensations, although not always; and the distinction between those where they give ease, and where they rather give pain, I have not been able to make out.

As an abscess of the healthy kind requires but little surgical treatment,

* Viz. if a venereal abscess has its specific quality destroyed, it admits of cure as readily as any other, and the same treatment becomes necessary.

† Vide Symptoms of Suppurative Inflammation.

‡ This very appearance makes a material difference between an abscess arising from brisk inflammation, and one that is slow in its progress; it is so remarkable, that I have seen this effect where the matter was at such distance as not to be felt in the least, and where I have doubted whether there was matter or not, almost conceiving that it preceded suppuration. It certainly has this effect long before there is any distention: besides this, of a pointing taking place, there is another effect of deep suppurations in consequence of inflammation, which is an œdematous appearance, or thickening of the superficial parts. This was taken notice of by Le Dran in internal abscess of the abdomen, where adhesions had taken place between the suppurating part and the parietes of the abdomen, and by Mr. Pott in suppuration of the brain; whether in such there is a pointing or not I do not know.

between its commencement and opening, it also requires but very little attention afterwards for the cure or the restoring the parts. This depends more on the operation of the powers or abilities the machine is in possession of, than on any assistance the surgeon can give; however, abscesses may have other circumstances attending them, besides soundness and unsoundness, which will require surgical treatment; such as the extraction of exfoliated bones, which by their stay retard the cure. Further, as few inflammations arise in perfectly sound parts and constitutions, it will generally be necessary to treat them in some degree as if they had an unsound tendency, and also according to other circumstances.

As no abscess can set about a cure till the matter is discharged, the first process, therefore, is the discharge of the matter; but simply discharge is not always sufficient; therefore it becomes necessary to consider whether or not, almost in every case it would not be proper to do more; and I am inclined to believe that whatever would in general assist an unsound abscess, would also do the same to a sound one; but this practice should be followed with great caution, and not carried too far, for in many it will be perfectly unnecessary, therefore it should not be practised; in others it will only be necessary in part; besides, in many cases it may do harm, for many abscesses may have tolerable dispositions under the present treatment, yet may be in such a state as very readily to fall into an unsound one, of some kind or other, when too much violence is committed; some having a tendency to irritability: on the other hand, our practice may fall short of the intention, as many parts have a strong tendency to indolence; and if the stimulating method is applied to the first it would be unlucky, and vice versâ.

It will be generally more in the power of the parts to perform a cure if certain operations are done, which even dispose the most active and healthy disposition, both of constitution and of parts to heal sooner; but this does not hold of the irritable. The first of these operations will be the mode of exposing abscesses, by opening them sufficiently, which will make any particular treatment afterwards, either less necessary, or more easy of application, if necessary; so that the first principle of the cure, even of sound abscesses, may be the freedom of opening them in the beginning; however, the more sound they are, there is the less necessity for such treatment; for if it does not give new powers to the parts, it keeps up those of which they are already in possession, and obliges them to go on towards a cure; for the living principle in parts, more especially sound parts, seems uneasy under the circumstance of exposure, and of having no skin, and therefore is roused to action, acting with a view to cover the part. It has no alternative; and, as I have just now observed that few spontaneous abscesses take place from so slight a cause as simple violence produces, there must be a something to be got the better of. This is, perhaps, as well illustrated in the fistula in ano, as in any other; for without dividing along the gut to the bottom, which is where the disease is, and where the abscess has formed, it seldom or never heals; however, all this will be according to circumstances, for if the suppuration is quick and comes fast to the skin, the parts will heal in the same proportion more readily, either with or without opening; therefore, in such instances, it is not so necessary to open freely, though as it is not the method nature commonly takes, it has by many been objected to; but let us observe, that where an abscess opens of itself by a small orifice, the parts are commonly very sound where the opening is, although the bottom may be diseased; but if it be diseased where it opens, then ulceration commonly takes place at this orifice, which effects what should be done by art.

To illustrate that a large opening is not detrimental to the healing of a sore, let us observe that there is no difference between an abscess opened largely, and a wound in consequence of an operation which is not healed by the first intention, such as an amputation, etc.; for in such cases there is a breach in the continuity of the parts communicating with the skin, as large, if not larger than at the bottom, and it heals readily. We endeavour, however, to remedy this as much as possible by saving skin, which, in some degree answers to a small opening; and we may also observe that where there is only a small opening leading to a large cavity, which is to suppurate, as in the case of a hydrocele treated by a caustic or seton, (which when come to suppuration is in all respects similar to an abscess,) the whole so far as suppuration extends, heals equally well with those that are wholly exposed; but I do not know that they do better: and where the sac is not very sound I do believe they do not so well as when more fully enlarged: and we may also observe, that opening largely into the scrotum is not subject to the same inconvenience as in many other parts, for here there is so much loose skin as to remove any retardment to the healing that might arise in other parts from opening largely: however, after viewing this in every light, there seems but little advantage gained in the one way or the other. The opening more or less freely must be directed by some other circumstance, by which the surgeon must be guided. But as most abscesses owe some of their size to distention, and as this will be more or less according to circumstances, it becomes necessary to distinguish the one kind from the other, for the one will require a freer opening than the other.

Abscesses in soft parts will owe more of their size to distention than those in hard parts, such as bones, joints, etc. Abscesses in soft parts, not connected with the hard, will owe more of their size to distention than those in soft parts connected with the hard; for instance, an abscess in the calf of the leg, thick of the thigh, buttock, etc., will owe more of its size to distention than an abscess on the shin-bone, on the head, etc. Therefore an abscess, whose size is in some degree owing to distention, need not be so freely opened as one that is not; because when the distention is taken off by the discharge of the pus, the parts will contract, or fall into their natural position, which cannot so easily happen in the other case. Besides, the granulations will also be allowed to contract in the one case, much more than in the other. However, we find many abscesses healing very readily without any other opening than what was at first made by ulceration, and this will be more readily effected if the abscess has been allowed to break of itself, which I shall now more fully explain.

§. 2. *Of the Time when Abscesses should be opened.*

The natural process that abscesses are obliged to go through for the discharge of their contents is in general the most proper, and it is so much so as to be in most cases allowed to go on; and this process becomes more necessary in unsound abscesses than in sound ones, as it exposes them more fully, from ulceration having destroyed more of the parts between the seat of the abscess and the external parts.

As abscesses, wherever formed, must increase as they approach the skin, and therefore increase that part of their cavity next to the skin faster than at the bottom, so that they become in some degree tapering towards the bottom, with a wide part immediately under the skin; and this will be more or less so, according to their depth, their meeting with different substances which give a resistance to the pus, or their coming fast or slowly to the skin.

This shape of the abscess, when allowed to take place, is well adapted for healing; for it puts the bottom, which is the seat of the disease, more upon a footing with the mouth of the abscess than it otherwise could be. When these two are not well proportioned there is a retardment in the cure; for as the bottom, or part where the abscess begun, is more or less in a diseased state, and as the parts between the seat of the abscess and the external surface are sound parts, having only allowed a passage for the pus, they of course have a stronger disposition to heal than the bottom has; and we commonly find this to be the case.

If there could be made at any time a difference in the powers of healing between the mouth of the abscess and its bottom, it ought to be made the most defective at the mouth of the abscess, as that part is the easiest of management. To have this effect produced as much as possible, abscesses should be allowed to go on till they break or open of themselves; for although abscesses in general only open by a small orifice, more especially when sound, yet it is to be remarked that the skin over the general cavity of the abscess is in such cases so much thinned as to have but very little disposition to heal, and is often so much so as to ulcerate and make a free opening; and if it does not, an opening is more easily procured by art.

It is a curious circumstance in the œconomy of abscesses that those that have the best dispositions to heal come fastest to the skin; the lead takes place almost at a point, it does not swell so much into that conical form above described, not being under the same necessity in point of healing, and it opens by a small orifice; while, on the other hand, if there is an indolence in the progress of the abscess it will spread more, or distend the surrounding parts, from their not being so firmly united by inflammation in the one as they were in the other; nor will ulceration so readily take the lead, and it will come to the skin by a broad surface, so as to thin a large portion of the skin. But abscesses should only be allowed to open of themselves where the confinement of the matter can do no mischief, which will generally be in such as ought to heal up from the bottom; but in the reduction of circumscribed cavities to the state of an abscess it will be in most cases proper to open early, as in abscesses of the abdomen or thorax, those within the cranium, those of the eye, and those in joints. In the abscess of the tunica vaginalis testis it would be better to let it open of itself, as it should be allowed to heal up from the bottom, similar to an abscess in the cellular membrane.

If it should be unnecessary to open freely, or if from circumstances this should be impossible, it will in either case be very proper to make the opening which is necessary or practicable at the most depending part, with a view to remove the pressure arising from the matter collected, which is commonly called confinement or lodgement of matter, which will otherwise happen; for I shall observe that a very small pressure on that side of the abscess next to the skin may produce ulceration there; and although this pressure in many cases might not be so great as to produce ulceration at the bottom of the abscess, yet it may be so great as to prevent granulations from forming on that side, and thereby retard the cure, as no union can take place but by means of granulations; or if it should not prevent granulations from forming, yet it might retard their growth, so that the cure would be more tedious than if the pressure did not exist; and this retardation will be greatest where the pressure is the greatest, which will be at the most depending part of the abscess; so that its upper part will readily heal to a small point, and be reduced to the state of a fistula. But it is not always possible to open at the most depending part of an abscess, and when possible often very improper. When impossible, perhaps nothing more can be done than to evacuate the matter as often as necessary, and by gentle pressure keep the sides of the sinus together, to allow their growing into one another; but the situation will not in all cases allow this.

The inexpediency of opening at the most depending part of an abscess will in general arise from the distance between the matter and the skin at this part; for if the abscess is pretty deeply seated, and points at a part superior to that of its seat, which it sometimes does from the parts above, being such as more easily give way, in such a case it will be proper to open it where it points. For instance, if an abscess is formed in the centre of the breast, and opens at the upper part, (which is often the case,) it would be improper to cut through the lower half to allow the matter to pass that way, although it may make its way there afterwards, from the pressure of the matter, as was just now observed; which I have seen happen more than once.

If an abscess forms on the upper part of the foot, it is improper to open through the sole of the foot to get at the most depending part of the abscess, for besides cutting such a depth of sound parts, which is an objection, it would be destroying a great many useful parts. It would also be impossible to keep it open, the sound parts having such a disposition to heal; and it would be contradictory to my first position, which was to have parts as thin as possible before they are opened, in order to destroy the healing disposition there*.

As in such cases the place where the matter threatens to open a passage for itself is where the future opening is most likely to be, and as the situation is disadvantageous to the healing of the seat of the abscess, it will be more necessary to let it first open of itself (because the abscess just under the skin will be increased in width, as was observed), and then to dilate it as freely as may be thought necessary; for by allowing abscesses to open of themselves the opening has a less disposition to heal than if it had been opened early by art; therefore [the former method] is more desirable in such situations.

* One would imagine that this last caution was hardly necessary, but I once saw a case where it was advised, upon the general principles of opening in the most depending part.

§. 3. *Of the Methods of opening Abscesses, and treating them afterwards.*

All abscesses I have already observed will open of themselves, excepting where the matter is re-absorbed; and I have also observed, that in general they ought to be allowed to open of themselves, excepting some particular circumstance calls for an early opening; but when the skin over the abscess is very thin, it is not of so much consequence whether it is allowed to open of itself, or is opened at first by art.

In large abscesses it will generally be necessary to open them by art, whether they have opened of themselves or not, for the natural opening will seldom be sufficient for the complete cure; and although it may be sufficient for the free discharge of the matter, yet they will heal much more readily if sufficiently opened, for the thin skin over the cavity granulates but indifferently, and therefore unites but slowly with the parts underneath. Where the skin is very thin, loose, and much of it, it may be necessary to remove an oval piece from the centre, where it is generally thinnest. A question naturally occurs, in what way should these be opened?

The methods recommended and used are by incision and caustic. Incision may or may not remove a piece of the skin, but the caustic always will. I believe, as a general practice, there is no preference to be given to either, but under circumstances the incision is best; for instance, where there is but little skin to spare, as on the shin, scalp, etc., but where there is skin to spare, either arising from situation, as in the scrotum, or where a great deal of skin was thinned, as in a great extent of inflammation and suppuration under the skin, a caustic will answer equally well; therefore I should be very apt to be directed by my patients if they had any fears or opinions about the matter, for some have a terror at the idea of a cutting instrument, while others hate the idea of a continued pain. If a caustic is approved of, then I should prefer the lapis infernalis vel septicus to the common caustic; the method of application I described when speaking of the methods of producing death by art: but if left entirely to myself, I should prefer the incision to the caustic, because it is immediately done.

If an abscess is allowed to open of itself, and this opening is not enlarged, no dressing is necessary, nor anything but to keep the surrounding parts clean; the continuation of the poultice, which was before applied (if convenient), is perhaps as good an application as any, and when the tenderness arising from inflammation is over, then lint and a pledget; but an abscess opened by a cutting instrument may be called a mixed case, being both a wound and a sore, and is more of the nature of a fresh wound in proportion to the thickness of the parts cut, and therefore the dressing should be somewhat similar to that of a fresh wound. It is necessary that something should be put into the opening, to keep it from healing by the first intention; if it is lint it should be dipt in some salve, which will answer better than lint alone, as it will allow of more early extraction; for such sores should be dressed the second time the next day, or the second day at latest, because there is a suppurating sore at the bottom, and the pus requires being discharged much sooner than if wholly either a fresh wound or a circumscribed cavity, which is to suppurate, as the tunica vaginalis in the case of the radical cure of the hydrocele. This pus keeps the lint (if dressed with lint) moist, so that it does not dry, as in fresh wounds in common. When the cut edges have come to suppuration, which will be in a few days, then the dressing afterwards may be as simple as possible, for Nature will in general perform the cure.

If the abscess has been opened by caustic, and the slough is either cut out or allowed to slough it, then it is to be considered as an entire suppurating sore, and may be dressed accordingly; perhaps dry lint is as good as anything, till the nature of the sore is known; if of a good kind, the same dressing may be continued, but if not, then it must be dressed accordingly; for Nature cannot always perform a cure; for parts which were at first sound, or appeared so, from their readiness to go through the first stages, will subsequently take on every species of disease, whether from indolence, from irritability, from scrofulous or other dispositions, which in some cases are produced from the nature of the parts diseased, such as bone, ligament, etc.

[The reciprocal effects of structure on inflammation, and of inflammation on structure, are two important subjects which are only incidentally noticed in the preceding pages. I propose therefore very briefly to notice these points.

1. To Haller is undoubtedly due the merit of having first analytically divided the animal body into its component tissues, and ascertained their distinctive physiological properties; while to Hunter we must accord the merit of applying this mode of inquiry to pathological investigations, conceiving that as each texture was endowed with peculiar properties in a state of health, it would likewise in the same manner be affected in a special manner by the causes of disease, and consequently, that the same modes of lesion would always produce similar effects on all the analogous structures of the body. Bichat still further extended this system in his *Anatomie Générale*, which appeared in 1801, but without acknowledgements to Hunter; and it is undoubtedly to this source that we must ascribe the great and rapid advances which have been made in pathological knowledge during the present century.

To suppose, however, as some have done, and as was first ably suggested by Dr. Carmichael Smyth in 1790, that the differences of inflammation essentially and almost exclusively depend on differences of structure, is pushing the principle too far: for, as

Mr. Hunter has justly observed, in the division of the leg in amputation a great many different structures are divided, and yet they all become affected by the same inflammation, and show no difference, except under peculiar circumstances, in this respect. In fact the same inflammation may affect different structures, or the same structure be affected by different inflammations, or inflammation may be transferred from one structure to another. Structure, therefore, is merely a modificatory cause, and often of the least consequence in giving a peculiar character to the inflammatory action.

Cellular Membrane.—This structure forms the basis of all the organs of the body, and therefore may not improbably constitute the proper seat of inflammation, as well as the proper generative tissue, in all cases; for we may observe that the lymph effused in inflammation is always the same, from whatever structure it proceeds; that the process of union is likewise similar for all parts; and that in the regeneration of tissues the production of cellular membrane is invariably the first effort of the organizing principle. It seems not unlikely, therefore, that this uniformity of effect is to be referred to the cellular structure being always affected. The cellular membrane is remarkably susceptible of inflammation, which is generally characterized by the sthenic type, acute throbbing pain, and the rapid and abundant effusion of coagulable matters. It readily passes into all the terminations of inflammation; that is, adhesion, suppuration, ulceration, and mortification. Inflammation of this structure in a healthy constitution shows little disposition to spread, in consequence of the cells being speedily united by coagulable lymph; but under certain states of impaired health, and in particular kinds of inflammation, as, for instance, of the veins, or that arising from the inoculation with morbid poisons, it spreads with great rapidity; not circumferentially, as in a state of health, but irregularly, attended with comparatively little pain. In consequence of adhesive matter not being poured out, the foul sanies, which is secreted instead of pus, easily pervades the cells of this membrane, and carries devastation before it, producing a quaggy state of the subjacent parts, arising from a mixture of pus with sloughy cellular membrane. The seat of this inflammation is usually the subadipose or subfacial cellular membrane; and though in its local and constitutional effects it closely resembles the erysipelas phlegmonoides, yet in the former case the skin remains unaffected, so as to conceal in great measure the mischief which has taken place. In these cases simultaneous purulent depositions not uncommonly take place in various situations of the body. (*Tr. of Med. and Chir. Soc. of Edin.*, vol. i.; *Edin. Med. and Surg. Journ.*, xxiv. 225.; *Travers on Constitutional Irritation*; *and Med. and Chir. Tr. of London*, vol. xvi.)

Dermoidal Tissue.—Inflammation of the skin affords the best type of inflammatory affections, for here it is that the external marks of inflammation are most conspicuously developed; the phenomena, however, are much diversified, according to the part of the skin which happens to be affected. If the external layer of the corion is affected, as in erythema and erysipelas, the inflammation is apt to spread; if the papillæ or muciparous follicles, or the bulbous roots of the hair, then the character of the inflammation is that of the circumscribed eruptive disorders; and if the internal and attached surface, then that of the boil, carbuncle, and phlegmon. The skin is easily inflamed by direct mechanical and chemical injuries, but in a state of health this inflammation is not apt to extend itself. It is also peculiarly accessible to inflammation from morbid poisons or vitiated states of the system, and hence the pathological conditions of this system have always afforded the chief arguments to the humoral pathologists. The dermoidal and mucous tissues offer many points of affinity, both in a physiological and pathological view. In both inflammation is apt to migrate from one part to another, overleaping the intermediate portion; in both pustular and follicular inflammations occur; ulceration and mortification take place in both with great facility, and in both it is observable that their morbid states reciprocally influence one another. It may also be noted, that neither of these tissues is subject to the ossific transformation. The regenerative powers of skin are only inferior to those of the cellular membrane, but the new cutis is different from the old, in being devoid of hairs, muciparous follicles, fat, papillæ, and epidermis, and sometimes of the rete mucosum, although the three latter are certainly reproduced in many cases after a certain lapse of time. The fibrinous contractile cicatrix, which is generated in burns, is not peculiar to this tissue, but occurs occasionally in mucous and serous membranes, producing in the one set of cases the worst forms of stricture, and in the other a more or less complete atrophy of the organs which it envelopes.

Mucous membranes. This structure, like the skin, is exposed to a variety of external influences and therefore is very subject to attacks of inflammation, which generally commence by separate raniform patches, which extend with some degree of capriciousness: the urethra, for example, becomes first inflamed towards the orifice, then the membranous portion or bladder, and lastly the kidneys or testicles; the intermediate continuous portions of the sound membrane not suffering. The same thing is observed of the air-passages and alimentary canal, the different portions of which become successively, but not continuously affected. The mucous membrane is at first dry, then swells, becomes intensely vascular, and often in a high degree villous, the follicles usually enlarge, and the secretion is gradually changed from a highly limpid mucus into genuine pus. There is a great difference, however, in this respect; for while some, as the urethra, secrete pus very readily and in great abundance without being prone to ulceration, others, as the intestines, are seldom found to produce this fluid without previous ulceration; while others again, as the fauces and tonsils, not unfrequently secrete a peculiar modification of albumen, which, although not organizable, adheres for a considerable length of time to the free surface, and assumes the appearance of an ash-coloured or greyish slough. The bladder and colon secrete a ropy tenacious mucus, especially in chronic inflammation, while the internal membrane of the stomach and small intestines is reduced, under the same circumstances, to a soft pulpy condition, so as easily to admit of being scraped off, or even to be removed by the natural actions of the part. Specific diseases and poisons are peculiarly apt to attack parts of this system, and at the same time to produce specific effects, as is seen in croup, dysentery, and scurvy; but in general the prevailing tendency of this system may be stated to be, suppuration, ulceration, and mortification. Occasionally, however, there is considerable submucous infiltration either of serum or lymph, producing in the former case œdema, and sometimes death, when it happens to occur in the larynx, and in the latter permanent cartilaginous strictures. The regenerative powers of this tissue differ in different parts; for in the bucco-pharyngeal portions they are very considerable, while in the enteric, laryngeal, and urinary portions they are very limited. In extensive regenerations, as at the back of the pharynx, the new membrane is of a different colour from the old, and unprovided either with follicles or villi, in consequence of which it is no longer a secreting surface; but in other cases, especially where a considerable time has elapsed, it is perfectly restored. The lining membranes of certain forms of gelatiniform encysted tumours and sinuses are the natural transition between the mucous and serous classes.

Serous membranes. Inflammations of this class are characterized by their tendency to spread and to exude a great abundance of the coagulable parts of the blood; they are also generally characterized by their acuteness, by the severe and rousing pain which they occasion, and by the great capability which the system evinces under their influence of enduring great losses of blood; in which respect, as well as by their indisposition to take on the suppurative form, they are remarkably contra-distinguished from those of the former class. Primary ulceration and mortification of this tissue are extremely uncommon; but in certain forms of secondary inflammations, which have been before adverted to, it gives rise to an abundant purulent secretion. Next to the fibrous class, the serous tissue is most subject to metastatic inflammations, as gout, rheumatism, syphilis, &c., and in such cases many parts are often simultaneously attacked. Pathologists are divided as to the proper seat of this inflammation, some considering it to be the serous membrane itself, and others the subserous cellular tissue, the proper serous membrane being regarded, like the epidermis, as extra-vascular. There is, however, no doubt of the former becoming visibly vascular in some stages of its progress, of the vessels thus formed being in communication with those which are generated in the effused lymph, and of all the other changes of inflammation being produced without visible vascularity, as in the arachnoid membrane; so that upon the whole there seems no reason to doubt that the serous membranes are themselves inflamed, especially as subserous infiltrations, whether of serum, lymph, or pus, are to be regarded as unfrequent occurrences. After removing a portion of the pleura pulmonalis, Dr. Thomson could not discover any visible cicatrix; from which, as well as from the frequent generation of this tissue in new situations, there is no reason to doubt that this membrane is readily reproduced.

The synovial and bursal structures resemble the serous in most leading respects; but the change of structure into a pulpy greyish substance, to which the former are subject, and the tendency to fungoid growths, to which the bursæ are liable, have not been observed in the serous membranes, although both are extremely prone to cartilaginous and ossific transformations, the result of chronic inflammation; neither are they equally liable to the production of loose cartilages and small ovoid bodies in the form of melon seeds, nor equally exposed to metastatic inflammations.

Fibrous tissue. Like other dense and unvascular parts, the fibrous tissue exhibits a comparative backwardness to inflammation, the processes of reparation are slowly effected, and ulceration, mortification, and even suppuration are seldom primarily induced. The differing degrees of vascularity, however, in different parts of this system occasion a great difference in this respect. In general there is an abundant effusion of coagulable lymph, which often under such circumstances becomes ossified; but, upon the whole, the reproductive powers of this system are not considerable, so that tendons which have sloughed are not renewed, and ruptures of the capsular ligament, in cases of dislocation, have remained unrepaired for several years. This system is peculiarly obnoxious to inflammation from constitutional causes, as gout, rheumatism, and syphilis, in which cases there is often a metastasis of the disease from one part to another in succession, attended with severe nocturnal exacerbations. The confinement of matter in some of these cases is often productive of great constitutional irritation.

Cartilaginous system. It has been doubted whether true cartilage is ever subject to inflammation, principally because it has never been observed to become vascular; but as the phenomena of normal ossification leave no doubt as to the vascularity of this substance in a state of health, there seems no just reason for doubting its capability to inflame, especially as in similar unvascular parts, as the cornea, the arachnoid membrane, and even the teeth, there is no question on this subject. Neither is there any question respecting the vascularity of the fibro-cartilages, although these structures are traceable by insensible degrees into true cartilage, from which indeed they are not essentially different. Still, however, there are some peculiarities respecting the pathology of cartilages which are not easily explained: as, for example, the extreme dissimilarity which they exhibit in regard to the two forms of ulcerative and progressive absorption; the former of which takes place with the greatest readiness, and the latter with the utmost difficulty. Ulceration of the harder cartilages is sometimes unaccompanied with suppuration. It is generally, however, attended with a high degree of irritative fever, as compared with the actual extent of the disease, and often with partial exfoliations. The reproductive powers of cartilage are very limited, and it is observable that this substance invariably unites by osseous union.

Osseous system. The peculiarities of ostitis are principally referrible to the peculiar hard texture of bone, which does not admit of that rapid extension of vascularity which the reparative processes of inflammation seem to require; consequently all the processes of bone are extremely tedious, so that in some cases several years are required for the complete disjunction of a dead from a living portion. The general principle, of parts being less accessible to inflammation in proportion as they are dense in structure and deficient in vascularity, holds good in respect to bones, which are rarely subject to idiopathic inflammation; the compacter portions being less subject than those which are more porous, although both are much more so than tendons, fasciæ, and cartilages. Still, however, bones are much exposed to chronic inflammation from mercury, syphilis, gout, rheumatism, scrofula, &c., giving rise to various forms of hyperostosis. Bones become very vascular when inflamed, and the harder parts readily perish. In nearly all cases the texture of the bone is much loosened by inflammation, and a part of the earthy matter is absorbed, so that when macerated and dried it exhibits a light and spongy fabric; in some rare cases it acquires unusual density, approaching to the nature of ivory. The union of bone is precisely similar to that of soft parts, while its reproductive powers are of a high order, leading not only to the complete regeneration of entire shafts of bone, but to the perfect restoration of the organization to the normal state: in which respect, perhaps, they are not equalled by any other structure of the body.

Muscular Tissue. This tissue appears to be the least liable to inflammation and its consequences of any structure of the body. When inflammation attacks this structure from wounds, &c., it becomes soft and lacerable, and of various shades of green, brown, and red; but in such cases it is not observed that the inflammation has any disposition to extend along the whole course of the muscle. I have sometimes seen a diffused suppuration in the substance of muscles in secondary inflammations, as well as in inflammations arising from wounds received in dissection, and circumscribed abscesses have occasionally been discovered in the substance of the heart in carditis. Muscle is never reproduced, but the union is invariably effected by a fibro-ligamentous structure.

Vascular System. The arteries differ very remarkably in their liability to inflammation as compared with the lymphatics and veins, as well as in their constitutional effects and morbid changes. Inflammation of the internal coats of arteries must be considered as very uncommon, and rarely advances to the suppurative stage, whereas nothing is more common than inflammation and suppuration of the veins and lymphatics, attended with low typhoid symptoms, secondary suppurations in various situations of the body, and very often death. Chronic inflammation also, leading to considerable thickening of the venous tunics, is sufficiently common. In inflammation of the veins and lymphatics the adjacent tissues are always more or less involved, so that their course is indicated by hard and painful lines. Mr. Hunter has remarked that this system resists the effects both of ulceration and mortification beyond all other tissues; and with regard to mortification they are not, I believe, ever primarily affected in this way. The reproductive powers of vessels are certainly of the highest order, although differing in some measure from other parts. In an instance already referred to (see *note*, p. 242.), new vessels were actually produced, capable of performing all the functions of the old; but in general when large vessels are obliterated their office is vicariously performed by the enlargement of others which had previously existed.

Nervous Tissue. Little is known respecting the nerves. That they become inflamed and thickened in certain cases of local neuralgic disease has been demonstrated by dissection, but in other cases no such appearances have been observed; neither is it known whether they are ever primarily affected by ulceration, suppuration, or mortification. The question as to the regeneration of the proper nervous tissue is still undecided.

The proper medullary matter of the brain and spinal marrow is subject to acute and chronic inflammation, like other parts; probably the former, however, never takes place idiopathically, but from injuries and poisons only, when it is generally limited in its extent and characterized by a red colour of various degrees of intensity, verging towards brown, green, or yellow, and terminating in a state of diffluence. Chronic inflammation is much more frequent, attended with increased vascularity at first, but as the brain becomes softened, with a red, yellowish, or whitish colour, marking three several kinds of mollescence, depending on the effusion of blood, pus, or serum. There seems reason, however, for believing that this pulpy disorganization of the brain may take place independently of inflammation. The most remarkable circumstance connected with this tissue is the occurrence of large chronic abscesses, generally inclosed in thick cysts, and unattended with any symptoms during life. These I have known to occupy one entire hemisphere of the brain. Ulceration sometimes occurs towards the surface of the convolutions, and by some the diffluent state of the brain before spoken of is thought to resemble mortification.

2. It has been before stated that all the functions of a part are modified by inflammation; of these, however, two only are susceptible of examination, viz. secretion, including the inflammatory effusions, and nutrition: the former of these has been already considered, and it only remains to make a few observations respecting the latter.

The effects of inflammation as regards nutrition may be divided into two primary classes, including, in the first place, those which have respect to the physical properties of parts; and, in the second place, those which have more immediate reference to their organical constitution. These, it must be obvious, often run up into each other, so as to render any satisfactory classification of the phenomena impracticable.

The *primary* effects of inflammation, or those which regard the physical properties of parts, are several.

Induration, as regards the soft parts, is one of the most universal effects of inflammation, and may be said to depend on the interstitial deposition of lymph in the interspaces of the natural organization, which in process of time becomes converted into the same nature as the part itself. These effects are more or less permanent in different cases. In general, parts are found to revert to their former state upon the subsidence of the inflammation; but in other cases this does not happen, in consequence it may be presumed of the normal organization of the part being permanently injured; as, for instance, in the iris, which is often irretrievably destroyed by acute iritis. Instances of induration remaining, after the augmentation of bulk has subsided, occur in the liver, brain, muscles, spleen, and particularly in the eburnation of the articular extremities of bones from which the cartilages have been denuded.

Softening also is a very frequent consequence of inflammation, particularly of the cellular membrane, as is evinced in the diminished cohesion of parenchymatous organs, and the weakened attachment of membranous expansions to the parts which they cover. The harder textures, as bone, tendon, cartilage, &c., are most frequently softened by inflammation, in the same manner as the softer textures are most frequently hardened; but these effects are sometimes reversed. Softening has been ascribed to the infiltration of serum and pus disintegrating the healthy organization, but as such effusions are not always, or even generally, attended with this consequence, it is probably referrible to some peculiar modification of the nutritive function, especially as this is known to be sufficient of itself to produce the effect independently of inflammatory action. The most remarkable examples of softening occur in the lungs, spleen, mucous membranes of the stomach and bowels, and in the brain and spinal marrow. The original organization in such cases is often irrecoverably destroyed.

Fragility must not be confounded with softening, although it is often found associated with it. An increased lacerability of parts is, upon the whole, much more general than softening, and occurs under both the conditions which have previously been considered. It is seen in the inflamed and hepatized lung, as well as in the common cellular membrane which has been hardened by the infiltration of recent lymph.

Hypertrophy consists in the undue development of parts beyond their normal proportions. Like every other change consequent on inflammation, hypertrophy may occur from other causes besides inflammation, because inflammation merely alters the nutrition of parts, which many other causes are equally capable of doing. It is always associated with a state of hyperemy, and most frequently with increased density of structure. When it arises from simply increased functions there seems to be no difference in the mode of growth from that of ordinary nutrition; but when it arises from inflammation the augmentation of bulk is effected by interstitial deposition, which afterwards becomes organized. In hypertrophy of the bladder, consequent on diseases of this part, both these causes concur to produce the effect; these distinctions, however, are not always apparent, especially in bones, which often enlarge under circumstances which fall short of inflammation, and yet are more or less connected with it. Exostoses, for example, which are partial hypertrophic developments, are often traceable to mechanical injuries; and in the same manner bones are often found to enlarge from constitutional causes, as gout, rheumatism, syphilis, &c., which in a more active form produce inflammation. A chronic ulcer of the surface may occasion an enlargement of the bone beneath, and a similar effect may be produced by the Barbadoes leg.

Atrophy is a vice of nutrition, the very reverse of the former. Both appear to have their analogues in the evolution of the fœtus, in which there is sometimes an arrest and sometimes a persistence of the formative principle, giving rise to two opposite forms of monstrosity. As in inflammation, therefore, the principle of growth or augmentation of parts, which seems natural to this state, is sometimes persistent beyond the due and regular period, so on the other hand the principle of absorption, by which this excess of growth is removed, is sometimes continued after the due and regular effect of the restoration of the parts to their natural condition has been accomplished. The excess of growth in an inflamed part being useless when the inflammation has subsided, and perhaps an incumbrance to the due exercise of its functions, is removed on the same principle as many parts, having a temporary use in fœtal life, or parts in the adult which have become disorganized and unfit for their office, are got rid of; for in general it may be observed that the use of a part, and consequently its necessity, are the only protection which it has against the operation of this law. Accordingly, it is observed that those parts which have only a temporary use in the economy, as the testicles, mammæ, ovaries, &c., are most liable to the effect of wasting, in consequence of inflammatory action.

The *secondary* effects of inflammation, or those which regard the organical constitution of parts, are coextensive with the whole range of pathology, and cannot be entered into in this place. The most general division of these formations is into the *analogous*, or those which have some analogue in the healthy body, and the *heterologous*, or those which have no resemblance to any healthy elementary tissue, as schirrus, melanosis, tubercle, &c., and which therefore are to be regarded in the highest sense as morbid productions. The former again have been subdivided by Heusinger into *new* or *analogous formations*, or accidental, parasitical, and adventitious tissues anormally developed in situations where they did not previously exist, as serous cysts, fatty tumours, &c.; and *analogous transformations*, or the conversion of existing parts into structures of a different kind from that which they originally possessed, as when serous and fibrous membranes are converted into bone, muscle into fat, &c. The former are nearly as extensive as the natural elementary tissues of the body, and, for the most part, are injurious. The latter are less numerous, being sometimes characterized by an elevation of the natural organization of the part, to answer some new and useful object in the economy, and sometimes, by a degradation of the original tissue, subversive of its peculiar function.

In the opinion of many modern physiologists, the whole of these anormal productions are referrible to an inflammatory cause; and undoubtedly such a cause, or some external injury almost equivalent to it, may often be detected in many individual cases; but still this is very far from being general, and therefore, for reasons which I have previously given (I. 367, note), I cannot concur in this opinion. Inflammation appears to produce morbid growths; first, by weakening the parts; and secondly, by inducing a temporary modification of the normal mode of nutrition, both which circumstances are the invariable consequents of inflammation, and may reasonably be presumed to predispose the affected parts to assume a new disposition, corresponding to any preexisting cause of disease which may be in the constitution at the time. Without the concurrence of some other cause, however, inflammation alone is insufficient for the effect, and when this cause actually exists inflammation is unnecessary, and the remedies for inflammation unavailing.

BIBLIOGRAPHY OF INFLAMMATION.

Alison, op. cit.* (vide *ante*, p. 138), p. 393, and *op. cit.* (vide *ante*, p. 233).——Andral, op. cit.* (v. a. p. 138,) i. 12. De l'Hyperémie.

Badham, D., M.D. Reflections on the Nature of Inflam. and its alleged consequences. 8vo. 1834.——*Baldwin, H.* (Th.) De Inflam. 1803.——*Balfour, W., M.D.* Observ. on Adhesion, &c. 8vo. 1814.——*Bargen.* De Inflam. ejusque Theoriis. 8vo. 1827. ——*Baronio, G.* Degli innesti Animali. 8vo. 1804.——*Bell, B.* On Ulcers, White Swellings, and Inflam. 2nd edit. 8vo. 1779.——*Bell, J.* Principles of Surgery, (vol. i. on wounds, ulcers, &c.) 3 vols. 4to. 1801–1808.——*Berlioz, A.* Propositions sur l'Inflam. 4to. 1814.——*Black, J. M.D., op. cit.* (v. a. p. 234.)——*Boerhaave, H.* Diss. de Inflam. in Genere. 4to. 1707.——*Bohn.* Diss. de Inflam. 4to. 1684.—— *Boyer, Le Baron,* Traité des Mal. Chir. (vol. i.) 3ème. édit. 11 vols. 8vo. 1822–6. ——*Brachet, J. L.* De l'Emploi de l'Opium dans les Phlegmasies des Memb. Muqueuses, séreuses et fibreuses, &c. 8vo. 1828.——*Bricheteau,* in Dict. des Sc. Méd., Art. INFLAMMATION et PHLEGMASIE.——**Broussais, F. J. V.* Hist. des Phlegmasies, &c. 2 tom. 8vo. 1808; and Hist. des Phlegmasies Chroniques, 3 tom. 8vo. 1822; and 4ème édit. 3 tom. 8vo. 1826. *tr.* by Hays. Phil. 1831.——*Brown, J.* Med. Essays on Fever, Inflam., &c. 8vo. 1828.——*Burdach, K. F.* Diss. Observ. nonnullæ Microsc. Inflam. spectantes. 1825; and *op. cit.* (v. a. p. 139.)——*Burns, J.* Diss. on Inflamm. 2 vols. 8vo. 1800; and Principles of Surgery, vol. i. (p. 24.) 8vo. 1831.

Caffin, J. F. Du Caractère de l'Inflam., de la Congestion, &c. 8vo. 1819.——*Caffort.* Memoir sur la Nature de l'Inflam. 8vo. 1829.——*Carpue, J. C.* An Account of two successful Operations for restoring a lost Nose, &c. 4to. 1816.——*Carus, C. G.* De Vi Naturæ Medicatrice in formandis Cicatricibus. Part i. 8vo. 1822.——*Chaufford, H.* Traité des Inflam. Internes. 8vo. 1831.——*Chomel,* in Dict. de Méd., Art. INFLAM. tom. xii. 1825.——*Chortet, J. F.* Traité de l'Inflam. et de ses Terminaisons. 8vo. 1808.——*Coxe, J. B.* (Th.) On Inflam. Phil. 8vo. 1794.——*Crawford* and *Tweedie, D.'s.,* in Cyclopædia of Pract. Med., Art. INFLAM. vol. ii. 1832.——*Cruveilhier, J.* in Dict. de Méd. et Chir. Prat., Art. ADHESION. 1829.——*Cullen, W., M.D.* First Lines, &c. (vol. i.) 4 vols. 8vo. 1789.

Delpech, J. Précis Elém. des Mal. Chir. (tom. i. c. i.) 3 vols. 8vo. 1816.——*Dohlhof.* De Phlegmone. 8vo. 1819.——*Dowler, T., op. cit.* (v. a. p. 140.) On the Products

* See p. 138 for the explanation of the star, and for the titles of those works which are here merely referred to. It may be proper to mention that the extensiveness of this subject has made it necessary to fix some limit; I have therefore seldom inserted the titles of works prior to the time of Hunter or Monographics on particular subjects.

of Acute Inflam.——*Duges, A.* Essai Phys.-Path. sur la Nature de la Fièvre, de l'Inflam., &c. 8vo. 1823.——*Dzondi, H. C.* Aphorismi de Inflam. lib. i. 8vo. 1814. ——*Dzondi, K. H.* Pathologia Inflammationis. 8vo. 1828.

Earle, J. W., in Med. Gaz., vol. xvi. 1834–5. On Inflam.——*Edden, H. A.* Die Theorie d. Entzundung. 8vo. 1811.——*Eggers.* Von der Wiedererzeugung. 8vo. 1821.——*Emiliani, L.* Dell' Infiam. Comm. 8vo. 1824; and Ricerche sul trattamento delle Malattie Infiammatorie. 8vo. 1829.

Fegelein, G. M. Versuch einer Nosologie und Therapei der Entzundungen. 8vo. 1804. ——*Filippi, G. de.* Nuovo Saggio Analitico sull' Infiam.

**Gendrin, op. cit.* (v. a. p. 141.)——*Gerardin,* Essai sur les Phlogoses Sarcopée et Osteopée, &c. 4to. 1823.——*Gibson, W., M. D.* The Institutes and Practice of Surgery, &c. 2nd edit. 2 vols. 8vo. Phil. 1827.——*Goeden, H. A.* Die Theorie der Entzundung. 8vo. 1811.——*Goldoni, A.* Sulle infiam. trattato diviso in tre parti. pt. i. 1825. Discorso in risposta alle cose a su riguardo stampata dal Sig. Prof. G. Tommasini nel vol. ii. sull' infiam. 8vo. 1829.——*Good, J. M., M.D.* Study of Med. (ii. 283.) 3rd edit. by *S. Cooper.* 5 vols. 8vo. 1829.——*Graefe, R. C. F.* De Rhinoplatice, &c. Lat. edidit *J. F. C. Hecker.* 4to. 1818.——*Gruithuisen, Fr.*, in Gaz. Méd.-Chir. de Salzbourg, ii. 129. (1816.)—Theorie der Entzundung. *ib.* ii. 298. (1811.); and Preface to his Organozoonomie. 8vo. 1811.

Harles, J. C. F. Pratische Bemerkungen über innere Entzundungen bey Kindern. 4to. 1810.——**Hastings, C., M.D., op. cit.* (v. a. p. 235.)——*Herdman, J.* Diss. on White Swelling and the Doctrine of Inflam. 8vo. 1802.——*Heffter, D. F.* Doctrinæ de Gangrena Brevis Expos. 4to. 1807.—On the subject of hospital gangrene consult Larrey, O'Halloran, Delpech, Hennen, and the military surgeons generally. See also Reuss and Plouquet, Art. GANGRENE and SPHACELUS.——*Henke, A.* De Inflam. internis Infantum comm. 1817.——*Hermann,* De Inflam. in Genere.——*Hildenbrand, J. V. N.* Instit. Pract.-Med., &c. (ii. De Inflam.) 4 tom. 8vo. 1816–25.——*Hoffmann, C. R.* Sententia de Inflam. Naturâ. 8vo. 1819.——*Hofrichter, B.* Versuch über das Entzundungsfieber und die Entzundung. 8vo. 1806.——*Hohnbaum,* über das Fortschreiten des Krankheits-processes insbesondere der Entzundung, &c. 1826. ——*Hunt, J.* On the Progress of Medical Science regarding Inflam., Gangrene, and Gunshot Wounds. 4to. 1801.

**James, J. H.* Observ. on the General Principles, &c. of Inflammation. 8vo. 1821. 2nd edit. 1832.

**Kaltenbrunner, G., op. cit.* (v. a. p. 142.)——*Koch, C. A.* Diss. de Observ. nonnullis Microsc. Sang. Cursum et Inflam. spectantes, &c. 1825.——*Kolk, J. L. C.* Schroeder van der, Observ. Anat-Path. et Prat. Argumenti. fasc. i. 8vo. 1826; and *op. cit.*, (v. a. p. 142.)——*König, G., op. cit.* (v. a. p. 142.)

Lalanne, P. quelques Consid. sur l'Inflam. en général et sur les différentes terminaisons. 4to. 1804.——*Langenbeck, C. J. M.* Nosologie, &c. der Chir. Krankheiten (1. 6.) 3 bde 8vo. 1822–25.——**Lawrence, W.*, in Med. Gaz. vol. v. p. 97. 1829–30. Lect. on Surgery.——*Liesseling, C. L. G.* de Gangræna, 4to. 1811.——*Lizars, J.* in Edin. Med. and Surg. Journ. xv. 369. (1819.) On the Pathology of the Nerves in Inflam. ——*Lobstein, J. F.* Traité d'Anat. Path. (§ 334.) 8vo. et fol. 1829.——*Lucas, C. E., M.D.* The Principles of Inflam. and Fever. 8vo. 1822.

Magenisie, D. The Doctrine of Inflam., &c. 8vo. 1768.——*Mantavoni, V.* Lezioni di Nosologia e terapia sulle Infiam. (vol. iii.) 12mo. 1820.——*Meier, J.* Versuch einer kritische Geschichte der Entzundung. 8vo. 1812.——*Meyer, Im.* ueber die Natur. d. Entzundung. 8vo. 1810.——Versuch e. krit. Geschichte d. Entzundung. 8vo. 1812. ——*Moore, J.* Diss. on the Process of Nature in filling up Cavities, healing of Wounds, &c. 4to. 1789.——*Morgan, G. T.* on Inflam. and its Effects. 8vo. 1837.

Naumann, M. zur Lehre von der Entzundung. 12mo. 1828.——*Nietsch, K. F.* ueber verborgene Entzundung, &c. 8vo. 1819.

Parry, C. H., M.D. Elem. of Path. and Therap. 8vo. 1815, and *op. cit.* (v. a. p. 236.) ——*Paul, Fr.* Comm. Phys. Chir. de Vulneribus sanandis, &c. 4to. 1825.——*Porret, S.* (Th.) Aperçu sur les Phénomènes généraux de l'Inflam. considérés dans les différens Systèmes. 8vo. an. xi.——*Pinel, P.* Nosographie Phil., &c. (tom. ii. PHLEGMASIE,) 3 tom. 1813, and 6me' édit. 3 tom. 8vo. 1818.——*Plouquet.* Diss. de multifariis Inflam. Terminationibus. 4to. 1803.——*Portel, P. J. P.* Diss. sur l'Inflam. 4to. 1803.——*Prevost, J. L.* in Mém. de la Soc. de Phy. de Genève, vi. 142. (1833.) note sur l'Inflam.——*Prus.* de l'Irritation et de Phlegmone. 8vo. 1825.

Roche, in Dict. de Med. Prat. art. INFLAM. vol. x. 1833.—— *Ronnefeld, C. H.* Animadv. nonnullæ ad Doct. de Inflam. 4to. 1817.——*Rogerson, G.* A Treatise on Inflam. vol. i. 8vo. 1832.

Salfender. Diss. de Reunione Partium Corp. Hum. Elementarium. 8vo. 1826.—— *Sanson, L. J.* de la Réunion Imméd. des Plaies, &c. 8vo. 1834.——*Scholefield.* de Theoria Inflam. 1822.——*Scott, J.* Surgical Observ. on the Treatment of Chron. Inflam. in various Structures, &c. 8vo. 1822.——*Sérre, M.* Traité de la Réunion Immédiate, &c. 8vo. 1830.——**Smyth, J. C., M.D.* Of the different Kinds and Species of Inflammation, and of the Causes to which these Differences may be ascribed: in Med. Communications. (1790.) II. 168.——*Sommé.* Etudes sur l'Inflam. 8vo. 1830.——*Spörer, G. M.* de Inflam. Morbo Anim. et Veget. 1824.——*Stahl, G. E.* Diss. de Inflam. vera Pathologia. 4to. 1698.——*Stevens, A. H.* A Diss. on the proximate Causes of Inflam. 8vo. 1811.——*Suchs, L. W.* Grundlinien zu einem Systeme der pratische Medicin. (Th. 1. Entzundungen.) 8vo. 1821.——*Suringar.* Comm. Med. de Modo, quo Natura versatur in restituendo omni quod in Corp. Hum. solutum sit. 4to. 1823.——*Syme, J.*, in Edinb. Med. and Surg. Journ. vol. xxx. (1828.) p. 316. On the Nature of Inflam.

**Thomson, John, M.D. op. cit.* (v. a. p. 144.)——*Tommasini, G.* Dell' Infiam., &c. 8vo. 1820. and 2da ediz. 2 vol. 8vo. 1826-7.——*Travers, B.* Inquiry into the Disturbed State of the Vital Functions, called Constitutional Irritation. 8vo. 1826.—Further Inquiry, &c. 8vo. 1835.

**Vacca, L.* Liber de Inflam. Morbosæ, quæ in Humano Corpore fit, Natura, Causis, Effectibus, et Curatione. 1765.

Waring, (Th.) de Inflam. 1823.——*Wedemeyer, V. G.* Untersuchungen über des Kreislauf des Blutes. 1828.——*Wendelstedt.* Diss. de Cognatione et Differentia inter Inflam. et Profluvia. 1809.——*Wendt, G.* Die alte Lehre von den Verborgenen Entzundungen bestätigt. 2te Aufl. 8vo. 1826.——*White,* in Mem. of the Soc. of Manchester. vol. i. (1785.) On the Regen. of Animal Substances.——*Wiesmann, J. H. F.*, de Coalitu Partium a reliquo Corpore prorsus disjunctarum Comm., etc. c. tab. æn.

4to. 1824.——*Willis, J. C.*, (Th.) de Inflam., 1802.——*Wilson, J.*, *op. cit.* (v. a. p. 144.)——*Wilson, Philip, M.D.*, on Febrile Diseases, 8vo. 1799, and 4th edit. 8vo. 1820, and *op. cit.* (v. a. p. 236.)——*Winterl. J. J.* Inflam. Theoria Nova. 8vo. 1767.

For a further account of the literature of this subject, particularly of specific inflammations and of the opinions of the older authors, consult the undermentioned works:

Bernstein, J. G. Medic. Chir. Bibliothek.——*Burdach, K. T.* Die Literatur der Heil-Wissenschaft. 3 Bde. 8vo. 1810–21.——*Creuzenfeld, S. H.* Bibliotheca Chir., &c. 2 vol. 4to. 1781.——*Haller, A.* Bibl. Chir. 2 tom. 4to. 1774–5.——*Langenbeck, C. J. M.* Bibliothek für die Chir. 4 Bde. 12mo. 1807–13, and Neue Bib. f. d. Chir. 4 Bde. 12mo. 1815–28.——*Otto, op. cit.* (v. a. p. 237.)——*Plouquet, op. cit.* (v. a. p. 237.)——*Puchelt, F. A. B.* Literatur de Med. 8vo. 1822.——*Reuss, op. cit.* (v. a. p. 237.)——*Scavini, J. M.* Précis Hist. de la Doct. de l'Inflam., &c. 2de édit. 8vo. 1811.——*Sprengel, K.* Literatura Med. Externa, &c. 8vo. 1829.

Suppuration and Ulceration.

Abernethy, J. Obs. on Tumours and Lumbar Abscesses. 8vo. 1810.——*Andral* (I. 189. De l'Ulceration, I. 388. Pus.), *ut supra.*——*Balfour, J. H.* Probationary Essay on Purulent Deposits after Wounds and Operations. 8vo. 1833.——*Bell, B.* and *I.*, *ut supra.*——*Blackadder, H. H.* on Phagadæna Gangrenosa. 8vo. 1818.——*Brande, T. W.* In Phil. Tr. 1809. p. 373.——*Brugmanns, S. I.* De Puogenia, &c. 8vo. 1785. ——*Callisen, H.* System der Neueren Chir. 1822. p. 559. note.——*Cooper, Sir A.* Lectures on Surg., by F. Tyrrell. (vol. i.) 3 vol. 8vo. 1824–7.——*Daucher.* Momenta circa variam Puris Indolem, &c. 1804. Dict. des Sc. Méd. (Petit.) *Art.* Depot.—Dict. de Méd. (Roux) *Art.* Abcès.—Dict. de Méd. et Chir. Prat. (Dupuytren) Art. Abcès.—Cycl. of Prat. Med. (Tweedie) and Encyel. Wörterb. (Richter) Art. Abscess.——*Dupuy, J. M.* Sur les Abcès ou Tumeurs Purulentes. 1804.——*Encycl.* Métho. *Art.* Abcès.——*Ford, Ed.* Obs. on the Dis. of the Hip-joints, (Ch. on Abscesses) 8vo. 1794.——*Goebel*, in Schweigger's Journ., vol. iv. part iv. p. 408.——*Grashuis, J.* Diss. on Suppuration. 8vo. 1747.——*Gruithuisen, P.* Untersuchung über den Unterschied zwischen Eiter und Schleim durch das Mikroskop. 4to. 1809. with Engr.——*Hendy, J.* Ess. on Glandular Secretion containing an exp. Enq. into the formation of Pus. 8vo. 1775.——*Hoffmann*, Sententia de Supp. Natura. 8vo. 1818.——*Home, Sir E.* on the Properties of Pus. 4to. 1788.—Phil. Tr. 1819. p. 1. on the Conversion of Pus into new Flesh,—also on Ulcers of the Legs. 8vo. 1797. 2nd edit. 1801.——*Kaltenbrunner, G.* in Heusinger's Zeitschrift f. Organ-Physik. vol. i. Pt. III. p. 314.——*Koch, ut supra.*——*Kupfer, H. E.* de Inflam. et præsertim de Puris Generatione. 1828.——*Langenbeck, J. M.* in neue Bibl. für die Chir. 12mo. 1817. —also his Nosologie der Chir. Krankheiten (2ter b.) 3 bde. 8vo. 1822–25. ——*Laurent, J.* Essai sur la Supp. 8vo. 1803.——*Pearson, G. M.D.* in Phil. Tr. 1811. p. 294–317. Obser. and Exp. on Pus.——*Petgold, V.* de Diagnosi Puris. 1827.——*Pramann, A.* de Puris Indole et Genesi. 8vo. 1828.——*Quesnay, F.* Traité de la Supp. 12mo. 1749.——*Richter, A. G.* Anfangsgründe der Wundarzneykunst (b. 1. Kap. 2.), 7 bde. 8vo. 4te Aufl. 1804–25.——*Rizzetti, Rossi* and *Michelotti*, in Mém. de Turin. vol. ii. and iii.—— *Waldmann*, Disquisitiones de Discrimine inter Pus et Pituitam. 1807.

On the Effects of Inflammation on Texture.

Andral, (I. 91-298.) *ut supra.*——*Boullaud, A.* in Journ. des Prog. des Sc. Méd. iv. 149. 1827. Rech. Hist. sur les Tissus Accidentels sans-analogues.——*Bugayski*,

Diss. de Part. Corp. hum. solid. simil. Aberrationibus. 4to. 1813.——*Carswell, op. cit.* (v. a. p. 140.) Fasc. xi. analogous tissues.—— *Clarus, A.* Quæstiones de Partibus Pseudo-Organicis. 8vo. 1805.——*Cruveilhier, op. cit.* (v. a. 140.)——Dict. Abrégé des Sc. Méd. *Art.* ANAT. PATH., par MM. *Bayle et Boisseau.*——*Dumas, C. L.* in Sedillot's Journ. Gén. xxiii–xxv. sur les Transformations des Organes.——*Gisbert Van Beers.* de Textura Organorum per Inflam. 1826.——*Hesse,* ueber die Erweichung der Gewebe und Organe des menschl. Körpers. 8vo. 1827.——*Heusinger,* System der Histologie, Pt. I. p. 87–103. 4to. 1822. and in the first Berichte von der Königl. Anthropotomischen Anstalt zu Würzburg, p. 1–41. 4to. 1826.——*Junge,* de Pseudo-Plasmatum in Corp. Hum. obviorum Natura et Indole. 4to. 1822.——*Laennec, R. T. H.* in Journal de Méd. de Corvisart. XI. 360. and Dict. des Sc. Méd. vol. ii. *Art.* ANAT. PATH.——*Martin,* in Mem. de la Soc. Méd. d'Emulation. vii. on Organic Diseases.——*Meckel, J. F. op. cit.* i. 531. des Formations Accidentelles. (v. a. p. 236.) ——*Napple, (Th.)* Sur les Fausses Membranes et les Adhérences. 1812.—— *Otto, A. W. op. cit.* (v. a. p. 237.)——*Villermé,* Essai sur les Fausses Membranes. 4to. 1814.——*Walther,* in Journ. der Chir. vol. v. Pt. II. p. 196.——*Wenzel, C.* ueber dei Induration, &c. 8vo. 1815.

Cellular Tissue.

Aitkin, T. J. Essay on the Effects of Puncture received in Dissection. 8vo. 1826.—— *Baillie,* in Lond. Med. Rep. 1826. on Inflam. of Cell. Tissue.——*Butter, J. M.D.* on Irritative Fever. 8vo. 1815.——*Creutzwieser,* in Rust's Magaz. f. d. Ges. Heilk. xxii. Pt. II. 338. Necrosis Telæ Cellulosæ.——*Craigie, D.* (Path. Anat. p. 32.) *ut supra.*——*Dohlhof, D.* de Phlegmon. 8vo. 1819.——*Duncan, A. M.D.* in Edin. Med. and Chir. Tr. vol. i. 1824. on diffuse Cellular Inflam.——*Kirkland, T. M.D.* An Enquiry into the present state of Med. Surgery. (ii. 282.) 2 vols. 8vo. 1783.——*Naumann, D.* De Inflam. Telæ Mucosæ. 1820.——*Otto,* (p. 91.) *ut supr.* and Selt. Beob. Pt. II. p. 41.——*Pauli,* in Rust's Magaz. f. d. Ges. Heilk. (1828) xxvii. 128.—— *Scott,* in Edin. Med. and Surg. Journ. xxiv. 225. on Diffuse Cellular Inflam.—— *Testa, A. J.* in Rœmer Dissert. Med. Ital. 8vo. note. de Cellulosæ Telæ Affectibus. ——*Travers, ut supra.*

Dermoidal Tissue.

Alibert, J. L. Déscriptions des Maladies de la Peau. 8vo. 1816. and fol. 1825. Monographie des Dermatoses 4to. 1832.——*Batemann, Th. M.D.* A Practical Synopsis of Cutaneous Diseases. 8vo. 1813–14. 6th edit. 1824. with Atlas of Delineations 1817. by Dr. A. T. Thompson. roy. 8vo. 1829.——*Craigie,* (Path. Anat. p. 604.) *ut supra.*——*Danzer,* Synopsis der Hautkrankheiten. 1808.——*Hutchison, C.* in Med. Chir. Tr. v. 278. and xiv. 213. on Erysipelas.——*Kieser,* über das Wesen und die Bedeutung der Exantheme. 1812.——*Lawrence, W.* in Med. Chir. Tr. xiv. 1. on Erysipelas.——*Lorry, A. C.* De Morbis Cutaneis Tractatus. 4to. 1777. ——*Marcus, A. F.* Die Exantheme ihre Esckenntriss und Heilart. 1812.——*Meckel,* (p. 472.) *ut supra.*——*Nasshard,* Skizze einer Dermatopathologie. 1816.——*Otto,* (p. 117.) *ut sup.*——*Plenck, J. J.* De Morb. Cur. &c. Edit. 2da, 8vo. 1783.—— *Plumbe, S.* on Diseases of the Skin. 8vo. 1824. 2nd edit. 1827.——*Rayer, P.* Traité Théor. et Prat. des Maladies de la Peau. 2 tom. 8vo. 1826–7. *tr.* by Dr. Willis. 8vo. 1835.——*Serre, M.* Nouveau Traitement Special d'Abortif de l'Inflam. de la Peau, du Tissu Cellulaire, &c. 8vo. 1837.——*Turner, D.* Treatise of Diseases incident to the Skin, &c. 8vo. 1723. and 4th Edit. 4to. 1731.——*Willan, R., M.D.* Description and Treatment of Cutaneous Diseases. 4to. 1798–1808.

Mucous Tissue.

Abercrombie, J., M.D. Path. and Pract. Researches on the Stomach, &c. 8vo. 1828.——*Bichat, X.* Traité des Membranes en général, &c. 8vo. 1802; *tr.* by J. Houlton. 8vo. 1821; and Anat. Gen. *supra cit.* (v. a. p. 139.)——*Billard, C.* De la Memb. Muquese gastro-intest. dans l'état sain et dans l'état inflam. 8vo. 1825.——*Bretonneau, P.* Rech. sur l'Inflam. spécial du Tissu Muqueuse. 8vo. 1826.——*Cabanis, P. J. G.* Observ. sur les Affections Catarrhales en général, 2de édit. 8vo. 1813.——*Craigie, D.* (Path. Anat. p. 667.) *sup. cit.;* and Practice of Physic, vol. i. (p. 727.) 8vo. 1836.——*Franc. ab Hildenbrand,* (Th.) De Catarrhis. 4to. 1812.——*Hastings, ut supra.*——*Hodgkin, F., M.D.* Lectures on the Mucous and Serous Membranes, vol. i. 8vo. 1837.——*Lejeune,* (Th.) Inflam. du Système Muqueux. 4to. 1806.——*Lelut,* in Répert. Gén. d'Anat. et de Phys. Path. iii. P. i. p. 145, sur le Muguet.——*Otto,* (p. 101.) *ut supra.*——*Meckel,* (p. 502, du Système Cutané Interne, état anormal) *ut supra.*

Serous Tissue.

Andral, (ii. 569, Maladies du Tissu Cellulaire et Membranes Séreuses,) *ut supra.*——*Belmas, D.* Récherches sur un moyen de déterminer des Inflam. adhésives dans les Cavités Séreuses. 8vo. 1831.——*Brodie, Sir B.* On the Joints, (ch. i. ii. iii., on Diseases of the Synovial Memb.; and ch. ix., on Inflam. of the Bursæ Mucosæ) 3rd edit. 8vo. 1834.——*Chomel, D. F* sur le Rheumatisme, 1813.——*Cloquet, J.* In Archiv. Gén. de Méd. sur les Ganglions.——*Craigie,* (Path. Anat. pp. 759, 807.) *ut supra.*——*Herwig, D.* De Morbis Bursarum Mucosarum. 4to. 1795.——*Koch,* De Morbis Bursarum Tendinum Mucosorum. 1790; and Untersuchung des natürl. Baues und der Krankheiten der Schleimbeutel. 8vo. 1795.——*Lahalle,* (Th.) sur l'Inflam. du Système Sereux. 8vo. 1802.——*Lorich.* De Signis Inflam. Memb. Serosarum. 4to. 1812.——*Meckel,* (i. 448., du Systeme Séreux, état anormal,) *ut supra.*——*Moffait,* Sur les Phlegmasies des Memb. Synov. des Articulations. 8vo. 1810.——*Otto,* (pp. 97, 373,) *ut supra.*——*Roche,* Phlegmasies du Syst. Fibro-séreux des Articulations. 4to. 1819.——*Sauveur De la Villeroye, J. T.* Essai sur les Inflam. du Système Séreux et du Système Synovial. 4to. 1812.——*Villerande, De la Fosse,* Dis. sur Rheumatisme. 1815.——*Zinc,* In Jour. Comp. du Dic. des Sc. Méd. xxi. 24. sur les Fungus des Memb. Séreuses.

Fibrous Tissue.

Craigie, (Path. Anat. pp. 505, 511.) *ut supra.*——*Crampton, P.* In Dubl. Hosp. Reports, i. 337, 397.—On Periostitis.——*Gotz, G.* De Morbis Ligamentorum, 4to.——*Huhn.* De rite cognoscenda et curanda System. Fibr. Inflam. 8vo. 1820.——*Meiselbach.* De Periostei Inflam. 8vo. 1824.—*Otto,* (pp. 233, 255.) *ut supra.*——*Rayer,* In Arch. Gén. de Méd. Mar. et Apr. 1823.

Osseous and Cartilaginous Tissue.

Bell, B. On the Diseases of Bones. 12mo. 1828.——*Boyer, M. Le Baron,* Lectures on the Diseases of Bones. *tr.* by Forrel, 2 vols. 8vo. 1804.——*Breschet, S.* (Th.) Sur la Formation du Cal. 4to. 1819.——*Brodie, ut supra.* and Med. Chir. Tr. XVII. 239.——*Charmeil,* De la Regen. des Os. 1821.——*Craigie,* (Path. Anat. p. 551.) *ut supra.*——*Cruveilhier,* In Arch. Gen. de Med. Feb. 1824. p. 161.——*Flormann,* De Inflam. Ossium. 1799.——*Goetz.* De Ostitide. 1822.——*Howship, I.* In Med. Chir. Tr. vi. 263. vii. 387–581. viii. 57. x. 176, 18; on the Morbid Appearances and Structure of Bones.——*Knox,* In Edinb. Med. and Surg. Journ. 1822, 1823.——*Koeler, G. L.*

Exper. circa Regenerationem Ossium. 8vo. 1786.——*Mayo, H.* In Med. Chir. Tr. vol. ii. 104, on Ulcer. of the Cartilages.——*Meckel,* (p. 327,) *ut supra.*——*Naumann, A. F.* De Ostitide. 4to. 1818.——*Otto,* (p. 145,) *ut supra.*——*Petit, J. L.* Traité des Maladies des Os, 2 tom. 8vo. 1723.—Le même, revu et augmenté, par Louis, 2 tom. 12mo. 1784.——*Sanson, J. L.* Exposé de la Doct. de Dupuytren, sur le Cal, in Journ. Univ. des Sc. Méd. xx. 131.——*Scarpa, A.* De Anatome et Pathologia Ossium. 4to. 1827.——*Scavini, J. M.* Observ. sur une Exostose particulière produite de cause externe, &c. 8vo. 1810.——*Schramm.* De Oss. Inflam. 1805.——*Syme, Jas.* On Necrosis. 8vo. 1823.——*Weidmann, J. P.* De Necrosi Ossium. fol. 1793.——*Wilson, J.* Lect. on the Bones, &c. 8vo. 1820.

Muscular Tissue.

Craigie, (Path. Anat. p. 493.) *ut supra.*——*Otto,* (pp. 250, 281.) *ut supra,* and in Selt. Beob. part II. 40.——*Plouquet,* De Myostitide et Nevritide. 1790.

Vascular Tissue.

Abernethy, J. Surg. and Phys. Essays, part II. 8vo. 1793-7.——*Alard.* De l'Inflam. des Vaisseaux Absorbens, &c. 2de édit. 8vo. 1824.——*Arnott, J. M.* In Med. Chir. Tr. xv. p. 1; a Pathological Enquiry into the Secondary Effects of Inflam. of the Veins.——*Breschet,* In Journ. Comp. du Dict. des Sc. Méd. ii. 325.——*Bright, Op. cit.* (*v. a.* p. 139.)——*Brodie, Sir B. C.* In Méd. Chir. Tr. viii. 195.——*Carmichael,* Observ. on Varix and Venous Inflam.——*Craigie,* (Path. Anat. p. 88, 128, 143.) *ut supra.*——*Fedeli, F.* De Lymphangiotide, &c. 8vo. 1825.——*Fricke,* Annalen des Hamburger Krankenhauses. 1826. *with plates.*——*Guthrie,* In Lond. Med. and Phys. Jour., July 1826.——*Hodgson, J.* On Diseases of the Arteries and Veins. 8vo. 1815.——*Lee, R., M.D.* In Cyc. of Pract. Med., *Art.* Veins; and Med. Chir. Tr. xv. 132, 369.——*Locatelli, B.* De Angiotide, &c. 1828.——*Longuet,* (Th.) Inflam. des Veines. 4to. 1815.——*Osiander,* Neue Denkwürdigkeiten, i. p. 57.——*Otto.* (p. 327, Arteritis; p. 345, Phlebitis; p. 358, Inflam. of Lymphatics,) *ut supra.*——*Ribes and Bouillaud,* In Rev. Méd. Fran. et Etrang. ii. 71, 448, and iii. Pt. iv. and vi.——*Sasse,* De Vasorum Sang. Inflam. 1797.——*Schmuck,* De Vasorum Sang. Inflam. 1793.——*Schwilgué,* In Bibl. Méd. xvi. 194; Hist. des Inflam. des Veines.——*Spangenberg,* In Horn's Archiv. für Med. Erfahrung. 1804. v. 269. Ueber die Entzundung der Arterien.——*Testa, A. J.* Delle Malattie del Cuosi, 3 vols. 8vo. 1826.——*Travers, B.* On Wounds and Ligatures of Veins, in Essays, by Cooper and Travers, part i. p. 227. 8vo. 1818.——*Velpeau,* In Arch. Gén. de Méd. Oct. 1824.

Nervous Tissue.

Abercrombie, J., M.D. Research. on the Dis. of the Brain and Spinal Cord. 8vo. and 2nd edit. 1829.——*Bayle, G. L.* Traité des Maladies du Cerveau, &c. 8vo. 1826.——*Craigie,* (pp. 281, 376,) *ut supra.*——*Graf.* De Myostitidis Nosographia. 4to. 1823. *Hooper, R., M.D.* The Morbid Anat. of the Human Brain. 4to. 1826.——*Klohss, K. L.* Diss. de Myostitide. 8vo. 1820.——*Lallemand, F.* Rech. Anat.-Path. sur l'Encephale, &c. 8vo. 1824-9.——*Mortinet, L.* Mém. sur l'Inflam. des Nerfs. 1824; and Rev. Méd. ii. 329, 354.——*Ollivier, C. P.* De la Moelle Epinière et de ses Maladies. 1824.——*Otto,* (pp. 407, 437, 452.) *ut supra.*——*Pinel, P.* in Journ. de Phys. i. 54. sur l'Inflam. de la Moelle Epinière.——*Rostan, L. N.* Rech. sur la Ramouillissement du Corveau. 8vo. 1820. and 2de édit. 8vo. 1823.——*Velpeau, M. A.* In Arch. Gén. de Med. vii. 52, 329, (1825.). Mém. sur une Altération de la Moelle allongée, &c.

PART IV.

CHAPTER I.

OF GUN-SHOT WOUNDS.

GUN-SHOT wounds may be said to be an effect of a modern improvement in offence and defence, unknown in the former mode of war, which is still practised where European improvements are not known; and it is curious to observe that fire-arms and spirits are the first of our refinements that are adopted in uncivilized countries; and, indeed, for ages they have been the only objects that have been at all noticed or sought after by rude nations. It was not till the fourteenth century that gunpowder was made, or rather compounded; but it was not till afterwards applied to the purpose of projecting bodies. But even now the wounds received in war are not all gun-shot wounds: some, therefore, are similar in many respects to those received in former times.

The knowledge of the effect of gunpowder, and its application to the art of war, or the projection of bodies for the destruction of men, has been in some degree accompanied by improvements in the arts and sciences in general, and among others that of surgery, in which art the healing of wounds so produced makes a material part. In France, more especially, the study of both were carried to considerable lengths; but though the art of destruction has been there improved and illustrated by writings, it is rather surprising that the art of healing should not have been equally illustrated in the same manner[a]. Little has been written on this subject, although perhaps, when we take every circumstance into consideration, it requires particular discussion; and what has been written is so superficial that it deserves but little attention. Practice, not precept, seemed to be the guide of all who studied in this

---

[a] [The illiberality of this sarcasm has been amply atoned for by the judicious Hennen, who, in his "Introductory Remarks" to Military Surgery, has not scrupled to assign the chief rank to the military surgeons of France, previous to the time of Hunter, at the same time that he pays a well-deserved compliment to the admirable "Memoirs of the French Academy of Surgery," which were published in 1743–57.—*Principles of Military Surgery, by John Hennen, M.D.*, p. 12.]

branch; and if we observe the practice hitherto pursued, we shall find it very confined, being hardly reduced to the common rules of surgery, and therefore it was hardly necessary for a man to be a surgeon to practise in the army.

§. 1. *The difference between Gun-shot Wounds and common Wounds.*

Gun-shot wounds are named, as is evident, from the manner in which they are produced; from the frequency of their happening in the time of battle to a set of men appropriated for war, both by sea and land: and from the appointment of particular surgeons for their cure, they have been considered apart from other wounds, and are now become almost a distinct branch of surgery.

Gun-shot wounds are made by the projection of hard obtuse bodies, the greatest number of which are musket-balls; for cannon-balls, pieces of shells and stones from ramparts in sieges, or splinters of wood, etc., when on board of a ship in an engagement at sea, can hardly have their effects ranked among gun-shot wounds; they will come in more properly with wounds in general. As the wounds themselves made by those very different modes will in general differ very considerably, any peculiarity that may be necessary in the treatment of gun-shot wounds from those made by cannon-balls, shells, etc., or even common wounds, will generally belong to those made by musket-balls.

The whole of gun-shot wounds will come within the definition of accidents. They are a recent violence committed on the body, but they often become the cause of, or degenerate into, a thousand complaints which are the objects of surgery or physic, many of which are common to accidents in general, and to many other diseases. Of this kind are abscesses, ulcerating bones, and fistulæ; but some are peculiar to gun-shot wounds, as calculi in the bladder from the ball entering that viscus, consumption from wounds in the lungs, which I believe rarely happens; for I cannot say I ever saw a case where such an effect took place. But it is the recent state in which they are distinguished, and in which they are to be considered as a distinct object of treatment.

Wounds of this kind vary from one another, which will happen according to circumstances: these variations will be in general according to the kind of body projected, the velocity of the body, with the nature and peculiarities of the parts injured. The kind of body projected, I have observed, is principally musket-balls, sometimes cannon-balls, sometimes pieces of broken shells, and very often, on board of ship, splinters of wood. Indeed, the effects of cannon-balls on different parts of the ship, either the containing parts, as the hull of the ship itself, or the contained, are the principal causes of wounds in the sailor; for a cannon-ball must go through the timbers of the ship before it can do more execution than simply as a ball, (which makes it a spent ball,) and which splinters the inside of the ship very considerably, and moves other bodies in the ship, neither of which it would do if moving with sufficient velocity; musket- or cannon-balls seldom doing immediate injury to those of that profession. The wounds produced by the three last bodies will be more like many common and violent accidents, attended with much contusion and laceration of parts.

Gun-shot wounds, from whatever cause, whether from a musket-ball, cannon-ball, shell, etc., are in general contused wounds, from which contusion there is most commonly a part of the solids surrounding the wound deadened, as the projecting body forced its way through these solids, which is afterwards thrown off in form of a slough, and which prevents such wounds from healing by the first intention, or by means of the adhesive inflammation, from which circumstance most of them must be allowed to suppurate. This does not always take place equally in every gun-shot wound, nor in every part of the same wound; and the difference commonly arises from the variety in the velocity of the body projected; for we find in many cases where the ball has passed with little velocity, which is often the case with balls even at their entrance, but most commonly at the part last wounded by the ball, that the wounds are often healed by the first intention.

Gun-shot wounds, from the circumstance of commonly having a part killed, in general do not inflame so readily as those from other accidents: this backwardness to inflame will be in the proportion that the quantity of deadened parts bears to the extent of the wound; from which circumstance the inflammation is later in coming on, more especially when a ball passes through a fleshy part with great velocity, because there will be a great deal deadened, in proportion to the size of the wound: therefore inflammation in gun-shot wounds is less than in wounds in general, where the same quantity of mischief has been done; and this also is in an inverse proportion to the quantity of the parts deadened, as I have already explained in my introduction to inflammation, viz. that inflammation is less where parts are to slough than where parts have been destroyed by other means. On the other hand, where the ball has fractured some bone, which fracture in the bone has done considerable mischief to the soft parts, independently of the ball, then there will be nearly as quick inflammation as in a compound fracture of the same bone, because the deadened part bears no proportion to the laceration or wound in general.

From this circumstance, of a part being often deadened, a gun-shot wound is often not completely understood at first; for it is at first, in many cases, impossible to know what parts are killed, whether bone, tendon, or soft part, till the deadened part has separated, which often makes it a much more complicated wound than at first was known or imagined; for it very often happens that some viscus, or a part of some viscus, or a part of a large artery, or even a bone, has been killed by the blow, which does not show itself till the slough comes away. If, for instance, it is a part of an intestine that has received a contusion so as to kill it, and which is to slough, a new symptom will most probably appear from the sloughs being separated, the contents of the intestine will most probably come through the wound, and probably the same thing will happen when any other containing viscus is in part deadened; but those cases will not be so dangerous as if the same loss had been produced at first, for by this time all communication will be cut off between the containing and contained parts: nor will it be so dangerous as when a considerable blood-vessel is deadened; for in this case, when the slough comes off, the blood, getting a free passage into the wound, as also out of it, probably death will immediately follow. If this artery is internal, nothing can be done; if in an extremity, the vessel may be either taken up, or probably amputation may be necessary to save the person's life; therefore an early attention should be paid to accidents where such an event is possible. In case of a bone being deadened an exfoliation takes place.

Gun-shot wounds are often such as do much mischief to vital parts, the effects of which will be according to the nature of the parts wounded and the violence of the wound; and also to parts, the soundness of which are essential either to the health of the whole, or to the uses of the parts wounded: such as some viscus, whose contents are voided through the opening or joints, the disposition of which is slow to heal, and whose uses are impeded when healed.

Gun-shot wounds often admit of being classed with the small and deep-seated wounds, which are always of a particular kind respecting the cure.

The variety of circumstances attending gun-shot wounds is almost endless: the following case may be given as an example.

An officer in the navy was wounded by a pistol-ball in the right side, about the last rib; it entered about five inches from the navel, and appeared on the inside of the skin about two inches from the spinal process, having passed in, I believe, among the abdominal muscles. The only remarkable thing that occurred was that the cellular membrane for some way about the passage of the ball was œdematous, and when I cut out the ball air came out with it.

§. 2. *Of the different Effects arising from the difference in the Velocity of the Ball.*

Many of the varieties between one gun-shot wound and another arise from the difference in the velocity of the body projected; and they are principally the following.

If the velocity of the ball is small, then the mischief is less in all of them, there is not so great a chance of their being compounded with fractures of the bones, &c.; but if the velocity is sufficient to break the bone it hits, the bone will be much more splintered than if the velocity had been very considerable, for where the velocity is very great, the ball as it were takes a piece out; however, all this will also vary according to the hardness of the bone. In a hard bone the splinters will be most frequent.

When the velocity is small, the direction of the wound produced by the ball will in common not be so straight, therefore its direction not so readily ascertained, arising from the easy turn of the ball.

When the velocity is small the deadened part or slough is always less; for with a small velocity a ball would seem only to divide parts, while when the velocity is great the contrary must happen. From this circumstance it is that the slough is larger at that orifice where the ball enters than where it comes out; and if the ball meets with a great deal of resistance in its passage through, there will very probably be no slough at all at its exit, which will be therefore only a lacerated wound.

The greater the velocity of the ball the cleaner it wounds the parts; so much so as almost to be similar to a cut with a sharp instrument, from which circumstance it might be imagined that there should be a smaller slough. But I suspect that a certain velocity given to the best cutting instrument would produce a slough on the cut edges of the divided parts; for the divided parts not giving way equally to the velocity of the dividing body, must of course be proportionally bruised.

Gun-shot wounds are attended with less bleeding than most others: however, some will be attended with this symptom more than others, even in the same part. This arises from the manner in which the wound is produced. Bleeding arises from a vessel being cut or broken; but the freedom of bleeding arises from the manner in which this is done;

if the artery is cut directly across, and it is done by a ball passing with a considerable velocity, it will bleed pretty freely; if bruised, and in some degree torn, then it will bleed less. When the velocity of the ball is small, the vessels will be principally torn, for they will have time to stretch before the continuity of their parts gives way; but if it is great they will bleed more freely, because velocity will make up for want of sharpness.

According to the velocity of the ball so is the direction. When the velocity is great, the direction of the ball will be in general more in a straight line than when it is small; for under such circumstances the ball more easily overcomes obstructions, and therefore passes on in its first direction.

Velocity in the ball makes parts less capable of healing than when it moves with a small velocity; therefore gun-shot wounds in pretty thick parts are in general later of healing at the orifice where the ball enters than at the orifice where it passes out, because it becomes in some degree a spent ball, the part having less slough, being only torn, which will often admit of being healed by the first intention.

In cases where the ball passes through, and in such a direction as to have one orifice more depending than the other, I have always found that the depending orifice healed soonest, and more certainly so if the ball came out that way, and also if the ball had been pretty much spent in its passage; therefore it will require art to keep the depending orifice open, if thought necessary. But this circumstance of its being a spent ball will not always happen; because if the person is near the gun when fired, the velocity of the ball will be very little diminished in its progress through the soft parts, and therefore it will have nearly the same velocity on both sides.

This fact of the lower orifice healing soonest is common to all wounds, and I believe is owing to the tumefaction which generally arises from the extravasated fluid always descending to the lower part; and being retarded at the lower orifice, it is as it were stopped there, and presses the sides of the wound together, obliging it to heal, if the parts have not been deadened. This is evidently the case after the introduction of the seton in the hydrocele, especially if the two orifices of the seton are at some distance; but in the hydrocele there is a more striking reason for it, for in this disease the extravasated fluids are wholly detained about the lower orifice, as there is no depending part for the fluid to descend to.

§. 3. *Of the different kinds of Gun-shot Wounds.*

Gun-shot wounds may be divided into the simple and the compound. Simple, when the ball passes into or through the soft parts only; the compound will be according to the other parts wounded.

The first species of compound are those attended with fractures of the bones, or with the wound of some large artery. The second species of compound wounds is, where the ball penetrates into some of the larger circumscribed cavities. This last, or penetrating wound, may be doubly complicated, or may be divided into two. First, simply penetrating; and, secondly, where some viscus or contained part, as the brain, lungs, heart, abdominal viscera, &c., is injured; all which cases will be taken notice of in their proper places.

CHAPTER II.

OF THE TREATMENT OF GUN-SHOT WOUNDS.

IT has been hitherto recommended, and universally practised by almost every surgeon, to enlarge immediately upon their being received, or as soon as possible, the external orifice of all gun-shot wounds made by musket-balls. So much has this practice been recommended, that they have made no discrimination between one gun-shot wound and another. This would appear to have arisen, and to be still continued, from an opinion that gun-shot wounds have a something peculiar to them, and of course are different from all other wounds, and that this peculiarity is removed by the opening. I own that I do not see any peculiarity. The most probable way of accounting for the first introduction of this practice is from the wound in general being small, and nearly of a size from one end to the other; also the frequency of extraneous bodies being forced into these wounds by the ball, or the ball itself remaining there; for the way in which these wounds are made is by the introduction of an extraneous body, which is left there, if it has not made its way through, so that the immediate cause of the wound makes a lodgement for itself, often carrying before it clothes, and even the parts of the body wounded, such as the skin, &c. From hence it would naturally appear at first view that there was an immediate necessity to search after those extraneous bodies, which very probably led the surgeon to do it; and in general the impossibility of finding them, and even of extracting them when found, without dilatation, gave the first idea of opening the mouths of the wounds. But from experience they altered this practice in part, and became not so desirous of searching after these extraneous bodies; for they found that it was oftener impossible to find them than could at first have been imagined, and when found, that it was not possible to extract them, and that afterwards these bodies were brought to the skin by the parts themselves, and those that could not be brought to the external surface in this way were such as gave little or no trouble afterwards, such as balls. Yet they altered this practice only so far as respected the attempt to extract extraneous bodies; for when they found from experience that it was not necessary nor possible to extract these immediately. yet they did not see that it therefore was not necessary to take the previous or leading steps towards it.

The circumstance I have mentioned of gun-shot wounds being contused obliges most of them to suppurate, because in such cases there is more or less of a slough to be thrown off, especially at the orifice made by the entrance of the ball: there is therefore a freer passage for the matter, or any other extraneous substance, than the same-sized wound would have if made by a clean cutting instrument, even if not allowed to heal by the first intention.

From all which, if there is no peculiarity in a gun-shot wound, I think this of dilating them, as a general practice, should be rejected at once; even if it were only for this reason, that few gun-shot wounds are alike, and therefore the same practice cannot apply to all.

This treatment of gun-shot wounds is diametrically opposite to a principle which is generally adopted in other cases, although not understood as a general rule, which is, that very few wounds of any kind require surgical treatment at their commencement, excepting with an opposite view from the above, viz. to heal them by the first intention. It is contrary to all the rules of surgery founded on our knowledge of the animal œconomy to enlarge wounds simply as wounds. No wound, let it be ever so small, should be made larger, excepting when preparatory to something else, which will imply a complicated wound, and which is to be treated accordingly; it should not be opened because it is a wound, but because there is something necessary to be done which cannot be executed unless the wound is enlarged. This is common surgery, and ought also to be military surgery respecting gun-shot wounds.

As a proof of the inutility of opening gun-shot wounds as a general practice, I shall mention the cases of four Frenchmen and a British soldier, wounded on the day of the landing of our army on the island of Belleisle; and as this neglect rather arose from accident than design, there is no merit claimed from the mode of treatment.

A. B. was wounded in the thigh by two balls: one went quite through, the other lodged somewhere in the thigh, and was not found while he was under our care.

B. C. was shot through the chest: he spit blood for some little time.

C. D. was shot through the joint of the knee: the ball entered at the outer edge of the patella, crossed the joint under that bone, and came out through the inner condyle of the os femoris.

D. E. was shot in the arm: the ball entered at the inside of the insertion of the deltoid muscle, passed towards the head of the os humeris, then between the scapula and ribs, and lodged between the basis of the scapula and spinal processes, and was afterwards extracted. The man's arm was extended horizontally when the ball entered, which accounts for this direction.

These four men had not anything done to their wounds for four days after receiving them, as they had hid themselves in a farm house all that time after we had taken possession of the island; and when they were brought to the hospital their wounds were only dressed superficially, and they all got well.

A grenadier of the 30th regiment was shot through the arm; the ball seemed to pass between the biceps muscle and the bone; he was taken prisoner by the French. The arm swelled considerably, they fomented it freely, and a superficial dressing only was applied. About a fortnight after the accident he made his escape, and came to our hospital; but by that time the swelling had quite subsided, and the wounds healed; there only remained a stiffness in the joint of the elbow, which went off by moving it.

§ 1. *Of the propriety of dilating Gun-Shot Wounds.*

It would be absurd for any one to suppose that there is never occasion to dilate gun-shot wounds at all; but it is certain there are very few in which it is necessary[a]. It will be impossible to determine by any general description what those are that ought to be opened, and what those are that ought not; that must be left in a great measure to the discretion of the surgeon, when once he is master of the arguments on both sides. Some general rules may be given with regard to the more simple cases; but with regard to the more complicated, the particular circumstances of each case are the only guide; and they must be treated according to the general principles of surgery.

Let us first give an idea of the wound that would appear to receive no benefit from being dilated; and first of the most simple wounds.

If a ball passes through a fleshy part where it can hurt no bone in its way, such as the thick of the thigh, I own, in such a simple wound, I see no reason for opening it; because I see no purpose that can be answered by it, except the shortening of the depth of the wound made by the ball, which can be productive of no benefit. If the ball does not pass through, and is not to be found, opening can be of as little service.

---

[a] [The practice of dilating gun-shot wounds was forcibly inculcated by Ambrose Paré and Wiseman, and afterwards, in 1792, by Baron Percy, who in his *Manuel de Chirurgien d'Armée*, says, " The first indication of cure is to change the nature of the wound as nearly as possible into an incised one." The judicious restriction of this practice to such cases as are pointed out in the concluding part of this section was fully borne out by the experience of our army surgeons during the late war.

If the opening in the skin should be objected to as being too small, and thereby forming an obstruction to the exit of the slough, etc., I think that in general it is not; for the skin is kept open by its own elasticity, as we see in all wounds: this elasticity muscles and many other parts have not; and in general the opening made by a ball is much larger than those made by pointed instruments; for I have already observed that there is often a piece of the skin carried in before the ball, especially if it passed with considerable velocity, besides the circular slough; so that there is really in such cases a greater loss of substance; therefore whatever matter or extraneous body there is, when it comes to the skin it will find a free passage out. Nor does the wound in the skin in general heal sooner than the bottom; and indeed in many cases not so soon, because the skin is generally the part that has suffered most.

However, this is not an absolute rule, for the skin sometimes heals first; but I have found this to be the case as often where openings had been made as in those where they had not; and this will depend upon circumstances or peculiarities; such as the bottom being at a considerable distance, with extraneous bodies, and having no disposition to heal, tending to a fistula; and I have observed in those cases, that the wound or opening made by the surgeon generally skinned to a small hole before the bottom of the wound was closed, which brings it to the state it would have been in, if it had not been dilated at all, especially if there are extraneous bodies still remaining; for an extraneous body causes and keeps up the secretion of matter, or rather keeps up the disease at the bottom of the wound, by which means the healing disposition of its mouth is in some degree destroyed.

Let me state a case of this last description. Suppose a wound made with a ball; that wound (from circumstances) is not to heal in six months, because the extraneous bodies, etc. cannot be extracted, or work out sooner, or some other circumstance prevents the cure in a shorter time: open that wound as freely as may be thought necessary, I will engage that it will be in a month's time in the same state with a similar wound that has not been opened, so that the whole advantage (if there is any) must be before it comes to this state; but it is very seldom that anything of consequence can be done in that time, because the extraneous bodies do not come out at first so readily as they do at last, for the inflammation and tumefaction, which extend beyond that very opening, generally keep them in; and if the wound is opened on their account at first, it ought to be continued to the very last. Upon the same principle, opening on account of extraneous bodies at first cannot be of so much service as opening some time after; for the suppuration, with its leading causes, viz. inflammation and sloughing, all along the passage of the ball, makes the passage itself much more determined and more easily followed; for the want of which few extraneous bodies are ever extracted at the beginning, excepting what are superficial, small, and loose.

If the extraneous bodies are broken bones, it seldom happens that they are entirely detached, and therefore must loosen before they can come away; also the bones in many cases are rendered dead, either by the blow or by being exposed, and must exfoliate, and this requires some time; for in gun-shot wounds, where bones are either bruised or broken, there is most commonly an exfoliation, because some part of the bone is deadened, similar to the slough in the soft parts.

A reason given for opening gun-shot wounds is, that it takes off the tension arising from the inflammation and gives the part liberty; this would be very good practice if tension or inflammation were not a consequence of wounds; or it would be very good practice, if they could prove that the effects from dilating a part that was already wounded were very different, or quite the reverse of those of the first wound; but as this [dilatation] must always be considered as an extension of the first mischief, we must suppose it to produce an increase of the effects arising from that mischief; therefore this practice is contradictory to common sense and common observation. They are principally the compound wounds that require surgical operations, and certain precautions are necessary with regard to them, which I shall here lay down.

As the dilatation of gun-shot wounds is a violence, it will be necessary to consider well what relief can be given to the parts or patient by such an operation; and whether without it more mischief would ensue; it should also be considered what is the proper time for dilating.

But it will be almost impossible to state what wound ought, and what ought not to be opened; this must always be determined by the surgeon, after he is acquainted with the true state of the case and the general principles; but from what has been already said, we may in some measure judge what those wounds are that should be opened, in order to produce either immediate relief, or to assist in the cure: we must have some other views than those objected to; we must see plainly something to be done for the relief of the patient by this opening, which cannot be procured without it, and if not procured, that the part cannot heal, or that the patient most probably must lose his life. The practice to be recommended here will be exactly similar to the common practice of surgery, without paying any attention to the cause as a gun-shot wound.

One of the principal points of practice will be to determine at what period of time the dilatation should be made.

1. If the wound should be a slight one, and should require opening.

it will be better to do it at the beginning before inflammation comes on; for the inflammation, in consequence of both, will be slight; but in slight cases dilatation will never be necessary, except to allow of the extraction of some extraneous body that is near. But if the wound is a considerable one, and it should appear upon consideration that you cannot relieve immediately any particular part or the constitution, then you can gain nothing by opening immediately, but will only increase the inflammation, and in some cases the inflammation arising from the accident and opening together may be too much for the patient: under this last circumstance it would be more advisable to wait till the first inflammation ceases, by which means the patient will stand a much better chance of a cure, if not of his life; therefore it is much better to divide the inflammations: however, it is possible that the inflammation may arise from some circumstance in the wound which could be removed by opening it; for instance, a ball or broken bone pressing upon some part, whose actions are either essential to the life of the part or the whole, as some large artery, nerve, or vital part; in such the case will determine for itself. On the other hand, it may in many cases be better to remove the whole by an operation, when in such parts as will admit of it, which will be taken notice of.

2. If an artery is wounded, where the patient is likely to become either too weak, or to lose his life from the loss of blood, then certainly the vessel is to be tied, and most probably this cannot be done without previously opening the external parts, and often freely.

3. In a wound of the head where there is reason to suspect a fracture of the skull, it is necessary to open the scalp, as in any other common injury done to the head where there was reason to suspect a fracture; and when opened, if a fracture is found, it is to be treated as any other fractured skull[a].

4. Where there are fractured bones in any part of the body, which can be immediately extracted with advantage, and which would do much mischief if left, this becomes a compound fracture wherever it is, and it makes no difference in the treatment whether the wound in the skin was made by a ball or the bone itself, at least where the compound fracture is allowed to suppurate; for there is often a possibility of treating a compound fracture as a simple one, which gun-shot fractures, if I may be allowed the expression, seldom will allow of; but where the compound fracture must suppurate, there they are very similar. However, there have been instances where a fracture of the thigh-bone made by a ball has healed in the same way as a compound fracture by other means.

---

[a] [See Vol. I. p. 496, *note.*]

5. Where there is some extraneous body which can with very little trouble be extracted, and where the mischief by delay will probably be greater than that arising from the dilatation.

6. Where some internal part is misplaced, which can be replaced immediately in its former position, such as in wounds in the belly, where some of the viscera are protruded, and it becomes necessary to perform the operation of gastroraphia; which is to be done in this case in the same manner as if the accident arose from any other cause; but the treatment should be different, for gun-shot cases cannot heal by the first intention, on account of the slough that is to ensue.

7. When some vital part is pressed, so that its functions are lost or much impaired, such as will often happen from fractures of the skull, fractures of the ribs, sternum, etc., in short, when anything can be done to the part after the opening is made for the present relief of the patient, or the future good arising from it. If none of these circumstances has happened, then I think we should be very quiet. Balls that enter any of the larger cavities, such as the abdomen or thorax, need not have their wounds dilated, except something else is necessary to be done to the contained parts, for it is impossible to follow the ball; therefore they are commonly not opened, and yet we find them do very well.

Balls that enter any part where they cannot be followed, such as into the bones of the face, need not have the wound in the skin in the least enlarged, as it can give no assistance to the other part of the wound, which is a bony canal. The following cases are strongly in proof of this, being respectively instances of both modes of practice.

I was sent for to an officer who was wounded in the cheek by a ball, and who had all the symptoms of an injured brain; upon examining the parts, I found that the ball had passed directly backwards through the cheek-bone; therefore, from the symptoms and from the direction of the wound, I suspected that the ball had gone through the basis of the skull into the brain, or at least had produced a depression of the skull there. I enlarged the external wound, and with my fingers could feel the coronoid process of the lower jaw; I found that the ball had not entered the skull, but had struck against it about the temporal process of the sphenoid bone, which it had broke, and afterwards passed down on the inside of the lower jaw. With a pair of small forceps I extracted all I could of the loose pieces of bone: he soon recovered from his stupor, and also from his wound. The ball afterwards caused an inflammation at the angle of the lower jaw, and was extracted. The good which I proposed by opening and searching for extraneous bodies and loose pieces of bone was the relieving of the brain; but as the ball had not entered the skull, and as none of the bones had been driven into the brain, it is most probable that I did no good by my opening; but that I could not foresee.

An officer received a wound by a ball in the cheek (which in this case was on the opposite side); the wound led backwards, as in the other; by putting my finger into the wound I felt the coronoid process of the lower jaw, as in the former; but he had no symptoms of an injured brain; I therefore advised not to open it, because the reason for opening in the preceding case did not exist here; my advice was complied with, and the wound did well, and rather better than the former, by healing sooner. The ball was never found, so far as I know.

The present practice is not to regard the balls themselves, and seldom or ever to dilate upon their account, nor even to search much after them when the wound is dilated, which shows that opening is not necessary, or at least not made upon account of extraneous bodies. This practice has arisen from experience; for it was found that balls, when obliged to be left, seldom or ever did any harm when at rest, and when not in a vital part; for balls have been known to lie in the body for years, and are often never found at all, and yet the person has found no inconvenience. This knowledge of the want of power in balls to promote inflammation when left in the body, arose from the difficulty of finding them, or extracting them when found, and therefore in many cases they were obliged to leave them.

One reason for not readily finding the ball at first is, because the parts are only torn and divided, without any loss of substance (till the slough comes off), by which means the parts collapse and fall into their places again, which makes it difficult to pass anything in the direction of the ball, or even to know its direction. The different courses they take, by being turned aside by some resisting body, add also to the difficulty, as will be explained.

But the course of a ball, if not perpendicular, but passing obliquely and not very deep a little way under the skin, probably an inch or more, is easy to be traced through its whole course, for the skin over the whole passage of the ball generally is marked by a reddish line. I have seen this redness, even when the ball has gone pretty deep; it has none of the appearances of inflammation, nor of extravasation, for extravasation is of a darker colour, and what it is owing to I have not been able to discover. I can conceive it to be something similar to a blush, only the small vessels allowing the red particles of the blood to flow more easily.

§. 2. *Of the strange Course of some Balls.*

The difficulty of finding balls, I have just observed, often arises from the irregular course they take. The regularity of the passage of a ball will in general be in proportion to its velocity and want of resistance, for balls are turned aside in an inverse proportion to the force that they come with, and this is the reason why we seldom find them take a straight course; for if they are spent balls, the soft parts alone are capable of turning them; and if they come with a considerable velocity it is a chance they may hit some bone obliquely, and then they are also turned aside, for any body that gives a ball the least oblique resistance throws it out of its direct course; therefore the balls that do not pass through and through (which are the only ones that are searched after), will be in general spent ones, excepting those that come directly against some considerable bone, as the thigh-bone, etc. As a proof that balls are easily thrown off obliquely, we often find that a ball shall enter the skin of the breast obliquely, and afterwards shall pass almost round the whole body under the skin. The skin here is strong enough to stop the ball coming out again, so that it turns it inwards, which, meeting with the ribs, it is again turned out against the skin, and so on alternately as long as it has force to go on; however, in many cases the ball goes a little way after it has passed through the skin, and when it meets with any hard body on that side next the centre of the body, such as a rib, its course is directed outwards, and it pierces the skin a second time; but the velocity of such balls must have been considerable.

I have seen a ball pass in at one side of the shin-bone, and run across it under the skin, without either cutting the skin across or hurting the bone, which shows that the velocity could not be great; for we know that there is not sufficient room between these two parts in a natural state for a ball to pass; but the ball, after it had got under the skin, where there was room for it to cover itself, then came against the tibia, which threw it outwards, and the skin counteracting, it only raised the skin from the tibia, and passed on between them; but if this ball had had a sufficient velocity it would have either cut the skin across, or taken a piece out of the bone, or most probably both.

Another circumstance in favour of the uncertainty of their direction is, that the parts wounded are often not in the same position that they were when they received the ball. The French soldier who was wounded in the arm was a striking instance of this. The ball entered the arm about its middle on the inside of the biceps muscle, and it was extracted from between the two scapulæ, close on one side of the spinal process of the back-bone. The reason of this strange course I have already observed in the case, was owing to his having had his arm stretched out horizontally at the time he was wounded, and the ball passed on in a straight line.

These uncertainties in the direction of the balls above mentioned have made the common bullet-forceps almost useless; yet forceps are not to be entirely thrown aside, for it will often happen that a ball will be found to lie pretty near the external wound, which, if the ball was removed, would probably heal by the first intention; for in such superficial wounds they must have passed with little velocity; or if there was a part killed, it would heal immediately; but if there is a slough, the extraction is best done after all inflammation, and the separation of the slough is over, for then the passage of the ball is better ascertained, in consequence of the surrounding adhesive inflammation; and moreover, the granulations are beginning to push the extraneous body towards the surface; but the operation of ulceration, which brings it to the skin, being often too slow, the ball, etc. had better be extracted, and even the part might be dilated. However, I would be very cautious how far I carried this practice, and only do it when all circumstances favoured.

For the same reasons probes are become of little use; indeed, I think that they should never be used but by way of satisfaction, in knowing sometimes what mischief is done; we can perhaps feel if a bone is touched, or if a ball is near, etc., but when all this is known it is a hundred to one if we can vary our practice in consequence of it. If the wound will admit of it, the finger is the best instrument.

In cases where the ball passes a considerable way under the skin, and near to it, I think it would be advisable to make an opening midway between the two orifices which were made by the ball (especially when the orifices are at a very great distance), that fractured bones, or extraneous bodies may now or hereafter be better extracted; for if this is not done we have often an abscess forming between them, which indeed answers the same purpose, and often better; but sometimes it should not be delayed for such an event to take place.

Where the ball has passed immediately under the skin, as in the case where the ball passed between the skin and tibia, it will be often proper to open the whole length of the passage of the ball, the necessity of which I think arises from the skin not so readily uniting with the parts underneath, as muscles do with one another.

Although we have given up in a great measure the practice of searching after a ball, broken bones, or any other extraneous bodies, yet it often happens that a ball shall pass on till it comes in contact with the skin of some other part, and where it can be readily felt; the question is, should such a ball be cut out? If the skin is bruised by the ball coming against it, so that we may imagine that this part will slough off, in that case I see nothing to hinder opening it, because the part is dead; therefore no more inflammation can arise from the opening than otherwise would take place upon allowing the slough to be thrown off; while, on the other hand, I should also suppose as little good to arise from it, because the ball will come out of itself when the part sloughs off; however, it may be suspected that before the slough falls off the ball may so alter its situation that it will be impossible to extract it by that opening; however, I should very much doubt the ball altering its course under such circumstances, for if the skin was so much bruised as to slough, inflammation would soon come on, and confine the ball to that place; however, it always gives comfort to the patient to have the ball extracted. But if the ball is only to be felt, and the skin quite sound, I would in that case advise letting it alone, till the wound made by the entrance of the ball had inflamed and was suppurating; my reasons for it are these:

First, we find that most wounds get well when the ball is left in, (excepting it has done other mischief than simply passing through the soft parts,) and that very little inflammation attends the wound where the ball lodges, only that where it enters; the inflammation not arising so much from the injury done by the ball as from the parts being there exposed to the suppurative inflammation, if it is immediately removed. There is always a greater chance of a slough where the ball enters than where it rests, arising from the greater velocity of the ball; for beyond where the slough is the parts unite by the first intention.

Secondly, in those cases where the ball passes through and through we have two inflammations, one at each orifice, instead of the one at the entrance; or a continued inflammation through and through, if the ball has passed with great velocity. Where the ball makes its exit, the inflammation passes further along the passage of the ball than when the wound has been healed up to the ball, and then cut out afterwards; so that by opening immediately the irritation will be extended further, and of course the disposition for healing will be prevented.

If this is the case, I think that two wounds should not be made at the same time; and what convinces me more of it is, that I have seen cases where the balls were not found at first, nor even till after the patients had got well of their wounds; and these balls were found very near the skin. They gave no trouble (or else they would have been found sooner); no inflammation came upon the parts, and they were afterwards extracted and did well. Again, I have seen cases where the balls were found at first and cut out immediately, which were similar to balls passing through and through; and in these the same inflammation came on the cut wounds that came on the wounds made by the entrance of the ball.

§. 3. *Penetrating Wounds of the Abdomen.*

Wounds leading into the different cavities of the body are very common in the army, and in a great measure peculiar to war. They are mostly gun-shot wounds, but not always, some being made with sharp-pointed weapons, as swords, bayonets, &c.; they are pretty similar, in whatever way they are made, and I have given them a name expressive of the nature of the wound. I shall not take notice of any of this kind but those which penetrate into the larger cavities, as the abdomen, thorax, and skull; but those into the skull are made most commonly by balls, shells, &c.

These wounds become more or less dangerous according to the mischief done to the contents of the cavity into which they penetrate.

These wounds may be distinguished according as they are simply penetrating, without extending to the contained parts, or as they affect these parts, and the event of these two kinds of wounds is very different; for in the first little danger is to be expected if properly treated, but in the second the success will be very uncertain, for very often nothing can be done for the patient under such wounds, and very often a good deal of art can be made use of with advantage.

Wounds of the parietes of the abdomen, not immediately inflicted on such a viscus as has the power of containing other matter, will in general do well, let the instrument that made the wound be what it will*. There will be a great difference, however, should that instrument be a ball passing with great velocity, for in this case a slough will be produced; but if it should pass with little velocity, then there will be less sloughing, and the parts will in some degree heal by the first intention, similar to those made by a cutting instrument. But although the ball has passed with such velocity as to produce a slough, yet that wound shall do well, for the adhesive inflammation will take place on the peritoneum all round the wound, which will exclude the general cavity from taking part in the inflammation, although the ball has not only penetrated but has wounded parts which are not immediately essential to life, such as the epiploon, mesentery, &c., and perhaps gone quite through

* What I mean by a containing viscus is a viscus that contanis some foreign matter, as the stomach, bladder, ureters, gall-bladder, &c., to which I may add blood-vessels.

the body; yet it is to be observed that wherever there is a wound, and whatever solid viscus may be penetrated, the surfaces in contact, surrounding every orifice, will unite by the adhesive inflammation, so as to exclude entirely the general cavity, by which means there is one continued canal wherever the ball or instrument has passed; or if any extraneous body should have been carried in, such as clothes, &c., they will also be included in these adhesions, and both these and the slough will be conducted to the external surface by either orifice.

All wounds that enter the belly, which have injured some viscus, are to be treated according to the nature of the wounded part, with its complications, which will be many, because the belly contains more parts of very dissimilar uses than any other cavity in the body, each of which will produce symptoms peculiar to itself and the nature of the wound.

The wounding of the several viscera will often produce what may be called immediate and secondary symptoms, which will be peculiar to themselves, besides what are common to simple wounds, such as bleeding, which is immediate, and inflammation and suppuration, which are secondary. Sensations alone will often lead to the viscus wounded, and this is frequently one of the first symptoms.

The immediate symptoms arising from wounds in the different viscera are as follows:

From a wound in the liver there will be pain in the part of the sickly or depressing kind; and if it is in the right lobe, there will be a delusive pain in the right shoulder, or in the left shoulder from a wound in the left lobe.

A wound in the stomach will produce great sickness and vomiting of blood, and sometimes a delirium; a case of which I once saw in a soldier in Portugal, who was stabbed into the stomach with a stiletto by a Portuguese.

Blood in the stools will arise from a wound in the intestines, and according to the intestine wounded it will be more or less pure. If the blood is from a high part of an intestine, it will be mixed with fæces and of a dark colour; if low, as the colon, the blood will be less mixed and give the tinge of blood; and the pain or sensation will be more or less acute according to the intestine wounded: more of the sickly pain the higher the intestine, and more of the acute the lower.

There will be bloody urine from a wound in the kidneys or bladder; and if made by shot or ball, and a lodgement made, these bodies will sometimes become the cause of a stone. The sensation will be trifling.

A wound of the spleen will produce no symptoms that I know of, excepting probably sickness, from its connection with the nerves belonging to the stomach, &c.

Extravasations of blood into the cavity of the abdomen will take place more or less in all penetrating wounds, and more especially if some viscus is wounded, as they are all extremely vascular; and this will prove dangerous or not, according to the quantity.

These are the immediate and general symptoms upon such parts being wounded; but other symptoms may arise, in consequence of some of those viscera being wounded, which require particular attention. There may be wounds of the liver and spleen which produce no symptoms but what are immediate, and may soon take on the healing disposition; but wounds in those viscera which contain extraneous matter, such as the stomach, intestines, kidneys, ureters, and bladder may produce secondary symptoms of a distinctive kind. If the injury is done by a ball to any of those viscera, the effect may be of two kinds: one where it makes a wound, as stated above, the other where it only produces death in a part of any of them; these will produce very different effects. The first will most probably be always dangerous: the second will hardly ever be so. The first is where the ball has wounded some one of the above-mentioned viscera in such a manner as not to produce the symptoms already described, but one common to them all, viz. their contents or extraneous matter immediately escaping into the cavity of the abdomen. Such cases will seldom or ever do well, as their effect will hinder the above-mentioned adhesions taking place; the consequence of which will be that universal inflammation on the peritoneum will take place, attended with great pain, tension, and death. But all this will be in proportion to the quantity of wound in the part, and quantity of contents capable of escaping into the cavity of the abdomen; for if the wound is small, and the bowels not full, then adhesions may take place all round the wound, which will confine the contained matter, and make it go on in its right channel. These adhesions may take place very early, as the following case shows.

The case of an officer who died of a wound which he received in a duel.

On Thursday morning, the 4th of September, 1783, about seven o'clock, an officer fought a duel in the Ring in Hyde-park, in which he exchanged three shots with his antagonist, whose last shot struck him on the right side, just below the last rib, and appeared under the skin on the opposite side, exactly in the corresponding place, and was immediately cut out by Mr. Grant.

About three hours after receiving this wound, I saw him with Mr. Grant. He was pretty quiet, not in much pain, rather low, pulse not quick nor full, and a sleepy languidness in the eye, which made me suspect something more than a common wound. He then had neither had a stool nor made water, and therefore it could not be said what viscera might be wounded. His belly had been fomented, a clyster of warm water was ordered, and a draught with confec. card. as a cordial, with twenty drops of laudanum, to procure sleep, as he wished to have some. We saw him again at three o'clock: the draught had come up. Had no stool from the clyster, nor any sleep; had made water, and no blood being found in it, we conjectured that the kidneys, &c. were not hurt. He was now rather lower, pulse smaller, more restless, a good deal of tension in the belly, which made him uneasy, and made him wish to have a stool. It was at first imagined that this tension might be owing to extravasated blood; but on patting the belly, especially along the course of the transverse arch of the colon, it plainly gave the sound and vibration of air; therefore we wished to procure a motion, to see if we could not by that means have some of that air expelled. We wished also to repeat the cordial and the opium, but the stomach was become now too irritable to retain anything, and was at times vomiting, independently of anything he took: a clyster was given, but nothing returned or came away. We saw him again at nine o'clock in the evening. His pulse was now low and more frequent, coldness at times, vomiting very frequent, which appeared to be chiefly bile, with small bits of something that was of some consistence; the belly very tense, which made him extremely uneasy; no stool. From nothing passing downwards, and the colon continuing to fill, we began to suspect that it was becoming paralytic, probably from the ball having divided some of its nerves.

Fumes of tobacco by clyster were proposed, but we were loath to use it too hastily, as it would tend to increase the disease, if it did not relieve; however, we were prepared for it.

Mr. Grant stayed with him the whole night; all the above symptoms continued increasing, and about seven o'clock in the morning he died, viz. about twenty-four hours after receiving the wound.

He was opened next day at ten o'clock, twenty-seven hours after death, when we found the body considerably putrid, although the weather was cold for the season, the blood having transuded all over the face, neck, shoulders and breast, with a bloody fluid coming out of his mouth, with an offensive smell: below this the body was not so far gone.

On opening the abdomen a good deal of putrid air rushed out; then we observed a good deal of fluid blood, principally on each side of the abdomen, with some coagulum upon the intestines; when sponged up it might be about a quart.

The small intestines were slightly inflamed in many places, and there adhered. We immediately searched for the passage of the ball.

On searching for the course of the ball we found that it had passed directly in, pierced the peritoneum, entered again the peritoneum where it attaches the colon to the loins, passed behind the ascending colon, and just appeared at the right side of the root of the mesentery where the colon is attached; passed behind the root of the mesentery, and entered the lower turn of the duodenum as it crosses the spine; then passed out of that gut on the left of the mesentery, and in its course to the left side it went through the jejunum, about a foot from its beginning; then through between two folds of the lower part of the jejunum, taking a piece out of each; then passed before the descending part of the colon, and pierced the peritoneum of the left side, as also some of the muscles, but not the skin, and was immediately cut out exactly in the same place on the left where it entered at the right; so it must have passed perfectly in a horizontal direction.

There was no appearance of extravasation of any of the contents of the intestines loose in the cavity of the abdomen. The intestines in many places were adhering to one another, especially near to the wounds, which adhesions were recent, and of course very slight; yet they showed a ready disposition for union to prevent the secondary symptoms or what may be called the consequent, which would also have proved fatal.

There was little or no fluid in the small intestines, but there was a good deal of substance in consistence like fæces, in broken pieces about the size of a nut, through the whole track of the intestine, even in the stomach, which he vomited up; but in the upper end of the jejunum, as also in the duodenum, there was some fluid mixed with the other; but that fluid seemed to be rather bile. If this solid part was excrement, then the valve of the colon must not have done its duty. Was all the thin part absorbed to hinder extravasation into the belly? or was it all brought back into the stomach to be vomited up? There was a good deal of air in the ascending, but more especially in the transverse turn of the colon.

This case admits of several observations and queries.

First, the lowness and gradual sinking, with the vomiting without blood, bespoke wounded intestines, and those pretty high up. It shows how ready Nature is to secure all unnatural passages, according to the necessity.

Query, what could be the cause of his having no stool, even from the clyster? Were the intestines inclinable to be quiet under such circumstances? Would he not have lived if the immediate mischief had not been too much? I think that if the immediate cause of death had not been so violent, Nature would have secured the parts from the secondary, viz. the extravasation of the fæces.

What is the best practice where it is supposed an intestine may be wounded? I should suppose the very best practice would be to be quiet and do nothing, except bleeding, which in cases of wounded intestines is seldom necessary.

As he was extremely thirsty, and could not retain anything in his stomach, which, if he could, would probably have been productive of mischief, by giving a greater chance of extravasation; would not the tepid bath have been of service, to have allowed of fluids to enter the constitution?

It is very possible that a wound of the gall-bladder, but more readily of the ductus communis, and also of the pancreatic duct, will produce the same effects, although not so quickly; and it may be observed, that a wound in them could not be benefited by any adhesions that could take place, because the secreted fluids could never, most probably, get into the right channel again, and would therefore be the cause of keeping the external wound open to discharge the contents, as we find to be the case in the disease called fistula lachrymalis, as also when the duct of the parotid gland is divided.

Wounds of parts that have been only deadened will be very similar to the above-stated penetrating wounds, but they will differ from them in effects, arising from a slough separating from a containing viscus; for whenever the slough comes away the extraneous or contained matter of that viscus will escape by the wound, such as the contents of the stomach, intestines, ureters, bladder, etc., the two last of which will be similar; or the slough may escape by either of these outlets; whereas in the former kind of wounds any of the contents that could possibly escape would immediately pass into the cavity of the abdomen. The periods of these symptoms appearing after the accident will be according to the time of separation, which may be in eight, ten, twelve, or fourteen days.

These new symptoms, although in general very disagreeable, will not be dangerous*, for all the danger is over before they can appear; but that the orifice should afterwards continue, and become either an artificial anus or urethra, is a thing to be avoided; though they commonly close up, and the contents are directed the right way: in such cases nothing is to be done but dressing the wound superficially, and when the contents of the wounded viscus become less, we may hope for a cure.

The following case explains the foregoing remarks:

A young gentleman was shot through the body. The musket was loaded with three balls, but there were only two orifices where they entered, and also only two where they came out, one of the balls having followed one of the others; that there were three that went through him

* How far the contents of the stomach escaping through a wound might not be attended with bad consequences I cannot pretend to say.

was evident, for they afterwards made three holes in the wainscot behind him, but two very near one another[a].

The balls entered upon the left side of the navel, one a little further out than the other, and they came out behind, pretty near the spinal processes, about the superior vertebræ of the loins. From the closeness of the gun to the man when fired, which of course made its contents pass with great velocity, as also from the direction of the innermost ball, which we supposed to be the double one, we were pretty certain that it had penetrated the cavity of the abdomen, but could not be so certain of the course of the other.

The first water he made after the accident was bloody, from which we knew the kidney was wounded; but that symptom soon left him. He had no blood in his stools, from which we concluded that none of the intestines were wounded; and no symptoms of extravasation of the contents of any viscus taking place, such as the symptoms of inflammation of the peritoneum, we were still more confirmed in our opinion.

The symptomatic fever did not run higher than could have been expected, nor was there more pain in the track of the ball than might be imagined.

These consequent symptoms of the immediate injury abated as soon as could be expected, and in less than a fortnight I pronounced him out of danger from the wound; for no immediate secondary symptoms having taken place, I concluded that whatever cavities the balls had entered, there the surrounding parts had adhered, so that the passage of the ball was by this means become a complete canal; and therefore, that neither any extraneous bodies that had been carried in with the balls, and had not been carried through, nor any slough that might separate from the sides of the canal, nor the matter formed in it, could now get into the cavity of the abdomen, but must be conducted to the external surface of the body, either through the wounds, or from an abscess forming for itself, which would work its own exit somewhere.

But this conclusion was supposed to be too hasty, and soon after a new symptom arose, which alarmed those who did not see the propriety of my reasoning; which was some fæces coming through the wound: this new symptom did not alter my opinion respecting the whole operations of Nature to secure the cavity of the abdomen, but it confirmed it (if a further confirmation had been necessary), and therefore I conceived it could not affect life; but as I saw the possibility of this wound becoming an artificial anus, I was sorry for it. It was not difficult to

---

[a] [Balls impinging on a sharp edge of bone have sometimes been known to be cut in two, and to take different courses in the body.]

account for the cause of this new symptom; it was plain that an intestine (the descending part of the colon most probably,) had only received a bruise from the ball, but sufficient to kill it at this part, and till the separation of the slough had taken place, both the intestine and canal were still complete, and therefore did not communicate with each other; but when the slough was thrown off, the two were laid into one at this part, therefore the contents of the intestine got into the wound, and the matter from the wound might have got into the intestine. However, this symptom gradually decreased, by (we may suppose) the gradual contraction of this opening, and an entire stop to the course of the fæces took place, and the wounds healed very kindly up.

But the inflammation, the sympathetic fever, the reducing treatment, and the spare regimen all tended to weaken him very much.

§. 4. *Of penetrating Wounds in the Chest.*

Little notice has been taken of wounds in the chest and lungs; indeed it would appear at first that little or nothing could be done; yet in many cases a great deal may be done for the good of the patient.

It is possible a wound in the chest may be of the first kind, viz. only penetrating, yet from circumstances may prove fatal, as will be explained in the second or complicated, viz. a wound of the lungs.

It is pretty well known that wounds of the lungs (abstracted from other mischief,) are not mortal. I have seen several cases where the patient has got well after being shot quite through the body and lungs, while from a very small wound made by a sword or bayonet into the lungs the patients have died, from which I should readily suppose that a wound in the lungs from a ball would in general do better than a wound in the same part with a pointed instrument; and this difference in effects would appear in many cases to arise from the difference in the quantity of blood extravasated, because the bleeding from a ball is very inconsiderable in comparison to that from a cut, and there is therefore a less chance of extravasated blood, either into the cavity of the thorax or into the cells of the lungs: another circumstance that favours gun-shot wounds in these parts is, that they seldom heal up externally by the first intention, on account of the slough, especially at the wound made by the entrance of the ball, so that the external wound remains open for a considerable time, by which means any extravasated matter may escape; but even this has often its disadvantages, for by keeping open the external wound, which leads into the cavity, we give a chance to produce the suppurative inflammation through the whole surface of that cavity, which most probably would prove fatal, and which would be equally so if no viscus was wounded; but it would appear that the cavity of the thorax does not so readily fall into this inflammation from a gun-shot wound as we should at first imagine; nor can we suppose that the adhesive inflammation readily takes place between the lungs and pleura round the orifice, as we described in the wounds of the abdomen, because these parts are not under the same circumstances that other contained and containing parts are; for in every other case the contained and containing have the same degree of flexibility or proportion in size. The brain and the skull have not the same flexibility, but they bear the same proportion in size. The lungs immediately collapse when either wounded themselves or when a wound is made into the chest, and, from this circumstance, are not allowed to heal by the first intention, but become by much too small for the cavity of the thorax, which space must be filled either with air or blood, or both, so that adhesion cannot readily take place: but it very often happens that the lungs have previously adhered, which will frequently be an advantage.

In the cases of stabs, especially if with a sharp instrument, the vessels will bleed freely, but the external wound will collapse, and cut off all external communication. If the lungs are wounded in the same manner, we must expect a considerable bleeding from them, and this bleeding will be into the general cavity of the thorax (if the lungs at this part have not previously adhered there), and likewise into the cells of the lungs or bronchiæ, which will be known by producing a cough, and in consequence of it a bleeding at the mouth; for the blood that is extravasated into the air-cells of the lungs will be coughed up by the trachea, and by that means will become a certain symptom of the lungs being wounded; but that which gets into the cavity of the thorax cannot escape, and therefore must remain till the absorbents take it up; which they will do if it is only in small quantity; but if in large quantity this extravasated blood will produce symptoms of another kind.

The symptoms of these accidents are: first, a great lowness, which proceeds from the nature of the parts wounded, and perhaps a fainting from the quantity of blood lost to the circulation; but this will be in proportion to the quantity and quickness with which it was lost. A load in the breast will be felt, but more from a sensation of this kind than from any real weight; and a considerable difficulty in breathing. This difficulty in breathing will arise from the pain the patient will have in expanding the lungs in inspiration, and will also proceed from the muscles of respiration of that side being wounded, and this will continue for some time from the succeeding inflammation: it will hinder the expansion of the thorax on that side, and of course in some degree of the other side, as we have not the power of raising one side without raising the other*; and if wounded by a cutting instrument, the lungs of that side not being able to expand fully, by the cavity of the thorax being in part filled with blood, will also give the symptoms of difficulty of breathing. The patient will not be able to lie down, but must sit upright, that the position may allow of the descent of the diaphragm, to give room in the chest; all which symptoms were strongly marked in the following case.

A person received a stab behind the left breast with a small sword; the wound in the skin was very small. He was almost immediately seized with a considerable discharge of blood from the lungs to near a quart, by the mouth, which showed that the lungs were considerably wounded, for from the situation of the external wound we were sure that the stomach could not be injured. His breathing soon became difficult and painful, and his pulse quick; he was bled; these symptoms increased so fast that every one thought him dying. He could only lie on his back; for if he lay on the sound side, he could not breathe in the least, and the pain would not let him lie on the unsound side; the easiest position was an erect posture, which obliged him to sit in a chair for several days; when he coughed he was in great pain; he very seldom spat with the cough, and never discharged any blood after the second day, by which we supposed that the bleeding was stopped in the lungs.

While the parts were in a state of inflammation he was in great pain, his breathing excessively quick, and his pulse hard and extremely quick; but as the inflammation went off, he drew his breath in longer strokes, his pain became less, and his pulse not so quick nor so hard; but this last circumstance varied as he moved his body, coughed, or put himself into a passion, which he often did.

I suspected from both the wound and its effects that there was a good deal of extravasated blood in the cavity of the thorax; for I considered that the blood which got out of the vessels of the lungs into the wound in the lungs would find a readier passage into the cavity of the thorax than into the cells of the lungs; and indeed every attempt to dilate the thorax would rather act as a sucker upon the mouth of the wound in the lungs, as the pressure of the external air was taken off by that means; I proposed the operation for the empyema, because the extravasated blood must compress the lungs of that side, and hinder their expansion, and likewise irritate, and at last might produce inflammation. He continued for some days with little variation, but upon the

* I have often thought it a great pity that we do not accustom ourselves to move one side of our thorax independently of the other, as we from habit move one eyelid independently of the other.

whole seemed getting better; but the day before he died, he became worse in his breathing, which we imputed to his stirring too much, and was rather better on the day that he did die: just before death he was taken with a sort of suffocation, and in half an hour he died.

Through his whole illness he had a moist skin, and sometimes sweated profusely; at last his legs swelled.

At first he only took a spermaceti mixture with a little opium, which gave him relief; I wanted to increase the opium, but it was objected to, for fear it should bind the chest too much, as it often does in asthmas, therefore it was given with the squills. On the day that he died, we ordered him the bark with a sudorific.

As this was very different from a common asthma, and the difficulty of breathing arose entirely from the inflammation of the intercostal muscles and lungs, and likewise from having but one lung, I thought it advisable to give opium in this case, as it would take off the irritation of the inflamed parts, and therefore allow a greater stretch or expansion; especially as we found whenever it was given that it gave relief and produced these effects.

One might at first wonder why he should breathe with such difficulty, as he had one side whole or sound; for I have seen people breathe pretty freely who have had but one side to expand; but when we consider the case, we can easily account for this.

After death we opened him. On raising the sternum I cut into the cavity of the thorax, and a great deal of blood gushed out at the incision; we sponged out of the left side of the thorax above three quarts of fluid blood; the coagulum appeared to have been attracted to the sides of the cavity everywhere, as if it had been furred over with the coagulating lymph, which was nowhere floating in the fluid; but most probably the extravasated blood had never coagulated, and this thick buffy crust was an exudation of coagulating lymph from the lungs and pleura, which covers the ribs as in all inflammations; if so, this is another instance, beside that of the inflammation of veins, in which the coagulating lymph coagulates immediately upon being thrown upon the surface; for if it had not, it then must have mixed with the blood in the chest, and only been found floating there. The lung was collapsed into a very small substance, and was therefore firmer than common; we observed the wound in it, which corresponded to the wound in the pleura; I introduced a probe into the wound in the lung, which passed near four inches, but was not certain whether it did not make some way for itself; however, I traced the wound by opening the lung, and could easily distinguish the wounded part by the coagulated blood that lay in it. I found the heart and inside of the pericardium inflamed, and their surfaces furred over with coagulating lymph, similar to that on the lung. The lung of the right side had also become a little inflamed on its anterior edges.

Wounds in the lungs generally become a cause of a quick pulse; this likewise may arise in some degree from the lungs being so immediately concerned in the circulation, that anything that gives a check to the blood's free motion through them may affect the heart. But the pulse becomes hard, which arises from the nature of the inflammation that attends, and also from the wound being in a vital part.

In the cases arising from balls, nothing in general is to be done but to keep quiet, and dress the wounds superficially; for any extravasated blood that might have got into the cavity of the thorax will generally make its escape by the external wound, as also any matter from suppuration. But in the cases of wounds made by cutting instruments, and where there is reason to suspect a considerable quantity of blood in the cavity of the thorax, then we may ask what should be done; and the natural answer is, that the operation for the empyema should be performed. This operation will relieve the patient and bring the disease to the [state of a] simple wound, and somewhat nearer to the gun-shot wound; it should be performed as soon as possible, before the blood can have time to coagulate; for the coagulum of the blood may be with difficulty extracted. The enlargement of the wound already made will often answer; but if that is in such a situation as to forbid dilatation, then the common directions for the empyema are to be followed here.

When all symptoms appear, and we have great reason to suppose a considerable extravasation of blood into the cavity of the chest, I think that we should not hesitate in performing the operation for the empyema.

§. 5. *Of Concussions and Fractures of the Skull.*

These injuries, in consequence of a musket-ball, differ in nothing from the same accidents arising from any other cause, excepting the lodgement of the ball, which I imagine will require no peculiar mode of treatment.

§. 6. *Of Wounds compounded with Fractured Bones, or containing Extraneous Bodies.*

The compound gun-shot wounds, where bones are broken, or where there are extraneous bodies that continue the irritation, similar to compound fractures, seldom if ever heal at once, or by regular degrees, as wounds of the former kind, but generally heal very quick at first, upon the going off of the inflammation, similar to the healing of simple gun-shot wounds; but when healed so far as to be affected by the extraneous bodies, then they become slow in their progress, till at last they come to a stand, or become fistulous; in which state they continue till the irritating cause is removed: and this takes place even if the dilatation should have been made at first as large as could be thought necessary; so that the opening at first, in such cases, can only let out those extraneous bodies or detached bones that are perfectly loose, or become loose while the wound continues large: however, even this can only take place in superficial wounds; but in those that are deep, or where there is an exfoliation to take place, the dilated part always heals up long before they are fit to make their exit; but before this happens the parts often acquire an indolent diseased state, and even when all extraneous bodies are extracted the parts do not readily heal.

When a wound comes to this stage, surgeons generally put in sponge or other tents into the opening, or apply some corroding medicine to keep it open, and also with a view to make it wider; but this practice is unnecessary, as a wound in such a state seldom heals entirely over, nor do tents add much to the width of the wound, and always confine the matter [for the time] between the two dressings.

Where an exfoliation is expected, it is generally better to expose as much of the bone as possible: it keeps up a kind of inflammation, which I imagine gives a disposition for this process. This can only be done where the bone is pretty superficial; but in cases where the separation has already taken place, and it is now to make its way to the skin, like any other extraneous substance, then, instead of the practice of sponge tents to keep the orifice in the skin open, it would be often better in such cases to let the whole heal over; because the extraneous body would form an abscess round itself, which would enlarge the cavity, and produce the ulcerative inflammation quicker towards the surface; and when that was opened, the extraneous body could be with more ease extracted, or would come out of itself: but this method of healing the mouths of fistulous sores is not always practicable.

If this last practice has no inconveniences attending it, it has this advantage, that the patient has not the disagreeable trouble of having a sore to dress every day till the extraneous body comes away, which I think is no small consideration. This practice, however, is not to be followed in every case: for instance, if the wound should communicate with a joint, as is common to most sores in the foot and hand where the bones are diseased, it would be in such cases very imprudent to allow the wound to heal, as the confined matter would get more readily into the different joints, and increase the disease: there may be other causes to forbid this as a general practice.

If wounds are to be kept open at their mouths, whose bottoms have not a disposition to heal, they should be kept open to that bottom; because, whenever they do heal at their mouths, it is most commonly owing to their sides underneath first uniting; for the skin will seldom unite when all beyond it is open.

In wounds that become fistulous, where there is no extraneous body, there is always a diseased bottom, which is to be looked upon as having the same effect as an extraneous substance. To alter this diseased disposition they should be opened freely, as large openings produce quick inflammation, quick suppuration, and quick granulations, which are generally sound when they arise from such a cause: on the other hand, letting such wounds heal at their mouths has often a salutary effect, as it becomes a means of destroying this diseased part by the formation of an abscess there, and in general there can be no better way of coming at a part or extraneous body than by the formation of an abscess there. It is a natural way of opening to relieve diseased parts; but we often find in practice that this method is not sufficient, either for the extraction of extraneous bodies, or to expose the diseased bottom, excepting these abscesses are opened very largely by art, so as to expose the whole of the diseased parts or extraneous body.

§. 7. *Of the Time proper for removing Incurable Parts.*

Many gun-shot wounds are at the very first evidently incurable, whether in a part that cannot be removed, or in one that will admit of being removed. When such wounds are in parts that will not admit of a removal of the parts injured, then nothing can be done by surgery; but when in a part that can be removed, then a removal of the injured part is to be put in practice; but even this is to be under certain restrictions: perhaps it should not be done immediately upon the receiving of the injury, excepting where a considerable blood-vessel is wounded, so as to endanger the life of the person, and that it absolutely cannot be taken up, or it is suspected that the inflammation in consequence of the accident will kill, by which means you have only the inflammation in consequence of the amputation; but this is a bad resource, especially if it is a lower extremity that is to be amputated, and which is perhaps the only part that can be removed of which the inflammation will kill.

How far the same practice is to be followed in cases which we may suppose will not kill, but that the part is so hurt as to all appearance not to be in the power of surgery to save, I will not now determine. This is a very different case from the former, and its consequences depend more upon contingencies, so that the part should be removed only when the state of the patient in other respects will admit of it; but this is seldom the case, for few people in full health are in that state, and still less so those who are usually the subjects of gun-shot wounds: the situation they are in at the time, from the hurry of mind, makes it here in general to be the very worst practice; it will in general, therefore, be much better to wait till the inflammation, and all the effects of both the irritation and inflammation, shall be gone off.

If these things are not sufficiently attended to, and the first inflammation, as in the first-stated case, (for instance, that which is likely to prove mortal,) is allowed to go on, the patient will most probably lose his life; or if the first inflammation is such as is likely to go off, according to the last-stated case, then we should allow it to go off before we operate, and not run the risk of producing death by an operation; for I have already observed, few can support the consequences of the loss of a lower extremity when in full health and vigour. We know that a violent inflammation will in a few hours alter the healthy disposition, and give a turn to the constitution, especially if a considerable quantity of blood has been lost, which most probably will be the case where both accident and operation immediately succeed one another. The patient under such circumstances becomes low, simply by the animal life losing its powers. and hardly ever recovers afterwards.

After considering the curative treatment of gun-shot wounds and other accidents common to the soldier as also the sailor, let us further consider the treatment of those patients whose wounds at the very first appear to be incurable when they are in parts that will admit of being removed.

The operation itself is the same as in other cases, and the only subjects of peculiar consideration here are the situation of the patient, and the proper time for performing the operation after the injury.

I have already given some directions with regard to the proper time of operating, in treating upon the dilatation of gun-shot wounds, which are in some degree applicable here; but we shall consider this now more fully, as the proper time of removing a part is often much shorter than that of dilating.

Amputation of an extremity is almost the only operation that can and is performed immediately on receiving the injury.

As these injuries in the soldier are generally received at a distance from all care, excepting what may be called chirurgical, it is proper we should consider how far the one should be practised without the other.

In general, surgeons have not endeavoured to delay it till the patient has been housed, and put in the way of a cure; and therefore it has been a common practice to amputate on the field of battle. Nothing can be more improper than this practice, for the following reasons; in such a situation it is almost impossible for a surgeon, in many instances, to make himself sufficiently master of the case, so as to perform so capital an operation with propriety; and it admits of dispute, whether at any time and in any place amputation should be performed before the first inflammation is over. When a case is so violent as not to admit of a cure in any situation, it is a chance if the patient will be able to bear the consequent inflammation; therefore in such a case it might appear, at first sight, that the best practice would be to amputate at the very first; but if the patient is not able to support the inflammation arising from the accident, it is more than probable he would not be able to support the amputation and its consequences. On the other hand, if the case is such as will admit of being brought through the first inflammation, although not curable, we should certainly allow of it; for we may be assured that the patient will be better able to bear the second.

If the chances are so even where common circumstances in life favour the amputation, how must it be where they do not? how must it be with a man whose mind is in the height of agitation, arising from fatigue, fear, distress, &c.? These circumstances must add greatly to the consequent mischief, and cast the balance much in favour of forbearance.

If it should be said that, agreeable to my argument, the same circumstances of agitation will render the accident itself more dangerous, I answer, that the amputation is a violence superadded to the injury, therefore heightens the danger; and when the injury alone proves fatal, it is by slower means. In the first case it is only inflammation; in the second it is inflammation, loss of substance, and most probably loss of more blood; as it is to be supposed that a good deal has been lost from the accident, not to mention the awkward manner in which it must be done.

The only thing that can be said in favour of amputation on the field of battle is, that the patient may be moved with more ease without a limb than with a shattered one: however, experience is the best guide, and I believe it is universally allowed by those whom we are to esteem the best judges, those who have had opportunity of making comparative observations on men who have been wounded in the same battle, some where amputation had been performed immediately, and others where it had been left till all circumstances favoured the operation; it has been found, I say, that few did well who had their limbs cut off on the field of battle; while a much greater proportion have done well, in similar cases, who were allowed to go on till the first inflammation was over, and underwent amputation afterwards.

There will be exceptions to the above observations, which must be in a great measure left to the discretion of the surgeon; but a few of these exceptions may be mentioned, so as to give a general idea of what is meant.

First, it is of less consequence, whichsoever way it is treated, if the part to be amputated is an upper extremity; but it may be observed, that there will be little occasion in general to amputate an upper extremity upon the field, because there will be less danger in moving such a patient than if the injury had happened to the lower.

Secondly, if the parts are very much torn, so that the limb only hangs by a small connection, then the circumstance of the loss of so much substance to the constitution cannot be an objection, as it takes place from the accident, and indeed everything else that can possibly attend an amputation: therefore, in many cases, it may be more convenient to remove the whole. In many cases it may be necessary to perform the operation to get at blood-vessels which may be bleeding too freely, for the searching after them may do more mischief than the operation.

I have already observed that gun-shot wounds do not bleed so freely as those made by cutting instruments, and are therefore attended with less danger of that kind: however, it may often happen that a considerable vessel shall be divided, and a considerable bleeding take place; in such cases no time is to be lost; the vessel must be taken up to prevent a greater evil. This operation may in many cases be attended with considerable trouble, especially as it will, in general, be on the field of action. Here the sailor has the advantage of the soldier.

It will also be immediately necessary on the field to replace many parts that would destroy the patient if their restoration was delayed, such as the bowels or lungs protruding out of their cavities, or to remove large bodies, such as a piece of shell sticking in the flesh, which would give great pain, and do mischief by moving the whole together.

Very little can be done to relieve the brain in such a situation[a].

---

[a] [It seems to be now universally admitted by the most esteemed army surgeons that amputation on the field, or very shortly after removal to some fixed hospital, is the most judicious practice, and that the danger is infinitely increased by extending the delay beyond twenty-four hours, with a view of obtaining a more favourable opportunity for its performance. The cases which, according to Dr. Hennen, require this relief, are, 1st, where an arm or leg is carried completely off by a round shot; 2nd, where

§. 8. *Of the Treatment of the Constitution.*

Bleeding is recommended in gun-shot wounds, and in such a manner as if of more service in them than wounds in general; but I do not see this necessity more than in other wounds that have done the same mischief, and where the same inflammation and other consequences are expected.

Bleeding is certainly to be used here, as in all wounds where there is a strong and full habit, and where we expect considerable inflammation and symptomatic fever; but if it is such a gun-shot wound as not to produce considerable effects, either local or constitutional, I would not bleed, merely because it is a gun-shot wound: and from what I have seen, I think that inflammation, &c. does not run so high in these wounds as I should have at first expected. I believe this is the case with all contused wounds where death in the part is a consequence: a contused wound is somewhat similar to the effects of a caustic; for while the separation of the dead part is forming, the suppurative inflammation is retarded, and therefore not so violent; but this can only be said of those wounds which are not complicated with any other injury except what is produced by the balls passing through soft parts; for if a bone is broken, it will inflame like any other compound fracture.

It is often of service, in the time of inflammation, to bleed in the part with leeches or by punctures with a lancet: this helps to empty the

---

there are extensive injuries of the joints; 3rd, where there are compound fractures close to the joints, especially if conjoined with lacerated vessels or nerves, or much comminution of the bone, particularly if the femur is the injured bone; 4th, where there is extensive loss of substance, or disorganization of the soft parts, by round shot; 5th, where the bones have been fractured or dislocated without rupture of the skin, or great loss of parts, but with great injury or disorganization of the ligaments, &c., and injuries of the vessels, followed by extensive internal effusions of blood among the soft parts.

From the returns of the British army in the Peninsula, Mr. Guthrie found that at Toulouse 38 cases out of 48 terminated favourably when amputation was immediately performed; 41 of these operations were of the thigh and leg, and 7 of the arm. Of the unfavourable cases, 3 were amputations of the thigh, performed as high up as is practicable by the common operation. Of 52 secondary operations, 15 of the superior extremity and 37 of the thigh, as many as 3 of the former were lost, and 8 of the latter; and altogether of 842 amputations performed at the Hospital Stations between the 21st of June and 24th of December, 1813, the comparative loss of secondary or delayed operations, and of primary or immediate operations, was as follows:

	Secondary.		Primary.
Upper extremities	12	to	1
Lower extremities	3	to	1

Guthrie on Gun-shot Wounds, 2nd edit., pp. 150, 220.]

vessels of the part, to lessen the inflammation sooner, and of course to promote suppuration; but I must own that bleeding must be used with great caution where inflammation and fever run very high, for to reduce the patient equal to the action at the time (which, whether an increased action or an acquired one, is only temporary) will be reducing him often too much for the constitution to support life when this action ceases; for the very worst thing that can happen is the patient's being reduced too low. We often afterwards find more difficulty in keeping up the strength with cordials, bark, &c. than we find in lowering it; and we may avail ourselves of observing those who have lost considerable quantities of blood from the accident, which is always immediate; for we find that a second bleeding, by some other accident, although very small in quantity, often destroys our patient very quickly: but this will in a great measure depend upon the seat of the injury; for in cases of great violence done to some parts of our body, bleeding answers better than in others, because the symptoms of dissolution, and dissolution itself, come on sooner from mischief done to some parts than when it is done to others. A man will bear bleeding better after an amputation of the arm than the leg; better after a compound fracture of the arm than the leg: he will bear bleeding better after an injury done to the head, chest, lungs, &c. than either to the arm or leg.

We find that injuries done to inactive parts, such as joints, do worse, and are more susceptible of irritation than those in fleshy parts of the same situation.

It would appear upon the whole that the decay of animal life is sooner brought on when the inflammation is in a part whose circulation is not so strong, and where the nervous influence or the force of the circulation is far removed.

Bark is greatly recommended in gun-shot wounds, and with good reason; but it is ordered indiscriminately to all patients that have received such wounds, whatever the symptoms or constitution of the patient may be. That there is no better medicine for wounds in general, not only when the inflammation is gone off, but in the time of inflammation, if the patient is rather low, and indeed before it comes on, experience daily shows. Bark is to be looked upon as a strengthener or regulator of the system, and an antispasmodic, both of which destroy irritation. The bark and gentle bleedings, when the pulse begins to rise, are the best treatment that I know of in inflammations that arise either from accidents or operations; one lessens the volume of the blood and the increased animal powers at the time, which makes the circulation more free, so that the heart labours less, and simple circulation goes on more freely; the other gives to the blood that which makes it less irritating, makes the blood-vessels do their proper offices, and gives to the nerves their proper sensations, which take off the fever.

BIBLIOGRAPHY OF GUN-SHOT WOUNDS.

Abernethy, J. Surg. Obs. on Tumours and Lumbar Abscesses. 8vo. 1810.——*Allan, Rob.*, A Syst. of Pathological and Operative Surgery, 3 vol. 8vo. 1821–7.——*Andouillé*, in Mém. de l'Acad. de Chir., 12mo. tom. vi.——*Arnal,* Mém. sur quelques Particularitées des Plaies par Armes à Feu. Univ. Hebd. de Méd., 8vo. 1831. tom. iii. ——*Assalini, P., M. D.* Manuale di Chirurgia. 12mo. 1812.——*Atkins, J.* The Navy Surgeon. 8vo. 1742.

Bagien. Examen des plusieurs parties de la Chirurgie. 8vo. 1756.——*Baldinger, E. G.* Introd. in Notitiam Scriptorum Medicinæ Militaris, cum Additamentis. 8vo. 1764. ——*Ballingall, Sir G.* Outlines of Military Surgery. 8vo. 1833.——*Bell, Charles.* Syst. of Operative Surgery, 2 vol. 8vo. 1807–9, and 2nd edit. 1814, in which is incorporated a Treatise on Gun-shot Wounds.——*Bell, John.* A Disc. on the Nature and Cure of Wounds, etc., 8vo. 1795. and 3rd edit. 1812. p. 169 et seq.——*Bilguer, I. U.* Dissert. de Membrorum Amputatione, 1761.——*Blane, Sir Gilbert, M.D.* Observ. on the Diseases incident to Seamen, 8vo. 1785.——*Boggie, Dr.* On Hospital Gangrene, in Med. and Chir. Tr. of Edin., vol. iii.——*Bordenave.* In Mém. de l'Acad. de Chir., 12mo, tom. vi.——*Botallus, Leonard.* De Curandis Vulneribus Sclopettorum, 8vo. 1575.——*Boucher.* Observ. sur les Plaies d'Armes à Feu, compliquées de fracture aux articulations des Extrem. &c., in Mém. de l'Acad. de Chir., 12mo. v. 279. vi. 109.——*Brown, John.* A Compleat Discourse of Wounds, etc. 1678.——*Brunswich, Hieron.* The noble Experience of the vertuous Handywarke of Surgerie, fol. 1525.

Cannac. Observ. sur les Plaies d'Armes à Feu, etc., in Mém. de l'Acad. de Chir. tom. vi. ——*Carcanus, J. B.* De Vulneribus Capitis, 1583.——*Chevalier, Thos.* On Gun-Shot Wounds, small 8vo. 1804.——*Clowes, W.* A Prooved Practice for all Young Chirurgians, concerning burning with Gun-Powder, and Wounds made with Gun-Shot, Sword, etc., 4to. 1588.——*Cooper, Sam.* Surgical Dict., 8vo. 1812. and last Edit. 1830.——Also, First Lines, etc., 8vo. 1813. and last Edit. 1836.

Duignau, M. G. Réflexions Importantes sur le Service des Hôpitaux Militaires, 8vo. 1785.——*De Conte.* In Prix de l'Acad. de Chir., 12mo. tom. viii.——*Desport.* Traité des Plaies d'Armes à Feu, 12mo. 1749.——*Dewar, H.* On a particular sort of Gun-shot Wound, 8vo. 1815.——*Dict.* des Sc. Méd. (Petit), Art. Depôt. Dict. de Méd. (Roux). Dict. de Méd. et Chir. Prat. (Dupuytren), Art. Abcès. Cyc. Pract. Med. (Froudie). Encyc. Wörterb. (Richter), Art. Abscess.——*Dupuy, J. M.* Sur les Abscès ou Tumeurs purulentes. 1804.——*Dupuytren, le Baron.* Traité Théoretique et Pratique des Blessures par Armes de Guerre, etc., par MM. Paillard et Marx. 2 tom. 8vo. 1834, et Leçons orales (ii. 417.) 4 tom. 8vo. 1832–4.

Encycl. Méthod., Partie Chir., Art. Plaies d'Armes à Feu.

Faure. In Prix de l'Acad. des Chir., 12mo.——*Ferrius, Alph.* De Tormentariorum sive Archibusorum Vulnerum Natura et Cur., 2da Imp., 8vo. 1577.——*Foudacq, C. F.* Réflexions sur les Playes, &c. 12mo. 1753.

Gale, Tho. An Institution of a Chirurgian, conteynynge the sure Grounds and Principles of Chirurgerie. 8vo. 1563.——Also an Enchiridion of Chirurgerie, &c. 8vo. 1563.——*Gerard.* In Mém. de l'Acad. de Chir. 12mo. tom. vi.——*Gesscher, Van.* Abhandlung von der Nothwendigkeit der Amputation. 1775.——*Graefe, R. C. F.* Normen für die Ablösung Grosserer Gleidmassen. 4to. 1812.——*Guthrie, J. C.* On Gun-shot Wounds of the Extremities, &c. 8vo. 1815. and 3rd Edit. 1827.

Heisterus, Laur. Chirurgie; in welcher Alles was zur Wund-Artzney Gehört, Gründlich abgehandelt ist. (the 3rd chap. is devoted to Gun-shot Wounds). 4to. 1719. *tr. Lat.* 4to. 1743.——*Hennen, John, M.D.* Principles of Military Surgery, 3rd Edit. 1829. ——*Home, Francis, M.D.* Medical Facts and Experiments (including a chap. on Gun-shot Wounds), 8vo. 1759.——*Hutchison, A. Copeland.* Some Practical Observ. on Surgery, 8vo. 1816. and 2nd Edit. 1826.—Some further Observ. &c. on Amputation. 8vo. 1817.——Histoire de l'Etat et des Prog. de la Chir. Militaire en France, pendant les Guerres de la Révolution, par M. Briot. 8vo. 1817.

Jobert, De Lambelle. Plaies d'Armes à Feu. &c. 8vo. 1833.——*Journal* de Méd. Militaire. 8vo. 1782 et ann. seq.

Klohss, K. L. Diss. de Myclitide. 8vo. 1820.

Larrey, Le Baron D. J. Relation Hist. et Chir. de l'Exped. de l'Armée en Egypt, &c. 8vo. 1803.—Mém. de Chir. Milit. 4 tom. 8vo. 1812. *tr.* by J. Waller, 1815. —Recueil des Mém. de Chir. 8vo. 1821.—Clinique Chirurg., &c. 4 tom. et Atlas. 8vo. 1829–32.—Mém. sur les Plaies Pénétrantes de la Poitrine, in Mém. de l'Acad. Roy. de Méd. 1828. I. 2.——*Laurent, J.* Essais sur la Supp. 8vo. 1803. ——*Léveillé, J. B. F.* Nouvelle Doct. Chir. (tom. i. chap. viii. p. 436.) 4 tom. 8vo. 1812.——*Le Dran, H. F.* Traité ou Réflexions tirées de la Pratique sur les Plaies d'Armes à Feu. 2de édit. 12mo. 1740.——*Lizors, I.* in Edin. Med. and Surg. Journ. xv. 396. (1819.) on the Pathology of the Nerves in Inflamm.——*Lombard, C. A.* Dissert. sur l'importance des Evacuans dans la Cure des Plaies. 8vo. 1783. —Clinique Chir. des Plaies, des Plaies Recentes et des Plaies d'Armes à Feu. 3 tom. 8vo. 1798–1804.——*Lowe, P., M.D.* A Discourse of the whole Art of Chyrurgerie. 4to. 1597.

Macgrigor, Sir Jas. On the Diseases of the Army, in Med. Chir. Tr. vi. 455.——*Maggius, Bart.* De Vulnerum Sclopetorum et Bombardarum Curatione Tractatus. 4to. 1552.——*Mann, James.* Med. Sketches of the Campaigns of 1812, 1813, 1814, &c. 8vo. 1816.——*Martiniere,* in Mém. de l'Acad. de Chir. 12mo. tom. xi.——*Méher, J.* Traité des Plaies d'Armes à Feu. 8vo. 1800.——*Millengen J. G. V., M.D.* The Army Medical Officer's Manual upon Active Service, &c. 8vo. 1819.——*Morand, Salv.* Opuscules de Chirurgie. 4to. 1768–72.——*Mursinna.* Neue Med. Chir. Beobachtungen. Zweiter Thiel, s. 138. 1796.

Neale, H. St. John. Chirurg. Instit. on Gun-shot Wounds, &c. 8vo. 1804.

Paré, Amb. Manière de traiter des Plaies d'Arguebusades et Fleches. 8vo. 1751. Et Opera, curâ Guillemeau. fol. 1582.——*Paroisse, J. B.* Opuscules de Chirurgie, &c. 8vo. 1806.——*Percy, Le Baron P. F.* Manuel du Chirurgien d'Armée, &c. 8vo. 1792. ——*Plazzonus, Fr.* De Vulneribus Sclopetorum, &c. 4to. 1618.

Quercetanus, Jos. Sclopetarius, sive de curandis Vulneribus, &c. 8vo. 1578.

Ranby, J. The Method of treating Gun-shot Wounds, &c. 8vo. 1744.——*Ravaton.* Chirurgie d'Armée, &c. 8vo. 1768.—Recueil d'Observ. de Méd. des Hosp. Militaires. 4to. 1766–72.——*Richerand, Ant.* Nosographie Chir. (tom. i.) 5ème edit. 4 tom. 8vo. 1821.—Recueil de Mém. de Méd. Chir. et Pharm. Milit., &c. rédigé par MM. Biron et Fournier et continue par MM. Bégin et Etienne. 32 tom. 8vo. 1816–32. ——*Richter, A. G.* Anfangsgründe der Wundarzneykunst (bande i.) 7 Bde. 8vo. 4te Aufl. 1804–25.——*Rota, J. F.* De Tormentariorum sive Archibusorum Vulnerum Natura et Cur. 4to. 1555.——*Roux, P. J.* Considérations sur les Blessés des Trois Jours. 8vo. 1830.

Schmucker, J. L. Chirurgische Wahrnehmungen. 8vo. 1774-89. Vermischte Chir. Schriften. 3 vols. 8vo. 1776–1782.

Theden, J. C. A. Unterricht fur die Unterwundarzte bey Armeen. 8vo. 1782.——*Thomassin, M.* Diss. sur l'Extraction des Corps étrangers des Plaies. 8vo. 1788.——*Thomson, John, M.D.* Report of the State of the Wounded in Belgium after the Battle of Waterloo. 8vo. 1816.——*Trotter, Thomas, M.D.* Medicina Nautica, &c. 3 vols. 8vo. 1797–1803.

Vacher. Sur quelques Particularités concernant les Playes faites par les Armes à Feu. in Mém. de l'Acad. de Chir., &c. 12mo. tom. xi.——*Vigo, John.* The most excellent Works of Chirurgerye; *tr.* by B. Traherom. fol. 1543.

Wedekind. Nachrichten über das Französische, Kriegspitalwesen, Erster Bde. 1797. ——*Wiseman, Rich.* Several Chirurgical Treatises (one of which is *ex professo* on gun-shot wounds). fol. 1676.——*Woodall, John.* The Surgion's Mate, &c. 1617. also Viaticum or Pathway to the Surgeon's Chest. 1628.

OBSERVATIONS ON THE INFLAMMATION OF THE INTERNAL COATS OF VEINS.

Read February 6, 1784.

[*From the Transactions of a Society for the Improvement of Medical and Chirurgical Knowledge, Vol. I. p.* 18. 1793.]

THE following observations will show that the inside of veins, as well as of all other cavities, is a seat of inflammation and abscess. I have found in all violent inflammations of the cellular membrane, whether spontaneous or in consequence of accident, as in compound fractures, or of surgical operation, as in the removal of an extremity, that the coats of the larger veins, passing through the inflamed part, become also considerably inflamed, and that their inner surfaces take on the adhesive, suppurative, and ulcerative inflammations; for in such inflammations I have found in many places of the veins adhesion, in others matter, and in others ulceration. Under such circumstances the veins would have abscesses formed in them, if the matter did not find in many cases an easy passage to the heart along with the circulating blood, so as to prevent the accumulation of the pus; but this ready passage of the matter into the common circulation does not always happen. It is in some cases prevented by the adhesive inflammation taking place in the vein between the place of suppuration and the heart, so that an abscess is formed, as will be further observed.

Where the inflammation is most violent there we find the vein most inflamed, there also after suppuration we find the purest pus; and as we trace the vessels from this part, either farther from or nearer to the heart, we find the pus more and more mixed with blood, and having more of the coagulated parts of the blood in it.

As these appearances are only to be seen in dead bodies, they cannot be described but from thence; but it is so common a case that I have hardly ever seen an instance of suppuration in any part furnished with large veins where these appearances were not evident after death. I have found them in the bodies of those who have died from amputations, compound fractures, and mortifications.

These circumstances all considered lead us to account for a very frequent complaint, that is, an inflamed arm after bleeding: a complaint which has by some been imputed to the wounding of a tendon, because the tendon of the biceps muscle lies under some of those veins in which we often bleed, and when the complaint occurs it is unjustly supposed to arise from want of skill in the operator; by others it has been supposed to arise from the wounding of a nerve; and again it has been laid to the charge of a bad constitution.

But if we consider more critically this consequence arising from bleeding, we shall find that it happens frequently after bleeding in veins where no tendon could possibly be wounded, and also where no particular nerve could be in the way. It seems likewise to happen as frequently in constitutions where there is no appearance of want of health, as in those disposed to disease. As a proof of this last, upon bleeding in another vein in the same person, perhaps with a view to assist in the cure of the inflammation arising from the first bleeding, the wound has healed very readily.

If we examine the proportion which the number of those inflammations that happen after bleeding bears to those which arise from as slight a wound where no large vein has been injured, and even perhaps where the wound has not been made by so clean a cutting instrument, and the same pains not taken to close it up, we shall find that those from wounded veins are much the most frequent, and that such inflammations seldom or ever happen under the last-mentioned circumstances: therefore we must look for some other cause to explain this effect of bleeding.

The manner in which those sore arms come on shows plainly that they arise from the wound not healing by the first intention: for the external wound in most cases first festers or inflames, then suppurates and ulcerates, so that the cavity of the vein becomes impervious. In some this suppuration is only superficial, the vein and parts below having united. In others the skin shall appear to be united, but not close to the vein, so that a small abscess shall form between the skin and the vein; it shall burst and discharge a thin watery fluid, and no further mischief happen; but when this imperfection of union is continued on to the cavity of the vein, then the vein inflames both upwards and downwards, and that often for a considerable way, and the surrounding parts join in the inflammation.

We find all these variations in different cases: for the disease sometimes goes no further than an inflammation in the vein near to the orifice, which is often resolved; at other times the inflammation is carried further, but suppuration is prevented by the adhesive inflammation taking place in the vein at this part, so as to exclude the suppurative inflammation, and the veins in such cases may be plainly felt, after the surrounding tumefaction has subsided, like hard cords. But this salutary effect is not always produced, and suppuration in the vein is the consequence; but often so confined, that only a small abscess forms in the cavity of the vein near to the orifice. The confinement of the matter in this part of the vein arises from adhesions in the vein a little above and below the orifice. But in many cases the inflammation and suppuration are not confined to this part, from the adhesions not having taken place; for it frequently happens that an abscess is formed, occupying a considerable length of the vein both ways; and we often have more than one abscess, nay at times there is a series of them, and generally in the direction of the vein, between the orifice and the heart; but not always in this course, for we find them sometimes between the wound and the extreme parts.

I have seen from a wound in the foot the vena saphæna inflamed all up the leg and thigh, nearly as high as the groin; and I have been obliged to open a string of abscesses almost through its whole course.

In cases where I have had opportunities of inspecting veins after death in which the inflammation had been violent, upon examining the vein at some distance from this violence, I found the inflammation in the adhesive state: in some places the sides of the vein were adhering, and in others the inner surface of the veins was furred over with a coagulable lymph. Where different abscesses had formed I have always found that the spaces of the vein between them had united by the adhesive inflammation, and it is this union which circumscribes the abscesses.

Upon examining the arm of a man who had died at St. George's Hospital, I found the veins, both below and above the orifice, in many places united by the adhesive inflammation. I also found in many parts of the veins that suppuration had begun, as we find, on an inflamed surface, but had not yet arrived at ulceration; and in several ether places ulceration had taken place, so as to have destroyed that surface next the skin, and a circumscribed abscess was formed. The vein near to the axilla had taken on suppuration, beyond which adhesions had not formed, and this had given a free passage for the matter into the circulation, of which most probably the patient died.

In those cases where larger abscesses have come on than those formed simply from the ulceration of the wound made by the lancet, I have always found that the vein was afterwards obliterated, having united and healed up as any other cavity does, so that such patients could never be bled in the same vein again, which is a proof that the sides of the vein can unite by the adhesive inflammation.

Inflammation of a vein is a common effect after bleeding horses, which is usually done in the neck. The operator on this animal does not always take sufficient care to close up the external wound; for although the method usually employed would at first sight appear to be a good one, that is, by a pin passed through the wound from side to side, as in the hare-lip, and over-tied by a thread or hair, yet, if not executed with sufficient attention, I should be inclined to believe that it is the very worst, as it very readily promotes inflammation in the cavity of the vein, either of the adhesive or suppurative kind, according as the ligature does or does not communicate with the cavity.

In some of these inflammations of horses I have seen the jugular vein inflamed through its whole length, and all the side of the head has been considerably swelled, and the inflammation carried along the vein quite into the chest. In these cases there is always an abscess formed at the wound, and often several along the vein, as in the human subject; and whenever the complaint is carried so far as this stage, the cavity becomes united at those places by granulations, and the vein is ever after impervious. Many horses die of this disease; but what is the particular circumstance which occasions their death I have not been able to determine. It may either be that the inflammation extends itself to the heart, or that the matter secreted from the inside of the vein passes along that tube in considerable quantity to the heart, and mixes with the blood.

I am inclined to believe that the exposure of cavities of the larger veins in cases of accidents, and also of operations, is often the cause of many of the very extensive inflammations which sometimes attend these cases, and indeed may be the reason why inflammations extend or spread at all beyond the sphere of continued sympathy[a].

In all cases where inflammation of veins runs high, or extends itself considerably, it is to be expected that the whole system will be affected. For the most part the same kind of affection takes place which arises from other inflammations, with this exception, that where no adhesions of the sides of the veins are formed, or where such adhesions are incomplete, pus passing into the circulation may add to the general disorder and even render it fatal.

In all cases of inflammation where adhesions take place they arise from an extravasation of coagulable lymph; but how such adhesions should take place on the internal surface of veins appears at first sight difficult to conceive, since it is most obvious that the coagulable lymph thrown out by the exhalants on the internal surface of the vein, mixing with the same fluid circulating with the other parts of the blood, would be swept

[a] [The frequency of phlebitis, not only after accidents and operations but in puerperal women, has fully confirmed the truth of this conjecture. Inflammation even of the veins of he bones, according to Cruveilhier, is a frequent consequence of operations on these parts.]

away without producing any effect. But since such adhesions do in fact happen, the coagulable lymph must undergo some change connected with the disposition which produces its extravasation.

Although the operation which is the most frequent cause of this complaint is to appearance trifling, yet as it is often of very serious consequence, both to the life of the patient and the character of the surgeon, it requires particular attention in the operator to prevent as much as possible an evil of such magnitude. With this view he will be particularly attentive to the mode of closing the wound and binding up the arm. This is to be done by bringing the two sides of the wound together, that they may unite by the first intention. To accomplish this, let the surgeon, with the thumb of that hand which holds the arm, push the skin towards the orifice, while he draws it on the other side to the same point with the compress: thus the skin will be thrown into folds at the wound over which he is immediately to apply the compress. The compress should be broad, to keep the skin better together; and thick, to make the compression more certain. Another advantage arising from this caution is the prevention of the vein bleeding a second time. I have known an inflammation attack the orifice, which appeared to have arisen from the first union having been broke through, and no second union formed; but this probably did not arise from the vein being opened a second time, but from the sides of the orifice not having been again brought together. I would recommend a compress of linen or lint, in preference to sticking plaster; for I imagine that the blood drying over, the orifice is a kind of bond of union more natural and effectual than any other application: and this conclusion is drawn from practice; for I have seen more sore arms in consequence of bleeding where plasters have been afterwards applied, than from any other; and in cases of the compound fracture, when attempted to be cured as a simple fracture, if the wound will allow of being scabbed over, I have seen it always do well; whereas if it has been kept moist, or prevented from evaporating by plasters or other applications, it has always suppurated.

When inflammation takes place beyond the orifice, so as to alarm the surgeon, he should immediately make a compress upon the vein at the inflamed part, to make the two sides adhere together; or if they do not adhere, yet simple contact will be sufficient to prevent suppuration in this part; or if inflammation has gone so far as to make the surgeon suspect that suppuration has taken place, then the compress must be put upon that part of the vein just above the suppuration. This I once practised, and, as I supposed, with success[a].

---

[a] [Few diseases possess more practical or theoretical interest than the subject of phlebitis; and yet, clear and satisfactory as Mr. Hunter's observations on the subject are,

they do not appear to have attracted much attention until comparatively a recent period. From 1784, the date of Mr. Hunter's paper, to 1815, when Mr. Hodgson's valuable treatise on the diseases of the arteries and veins appeared, only a very few cases are recorded in the literature of this country. Bichat, in his *Anatomie Générale*, does not appear to have been acquainted with the complaint, at least with that peculiar form of suppurative inflammation to which the veins are liable, while the French journals, with one single exception, are equally silent on the subject. The successive publications, which have since appeared, of Abernethy, Hodgson, Travers, Carmichael, Arnott, &c., have thrown much light on the pathology of phlebitis, while they have at the same time not only pointed out the frequent complication of phlebitis with other affections, as, for example, accidents and surgical operations, but also that it is often the cause of death in other cases where it was not previously suspected, especially in puerperal women. Among the most remarkable circumstances brought to light in the course of these investigations, must be mentioned the resemblance which the constitutional symptoms attending this form of inflammation, bear to those produced by injection of putrid or infectious matters into the current of the blood, and also the frequent occurrence of secondary suppurations in various parts of the body and often in many parts of the same body. The cause of these peculiarities has not yet been satisfactorily determined, nor has it yet been decided what mode of treatment is most generally eligible. Experience has shown that little reliance is to be placed on the application of compresses above the inflamed part, as advised by the author.]

ON INTROSUSCEPTION.

[Read August 18, 1789.]

[*From the Transactions of a Society for the Improvement of Medical and Chirurgical Knowledge, Vol. I. p.* 103. 1793.]

INTROSUSCEPTION is a disease produced by the passing of one portion of an intestine into another, and it is commonly, I believe, from the upper passing into the lower part.

If the mode of accounting for introsusception, which I am going to offer, be just, it will most frequently happen in the way I have stated, although there is no reason why it may not take place in a contrary direction, in which case the chance of a cure will be increased by the natural actions of the intestinal canal tending to replace the intestine; and probably from this circumstance it may oftener occur than commonly appears.

When the introsusception is downwards it may be called progressive, and when it happens upwards, retrograde. The manner in which it may take place is, by one portion of a loose intestine being contracted, and the part immediately below relaxed and dilated, under which circumstances it might very readily happen, by the contracted portion slipping a little way into that which is dilated; not from any action in either portion of intestine, but from some additional weight in the gut above. How far the peristaltic motion, by pushing the contents on to the contracted parts, may force them into the relaxed, I will not determine, but should rather suppose that it would not.

By this mode of accounting for an accidental introsusception, it may take place either upwards or downwards; but if a continuance or an increase of it arises from the action of the intestine, it must be when it is downwards, as we actually find to be the case; yet this does not explain those in which a considerable portion of intestine appears to have been carried into the gut below: to understand these we must consider the different parts which form the introsusception. It is made up of three folds of intestine; the inner, which passes down, and being reflected upwards, forms the second or inverted portion, which being reflected down again, makes the third or containing part, that is, the outermost, which is always in the natural position.

The outward fold is the only one which is active, the inverted portion being perfectly passive, and squeezed down by the outer, which inverts more of itself, so that the angle of inversion in this case is always at the angle of reflection of the outer into the middle portion or inverted one, while the innermost is drawn in. From this we can readily see how an introsusception, once begun, may have any length of gut drawn in.

The external portion acting upon the other folds in the same way as upon any extraneous matter, will, by its peristaltic motion, urge them further; and, if any extraneous substance is detained in the cavity of the inner portion, that part will become a fixed point for the outer or containing intestine to act upon. Thus it will be squeezed on, till at last the mesentery, preventing more of the innermost part from being drawn in, will act as a kind of stay, yet without entirely hindering the inverted outer fold from going still further. For it being the middle fold that is acted upon by the outer, and this action continuing after the inner portion becomes fixed, the gut is thrown into folds upon itself; so that a foot in length of intestine shall form an introsusception of not more than three inches long.

The different appearances which I have described as taking place in an introsusception are distinctly seen in Plate XXIV., fig. 4., in which the different folds of intestine are exposed.

I have asserted that the outer portion of intestine was alone active in augmenting the disease when once begun, but if the inner one was capable of equal action in its natural direction, the effect would be the same, that of endeavouring to invert itself, as in a prolapsus ani; the outer and inner portions, by their action, would tend to draw in more of the gut, while the intermediate part only would, by its action, have a contrary tendency.

The action of the abdominal muscles cannot assist in either forming or continuing this disease, as it must compress equally both above and below, although it is capable of producing the prolapsus ani.

In cases where introsusception begins at the valve of the colon, and inverts that intestine, we find the ileum is not at all affected, which proves that the mesentery, by acting as a stay, prevents its inversion.

From the natural attachment of the mesentery to the intestines, one would, at the first view of the subject, conceive it impossible for any one portion of gut to get far within another, as the greater extent of mesentery that is carried in along with it would render its further entrance more and more difficult, and we should expect this difficulty to be greater in the large intestines than in the small, as being more closely confined to their situation: yet the largest introsusception of any known was in the colon, as related by Mr. Whately*.

* Vide Philos. Trans., vol. lxxvi. page 305.

The introsusception appeared to have begun at the insertion of the ileum into the colon, and to have carried in the cæcum with its appendix. The ileum passed on into the colon, till the whole of the ascending colon, the transverse arch and descending colon, were carried into the sigmoid flexure and rectum. The valve of the colon being the leading part, it at last got as low as the anus; and when the person went to stool he only emptied the ileum, for one half of the large intestines being filled up by the other, the ileum alone, which passed through the centre, discharged its contents.

Since that time the following case has occurred, which is in many respects similar; the patient was attended by Dr. Ash, and the body inspected after death by Mr. Home.

A. B. aged nine months, a large healthy well-looking child, who, as far as appeared, had never been indisposed from his birth, was seized with a strong spasm, stretching himself out suddenly, without having had any symptoms of previous ailment. Either during the spasm, or immediately after it, he passed a very large loose stool, and after that discharged at intervals small quantities of mucous slime, covered over with little specks of recent fluid blood. Dr. Ash visited him four or five hours after this attack, and found him in all other respects perfectly well; the child sucked heartily, but Dr. Ash, on observing his pulse to be less quick than is usual in children so young, his heat to be rather below the common standard, and, added to these, the small mucous and bloody discharges, suspected that mortification had taken place in the bowels, without being able to guess at the cause, as the child had laboured under no previous indisposition. In this uncertain situation various means of relief were attempted by purgatives, fomentations, the warm bath, and different kind of clysters, but without any good effect. On his first examination of the abdomen he felt (or thought he felt) a deap-seated fulness or hardness under the left hypochondrium; blisters were applied to the part, and every possible means attempted, without obtaining any evacuation by stool, or any other apparent relief; his strength gradually sunk, and his pulse became gradually weaker, although he continued to take the breast eagerly till within a few hours of his death, which happened just sixty hours after the first spasmodic attack.

The following were the appearances found in the dead body. Upon opening the abdomen the small intestines, considerably distended with fluid contents, occupied so much of the cavity as to prevent any of the other viscera from being seen, and the mesentery was so much confined that the convolutions of the small intestines could not be readily followed. This confinement was found to arise from an introsusception of the ileum and its mesentery, together with the cæcum and ascending colon into the descending part of the sigmoid flexure of the colon, the mesentery of the ileum being drawn up so obliquely across the root of the mesentery, as to prevent the jejunum from having its usual freedom of attachment.

The only part of the colon which could be seen was the sigmoid flexure, in which was distinctly to be felt a hard substance, consisting of the ileum and inverted colon. These parts being removed, for the purpose of a more accurate inspection of them, the sigmoid flexure of the colon was laid open, and was discovered to contain the cæcum and colon in an inverted state. The internal surface of these, when exposed, were found to have put on a dark red appearance, approaching to black; the whole appearing like a solid substance, rounded at the end, hanging loose into the descending colon, and about four inches long. Upon dividing the inverted colon, the ileum and appendix cæci were seen lying close to each other, and their two openings found on the rounded end of the inverted colon, leading directly into the sigmoid flexure; the portion of the ileum was a little twisted, but not in the least corrugated, it was rather stretched, and much pressed against the appendix cæci and its own mesentery by the surrounding colon, and a convolution of the appendix near the termination was so much pressed against the ileum as to make a mark upon it, and probably had compressed its sides so as to prevent anything from passing. The portion of ileum was about four inches long.

The inverted colon had drawn in the meso-colon, and a portion of the omentum that was attached to the transverse arch. The portion of the colon near the valve, which formed the extremity of the inverted part, was much thickened in its substance by the effects of inflammation, being four or five times its natural thickness; it was a good deal corrugated, or folded upon itself, the folds at this part seemed to adhere to one another, and form one mass. The inflammation and thickening only extending two inches, the gut becoming gradually thinner till it was of its natural thickness and appearance; so that what was only four inches in length of introsusception, contained a considerably greater length of intestine.

The sigmoid flexure, which was the containing intestine, had the natural appearance, but was dilated or relaxed; and the other contents of the abdomen were in a natural state, nor had the child any other apparent disease. A representation of the parts may be seen in Pl. XXIV.

From the account I have given of introsusception, it does not seem probable that it should be of the retrograde kind, unless from an inversion of the peristaltic motion, which could only continue for a short time, and the natural motion being restored, a cure would probably be performed.

This disease happens most frequently in the first fifteen years of life, not occurring so commonly in older people, neither does it, I believe, ever take place in the colon itself, although we find that gut affected by it*.

An introsusception can never be perfectly known till after death; but where there are violent affections of the bowels, attended with constipation, we have reason, from the cases which have been examined in the dead body, to suppose that this disease may be the cause of them: there are, however, so many other diseases which produce the same symptoms, that nothing can be ascertained. But if an introsusception is suspected, it will be proper in the mode of treatment to suppose it to be of the progressive kind.

In the treatment of this disease various methods have been proposed: bleeding, to lessen the inflammation that might be brought on, and quicksilver, to remove the cause, are the most obvious, and the means that are usually recommended.

Quicksilver would have little effect, either in one way or other, if the introsusception was downward; for it is to be supposed that it would easily make its way through the innermost contained gut, and if it should be stopped in its passage, it would, by increasing its size, become a cause (as before observed) of assisting the disease. In cases of the retrograde kind, quicksilver, assisted by the peristaltic motion, might be expected to press the introsusception back; but even under such circumstances it might get between the containing and inverted gut into the angle of reflection, and by pushing it further on increase the disease it is intended to cure.

From the account I have given of the manner in which it is produced, I should propose the following treatment in cases of progressive introsusception.

Everything that can increase the action of the intestine downwards is to be particularly avoided, as tending to increase the peristaltic motion of the outer containing gut, and thus to continue the disease. Medicine can never come in contact with the outer fold, and having passed the inner, can only act on the outer below, therefore cannot immedi-

* A prolapsus ani is, in some respects, similar to an introsusception, and may possibly begin in the same way, but is continued by the action of the abdominal muscles, never by the action of the gut itself. It differs from introsusception as not being contained in a gut; for, instead of having an inclosing gut inverting itself by its own action, there is an inclosed gut protruded by the action of the abdominal muscles and the passing of the fæces through it, and the point of inversion is at the extremity of the protrusion, and as it inverts it pushes out of the body.

ately affect that portion of the outer which contains the introsusception; but we must suppose that whatever affects or comes in contact with the larger portion of the canal, so as to throw it into action, will also affect by sympathy any part that may escape such application. I should therefore advise giving vomits, with a view to invert the peristaltic motion of the containing gut, which will have a tendency to bring the intestines into their natural situation.

If this practice should not succeed, it might be proper to consider it as a retrograde introsusception, and by administering purges endeavour to increase the peristaltic motion downwards.

SUPPLEMENT TO THE PAPER UPON INTROSUSCEPTION.

By Sir Everard Home, Bart.

The following case of introsusception upwards has been communicated to me by the late Mr. Smith, surgeon at Bristol; in whose collection of morbid preparations I saw the parts, which had been removed from the dead body, and preserved in spirits. That the introsusception was upwards is sufficiently ascertained from the preparation.

The particulars of the case, as far as they came to the knowledge of Mr. Smith, who examined the body after death, were as follow:

A cabin-boy, belonging to one of the ships lying in Bristol harbour, was corrected by his master for some misconduct, at which the boy was very much exasperated, and in the heat of his passion swallowed some arsenic, which had been laid in different parts of the ship to poison rats. He was attacked with violent pain in the stomach and intestines, attended with excessive vomiting, and expired before any medical assistance could be procured.

Upon inspection of the body, the internal surface of the stomach was found inflamed to a very great degree, the inflammation extending a considerable way along the track of the small intestines, and in the ileum there was discovered an introsusception of above two inches long, formed by a portion of the lower part of the gut having been inverted, and pushed into that immediately above it.

On slitting up the intestine, to examine the introsusception more accurately, a long round worm was found coiled round the projecting introsuscepted part, and is preserved in that situation in the preparation.

The circumstances under which the round worm was found determines the kind of introsusception, since I have observed that species of worm more commonly in the upper portion of the small intestines, in which situation having been disturbed by the effects of the arsenic, it had consequently moved, to get at a greater distance from the poison. It is likewise probable, from the coming on of inflammation, that vomiting, an immediate effect of the poison, by which the peristaltic motion was inverted, and the introsusception produced, had been followed by a contrary action, or disposition to purging, by which the worm being hurried along till it came to the introsuscepted part, was there stopped, and in the endeavour to extricate itself had twined round the projecting part, in which situation it died. If the introsusception had been downwards, the worm could not have been in that situation.

It is probable that if the boy had outlived the immediate effects of the arsenic, and the peristaltic motion had perfectly recovered itself, the introsusception would have been by that means unfolded.

AN ACCOUNT OF MR. HUNTER'S METHOD OF PERFORMING THE OPERATION FOR THE CURE OF THE POPLITEAL ANEURISM[a].

By SIR EVERARD HOME, Bart.

[*From the Transactions of a Society for the Improvement of Medical and Chirurgical Knowledge, Vol. I., p.* 138. 1793.]

THE popliteal aneurism being a disease which frequently occurs and generally proves fatal, unless some means are taken to prevent it, we cannot be surprised that it has attracted the attention and called forth the exertions of the ablest surgeons in this country to discover some method of cure.

Experience has shown that all the modes hitherto practised are exceedingly precarious, being rarely attended with success, and the death of the patient being commonly a consequence of a failure of the operation: a circumstance which has led some surgeons of great eminence to prefer the amputation of the limb in all such cases.

Mr. Hunter, who has repeatedly performed the operation for the aneurism, finding that it in general fails, and having likewise observed that the removal of a limb so high up, from a person in health, seldom succeeds in preserving life, and when it does, leaves the patient disabled, was excited to consider this disease with more than ordinary attention. The result has been a mode of practice that appears to possess many advantages over those hitherto recommended, and to be an improvement in the practical part of surgery; at least it is from this idea being strongly impressed on my mind that I am induced to communicate it to this Society, as Mr. Hunter is too much engaged to permit his taking that task upon himself.

An aneurism is a preternatural dilatation of a portion of an artery, and in general it is a very small part of the arterial coats which is thus affected. The dilatation is commonly on one side only, and when once begun gradually enlarges, from the force of the heart propelling the blood against the dilated part. Thus in time a sac is formed, which being in some measure out of the direct course of the circulation, the blood, where it is at the greatest distance from the channel of the artery, coagulates

[a] [Mr. Hunter's claim to the merit of this discovery has been fully vindicated in the course of his Life. Vol. I. p. 96. See also the description to Pl. XXIV. fig. 1 and 2; and the London Medical Journal, vol. ix.]

and forms layers or strata upon the inside of this sac. As the enlargement of the sac depends entirely on the force with which the blood is acted on by the heart, it does not, as at first, continue to swell out at right angles from the side of the artery, but is increased in a diagonal line between that and the course of the artery itself, from the force of the blood being applied in that direction; so that the sac is protruded along the outside of the artery, and by its pressure upon it obliterates, in many instances, the lower orifice, which communicates with the artery, and produces a total stagnation of the blood in the sac.

If the coats of an artery are examined in the commencement of this disease, the first appearance is a loss of the natural lustre and transparency of its internal membrane, that becoming opake, afterwards thicker, acquiring a leather-like appearance; and when the sac becomes larger the coats retain no longer a resemblance to those of an artery, but have more that of a membranous bag, communicating laterally with the artery by a rounded orifice, of different sizes, the margin of which resembles the internal membrane of an artery, in a thickened state; but beyond that gradually degenerates into a membranous substance.

The popliteal aneurism, which we are at present to consider, is the disease above mentioned, affecting the trunk of the popliteal artery, which runs down between the two hamstrings of the thigh. From the situation of the tumour, on whatever side of the artery the dilatation is produced, it will be distinctly felt in the hollow between the hamstrings, and will be readily ascertained by a pulsation to be felt in every part of the tumour: it seems to be one of the most frequent situations of aneurism; and though it may be difficult to ascertain whether it occurs so commonly as in the aorta itself, it is certainly found oftener in this artery than in any other branch which the aorta sends off[a]. This circum-

[a] [The following table*, from Mr. Hodgson's Treatise on the Diseases of Arteries and Veins, p. 87, exhibits the comparative frequency of aneurisms in the different arteries of the body:—

	Males.	Females.	Total.
Of the ascending aorta, the arteria innominata, and the arch of the aorta	16	5	21
Arch of the descending aorta	7	1	8
——— carotid artery	2	...	2
——— subclavian and axillary arteries	5	...	5
——— inguinal arteries	12	...	12
——— femoral and popliteal arteries	14	1	15
	56	7	63

* [This table does not include aneurisms arising from wounded arteries, or aneurisms from anastomosis.]

stance, as far as I know, has not hitherto been accounted for, and what is rather curious, in many recent instances of this disease, the patients have been coachmen and postilions*. The popliteal aneurism has been in general supposed to arise from a weakness in the coats of the artery, independent of the presence of disease: if this were true, we might reasonably conclude that, except in the part preternaturally dilated, the vessel remained in a sound state, which would naturally suggest the mode of practice generally recommended, viz. opening the sac, tying up the artery above and below it, leaving the bag to suppurate, and afterwards heal up like any common sore.

Mr. Hunter finding an alteration of structure in the coats of the artery previous to its dilatation, and that the artery immediately above the sac seldom unites when tied up in the operation for the aneurism, so that as soon as the ligature comes away, the secondary bleeding destroys the patient, was led to conclude that a previous disease took place in the coats of the artery, in consequence of which it admitted of dilatation capable of producing aneurism. But not satisfied with the experiments on frogs, given by Haller in support of the opinion that weakness alone was sufficient to produce the dilatation, he resolved to try the result in a quadruped, which, from the vessels being very similar in their structure to those of the human subject, would be more likely to ascertain the truth or fallacy of Haller's opinion. That the experiment might have as much as possible the chances most likely to produce aneu-

* Morgagni and his friends found aneurisms of the aorta more frequently in guides, post-boys, and other persons who sit almost continually on horseback, which is attributed to the concussion and agitation.—Vide Letter xvii. Art. 18.

When we consider the popliteal artery as affected by the different positions of the leg and thigh, and the obstruction which the circulation must inevitably meet with in that artery, when the limb is bent, we see a probable reason why it should be more liable to disease than any of the other ramifications of the aorta; especially when it is found that aneurisms in the aorta itself are most frequent at the curve of that artery.

If this observation is allowed to have any weight, the reason will be evident why the disease should occur more frequently in coachmen and postilions; for their knees being almost constantly in a bent state, from the necessary exertions of their bodies in their different occupations, and from the violent motion of their horses and carriages, the circulation must often be considerably increased; while the branches immediately below the popliteal artery will be in some measure obstructed by the action of the gastrocnemii and solæi muscles, in steadying the body in the stirrup, or against the footboard of the carriage.

The unfavourable circumstances respecting the popliteal artery, do not in common life seem of themselves capable of producing disease, but when increased to a great degree, as in the occupations of coachmen and postilions. They, at the same time, from want of sufficient exercise, have their legs weaker and less healthy than the rest of the body; and the cases to be mentioned appear still further to prove, that these circumstances may produce such a state of the artery at this part, as to dispose to the formation of aneurism.

rism, the carotid artery, as being near the heart, was selected for that purpose.

Mr. Hunter having laid bare the carotid artery of a dog, for above an inch in length, having removed its external coat, and afterwards dissected off the other coats, layer after layer, till what remained was so thin that the blood was plainly to be seen through it, left the dog to himself.

In about three weeks the dog was killed and the parts examined, when it appeared that the two sides of the wound having closed upon the artery, the whole of the surrounding parts were consolidated, forming a strong bond of union, and the artery itself was neither increased nor diminished in size.

This experiment appeared very conclusive, as the coats of the artery were weakened to a much greater degree, without dilatation, than can ever happen from accident in the living body, independent of morbid affection. But it was objected, on the other hand, that the parts having been left to themselves, immediately closed upon the weakened portion of the artery, and, being cemented together by the coagulated blood, effectually secured it against any dilatation. To try the force of this objection, I made the following experiment.

I laid bare the femoral artery of a dog, about two inches below Poupart's ligament, for about an inch in length, and dissected off the coats, till the hæmorrhage from the vasa vasorum was considerable, and the circulating blood was distinctly seen through the internal membrane of the artery. The hæmorrhage soon stopped by exposure, the surface was wiped dry, and afterwards covered with a dossil of lint, to prevent the sides of the wound from uniting. The dog continued very well, and the wound healed up from the bottom; after six weeks the dog was killed, and the artery was injected, that it might be examined with greater accuracy. It was not perceptibly enlarged or diminished, and its coats at this part had recovered their natural thickness and appearance.

The results of these experiments confirmed Mr. Hunter in his opinion that the artery, in cases of aneurism, is in a diseased state, and led him to believe that the disease often extends along the artery for some way from the sac; and that the cause of failure in the common operation arises from tying a diseased artery, which is incapable of union, in the time necessary for the separating of the ligature.

The femoral and popliteal arteries are portions of the same trunk, presenting themselves on different sides of the thigh, and are readily come at in either situation; but where the artery is passing from the one side to the other, it is more buried in the surrounding parts, and cannot be exposed without some difficulty.

In performing the operation for the popliteal aneurism, especially when the tumour is large, the ligature is commonly applied on the artery at that part where it emerges from the muscles. This mode of performing the operation will be found inadequate, if the disease of the artery extends above the sac; for if the artery should afterwards give way, there will not be a sufficient length of vessel remaining to allow of its being again secured in the ham. To follow the artery up, through the insertion of the triceps muscle, to get at a portion of it where it is sound, becomes a very disagreeable part of the operation; and to make an incision upon the fore part of the thigh, to get at and secure the femoral artery, would be breaking new ground: a thing to be avoided, if possible, in all operations.

Mr. Hunter, from having made these observations, was led to propose, that in this operation the artery should be taken up in the anterior part of the thigh, at some distance from the diseased part, so as to diminish the risk of hæmorrhage, and admit of the artery being more readily secured, should any such accident happen. The force of the circulation being thus taken off from the aneurismal sac, the progress of the disease would be stopped; and he thought it probable, that if the parts were left to themselves, the sac, with its contents, might be absorbed, and the whole of the tumour removed, which would render any opening into the sac unnecessary.

Upon this principle Mr. Hunter performed the operation at St. George's Hospital.

The patient was a coachman, forty-five years of age; he was admitted into the hospital in December 1785, with a popliteal aneurism, which he had first perceived three years previous to his admission, and had observed it gradually to increase during the whole of that period. It was so large as to distend the two hamstrings laterally, and make a very considerable rising between them; the pulsation was very distinct, and to be felt on every side of the tumour. The leg and foot of that side were so swelled as to be much thicker than the other, and were of a mottled brown colour; the swelling was not of the œdematous kind, but felt firm and brawny, probably from the extravasation of coagulable lymph; the leg retained its natural shape, excepting that it was larger. Previous to performing the operation, a tourniquet was applied upon the upper part of the thigh, but not tightened, that the parts might be left as much in their natural situation as possible.

The operation was begun by making an incision on the anterior and inner part of the thigh, rather below its middle, which incision was continued obliquely across the inner edge of the sartorius muscle, and made large, to give room for the better performing of whatever might be thought necessary in the course of the operation. The fascia which covers the artery was then laid bare about three inches in length, after which the artery itself was plainly felt. A slight incision, about an inch long, was then made through this fascia, along the side of the vessel, and the fascia dissected off; by this means the artery was exposed. Having disengaged the artery from its lateral connections by the knife, and from the other adhering parts by the help of a thin spatula, a double ligature was passed behind it, by means of an eyed probe. The doubling of the ligature brought through by the probe, was cut so as to form two separate ligatures. The artery was now tied by both these ligatures, but so slightly as only to compress the sides together. A similar application of ligature was made a little lower. The reason for having four ligatures was to compress such a length of artery as might make up for the want of tightness, it being wished to avoid great pressure on the vessel at any one part. The ends of the ligatures were carried directly out at the wound, the sides of which were now brought together, and supported by sticking-plaster and a linen roller, that they might unite by the first intention.

The limb was found, some hours after the operation, not only to retain its natural heat, but even to be warmer than the other leg. The second day after the operation the brawny firmness of the leg was considerably diminished, it was become soft, loose, and a good deal smaller, and the aneurismal tumour had lost more than one third of its size.

Nothing could show more plainly the action of the absorbents than the change the leg had undergone in so short a time; the diminution of the tumour probably arising from the fluid blood which it contained having passed into collateral branches, or into the tibial artery.

The fourth day, on the removal of the dressings, the edges of the wound were found united through its whole length, excepting where prevented by the ligatures; there was neither pain nor tumefaction in the part; but the aneurismal tumour was the same as on the second day.

On the ninth day after the operation there was a considerable discharge of blood from the part where the ligatures passed out; a tourniquet was therefore applied on the artery above, which stopped the bleeding; and although the tourniquet was taken off a few hours after, no blood followed. The head of a roller was then placed upon the wound, in the direction of the artery, and over that the tourniquet, which was not, however, tightened more than was thought sufficient to take off the impetus of the blood in that portion of the artery.

On the tenth day appearances were much the same, only that between the compress and the knee there appeared a little fulness, like beginning inflammation. On the eleventh day this was gone off, and on the fifteenth some of the ligatures came away, followed by a small discharge of matter, the tumour in the ham being lessened. On the seventeenth day the parts surrounding the aneurismal tumour were more reduced and pliable, so that it was distinctly to be felt.

About the latter end of January 1786, six weeks after the operation, the patient went out of the hospital, the tumour at that time being somewhat lessened, and rather firmer to the feel. He was ordered to come to the hospital once every week, and, in the mean time, to make some degree of pressure, by application of a compress and bandage, with a view to excite the absorbents to action, which in most cases has a good effect.

About the middle of February the tumour had decreased, and was become still firmer. March the 8th the wound, which had cicatrized, broke out again, and the patient was taken into the hospital. About the 8th of April some of the remaining thread of the ligature came away, and an inflammation appeared upon the upper part of the thigh. In the middle of May a small abscess broke at some distance from the old cicatrix, at which opening some matter was discharged, but no pieces of ligature were observed. Several small threads were, at different times, discharged from the old sore, and the swelling subsided; but the thigh soon swelled again to a greater size than before, attended with considerable pain. In the beginning of July, a piece of ligature, about one inch in length, came away, after which the swelling went off entirely, and he left the hospital the 8th of July, at which time there remained no appearance of tumour in the ham, he being in every respect well.

After leaving the hospital the man returned to his usual occupation of driving a hackney coach, and being, from the nature of his employment, much exposed to cold, in March 1787 he was seized with a fever of the remittent kind, which carried him off. He had not made any complaint of the limb on which the operation had been performed from the time of his leaving the hospital.

He died on the 1st of April, 1787, fifteen months after the operation, and leave was procured, with some trouble and considerable expense, to examine the limb seven days after death, at which time it was entirely free from putrefaction.

The cicatrix on the anterior part of the thigh was scarcely discernible, but the parts under it felt hard. The ham had no appearance of tumour, and was to the eye exactly like that of the other limb; there was, however, a solid tumour perceptible to the touch, filling up the hollow between the two angles of the thigh-bone.

The femoral artery and vein were taken out above the giving off the branch called profunda, and a little below the division into the arteriæ tibiales and interossea. The arteries and veins that were pervious being injected, the whole was carefully dissected.

The femoral artery was impervious from its giving off the arteria profunda as low as the part included in the ligature, and at that part there was an ossification for about an inch and an half along the course of the artery, of an oval form, the rim of which was solid, becoming thinner towards the centre, and not bony, but ligamentous. Below this part the femoral artery was pervious down to the aneurismal sac, and contained blood, but did not communicate with the sac itself, having become impervious just at the entrance.

What remained of the aneurismal sac was somewhat larger than a hen's egg, but more oblong, and a little flattened, extending along the artery below for some way, the blood pressing with greater force in that direction, and distending that part so as in some measure to give the appearance of a separate bag. The sac was perfectly circumscribed, not having the smallest remains of the lower orifice into the popliteal artery; whether this arose from the artery being pressed upon by the inferior portion of the sac, as appears to be the case in common, or was in consequence of the sac contracting after the operation, I will not pretend to determine; but it contained a solid coagulum of blood, which adhered to its internal surface. A section made of this coagulum appeared to be composed of concentric lamellæ, uniform in colour and consistence.

The popliteal artery, a little way below the aneurismal sac, was joined by a small branch, very much contracted, which must have arisen either from the profunda, or the trunk of the femoral artery. About two inches below the sac, the popliteal gave off, or divided into the tibiales.

The profunda was of the usual size, but a good deal ossified for some length after leaving the femoral artery; the two tibials, where they go off from the popliteal, were in the same state.

The trunk of the femoral vein, where it passed along the side of the tumour, must have been obliterated, for at this part it appeared to send off three equal-sized branches, passing over different parts of the aneurismal sac: these must have been dilated branches, none of them having the course which the trunk of the vein should have pursued.

These appearances throw some light upon the changes which took place in the limb after the operation. The ligature upon the femoral artery impeded the passage of the blood into the sac so much as to allow its contents to coagulate, and render the opening into it from the artery impervious. By this a stop was only put to the increase of the tumour; its reduction to the size met with in the dead body, must have been the effect of absorption.

The conclusion to be drawn from the above account appears a very important one, viz. that simply taking off the force of the circulation from the aneurismal artery, is sufficient to effect a cure of the disease, or at least to put a stop to its progress, and leave the parts in a situation from which the actions of the animal œconomy are capable of restoring them to a natural state.

In confirmation of the cure of aneurism depending on taking off the force of the circulation, I shall mention a case of aneurism that recovered without an operation, and in which the mode of recovery depended upon the same principle.

The aneurism was in the femoral artery, and the swelling appeared upon the anterior part of the thigh, a little above the middle, extending upwards nearly to Poupart's ligament; an attempt was made, by compressing the artery above the tumour, by means of an instrument somewhat resembling a steel truss, to give the blood in the sac a chance of coagulating, and by that means put a stop to the progress of the disease. But, from the pain which it occasioned, every attempt to make a permanent compression on the artery proved ineffectual. The tumour increased to a very considerable size, a great degree of inflammation and swelling took place in the sac and common integuments, and mortification appeared to be coming on the skin. While in this state no pulsation could be felt in the tumour, or the artery immediately above it, so that the steps preceding mortification had taken place*, which put a stop to the dilatation of the sac, and all its consequences. From the time the pulsation in the sac stopped, the inflammation and swelling subsided, although very slowly; and as the tumour diminished it became firm and solid, and the patient got perfectly well.

It appears from these cases that surgeons have laid too much stress upon the supposed necessity of large collateral branches, to insure the success of this operation: an opinion which must have arisen from anatomical knowledge, rather than observations made from practice.

The second time Mr. Hunter performed this operation was upon a trooper about forty years of age.

A tourniquet having been loosely applied upon the thigh, the operation was begun by a longitudinal incison through the integuments, and the artery and vein were exposed, as in the former case, but not taken up with a number of ligatures, for nothing appeared to have been gained by such practice, and the bad effects of it were obvious in the progress

* On examining the bodies of those who die in consequence of mortifications, the artery leading to the mortified part is completely stopped up with a firm coagulum for several inches in length; this must precede the mortification, and seems intended to prevent hæmorrhage.—*From Mr. Hunter's Lectures.*

of the cure; they were included in one strong ligature, sufficiently tight to prevent the pulsation in the sac without injuring the coats of the vessels. The ends of the ligature were brought out at the wound, which was in this case dressed from the bottom. The advantages proposed by this treatment were, to be able to see the progress of the cure, and to come readily at the artery, if any unfavourable circumstance occurred, since the abscesses in the former case were suspected to have arisen from the mode of healing.

After the operation, the superficial veins of the leg became exceedingly turgid and numerous, and the limb, although warm, became rather less so than the other, particularly the foot.

The next day the leg was swelled, and the heat 12° lower than the other; the second day it exceeded the other 5°; and on the fourth day the two limbs were equally warm: the patient was free from fever.

On the fourteenth day the ligature came away, and the torniquet was loosely applied, as a precaution against bleeding; the sartorius muscle was a good deal enlarged, and covered the passage down to the artery, so as to prevent the matter from having a free discharge, a good deal being confined behind it, and with difficulty squeezed out at each dressing.

On the nineteenth day there was a hæmorrhage from behind the muscle, the swelling of which rendered it nearly as difficult to come at the vessel, as if the parts had healed by the first intention: the bleeding was stopped by applying pressure, after having lost about ten or twelve ounces.

On the twentieth there was a slight bleeding, which was readily stopped: yet five hours afterwards the femoral artery gave way, and he lost about one pound of blood before the tourniquet was applied. The artery was laid bare, and tied a little higher up, the patient being very weak and low: in this state he continued till the twenty-third day without bleeding, when it bled again from a small vessel. On the twenty-sixth, a considerable hæmorrhage having taken place, he became faint, then delirious, had vomiting with hiccough, and died the same day.

Upon examining the limb, sinuses were discovered, both upwards and downwards, in the direction of the artery and sartorius muscle, besides smaller ones in different directions.

In this case the bad consequences and death of the patient do not appear to have arisen from the operation, but were entirely the result of the mode of treatment afterwards, as will appear from the following cases.

The third patient operated upon by Mr. Hunter was a postilion, thirty-five years old. Compression upon the femoral artery was attempted, but the pain was so great that it could not be continued.

In performing the operation only one ligature was used, and the parts healed by the first intention.

On the seventh day after the operation the first dressings were removed, and a good deal of matter came out by the side of the ligature. On the fourteenth the ligature came away, and in four weeks the wound healed.

The sac in the ham, from being chafed previous to the operation, burst at this time, but healed up like any other sore, and at the end of three months he was perfectly recovered.

Mr. Hunter's fourth patient was a coachman, thirty-six years old.

The tumour in the ham was not very large, and situated lower down than usual, the whole leg being swelled, and the veins turgid. The pain he complained of was exceedingly violent, but being in a very bad state of health an operation was not thought advisable, and gentle pressure on the tumour was attempted; but, from the pain it occasioned, the operation was had recourse to, as the only chance of saving his life, although, from the irritable state in which he then was, even that seemed a forlorn hope.

In performing the operation the vein was not included in the ligature; but in other respects it was similar to the former[a].

Immediately after the operation the limb was benumbed, and continued so for some time, which was singular, as the nerve had not been included. It became, on the same day, four or five degrees hotter than the other leg, and continued so for the first fourteen days, when the temperature became the same as that of the other limb.

The sixth day the first dressings were removed, and the skin was united everywhere except at the passage of the ligature. It remained in this state till the twenty-first, when the cicatrix inflamed and ulcerated, with a sloughy appearance, and hardness up the thigh.

On the twenty-ninth day the ligature came away; the sore now put on a better appearance, suppuration took place where the hardness had been in the course of the artery, and the parts became softer, the discharge gradually diminished, and in the seventh week the wound was healed.

But it did not continue so: for in three days an inflammation took place, and an abscess formed, and burst at the cicatrix, which also healed up.

---

[a] [If from this expression we are to infer that the artery and vein were included in the same ligature in the other cases, it readily accounts for the troublesome effects which ensued in those operations.]

About the end of the tenth week he was attacked with a very severe remitting fever, which lasted fourteen days, and left him much reduced; but in the fourteenth week he was so far recovered as to leave the hospital, and go into the country for the recovery of his health.

The fifth patient upon whom Mr. Hunter performed this operation was Joseph Caswell, aged forty-two, a man not accustomed to horse exercise or any mode of life which could in the least assist in producing the disease. The aneurism was in the ham of the left leg.

In performing the operation the artery alone was included in a strong single ligature, and the wound was healed by the first intention, leaving a passage for the ligature. The local inflammation was extremely small, and consequently attended with little sympathetic fever. The ligature came away the eleventh day, and in five weeks he went into the country, able to walk with a stick, the wound perfectly healed.

In this case the heat of the two legs was carefully examined twice a day, from the second to the ninth after the operation, and the limb operated upon was uniformly colder than the other.

He came to town six months after the operation, and said that the left leg was fully as strong as the right, but when exposed to cold he was more sensible of its effects upon that leg. About two months after the operation he had a violent pain in the upper part of the left foot, similar to what is felt when a nerve is pressed: this lasted for about six weeks, and afterwards went entirely off. As no nerve was included in the ligature, this affection probably arose from the nerve in its passage through the consolidated parts being deprived of its natural freedom. There was a small tumour, the remains of the aneurismal sac, very distinctly to be felt in the ham, but without pulsation, and to the feel perfectly solid.

The following case was operated upon by Mr. Lynn, surgeon of the Westminster Hospital, in the same manner as above mentioned; and the account of the operation is given in his own words:—

"Samuel Smart, a hackney-coachman, twenty-five years of age, had a popliteal aneurism, for which I performed the operation in the following manner. I made an incision down to the femoral artery, a little below the middle of the thigh, and having separated the artery from the contiguous parts, I passed under it, by means of an eyed probe, a broad ligature, which was tied so as to cut off all communication with the tumour, and the lips of the wound were brought together and retained by sticking-plaster, and the patient put to bed: this leg was rather colder than the other, and ordered to be fomented. The next day he was free from pain, and the limb was warmer than the other.

"On the fourth the dressings were removed, and the parts were found united, except at the ligature.

"On the thirteenth the ligature came away, and in the course of the month the whole was healed, and the patient soon afterwards perfectly recovered. WILLIAM LYNN."

This operation of Mr. Hunter's having succeeded in the first instance, surgeons of different hospitals were led to adopt it, but with some variation, according to their own judgment and the circumstances of the respective cases. These I did not introduce in the order in which they took place; for not being performed exactly in the same manner, they would have interrupted the regular series of those cases above related. But I shall now give them either in the words of the surgeons who performed the operations, or as correctly as I can from having myself been an eye-witness; and although they were not attended with success, that circumstance will not be found to affect the propriety of the mode of performing this operation which has been recommended above.

In a case of aneurism of the femoral artery, the operation was performed by Mr. Birch, surgeon to St. Thomas's Hospital, who relates the history as follows:

"John Lewis, a negro, aged forty-three, received a blow on the anterior part of the right thigh; about a month after he perceived a small tumour, which gradually increased, and his own expression was that he could feel it thump, thump.

"As the tumour enlarged, he came to London for advice, applied at St. Thomas's Hospital, on Thursday, the 26th of October, and was directly admitted. On examination I found a large tumour, extending within two inches of Poupart's ligature upwards, and occupying two thirds of the thigh: a pulsation could be felt, and there was no doubt of the disease being an aneurism of the femoral artery.

"I directed seven ounces of blood to be taken from the arm, and an opiate to be given at night; the patient rested well, and the next day a consultation was held, in which it was proposed to perform an operation, and endeavour to pass a ligature round the femoral artery, giving the patient the chance of nourishing the limb by the arteria profunda and other anastomising vessels.

"On Friday, the 3rd of November, it was determined to perform the operation. Mr. Cline undertook to compress the artery as it passes through Poupart's ligament, which he easily effected with a hard compress, in the shape of a T, with a broad basis.

"It was agreed, previous to the operation, that an incision should be carried in a semilunar form round the upper part of the aneurismal sac, in order to make room for the longitudinal incision necessary to dissect down to the artery. This was accordingly done, and the integuments raised, so as to make room to feel for the pulsation of the artery; some portion of cellular membrane and lymphatic glands were necessarily dissected and removed. With my fingers I then separated the muscular fibres, and tore away the connecting parts till the artery could be plainly felt in pulsation: it was then necessary to divide a part of the fascia covering the artery, which was done by carrying the back of the knife on Mr. Cline's nail, while his finger pressed upon the naked artery; after which the finger and thumb could surround and compress the vessel: an eye-probe, armed with a strong flat ligature, was then pushed through the cellular membrane, and carried under the artery. This being effected, we had such command of the vessel as to be able to strip it down, and pass another ligature somewhat lower. This last ligature was then tied, the first being left loose, to secure us against accident.

"The threads being separated and secured, the wound was lightly dressed, the tumour left in its natural situation, and the patient put to bed, with the loss of only four or five ounces of blood during the operation. No pulsation could be perceived in the tumour after the ligature was tied.

"On Saturday, November 4th, he had slept well, was easy, and there was sufficient warmth in the extremity to assure me of some circulation. On the 5th, the discharge from the wounded lymphatics was so abundant as to make it necessary to remove the superficial dressings; the tumour was rather softer to the touch, and the skin about the apex of it began to shrivel.

"The discharge of lymph continued till the 9th, and then the wound began to digest; affording, however, a very small quantity of pus. The tumour grew thinner at one point, and seemed as if disposed to ulcerate the integuments. This day I passed a bleeding-ligature round the leg, just below the knee, and the veins tumefied sufficiently to have bled freely if they had been punctured.

"10th. He was feverish in the evening.

"11th. He had stools from some laxatives I had directed and was better.

"12th. The tumour was very thin at one part, and a fluctuation evidently to be felt. The limb was warm and moveable, but the patient was feverish, and delirious at night. A decoction of bark, with a sedative bolus, was directed for him; but he would not take them.

"13th. The wound looked florid, and afforded good pus; the patient was feverish and delirious; the tumour was threatening to burst. This day he took his medicines.

"14th. He became sensible, but was languid and hot; the tumour burst, and discharged serum and grumous blood; he fainted; the dressings were not disturbed, he slept composedly; fainted again about six o'clock in the evening, and expired. I saw him at seven, when the limb was still warm; I removed the dressings, and found a small stream of fresh arterial blood, which had issued from the wound.

" It appears probable that if the patient had applied for relief before the tumour was so much enlarged, the operation might have succeeded, as we should then have been able to have tied the sound artery so much lower down. J. BIRCH."

The body was examined the morning after the patient's death by Mr. Cline.

" The integuments on the middle of the tumour were mortified. The blood contained in the tumour was very putrid, and the greater part of it fluid, it appearing to have been dissolved by putrefaction.

" Water injected by the external iliac artery escaped freely from the wound at the ligature where the artery was open, which appeared to have ulcerated at that part.

" In laying open the artery from the ligature to the heart, its internal surface appeared of a bright red. This appearance lessened at the curvature of the aorta, yet it was very evident in its semilunar valves.

" The arteria profunda, which passed off from the femoral artery rather less than half an inch above the ligature, was also inflamed within. There were near two inches of the femoral artery between the ligature and the aneurismal sac, the internal surface of which was of the usual white colour; from this a membranous-like substance could be peeled off, that seemed to resemble coagulable lymph.

" The opening where the artery passed out of the aneurismal sac was near three inches below the part where it entered. In opening this part of the artery from the sac to the ham it appeared quite sound, and of its natural colour. H. CLINE."

This mode of operating was adopted by Mr. Pott in a case of popliteal aneurism in St. Bartholomew's Hospital, which operation having been the object of medical attention for some time, I shall give a brief account of it, as I was present at the time it was performed.

Mr. Pott began the operation by making an incision about five inches in length upon the posterior part of the thigh, through the common integuments, a little higher than the tumour, and in the direction of the thigh, between the two hamstrings; he then dissected down to the vessels at the upper end of the incision, which being there deep seated, proved both tedious and difficult. Having come to the vessels, a double ligature was passed, and the two portions tied separately, at nearly half an inch distance. The depth of the incision made it difficult for any but the operator and those immediately assisting him to see what was included in the ligature, and at the time the popliteal artery was supposed to be secured by it. The wound was dressed up in the common way.

The second day after the operation a pulsation was felt in the tumour, which afterwards enlarged so much that Mr. Pott amputated the limb.

It is said that the aneurism appeared, upon an examination of the limb, to have been in an anastomising branch, not in the trunk of the artery.

The following remarks upon this operation will tend in some measure to illustrate the method recommended and practised by Mr. Hunter.

The mode of taking up the artery in the ham must be always unfavourable to the future success of the operation, if either the artery itself should be diseased, or if the tumour, by being so contiguous to the violence done in the operation, should be affected by the consequent inflammation, which seems to have been the case in Mr. Pott's operation, as I understand two abscesses were formed close to the sides of the sac.

Had the aneurism been situated in an anastomising branch of the popliteal artery, given off below the ligature, there should have been no pulsation afterwards in the tumour; and were it in a branch going off above the ligature, the pulsation in the tumour should have continued immediately after the operation, and should have been increased by it, neither of which effects appear really to have taken place, which throws a doubt upon the situation of the aneurism if the popliteal artery was rendered impervious by the compression of the ligature.

Mr. Cline, surgeon to St. Thomas's Hospital, performed the operation for the popliteal aneurism in the following manner, at which I was present; and although not exactly as recommended by Mr Hunter, it was very nearly so. The particulars of the case I have not received from Mr. Cline, but have taken them from my own observation, and the information of gentlemen who attended the patient, and were present at the examination after death.

The patient was a sailor, who came into St. Thomas's Hospital to undergo the operation for the popliteal aneurism.

Mr. Cline made a longitudinal incision on the anterior part of the thigh, and having laid bare the artery, passed, by means of a tin instrument, a double tape, about one inch broad, behind the artery, the two pieces of tape lying one over the other; the piece of tin which conducted the tape was cut off, and a cork nearly an inch long was laid upon the artery, and confined to its situation by means of the upper tape, producing in this way a sufficient pressure upon the vessel included between the ligature and cork to stop the circulation, and consequently the pulsation in the tumour in the ham; the other portion of tape was left loose. The intention of securing the artery in this way was to compress the sides of the vessel together, and produce an union without ulceration.

The patient went on very well, and the ninth day the tapes were removed, and everything seemed to be going on very favourably, when the patient was attacked by a fever (which was supposed to be caught from another patient in the same ward), of which he died.

Upon examining the state of the limb after death, it was found that ulceration had taken place through the whole extent of the artery included in the tape, and sinuses were formed both upwards and downwards, in the course of the thigh, to some distance.

I cannot conclude this paper without observing that it is seldom in giving an account of a new operation we are able to collect materials sufficient to render it so satisfactory as the present, having in our possession not only the successful and unsuccessful cases, but also an account of the appearances after death, under both circumstances, so that the causes of failure are rendered evident in those instances in which it did not succeed, and the means that are likely to insure future success are clearly pointed out.

The operation is in itself simple; it requires but a short time in the performance, and produces little, if any, affection of the constitution; but its advantages are more clearly seen by contrasting it with the common mode of operating for the popliteal aneurism. This is by exposing the sac in the ham through its whole extent, laying it open, scooping out the blood, searching for the two orifices leading into it, and taking up the artery with a ligature both above and below the sac. When this operation is over there remains a large deep-seated sore, composed of parts not perfectly in a natural state, and in a most disadvantageous situation, which sore is to suppurate, granulate, and heal, a process that is not soon performed, and which must leave a stiff knee for some time afterwards. Yet this is considering the operation in the most favourable view, since there is always a risk, from the artery being diseased so close to the sac, of the patient dying from a secondary bleeding; and when that does not happen there is still some danger of not being able to support the constitution during the healing of so large a sore, under circumstances so very unfavourable.

It is in comparison with this operation, the only one before in use, that the present improvement is to be considered, and it is in this view that I have thought it deserving the attention of the Society.

I cannot close this account without inserting the following case, in addition to those already stated, in favour of this operation. I have received it just time enough to give it a place, as the paper was in the press before it came to hand, and feel myself obliged to Mr. Earle for his readiness in communicating it.

"Hanover-Square, March 10, 1792.

"SIR,

"At your request I send you some account of the following case, and am Your most obedient Servant,

"JAMES EARLE.

"John Smith, about fifty years of age, was received into St. Bartholomew's Hospital on account of a fever. After having been under the care of the physician some time, he complained of a swelling and pain in his left leg, for which I was desired to visit him. He said, about six months before he had fallen from a scaffold; that his leg was caught between the rounds of a ladder, which broke his fall; that he felt immediately pain in the upper part of his leg; soon after it began to swell, and had gradually increased to its present size. On examination there appeared a large hard swelling under the heads of the gastrocnemii muscles, reaching up to the bend of the leg. A pulsation was plainly to be felt in it, and there was no doubt of its being an aneurism. It was now increasing very fast in size; the tumour, by its pressure, caused exquisite pain, all the lower part of the leg was loaded with œdematous swelling, and it became absolutely necessary to perform some operation to prevent a mortification taking place.

"Having noticed with much satisfaction the success which attended Mr. Hunter's method of tying the artery in the thigh, in a similar case, I decided in favour of that operation; but as, in the present instance, the artery appeared to be in its natural and perfect state in the ham, and in its whole course, till it reached the dilatation below the knee, I preferred taking it up in that part, rather than to tie it in the middle of the thigh, under the sartorius muscle, though it lies there more superficial, and more easily to be got at; because I thought the chance of the circulation being carried on was equal, if not greater, and if it should fail, and symptoms should occur to create a suspicion of an impending mortification, there might be an opportunity of removing the limb above the ligature, which would be impracticable if the artery was tied in the middle of the thigh.

"Jan. 28, 1792. The patient being laid on his face, and the tourniquet loosely applied, I made an incision about five inches long, in the direction of the artery, within those tendons which compose the inner ham-string. I then gradually separated the cellular substance; in doing this the nerve was exposed, which ran in its usual course, external to the artery, and much more superficial. In finding the artery some difficulty occurred, on account of the tumefaction of all the parts, affected by their vicinity to the aneurism, and from the imperceptibility of pulsation in the artery till it was actually laid bare: however, having discovered it in its usual situation near the bone, and in its natural undilated state, I passed a ligature round it, about two inches above the tumour. I now again examined, and being convinced that the artery was included alone in the ligature, I gradually made it tight, till I felt a pulsation above it, and none below, when I desisted, concluding that any pressure beyond this degree would be useless and dangerous.

"I will just observe here, that I found the common aneurismal needle with a handle very inconvenient, and would recommend in this case, where the artery lies so deep, a blunt semicircular needle, with the eye about half an inch from the end, without any handle.

"The wound was closed in the usual manner, and the edges brought together by sutures. On the following day the man was free from pain, the tumour much less tense or hard, and the whole leg greatly unloaded. No perceptible alteration in the heat of the limb could be remarked; when the current of blood was obstructed in the superficial veins by pressure, on its removal they immediately again became turgid, and in short every appearance indicated a continuance of perfect circulation.

"On the fifteenth day succeeding the operation the ligature came away, the limb was soft and unloaded, and the incision nearly healed; at the distance of six weeks there remains a small tumour, with some perceptible fluctuation. The patient cannot perfectly extend his leg; but is able to walk with the assistance of crutches."

ADDITIONAL CASES TO ILLUSTRATE MR. HUNTER'S METHOD OF PERFORMING THE OPERATION FOR THE CURE OF THE POPLITEAL ANEURISM.

BY SIR EVERARD HOME, BART., F.R.S.

Read June 5, 1798.

[*From the Transactions of a Society for the Improvement of Medical and Chirurgical Knowledge, Vol. II. p.* 235. 1800.]

IN a former paper published in the first volume of the Transactions of this Society, I stated the reasons that induced the late Mr. Hunter to propose this operation, and mentioned all the cases in which it had at that time been performed, either by himself or others.

Since Mr. Hunter's death two cases have occurred in which the patients had aneurisms in both popliteal arteries, and others where the disease was only in one. In these cases this operation was performed, and the intention of the present paper is to communicate to the Society these new facts.

CASE I. John Clegg, aged 33 years, a tobacco-pipe maker, was admitted into St. George's Hospital May 29th, 1797, with two popliteal aneurisms.

It appeared that about eight weeks before his admission, while walking, he felt, for the first time, an acute pain in the calf of the right leg, extending downwards, which gradually increased. Three weeks afterwards he perceived a swelling in the ham, which enlarged, and in a week more had an evident pulsation in it: this swelling proved to be an aneurism of the popliteal artery.

The knee also swelled, and was painful. When he came into the hospital the aneurismal tumour in the right ham appeared externally through the skin, of the size of a large hen's egg: there was also at that time a small aneurism in the popliteal artery of the other leg. He had thick lips, a very red nose, and a pale complexion; and for some months past had experienced frequent bleedings from the nose.

The nature of his business obliged him to walk, upon an average, 16 or 17 miles a day, carrying pipes to his respective customers, with the greater part of whom he was compelled to drink porter, which, in the course of the day, did not amount to less than 8 or 10 pints. There seemed to have been no other particularity in his mode of life.

After he had remained in the hospital a few days, on June 9th I performed the operation of taking up the femoral artery of his right thigh. In doing this I laid bare the fascia which covers the vessels, and made an opening through it large enough to expose the whole diameter of the artery. I passed a crooked silver needle, with a rounded point, behind it, taking care not to include the vein and nerve; in this way the needle and ligature were readily brought out on the other side. The ligature was tied, and immediately the pulsation in the tumour ceased. The wound was united by slips of adhesive plaster and a bandage. About two hours after the operation he complained of considerable pain in the sac, and in the course of the femoral artery, even to the toes.

He took thirty drops of tincture of opium, which dose was repeated at bed time.

June 10th. His skin was hot, and his pulse above 100 in a minute; ten ounces of blood were drawn from the arm, and he was ordered to take the saline mixture: the blood, on standing, showed no buff. Two hours afterwards his pulse was 96 in a minute, and softer; he complained of numbness in the leg, with a tingling sensation in about the middle of the sole of the foot; the heat was the same as in the other leg.

11th. His pulse was 120 in a minute, and strong; there was little moisture on the skin, and great pain in the leg and foot.

13th. The wound was dressed for the first time since the operation; it had a healthy appearance, and the parts were united by the first intention; the tumour in the ham was somewhat diminished, while that in the other leg rather increased since the operation.

16th. He was perceptibly better; the pain in the limb was much abated: the ligature was removed. This was the 12th day from the operation.

27th. The wound was nearly cicatrized, and the aneurism in the other ham was increasing very fast; he was therefore removed from the hospital for a fortnight to reestablish his health, that he might undergo the second operation with greater security.

July 11th. He returned to have the operation performed on the other femoral artery; which at his desire was done on the same day of the week as the former operation, and exactly five weeks after it.

14th. The operation was conducted in every respect in the same manner as the preceding; and the pulsation in the tumour ceased as soon as the ligature was tied upon the artery.

15th. His pulse was 100 in a minute, and full: he passed a restless night, and complained of great pain in the limb, and a slight pulsation was felt in the aneurismal sac.

16th. The pulsation in the sac was more distinct; this I imagined arose from some collateral branch having a communication with the sac. A compression was made upon the tumour by means of a circular bandage, to prevent the influx from any collateral branch.

17th. His pulse was about 96 in a minute, strong and full; he had little sleep during the night; the pulsation in the sac was rather less than the day before. He complained of pain about the wound, but not so much in the foot as after the first operation.

18th. His pulse was 73 in a minute: the pulsation in the sac was less; he had a very good night, but now complained of considerable pain in both feet.

24th. He had a slight hæmorrhage from the wound, which was brought on by his mind being agitated in consequence of some improper treatment his wife had received: it stopped of itself, but the tourniquet was loosely applied in case of a return. He complained of heat where the ligature was made; there was no difference in the pulsation of the sac.

26th. A second hæmorrhage took place from the wound, to the amount of three or four ounces, and then stopped. His pulse was about 108 in a minute; he complained of being faint and languid. I removed the dressings, and upon endeavouring to bring away the ligature, some blood escaped from the wound, per saltum, of a florid colour, supposed to be from the rupture of a small artery; a compress was immediately applied to the part, which stopped the bleeding. I removed the compress from the ham, the pulsation in the sac being much abated; eight ounces of blood were drawn from the arm, and he took the saline mixture. The hæmorrhage returned about seven in the evening, but was immediately stopped by increasing the compression.

27th. He was very restless all night, and had acute shooting pains in the wound; the bandages were slackened.

28th. He slept well during the night, and had a greater degree of moisture on the skin, and the pains in the limb were not so violent; the dressings were removed, and the wound appeared disposed to slough; the pulsation in the sac was scarcely perceptible.

29th. His spirits were much better; there was an appearance of swelling and inflammation between the wound and the knee; the pressure was therefore removed from the artery, and applied more uniformly over the whole limb.

30th. The ligature was removed without hæmorrhage; this was the sixteenth day after the operation.

August 6th. The hæmorrhage returned at five o'clock in the morning, to the amount of four ounces; a compress was applied to the wound, and kept on by a bandage; he was very restless during the night.

8th. His pulse was 110 in a minute, and felt hard and contracted.

He was ordered to take a bolus, containing three grains of camphor, every six hours.

10th. Had a bleeding from his nose, amounting to two ounces; he was ordered to lose four ounces of blood from the arm; the dose of camphor was increased to five grains; the pulse was 108 in a minute, and quick before the bleeding, but about twenty minutes afterwards the pulse was reduced to 96 in a minute, and he complained of faintness.

14th. The tourniquet was totally removed.

16th. He felt great pain upon touching the skin of any part of the limb, but particularly at the ham.

18th. Had a very good night, and the wound was superficial, and reduced to the size of a sixpence: it was now exactly five weeks from the operation; a circular bandage was still applied, and the sore dressed with ungt. hydrarg. nitrat. and hog's lard in equal proportions; there still remained great sensibility in the skin.

26th. The pain in the limb was much abated; the leg had been fomented with tepid salt water for several days, which gave him a great deal of ease; the wound was nearly healed, and the limb admitted of motion without uneasiness.

September 18th. He was quite well.

The pulsation being felt in the aneurismal sac the evening after the femoral artery was tied, its continuance for several days, and then ceasing altogether, are circumstances so curious, that it may be right to give some explanation of them.

The only way in which the pulsation could recur in the tumour, after it had been stopped, must be by means of anastomosing branches; and if the branch which renewed the communication had its origin near the ligature, it is probable that in the progress of the cure the femoral artery became obliterated higher up than the origin of this branch, and shut it up.

The extent of the artery rendered impervious above the ligature, in the first case operated upon by Mr. Hunter, in which there was an opportunity of examining the parts after death, makes this more probable.

A case of aneurism of both popliteal arteries occurred to Mr. Joseph Harris, surgeon, at Whitehaven, in the year 1796, of which he has favoured me with the following account, as an addition to the facts in favour of Mr. Hunter's mode of operating in cases of this disease.

Case II. William Spencer, a corporal in the Cumberland militia, in the thirty-second year of his age, of a tall and muscular make, was admitted a patient into the Whitehaven Hospital in June, 1795. He had a firm inelastic swelling, extending from the middle of the left thigh down to the toes, and attended with most excruciating pain. He gave the following account of his case. Fifteen months ago he wore for two months together a pair of tight leather breeches, which made his legs swell, and become so painful that he was obliged to leave them off; after which time the swelling in the leg subsided, and he suffered no further inconvenience. About a month after this, on his return from a journey on foot of ten miles, on a very hot day, he felt uneasiness in the hams of both legs, but went to bed in good health. In the course of the night he had a very profuse sweat, and the next day he discovered a small swelling in each ham; that on the left side continued gradually to increase, and had a pulsation in it, which was sensible to the touch for many months, but afterwards was not to be distinguished; the swelling diffused itself over the limb till it arrived at its present size. Upon examining the other ham, I found an aneurismal tumour about the size of a nutmeg, which he said had remained stationary from the time of its first appearance. The left leg seemed to be too much diseased to give the smallest hopes of saving it; the limb was therefore amputated. Upon examining the parts in the amputated limb, the aneurismal sac in the ham was found to have been burst, and eleven pounds and a half of coagulated blood had been diffused among the muscles, which were in a state approaching to mortification. The stump healed kindly, and he continued well for three months, without any apparent enlargement of the aneurism in the right ham; but at the end of this time it began to increase in size, and one day, after a violent exertion on his crutches, he had considerable pain in it, with an evident increase of the swelling, which now stretched both the ham strings; there was also a diffused swelling extending over the joint of the knee. From the history of the aneurism in the other leg, there was reason to expect that this was now burst, and would go on in exactly the same way; it was therefore determined to perform the operation for the aneurism immediately according to Mr. Hunter's method: this was done on the 15th of November, 1795. The artery alone was included in a single ligature, and the skin with the other parts brought together, and retained by adhesive plaster. For about two hours after he was put to bed he complained of coldness in the foot, but on covering it with flannel it felt as warm as the leg, which was of the natural heat of the body.

On the second day the swelling of the leg was a good deal abated, and the tumour itself softer.

On the third day the swelling of the leg was entirely gone, and the tumour more diminished.

On the sixth day the dressings were removed, and the wound had healed by the first intention, except an inch at the lower part, where the ligature passed out. There had been no pain, or swelling of the parts, since the operation, and the limb continued of the natural temperature, except on the fourth day, when it was two degrees hotter by Fahrenheit's thermometer.

On the eleventh day the ligature came away, attended with a considerable discharge of matter; this continued on the twelfth: I therefore made compression on the sides of the wound throughout its whole length, by compresses and a tight roller.

On the fifteenth the discharge scarcely moistened the dressings. He was attacked with a purging, attended with disorder of the whole system and loss of appetite, which lasted for a fortnight. During this time the superficial sore remained stationary; but it was completely healed, and the patient discharged from the hospital at the end of the fifth week.

The two following Cases contain nothing remarkable; but as they were both operated on in exactly the same manner as the first Case in the present paper, they increase the number of instances in which the most simple mode of performing this operation has been attended with success. I have therefore thought that they will appear to the Society of sufficient importance to be inserted in this place.

Case III. A. B., a dragoon, near six feet high, about thirty-six years of age, came into St. George's Hospital in the year 1794, on account of a popliteal aneurism, for which I performed the operation.

In making the external incision I was desirous of keeping it in a line with the edge of the sartorius muscle, that the muscle and skin might not form a double valve, and prevent the ready discharge of any matter that should be formed, which I had found to be the case in some instances above mentioned. As soon as the artery was exposed I did not attempt to disengage it laterally, but made a small opening on each side of it, just large enough to admit the end of the instrument, conveying the ligature, which was in this way passed round the artery, the nerve and vein being pushed on one side; the ligature was secured, and the wound brought together by means of adhesive plaster.

The man had no fever; little, if any, inflammation came upon the limb; the ligature came away the twelfth day; and in three weeks he went to his own house, there being only a superficial sore on the skin, which in a week more was entirely healed.

Case IV. George Pile, thirty-five years of age, butler to His Royal Highness the Duke of Clarence, a stout man, of a sallow complexion, and a hard drinker, had been sensible of the feeling of weakness in his left leg for two or three months, when he perceived a tumour of the size of a pigeon's egg in the ham: ten weeks after he applied to Mr. Knight. The tumour had been enlarged, after a journey from Margate upon the top of a stage-coach, about a fortnight before, so that now he could not button the knee of his breeches; there was a strong and equal pulsation in every part of the tumour, which left no doubt of its being aneurismal; the leg was swelled and felt hard, the pulse was quick, and at times intermitted; his general health, however, was tolerably good. Mr. Knight proposed performing the operation according to Mr. Hunter's method; and, knowing that I had lately performed it in that way with success, requested that I would assist him. The operation was performed on the 29th of September, 1797, by Mr. Knight, nearly in the same way that I have described in the case last related: the silver needle was passed behind the artery, without including the vein or nerve, or detaching it for more than a quarter of an inch from its lateral connections; the pulsation in the ham ceased the moment the ligature upon the artery was tied. The cut edges of the wound were brought together, except where the ligature passed out. On the 30th, the pulse was full and quick; he was therefore ordered to lose ten ounces of blood. August 3rd, the dressings were for the first time removed, and the wound was found united by the first intention: a small quantity of matter was pressed out by the side of the ligature. The wound was now dressed every day, and on the 18th he was allowed to get up; the ligature was examined at each dressing, but could not be brought away without using more force than it was prudent to employ. On the 22nd, there was a slight hæmorrhage from the wound, which was readily stopped by compression. On the 30th, the ligature came away with great ease. November 11th, the wound was completely healed; the tumour in the ham was nearly gone; the patient in perfect health, and daily gaining strength, and the use of his limb.

Case V. Mr. Marshal, a gentleman about fifty years of age, consulted me, in May, 1798, on account of a popliteal aneurism. The tumour in the ham, at the time I saw it, was considerably larger than a hen's egg. After examining the case, I gave it as my opinion that an operation was absolutely necessary to prevent a fatal termination of the disease; and that the chance of recovery depended wholly on the state of the femoral artery: if that was healthy, the operation which I intended to perform would succeed; and if it was not, even amputation of the limb would fail, as the divided artery could not be made to unite.

Dr. Marshal's opinion was taken whether it was advisable to try compression upon the aneurismal tumour; this he did not approve of, and the patient determined to submit to the operation.

He walked about, and drank a pint of wine daily, till the operation was performed; although I had urged him in the strongest manner to remain perfectly quiet in a horizontal posture, and to live sparingly.

The operation was performed on the 22nd of May; I was assisted by Dr. Marshal, and Dr. Wallis was present. When the incision through the skin had exposed the sartorius muscle, it appeared unusually large, and the fascia covering the artery was got at with difficulty, and was indistinctly seen: this I attributed to the state of the muscles, induced by the exercise which the patient had continued to use.

My first attempt to secure the artery failed, from the needle passing over it, and only including a portion of the fascia. I therefore exposed the artery more completely, about an inch higher up the thigh, and surrounded it by a ligature: the pulsation in the tumour immediately ceased, and the wound was dressed as in the former cases. The leg continued colder than the other for two days, and then regained its usual heat.

On the fourth day, the dressings were removed, and the wound had a healthy appearance; at this time there was a pulsation in the tumour.

On the seventh day, he bore being moved to have his bed made, and was considered to be going on perfectly well. From some mistaken notion he now indulged himself in the use of wine, without my knowledge.

On the ninth day, he had a violent shivering fit, which was not mentioned to me; and the use of wine was, notwithstanding, persisted in.

On the tenth day, the discharge from the wound was much increased, and the thigh and leg were swelled.

On the eleventh day, there was a slight bleeding from the wound, and in the evening a similar bleeding also took place. Alarmed at this circumstance, I left an assistant with the patient. The tourniquet likewise, which had remained on the thigh, was now adjusted, in case it should be necessary to use it.

On the twelfth day, at four in the morning, a violent hæmorrhage came on, and at nine he died.

The limb was examined next day, in the presence of Dr. Marshal, Dr. Wallis, and Mr. Colthurst. The ligature was found to have included the artery without the vein, and when the artery was laid open the space embraced by the ligature was quite white, and the coats at that part so thin as to be almost transparent; and there were also several small ulcerations through the coat by which the blood had escaped: there was not the smallest union of the sides of the artery; but immediately above and below the ligature the inner membrane had an unusual red appearance.

The inner membrane had lost its usual polish, and had its surface covered with opaque white spots; the same appearance, in a less degree, was seen in the artery near the groin.

The aneurismal tumour proved to be a diseased dilatation of the popliteal artery, of an oval form, situated between the heads of the gastrocnemius muscle.

In this case the femoral artery was so much diseased that probably neither amputation nor any other operation with which we are acquainted would have been attended with success. But as that is a circumstance which rarely happens, and can never be ascertained during the person's life, it ought not to be considered as an objection to the operation, though its possible existence must always render the event somewhat uncertain.

The internal surface of the artery in the present case became inflamed, without admitting the union of its sides, as happens when the operation succeeds. This inflammation, although probably owing chiefly to the diseased state of the artery, may yet in part have been produced by the neglect of proper attention in regard to diet and rest previous to the operation, and more particularly by the indulgence in wine after it.

A CASE OF PARALYSIS OF THE MUSCLES OF DEGLUTITION, CURED BY AN ARTIFICIAL MODE OF CONVEYING FOOD AND MEDICINES INTO THE STOMACH.

Read September 21, 1790.

[*From the Transactions of a Society for the Improvement of Medical and Chirurgical Knowledge, Vol. I. p.* 182. 1793.]

DISEASES which are not mortal in themselves may often, from their secondary effects, become the cause of death; but if these secondary effects are removed, the disease frequently admits of a cure, or even ceases of itself. Thus diseases, when they attack the vital organs, may, from the nature of the parts alone, prove fatal; and this will be sooner or later, according to the particular functions of the parts diseased.

Obstructions to breathing, to the passing of the urine, to the act of swallowing, or the discharge of the fæces, will all terminate in death, if continued for a certain length of time, whatever be the nature of the disease.

Difficulty in swallowing, the subject of the present paper, may arise from a variety of causes, since an obstruction in any part of the canal leading from the mouth to the stomach will produce that complaint.

The swallowing our food is a complicated operation, and includes two different actions. The first of these conveys it into the œsophagus; the second carries it along that canal into the stomach: and the parts which perform these two actions are in themselves distinct, so that one may be obstructed or diseased while the other remains perfectly sound.

The first action is often impeded, or wholly prevented, by inflammation; but this is seldom of long continuance, and the cure is probably promoted by the patient's being obliged to abstain from food. It is also impeded by swellings in the neighbouring glands, but this will commonly be in a less degree; and where it threatens suffocation, or a total prevention of deglutition, the patient can often be relieved by an operation.

The second action is sometimes obstructed by ulcers in the œsophagus, which have a cancerous appearance; sometimes strictures in that canal, which are of a permanent nature; also spasmodic contractions, which are commonly confounded with strictures, but may, I believe, be readily distinguished both from strictures and ulcerations.

Ulcers and strictures, from being permanent diseases, in the end destroy the patient; but spasmodic contractions admit of being cured. I have known a case of this kind get well in a fortnight from the use of electricity, which had not been at all relieved by mercury, although the mouth was affected by it for a month.

There is another cause of difficulty in swallowing, which is the reverse of contraction, viz. paralysis. Whether the muscular coats of the œsophagus are ever affected by it I cannot determine; but the muscles of the pharynx have become paralytic, and the patient has died of hunger.

As this disease is only rendered dangerous from the want of a substitute for deglutition, it becomes our duty to adopt some artificial mode of conveying food into the stomach, by which the patient may be kept alive while the disease continues, and such medicines may be administered as are thought conducive to the cure.

A successful instance of this practice is given in the following Case of well-marked paralysis in the muscles of the pharynx; the relation of which is given by the patient.

John S——l, about fifty years of age, became hypochondriac and attacked by what are called nervous disorders, in consequence of anxiety of mind, brought on by various distresses. In the beginning of his complaints he felt something crack within his head, and from that period his sensations became very acute, his passions, sympathies, and aversions exceedingly strong.

December 28, 1786, while under the influence of an uncommon degree of hypochondriasis, about one o'clock in the morning, he brought up a glutinous substance from his stomach, like the white of an egg, which seemed to relieve him, but did not remove an aversion which he had taken to his relations, his children, and even to life itself, of which he was tired.

He afterwards continued affected with low spirits and pains in the head, became restless, and turned his mind to religious subjects; as these affections either increased or diminished, he had frequent and severe fits of crying.

About the 21st of February, 1790, he had a violent cold in his head, with a considerable running from the nose; and on the 7th of March, between one and two in the morning, awoke with a sense of choking, and felt soon after a numbness in the whole of his right side, together with a paralysis of the muscles of deglutition, which deprived him of the power of swallowing.

By the advice of a physician he was cupped, blistered round the throat, and electrified; he was, in the mean time, supported by nourishing clysters. March the 9th, finding no benefit from this plan, he waited upon Mr. Hunter, with a letter from Mr. Cumming, watchmaker, accompanied by Mr. Duncan the surgeon.

Mr. Hunter, considering the support of the patient, and some mode of administering medicine, to be the first object, proposed that a hollow flexible tube should be passed down into the stomach, through which he might receive nourishment and medicines; and mentioned his having an instrument of that kind, made of spiral wire, covered with gut for the purpose of injecting liquids into the stomachs of animals, which might be applied to the present case; but that Mr. Cumming was better able to assist them in getting a tube that would answer that purpose. He also recommended, when the tube was made, to inject jellies, eggs beat up with a little water, sugar, and milk, or wine, by way of food, and that the medicines might be mixed with it.

In compliance with these directions they contrived a tube, and injected into the stomach some of the above-mentioned substances twice a-day: three drams of valerian were mixed with this food, increasing the dose to six drams. Laudanum was given in the dose of forty drops by clyster, and afterwards thirty drops by the mouth; but both doses affected the head, without procuring rest. The valerian was continued till the 26th of March, at which time he had taken four ounces, and had evidently recovered a degree of sensation in his throat. Mr. Hunter was again consulted, and ordered two scruples of flour of mustard, and one dram of tincture of valerian, twice a-day: under this treatment the power of swallowing gradually returned, and on the 29th the use of the tube was no longer necessary. The natural sensation of the throat and right arm had not returned in the month of April.

The instrument made use of was a fresh eel-skin, of rather a small size, drawn over a probang; and tied up at the end where it covered the sponge, and tied again close to the sponge where it is fastened to the whalebone, and a small longitudinal slit was made into it just above this upper ligature. To the other end of the eel-skin was fixed a bladder and wooden pipe, similar to what is used in giving a clyster, only the pipe large enough to let the end of the probang pass into the bladder without filling up the passage. The probang, thus covered, was introduced into the stomach, and the food and medicines were put into the bladder, and squeezed down through the eel-skin.

The instrument did not produce irritation in the fauces or œsophagus: in such cases, the parts losing their natural sensibility, allow greater liberties to be taken with them. An eel-skin seems very well adapted for this purpose, being smooth, pliable, and readily passed into the stomach; but as cases of this kind may occur where eels cannot be procured, a portion of the gut of any small animal, as a cat or lamb, will make a very good substitute.

SOME OBSERVATIONS ON THE LOOSE CARTILAGES FOUND IN JOINTS, AND MOST COMMONLY MET WITH IN THAT OF THE KNEE.

By Sir Everard Home, Bart., from Materials furnished by Mr. Hunter.

[*From the Transactions of a Society for the Improvement of Medical and Chirurgical Knowledge, Vol. I. p.* 229. 1793.]

SUCH detached and moveable cartilages as are the subject of the following observations, are not peculiar to the joint of the knee; they occasionally occur in other joints of the body; but as they are most frequently met with in the knee, and it is in that joint they produce symptoms which render them the object of a chirurgical operation, I shall consider them more particularly when situated in that cavity.

These substances in their structure are analogous to bone, but in their external appearance bear a greater resemblance to cartilage; they are not, however, always exactly of the same structure, being in some instances softer than in others. Their external surface is smooth and polished, which, being lubricated by the synovia, allows them to be moved readily from one part of the joint to another, seldom remaining long at rest, while the limb is in motion; when they happen to be in such situations as to be pressed upon with force by the different parts of the joint, they occasion considerable pain, and materially interfere with its necessary motions.

The circumstance of their being loose, and having no remains of a visible attachment, made it difficult to form conjectures respecting their formation; and I believe that no satisfactory account of their origin had been given, till Mr. Hunter's observations threw light upon the subject. The circumstances which led him to the investigation of this subject, appear at first sight so foreign to the purpose, that they require some explanation.

In the course of his experiments and observations, instituted with a view to establish a living principle in the blood, Mr. Hunter was naturally induced to attend to the phænomena which took place when that fluid was extravasated, whether in consequence of accidental violence, or other circumstances. The first change which took place he found to be coagulation; and the coagulum thus formed, if in contact with living parts, did not produce an irritation similar to extraneous matter, nor was it absorbed and taken back into the constitution, but in many instances preserved its living principle, and became vascular, receiving branches from the neighbouring blood-vessels for its support; it afterwards underwent changes, rendering it similar to the parts to which it was attached, and which supplied it with nourishment.

In attending to cases of this kind, he found that where a coagulum adhered to a surface, which varied its position, adapting it to the motions of some other part, the attachment was necessarily diminished by the friction, rendering it in some instances pendulous, and in others breaking it off entirely. To illustrate this by an example, I shall mention an instance which occurred in the examination of a dead body. The cavity of the abdomen was opened, to examine the state of its contents, and there appeared lying upon the peritoneum a small portion of red blood, recently coagulated; this, upon examination, was found connected to the surface upon which it had been deposited, by an attachment half an inch long, and this neck had been formed before the coagulum had lost its red colour. This steeped in water, so as to become white, appeared like a pendulous tumour.

From this case it became easy to explain the mode in which those pendulous bodies are formed, that sometimes occur attached to the inside of circumscribed cavities; and the principle being established, it became equally easy for Mr. Hunter to apply it under other circumstances, since it is evident, from a known law in the animal œconomy, that extravasated blood, when rendered an organized part of the body, can assume the nature of the parts into which it is effused; and consequently the same coagulum which in the abdomen formed a soft tumour, when situated on a bone, or in the neighbourhood of bone, forms more commonly a hard one. The cartilages found in the knee-joint, therefore, appeared to him to originate from a deposit of coagulated blood upon the end of one of the bones, which had acquired the nature of cartilage, and had afterwards been separated. This opinion was further confirmed by the examination of joints which had been violently strained, or otherwise injured, where the patients had died at different periods after the accident. In some of these there were small projecting parts, preternaturally formed, as hard as cartilage, and so situated as to be readily knocked off by any sudden or violent motion of the joint.

This opinion Mr. Hunter has mentioned for many years in his lectures, and his arguments in favour of it are so consonant to the general laws by which the operations of an animal machine are regulated, as scarcely to require further evidence: but the following case exhibits so many facts in confirmation of this theory, that it appears to me to afford a full explanation of the process above mentioned, and completely to establish the opinion.

A man, sixty-eight years of age, was brought into St. George's Hospital, on the 20th of March, 1791, with a simple fracture of the right thigh-bone. The fracture was situated about three inches below the great trochanter; it was treated in the usual manner, but no bony union had taken place in the beginning of June, about eleven weeks after the accident, the portions of bone at that time being readily moved on each other. There being nothing in the man's general health to account for this backwardness in the parts to unite, he was desired to explain whatever circumstance he was acquainted with respecting himself, likely to throw any light upon it. This inquiry led the patient to mention, that his right os humeri had been broken three years and nine months before, but that the bones had continued disunited, and admitted of motion more freely at that time than immediately after the accident.

Rest having proved ineffectual in producing union in the thigh, and it being evident, from the circumstance of the arm, that there was a natural backwardness in the constitution to form bony union, he was directed to walk upon crutches, and to press as much upon the broken thigh as the state of the parts would admit, without considerable pain, with a view to rouse the parts to action, forcing them by a species of necessity to strengthen the limb. In the course of a fortnight there was an evident firmness in the bone, and in less than two months the patient could walk with the assistance of a stick. As there was something uncommon in the case, he was allowed to remain in the hospital to acquire strength; in this convalescent state he was seized with a complaint in his bowels, which was very violent, and carried him off.

After death the thigh-bone was found firmly repaired by bony union, but the bone of the arm, an account of which is more immediately to the present subject, admitted of motion in every direction at the fractured part.

The arm was carefully dissected, to examine the state of the fractured parts, between which there was no callus, but a large bag filled with a glary fluid, resembling synovia. (See Plate XXIV. fig. 3.) The internal surface of this bag was smooth, like a capsular ligament, and its attachment to the bones was of the same kind: it adhered firmly to the surrounding parts, which were thickened and consolidated, rendering it very strong. The two ends of the bone were adapted to each other, all the irregularities having been absorbed; and their surfaces were of considerable extent, from the fracture being oblique; the upper one was slightly concave, or rather had two depressions, with a middle ridge; the lower one was smaller and rounded, and was adapted to both concavities, which received it in the different motions of the parts.

The surfaces of the bones fitted for motion were not completely covered with cartilage, but studded over with it, and the bone was exposed in the interstices; a number of projecting parts, covered with cartilage, grew out from the surfaces, some exceedingly small, others large. From the edges of the bones and the capsular ligaments these excrescences were larger, extremely irregular in their shape, broader in their attachments, softer in their texture, and serrated upon the external edge.

Thirty or forty small substances, similar to these above mentioned, were found loose in the cavity, varying in size from that of millet-seed to that of a barley-corn, of a roundish form, and smooth on the surface; the largest of them were more flattened and serrated. Their hardness varied considerably, some of them being as soft as cartilage, others so solid as not to be pierced by a needle. Those bodies must have been originally attached, and broken off by the friction of the parts on one another.

The preternatural cavity which I have described was in its nature and use similar to the naturally formed joints of the body; these excrescences and loose bodies were its principal peculiarities, the formation of which appears to have been the result of the violence committed on the parts previously to the formation of the joint, and may be explained in the following manner.

When the bone was broken the ruptured vessels poured out their contents into the interstices of the lacerated parts, for the purpose of uniting them again; this, however, not taking place, it was necessary to accommodate the parts to their disunited state; to this end the blood, which had now become useless, was in part absorbed, and the new joint formed. The remains of the coagulated blood, which had not given the stimulus for its own absorption, underwent changes in its nature, assimilating it as much as possible to that of the surfaces to which it was attached, in some parts its texture resembling ligament, in others being more allied to cartilage or bone.

When we compare these substances with the loose cartilages found in the knee-joint, which are also produced in consequence of accidental violence, and similar in their appearance, we are naturally led to conclude that the latter originate from extravasations of blood, altered in its nature by the parts in which it is deposited, similar to those in the artificial joint above described. In both cases they are evidently new-formed substances, and the readiest mode by which we can account for their production is to refer them thus to the blood, from which fluid every part of the body was originally formed.

These loose cartilages, as they have been commonly called, although they may occur in any joint of the body, are found most frequently in the knee; and in this joint, from the pain and inconveniences they produce, have become the object of an operation in surgery.

One or more of them may be formed in the same joint; I have known one instance in which there were three; they are commonly about the size of a horse-bean, often much smaller, and sometimes considerably larger; when very large they do not give so much trouble to the patient as the smaller kind. A soldier in the 56th regiment has one nearly as big as the patella, which occasions little uneasiness, being too large to insinuate itself into the moving parts of the joint.

In this disease the removal of the loose bodies is the only mode of relief, and it is fortunate for those who are afflicted with it that the knee-joint is the most favourable in the body for such an operation; for the cavity extends a considerable way beyond the moving parts of the joint, and is continued into parts, which, when divided, will more readily unite than the common capsular ligaments, and be less liable to communicate the inflammation that comes upon the wound to the general cavity.

As these loose bodies cannot always be found, no time can be fixed for the operation; but the patient, who will soon become familiar with his own complaint, must arrest them when in a favourable situation, and retain them there till the surgeon can be sent for.

Before the operation the limb should be extended upon a table in an horizontal position, and secured by means of assistants; the loose cartilages are to be pushed into the upper part of the joint above the patella, and then to one side; the inner side is to be preferred, as in that situation only the vastus internus muscle will be divided in the operation. Should there be several of these bodies they must be all secured, or the operation should be postponed till some more favourable opportunity, since the leaving of one will subject the patient to the repetition of an operation not only painful, but attended with some degree of danger.

The loose bodies are to be secured in the situation above mentioned, by an assistant, a task not easily performed while they are cut upon, from their being lubricated by the synovia; and if allowed to escape into the general cavity, they may not readily, if at all, be brought back into the same situation.

The operation consists in making an incision upon the loose cartilage, which it will be best to do in the direction of the thigh, as the wound will more readily be healed by the first intention. If the skin is drawn to one side previously to making the incision, the wound through the parts underneath will not correspond with that made in the skin, which circumstance will favour their union. The incision upon the cartilage must be made with caution, as it will with difficulty be retained in its situation if much force is applied. The assistant is to endeavour to push the loose body through the opening, which must be made sufficiently large for that purpose; but as this cannot always be done, the broad end of an eyed probe may be passed under it, so as to lift it out; or a sharp-pointed instrument may be stuck into it, which will fix it to its situation, and bring it more within the management of the surgeon.

The cartilages being all extracted, the cut edges of the wound are to be brought together, and, by means of a compress of lint, not only pressed close to one another, but also to the parts underneath, in which situation they are to be retained by sticking-plaster and the uniting bandage.

As union by the first intention is of the utmost consequence after this operation to prevent an inflammation upon the joint, the patient should remain in bed with the leg extended till the wound is perfectly united, or at least all chance of inflammation at an end.

OBSERVATIONS ON CERTAIN HORNY EXCRESCENCES OF THE HUMAN BODY.

By Sir Everard Home, Bart., from Materials furnished by Mr. Hunter.

Read February 17, 1791.

[*From the Philosophical Transactions*, Vol. LXXXI., p. 95.]

THE history of diseases belongs not properly to the province of the naturalist or philosopher; it is intimately connected with the inquiries of the physician and anatomist; but when disease becomes a cause of the formation of parts similar to others existing in nature, but rendered uncommon by novelty of situation, or produced in animals to which they are not naturally appropriated, it may be considered as having instituted a monstrous variety, highly deserving of attention from the naturalist.

To describe such varieties is indeed more fully the office of natural history than of medicine; but the investigation of diseases which are found to subvert the ordinary laws of nature respecting the situation or production of parts in an animal body, undoubtedly belongs to the medical practitioner.

By these considerations I have been induced to lay before the Royal Society the following account of a disease which occurs sometimes in the human body, very remarkable in its effects, but very little understood as to its cause, namely, the production of an excrescence similar to a horn. So curious a phenomenon has naturally attracted the attention of the ignorant as well as the philosopher; and the individuals who have had the misfortune to be subject to this disease have been considered as monsters.

Horny excrescences arising from the human head have not only occurred in this country, but have been met with in several other parts of Europe; and the horns themselves have been deposited as valuable curiosities in the first collections in Europe.

In giving the history of a disease so rare in its occurrence, and in its effects so remarkable as almost to exceed belief, it might be thought right to take some pains in bringing proofs to ascertain that such a disease does really exist: I consider the doing so as less necessary at present, there being two women now alive, and residing in England, who are affected by the complaint. I shall, however, in the course of this Paper, bring other evidence from the testimony of the most respectable authors who have considered this subject.

The two following cases contain a very accurate and distinct history of the progress of the disease through its different stages, and make any further detail of the symptoms entirely unnecessary.

Mrs. Lonsdale, a woman fifty-six years old, a native of Horncastle in Lincolnshire, fourteen years ago observed a moveable tumour on the left side of her head, about two inches above the upper arch of the left ear, which gradually increased in the course of four or five years to the size of a pullet's egg, when it burst, and for a week continued to discharge a thick gritty fluid. In the centre of the tumour, after the fluid was discharged, she perceived a small soft substance, of the size of a pea, and of a reddish colour on the top, which at that time she took for proud flesh. It gradually increased in length and thickness, and continued pliable for about three months, when it first began to put on a horny appearance. In two years and three months from its first formation, made desperate by the increased violence of the pain, she attempted to tear it from her head, and with much difficulty, and many efforts, at length broke it in the middle, and afterwards tore the root from her head, leaving a considerable depression, which still remains in the part where it grew. Its length altogether is about five inches, and its circumference at the two ends about one inch, but in the middle rather less. It is curled like a ram's horn contorted, and in colour much resembling isinglass.

From the lower edge of the depression another horn is now growing, of the same colour with the former, in length about three inches, and nearly the thickness of a small goose quill; it is less contorted, and lies close upon the head.

A third horn, situated about the upper part of the lambdoidal suture, is much curved, above an inch in length, and more in circumference at its root: its direction is backwards, with some elevation from the head. At this place two or three successive horns have been produced, which she has constantly torn away; but, as fresh ones have speedily followed, she leaves the present one unmolested, in hopes of its dropping off.

Besides these horny excrescences, there are two tumours, each the size of a large cockle; one upon the upper part, the other about the middle of the left side of the head; both of them admit of considerable motion, and seem to contain fluids of unequal consistence, the upper one affording an obscure fluctuation, the other a very evident one.

The four horns were all preceded by the same kind of incysted tumours, and the fluid in all of them was gritty; the openings from which the matter issued were very small, the cysts collapsed and dried up, leaving the substance from which the horn proceeded distinguishable at the bottom. These cysts gave little pain till the horns began to shoot, and then became very distressing, and continued so, with short intervals, till they were removed. This case is drawn up by the surgeon who attended the woman for many years, which gave him frequent opportunities of seeing the disease in its different stages, and acquiring an accurate history of its symptoms.

Mrs. Allen, a middle-aged woman, resident in Leicestershire, had an incysted tumour upon her head, immediately under the scalp, very moveable, and evidently containing a fluid. It gave no pain unless pressed upon, and grew to the size of a small hen's egg. A few years ago it burst, and discharged a fluid: this diminished in quantity, and in a short time a horny excrescence, similar to those above-mentioned, grew out from the orifice, which has continued to increase in size; and in the month of November 1790, the time I saw it, was about five inches long, and a little more than an inch in circumference at its base. It was a good deal contorted, and the surface very irregular, having a laminated appearance. It moved readily with the scalp, and seemed to give no pain upon motion; but when much handled the surrounding skin became inflamed. This woman came to London, and exhibited herself as a show for money; and it is highly probable that so rare an occurrence would have sufficiently excited the public attention to have made it answer her expectations in point of emolument, had not the circumstance been made known to her neighbours in the country, who were much dissatisfied with the measure, and by their importunity obliged her husband to take her into the country.

That the cases which I have related may not be considered as peculiar instances from which no conclusions can be drawn, it may not be amiss to take notice of some of the most remarkable histories of this kind, mentioned by authors, and see how far they agree with those I have stated in the general characters that are sufficiently obvious to strike a common observer; for the vague and indefinite terms in which authors express themselves on this subject show plainly that they did not understand the nature of the disease, and their accounts of it are not very satisfactory to their readers.

In the *Ephemerides Academiæ Naturæ Curiosorum* there are two cases of horns growing from the human body. One of these instances was a German woman*, who had several swellings, or ganglions, upon differ-

* Ephem. Acad. Nat. Cur. Dec. iii. An. V. Append. p. 148.

ent parts of her head, from one of which a horn grew. The other was a nobleman*, who had a small tumour, about the size of a nut, growing upon the parts covering the two last or lowermost vertebræ of the back. It continued for ten years without undergoing any apparent change; but afterwards enlarged in size, and a horny excrescence grew out from it.

In the History of the Royal Society of Medicine† there is an account of a woman, ninety-seven years old, who had several tumours on her head, which had been fourteen years in growing to the state they were in at that time; she had also a horn which had originated from a similar tumour. The horn was very moveable, being attached to the scalp, without any adhesion to the skull. It was sawn off, but grew again; and, although the operation was repeated several times, the horn always returned.

Bartholine, in his Epistles‡, takes notice of a woman who had a tumour under the scalp, covering the temporal muscle. This gradually enlarged, and a horn grew from it, which had become twelve inches long in the year 1646, the time he saw it. He gives us a representation of it, which bears a very accurate resemblance to that which I have mentioned to have seen in November 1790. No tumour or swelling is expressed in the figure; but the horn is coming directly out from the surface of the skin.

In the Natural History of Cheshire§, a woman is mentioned to have lived in the year 1668, who had a tumour or wen upon her head for thirty-two years, which afterwards enlarged, and two horns grew out of it: she was then seventy-two years old.

There is a horny excrescence in the British Museum, which is eleven inches long, and two inches and a half in circumference at the base, or thickest part. The following account of this horn I have been favoured with by Dr. Gray, taken from the records of the Museum. A woman, named French, who lived near Tenterden, had a tumour or wen upon her head, which increased to the size of a walnut; and in the forty-eighth year of her age this horn began to grow, and in four years arrived at its present size‖.

There are many similar histories of these horny excrescences in the authors I have quoted, and in several others; but those mentioned above

* Ephem. Acad. Nat. Cur., Dec. i. An. i. Observat. 30.

† Histoire de la Société Royale de Médecine, 1776, p. 316.

‡ Epistol. Thom. Barthol.

§ Lee's Natural History of Lancashire and Cheshire.

‖ The following extract is taken from the Minutes of the Royal Society, February 14, 1704–5:—

"A letter was read from Dr. Chariere, at Barnstaple, concerning a horn, seven

are the most accurate and particular with respect to their growth; and in all of them we find the origin was from a tumour, as in the two cases I have related; and, although the nature of the tumour is not particularly mentioned, there can be no doubt of its being of the incysted kind, since in its progress it exactly resembled them, remaining stationary for a long time, and then coming forwards to the skin; and the horn being much smaller than the tumour previously to the formation of the horn is a proof that the tumour must have burst and discharged its contents.

From the foregoing account it must appear evident that these horny excrescences are not to be ranked among the appearances called *lusus naturæ;* nor are they altogether the product of disease, although undoubtedly the consequence of a local disease having previously existed. They are, more properly speaking, the result of certain operations in the part for its own restoration; but the actions of the animal œconomy being unable to bring them back to their original state, this species of excrescence is formed as a substitute for the natural cuticular covering.

To explain the manner in which these horns are formed it will be necessary to consider the nature of incysted tumours a little more fully; and in doing so we shall find that this particular species does not differ in its principle, nor materially in its effects, from many others which are not uncommonly met with in the human body, as well as in those of many other animals, which, as they are more frequent in their occurrence, are also much better understood.

Incysted tumours differ exceedingly among themselves, both in the nature of their contents, and in their progress towards the external surface of the body. Many of them have no reference to our present purpose; it is only the more indolent kind to which I mean now to advert: some of these, when examined, are not found to contain a fluid, but a small quantity of thick, curd-like matter, mixed with cuticle broken down into small parts; and upon exposing the internal surface of the cyst, it is found to have a uniform cuticular covering adhering to it, similar to that of the cutis on the surface of the body, from which it only differs in being thinner, and more delicate, bearing a greater resemblance to that which covers the lips. Others of this kind, instead of having cuticle for their contents, are filled with hair mixed with a curdled

inches long, cut off the second vertebra of the neck of a woman in that neighbourhood.

"Dr. Gregory said that one of seven inches long, and of a dark brown colour, was cut off from a woman's temple at Edinburgh.

"Dr. Norris said that two horns had been cut off from a woman's head in Cheshire."

substance, or hair without any admixture whatever, and have a similar kind of hair growing upon their internal surface, which is likewise covered with a cuticle. These cuticular incysted tumors were, I believe, first accurately examined by Mr. Hunter, to whom we are likewise indebted for an explanation of the mode in which the parts acquire this particular structure.

Mr. Hunter considers the internal surface of the cyst to be so circumstanced respecting the body, as to lose the stimulus of being an internal part, and receive the same impression from its contents, either from their nature, or the length of application, as the surface of the skin does from its external situation. It therefore takes on actions suited to such stimuli, undergoes a change in its structure, and acquires a disposition similar to the cutis, and is consequently possessed of the power of producing cuticle and hair. What the mode of action is, by which this change is brought about, is not easily determined; but from the indolence of these complaints, it most probably requires a considerable length of time to produce it. That the lining of the cyst really does possess powers similar to cutis, is proved by the following circumstances: that it has a power of forming a succession of cuticles like the common skin; and what is thrown off in this way is found in the cavity of the cyst. It has a similar power respecting hair, and sometimes the cavity is filled with it, so great a quantity has been shed by the internal surface. Besides these circumstances, the hair found in the cyst corresponds in appearance with that which grows upon the body of the animal; and when incysted tumours of this kind form in sheep, they contain wool. What is still more curious, when such cysts are laid open, the internal surface undergoes no change from exposure, the cut edges cicatrize, and the bottom of the bag remains ever after an external surface. Different specimens, illustrative of the above-mentioned circumstances, are preserved in Mr. Hunter's collection of diseases.

The cysts that produce horny excrescences (which are only another modification of cuticle) are very improperly considered as giving rise to horns; for if we examine the mode in which this substance grows, we shall find it the same with the human nails, coming directly out from the surface of the cutis. It differs from the nails in not being set upon the skin by a thin edge, but by a surface of some breadth, with a hollow in the middle exactly in the same manner as the horn of the rhinoceros*; at least this is evidently the case in the specimen preserved in the Bri-

* The horn of the rhinoceros is a cuticular appendage to the skin, similar to nails and other cuticular excrescences, being in no respect allied to horns but in the external appearance.

tish Museum, and in one which grew out from the tip of a sheep's ear; they are also solid, or nearly so, in their substance.

This mode of growth is very different from that of horns, which are all formed upon a core, either of bone or soft parts, by which means they have a cavity in them; a structure peculiar to this kind of cuticular substance.

Incysted tumours in different animals would appear, from these observations, to be confined in their production to the cuticular substance proper to the animal in which they take place; for, although cuticle, hair, nail, hoof, and horn, are equally productions of animal substance, only differing in trivial circumstances from each other, we do not find in the human subject any instance of an incysted tumour containing a substance different from the cuticle, hair, and nails of the human body; to which last the horny excrescences, the subject of the present Paper, are certainly very closely allied, both in growth, structure and external appearance; and when of some length, they are found to be so brittle as to break in two, upon being roughly handled, which could not happen either to hoof or horn. In the sheep they produce wool instead of hair; and in one instance in that animal, where they gave rise to horny excrescence, it was less compact in its texture, and less brittle than similar appearances in the human subject; upon being divided longitudinally, the cut surface had more the appearance of hoof, and was more varied in its colour than nail.

Incysted tumours being capable of producing horns, upon the principle we have laid down, is contrary to the usual operations of nature; for horns are not a production from the cutis, and, although not always formed upon a bony core, but frequently upon a soft pulp, that substance differs from common cutis in its appearance, and extends a considerable way into the horn: it is probable, that this pulp requires a particular process for its formation*.

I shall conclude this paper by observing, that the cases of horns, as they are commonly termed, upon the human head, are no more than cuticular productions arising from a cyst, which in its nature is a variety of those tumours described by Mr. Hunter under the general name of cuticular incysted tumours†.

* A sheep, about four years old, had a large horn, three feet long, growing upon its flank. It had no connection with bone, and appeared to be only attached to the external skin. It dropped off in consequence of its weight having produced ulceration in the soft parts to which it adhered. Upon examining it there was a fleshy substance, seven inches long, of a fibrous texture, filling up its cavity upon which the horn had been formed.

† The principle upon which the production of these excrescences depends being once explained, the modes of preventing their formation, and removing them when formed,

These incysted tumours, when considered as varieties of the same disease, form a very complete and beautiful series of the different modes by which the powers of the animal œconomy produce a substitute for the common cuticle upon parts which have been so much affected by disease as to be unable to restore themselves to a natural state.

will be readily understood, the destruction of the cyst being all that is required for that purpose. This may be done before the tumour opens externally, or even after the excrescence has begun to shoot out, and will be better effected by dissection than escharotics, since the success of the operation depends upon the whole of the bag being removed.

END OF THE THIRD VOLUME.

Printed by Richard and John E. Taylor, Red Lion Court, Fleet Street.

INDEX TO THE FIRST THREE VOLUMES.

ABDOMEN, penetrating wounds of, iii. 559.

Abernethy, J. i. 86. Case related by, in which the vena portæ did not terminate in the liver, ii. 86, note. Erroneous interpretation of Hunter's doctrine of life, iii. 122, note. On a new method of opening lumbar abscesses, iii. 424, note.

Abscesses, i. 409; iii. 403. Treatment of, i. 412; iii. 411, 518. Methods of opening, iii. 526. The process of cure described, i. 414. Large do not produce hectic fever until they are opened, iii. 423. Constitutional effects of, iii. 424. The approach of to the surface described and explained, iii. 284, 300, 467, 479, 520. (See *Suppuration. Pus.*)

———, *near the anus*, iii. 401.

———, *chronic*, i. 413; iii. 422. Sometimes mistaken for tumours, i. 576.

———, *critical*, i. 370; iii. 303. The question whether they ought to be encouraged, i. 401. Are sometimes absorbed, iii. 417.

———, *in the antrum maxillare*; symptoms and causes of, ii. 77. Treatment of, ii. 78.

———, *in the jaws*; when deeply seated, how to be treated, ii. 76. (See *Gum Boils.*)

———, *lumbar*; i. 554, 596; iii. 423. The propriety of opening, i. 554, 600; iii. 526. The reason of their being so slow, iii. 422.

———, *milk*, iii. 485.

———, *scrofulous*, iii. 419.

———, *near the urethra*; treatment of, ii. 264. In the perinæum, are very apt to return on contracting a fresh gonorrhœa, ii. 271. Venereal, when obstinate, their treatment, ii. 458.

Absorbents, uses of discovered, i. 18, 237; ii. 354. Proposed work on, by Hunter, i. 20. Preparations of, i. 160. Description of, i. 250. The modellers of the body, i. 252. Their functions in health and disease, i. 255, 420; ii. 237; iii. 459, 481. Inflammation of, iii. 319, note. Inflam. of on the back of the penis, ii. 358. Resolution of, ii. 370.

Absorption, experiments on, i. 18. Organs of, i. 160. Function of, i. 247. Old notion respecting, i. 250. Interstitial, i. 253, 421; iii. 469. Of whole parts, i. 254. Progressive, i. 256, 421; iii. 471. The mode in which it is effected unknown, i. 257; but is not mechanical, i. 481. Table of, i. 258; iii. 460. Is sometimes a substitute for mortification, i. 255, 420. Progressive absorption of diseased parts similar to the healthy processes, *ib.* Remote causes of, i. 420; iii. 464. Immediate causes of, i. 481. General views of, iii. 459. Modes of producing, iii. 482. The external parts more prone to this action than the internal, iii. 467. Of matter, i. 413; iii. 417, 512.

——— *of foreign substances*, rapidity of, iii. 38, note; of matter, how prevented in a gonorrhœa, ii. 207; of venereal matter is of three kinds, ii. 356.

Accidents, the different kinds of, i. 388; iii. 240. (See *Wounds.*)

Acid carbonic, in venous blood, iii. 28, note. Whether the evolution of is the cause of the coagulation of the blood and of its black colour, iii. 94, note.

—— *prussic*, does not prevent the contraction of the clot, iii. 43, note.

—— *uric*, secreted in superabundance in gout, i. 353, note.

Action, the meaning of this term, ii. 396; iii. 3. Occasions waste and exhausts life, i. 214, 224, 345, 603. The power of, dependent on organization, i. 222, 241. Supports life, although not necessary to it, i. 224; iii. 124, note. Should always be in proportion to the powers of a part, i. 312, 479, 603; iii. 8. Action and disposition, the difference between, ii. 396. The former more easily cured than the latter, ii. 401.

——— *of the heart*, cause of, iii. 188, 189, note. (See *Heart.*)

Actions, of two kinds, i. 243, 318. Those which are vital are uninterrupted, i. 244. The involuntary arise from the brain, i. 263. Sometimes cease during sleep, i. 266. Critical, what meant by, i. 306. Preternatural, i. 308. Are the consequence of unnatural impressions, i. 299. Sometimes wear themselves out, i. 300. The weak destroyed by the strong, i. 310, 388. Scrofulous, remarkable for their tardiness, i. 593. Diseased, incompatible with each other, ii. 132; iii. 3.

Adair, Mr. i. 20, 25.

Adams, Dr. i. xxi. 28.

Addison, Dr. iii. 427.

Adhesion, may take place without inflammation or pain, iii. 299, 332. (See *Union by the First Intention* and *Adhesive Inflammation.*)

Adults, sympathies of, more determinate than in young children, i. 324.

Adult Teeth, progress of their formation, ii. 35. The first grinder decaying at an early age, ought to be removed, ii. 92.

Age, its effects on disease, i. 243, 484; and particularly as it respects cancer, i. 622.

Ague, iii. 432. Illustrates the doctrine of susceptibilities, i. 306. Ill-formed, i. 307.

Air; in the veins, the effects of, i. 350; iii. 28, note. Whether it ought to be regarded as an irritant, exciting to suppuration, i. 410; iii. 405. Coming in contact with the nerve of a tooth, the cause of the pain in, ii. 53. Means for excluding it, ii. 54. Effect of on the coagulation of the blood, iii. 27, note.

Albumen, in the serum, properties of, iii. 45, note. Circumstances which increase or diminish its amount, *ib.* Conversion of, into fibrin or oleaginous matter, iii. 37, note. Coagulation of, iii. 49, note. Test of, *ib.*

Aldini, Professor, i. 146.

Alison, Dr., his experiments on the tonicity of inflamed arteries, referred to, iii. 328, note.

Alveolar Process, in the upper jaw, described, ii. 1. In the lower jaw, ii. 2. Of the upper and lower jaw compared, *ib.* The sockets of the teeth, how formed, ii. 3. In both jaws, are rather to be considered as belonging to the teeth than as parts of the jaw, *ib.* Absorption of, always keeps pace with the gum, ii. 5, note. The formation of, traced from early infancy to adult age, ii. 32. Decay of, by wasting, ii. 79. A filling up of the socket and protrusion of the tooth, *ib.* The cause of these two disorders inquired into, ii. 80. Effects of the scurvy on, *ib.* Decay of, by what is called the scurvy of the gums, ii. 82.

Amputation; often immediately removes hectic fever, i. 324; iii. 513. The question of, in severe accidents and compound fractures, i. 510; iii. 281, note. In gun-shot wounds, iii. 572, 575, note.

Amusements, Mr. Hunter's, i. 10, 32, 55.

Analogy; often an unsafe mode of argument on physiological subjects, ii. 24, note; and also on disease, ii. 62, note.

Analyses of the blood and serum, iii. 18, note.

Anasarca, the punctures made in, do not always heal, iii. 280.

Anastomoses; uses of, iii. 207.

Anatomy; lectures on, i. 4. State of, before the time of Hunter, i. 5. Pursuit of and disputes in, i. 17.

Anatomy Comparative; Hunter enters on the study of, i. 20. Recommends, i. 29. MSS. volume of, i. 152.

Anchylosis; the different kinds of, i. 521.

Andral; on the power of effused blood to become vascular, iii. 269; which he compares to the development of the embryonic germ, iii. 457.

Angina Pectoris, i. 443, 444; iii. 79.

Anecdotes; of Cheselden, i. 9. Of Mr. Christie, i. 138. Of Dr. William Hunter, i. 4. Of Dr. Johnson's friend, i. 5. Of Linnæus, *ib.* Of Pitt, i. 135, 137. Of Pott, i. 5.

——— of John Hunter, i. 28, 57. Of J. H. at home, i. 41. Of J. H. in the lecture room, i. 47, 49. Of J. H. and Byrne, i. 166. Of J. H. and Sir A. Carlisle, i. 14, 115. Of J. H. and Dr. Clarke, i. 75. Of J. H. and Mr. Cline, i. 53. Of J. H. and Mr. Jesse Foot, i. 22. Of J. H. and Dr. Garthshore, i. 28, 114. Of J. H. and Mr. Lynn, i. 116. Of J. H. and Mr. G. Nicol, i. 29. Of J. H. and Sir Joshua Reynolds, i. 108, 121. Of J. H. and Taylor, i. 87. Of J. H. and Mr. Thomas, i. 114. Of J. H. and a would-be Lecturer, i. 56.

Anel; his claims to Hunter's operation for aneurism examined, i. 98.

Aneurism; Hunter's operation for, i. 96, 117, 543. Paper on, iii. 594. Anel's claims to, examined, i. 98. True and spurious aneurisms, i. 543. Causes of, i. 544. Na-

tural cure of, i. 546. Treatment of, *ib.* Necessity for operating early, i. 548. Arteries, on which the operation for may be practised, i. 549. Operation, i. 550, 551. Cases of, i. 551. The progress of, towards the surface, described, iii. 472. Comparative frequency of aneurism in the different vessels, iii. 595.
Animals, lower; the simple condition of, i. 247. Possess little power of resisting changes of temperature, i. 288. Compared in this respect to vegetables, i. 329. Some are not susceptible of venereal irritation, ii. 151.
Animal Œconomy; Hunter's work on, i. 103.
——— *Heat.* (See *Heat.*)
——— *Life*; the power which it possesses of existing under great extremes of temperature, i. 284, 293, notes.
——— *Substances*; instances, showing their disposition to unite, ii. 56.
Animalculæ, in scabies, i. 618.
Animalization, i. 215, note, 230.
Ankle, compound fractures of, i. 510.
Anson's Voyage, referred to, iii. 487.
Anthrax, i. 607.
Antimonial Medicines, and particularly the *Antimonium tartariz.*, in Inflammation, iii. 387, 388.
Antrum maxillare; abscess of, ii. 77. Method of puncturing, ii. 78, note.
Anus; fistula of, i. 579. Diffuse suppuration near the verge of, iii. 401.
Aorta; arch of, particularly subject to variation from the normal type, iii. 208, note. Action of the valves of, iii. 203, note.
Applications, external; in inflammation, i. 406, 480, 565. In scrofula, i. 600.
Apoplexy and *Hemiplegia*; proceed from the same cause, iii. 261. The mode of treatment generally adopted not judicious, *ib.*
Aristotle; believed that the blood was alive, iii. 105, note.
Arsenic; its action on living parts, i. 604, 605. Enters into most of the empirical nostrums for the cure of cancer, i. 625. Alters the diseased action of cancer, i. 626.
Arteries; structure of, i. 250; iii. 156. Elasticity of, *ib.* Muscularity of, iii. 157, 162. Not equally muscular in every part, iii. 160. Contractility of in animals is greater than in man, i. 538. Of the effect of these two properties on the circulation, iii. 169. Considered as a sort of supplemental heart, iii. 171. Of the vasa arteriarum, *ib.* Valves of, iii. 202. Ramification of, iii. 205. Anastomoses of, iii. 207. Experiments to prove that the area of an artery increases as it proceeds from the heart, iii. 211; so as to form a cone whose apex is at the heart, iii. 213. Action of, iii. 216. Regeneration of, iii. 242, 531, notes. The proper treatment when large arteries are wounded, i. 540; iii. 246.
Arteritis, i. 453; iii. 531.
Artery Carotid; peculiar arrangement of, in some animals, iii. 321.
——— *Crural*; case of wound of, iii. 89. Aneurism of, iii. 88.
Arterialization of the blood, iii. 92, note.
Articulation; of the lower jaw, described, ii. 6. Of the teeth, ii. 28.
Asphyxia, iii. 32, note. The order in which the vital functions cease in, iii. 78, note.
Astringents; their use in hardening the gums, ii. 81. (See *Gums.*)
Atmosphere; the most wholesome temperature of, i. 292. The state of, affects wounds, i. 297.
Atrophy; one of the effects of inflammation, iii. 533, note; and particularly of the testicle, ii. 311, 315; iii. 533, note.
Attraction; elective, i. 212. Of cohesion, i. 213. Of gravitation, *ib.*
Auckland, Lord; obtains a pension for Mrs. Hunter, i. 137. His letter to Sir J. Banks respecting the Hunterian Museum, i. 139, 141.
Auricles, to be considered only as reservoirs of the blood, iii. 177, 178, note.

B.

Babington, Dr., on the liquor sanguinis, iii. 331, note.
Baillie, Dr.; relationship to the Hunters, i. 2. Professional punctuality of, i. 53. Resigns Kilbride estate, i. 80. Executor to Hunter, i. 137. And Home, establish the Hunterian Oration, i. 146.
———, *Joanna*, i. 3.
Balls, Musket, of the strange course which they sometimes take, iii. 556.

Balsams, terebinthinate; in mortification, i. 604; ii. 222; iii. 8.
Bandages, remarks on, iii. 257.
Banks, Sir J.; Letters of, to Hunter, i. 83, 84. Letters of Lord Auckland to, i. 139. Letters from, to Lord A., i. 141. How affected with cold, i. 286.
Barber Surgeons, i. 5.
Bathing, Cold, i. 48. In the sea, in scrofula, i. 598, 599; ii. 83, note.
Bark; its use in scrofula, i. 598. In mortification, i. 604; ii. 137; iii. 8, 377. In gonorrhœa and gleet, ii. 205, 222. In mortification arising from the effusion of urine, ii. 268. In phimosis, ii. 339. In erysipelas, ii. 370. In inflammation, iii. 278, 284. In gunshot wounds, iii. 577.
Barruel; on the halitus of the blood, iii. 54, note.
Bartholomew's Hospital; Hunter a pupil at, i. 12.
Bath; Hunter visits, i. 64, 95.
Bats; torpid, whether the blood in, loses its fluidity, iii. 33, note.
Bayford, Mr., i. 34.
Bees; Mr. Hunter's paper on, i. 121. Require a high temperature, i. 285, note. The larvæ of, said to survive boiling, i. 294, note. Hunter's fondness for, i. 337.
Bell, Mr.; engaged by Mr. Hunter, i. 51. His drawings, i. 177.
——, *Mr. B.*, ii. 148, note.
Belladonna, extract of; does not prevent the contraction of the clot, iii. 43, note.
Bellows; Hunter's double, for artificial respiration, iii. 76.
Belleisle, siege of, i. 20.
Berzelius, his analysis of the blood, iii. 18, note.
Bibliography; of the blood, iii. 138. Of the vascular system, iii. 233. Of inflammation, iii. 534. Of gunshot wounds, iii. 578.
Bicuspides; particular description of that class of teeth, ii. 24. Their use, ii. 25.
Bichat, X.; quoted, i. 240, 242. On the effects of black blood on the system, iii. 78, 87, note. His definition of life, iii. 126.
Bile; in the blood, i. 353. Depositions of, in various parts, *ib.* Prevents the coagulation of the blood, iii. 35. Sometimes secreted from arterial blood, iii. 86, note.
Birds; the temperature of, i. 288. Of passage, i. 294.
Birthday; Hunter's, i. 1.
Black, Dr.; his discoveries on latent heat, i. 279.
Bladder; wounds of, i. 448. Affected in gonorrhœa, ii. 178, 188, 205. Treatment of, ii. 211, 225. Its strength increased in stricture, ii. 241. Diseases of, from obstructions to the urine, ii. 284. Increased irritability of, *ib.* And urethra, contract and relax alternately, *ib.* Inconveniences which arise when these actions do not take place regularly, ii. 285. Their treatment, ii. 286. Paralysis of, from obstruction to the passage of urine, ii. 287. Cure of paralysis of, when it arises from obstruction, owing to pressure or spasm, ii. 289. Puncture of, above the pubes, ii. 290. By the rectum, ii. 292. In the perinæum, ii. 296. Of the increased strength of, ii. 299. Irritability of, independent of obstructions to the urine, ii. 300. The cure of simple irritability of, *ib.* Reason why its contraction in inflammation is so painful, iii. 332.
Blane, Sir G., i. 295.
Bleeding; effects of, i. 537. Its use in gonorrhœa, ii. 205. In chordee, ii. 210. (See *Venesection.*)
Blisters; applied to the perinæum, their use in removing disagreeable sensations which remain after the cure of a gonorrhœa, ii. 218. In strangury, *ib.* In gleet, ii. 223. In spasmodic affections of the urethra, ii. 275. In paralysis of the urethra, ii. 276. In paralysis of the bladder, ii. 289. In spasmodic affections of the urethra, accompanied by a paralysis of the bladder, ii. 290. In simple irritability of the bladder, ii. 195. In paralysis of the acceleratores urinæ, ii. 301. In nodes, ii. 447.
Blizard, Mr. Thomas, i. 255, note.
———, *Sir William*, and Hunter, i. 54.
Blood; general principles of, iii. 10. Erroneous views respecting, i. 229. Life of, when communicated, i. 231. Proofs of its vitality, i. 231; iii. 103. The use of extraneous matters in, i. 232. Harmonizes with the solids, i. 233, note, 381; iii. 115. Coagulation of, i. 233; iii. 41, note. Buffy and cupped, i. 233, 383; iii. 38, note. Inflammation of, i. 234. Sensible changes in, i. 235. Foreign substances in, i. 347. Vitiations of, i. 352, note. Of the power of coagulated blood to become vascular, i. 236, 238, 368, 439; iii. 34, 115, 119, 243, 268, 350. Milky i. 353,

note; iii. 55, note. Death of, i. 381, 382. Disease throws great light on its natural history, iii. 12, 15. Nearly uniform in its composition, in different animals, iii. 13. The colour of, iii. 16, 58, note. Whether its constitution is always globular, iii. 16. Its various parts, and the uses which they fulfil in the animal œconomy, iii. 17. Analysis of, iii. 18. Specific gravity of, iii. 22, note. Standard heat of, iii. 338. Fluidity of, depends on the vitality of the vessels, iii. 29, note, 130. Does not always coagulate on extravasation, iii. 33. Has the power of action within itself, iii. 34, 115, 243, 350. Cases in which it does not coagulate after death, iii. 34, 42, 114, 357. Serum of, iii. 39. Observations to prove that the albuminous principles of the blood are distinct in their nature, iii. 37, note. Of the red globules, iii. 57. Difference between arterial and venous, iii. 73, note; the respective colours of which are sometimes reversed, iii. 91. Effects of respiration on, iii. 74, 92, note. Venous blood not poisonous, iii. 87, note; nor essential to the secretion of bile, iii. 86, note. Cause of the change of colour of the two bloods, iii. 97. The blood the same in all the arteries, iii. 101, 102: but different in the different veins, iii. 73, 102. Effects of various agents on, iii. 121. Whether the quantity of, or the velocity of its circulation is increased in inflammation, iii. 325, note. State of, in inflammation, iii. 354. Of a person having the lues venerea, will not communicate the disease to a sound person by inoculation, ii. 385. (See *Coagulation, Serum, Globules, Buff.*)

Bloodletting. (See *Bleeding, Venesection.*)

——— *local*, iii. 376.

Bloodvessels, preparations of, i. 169.

Blotches venereal, described, ii. 407. (See *Eruptions.*)

Blows, on the stomach, destroy the coagulability of the blood and the contractility of muscles after death, iii. 114.

Blumenbach, Professor, i. 284, 353, notes.

Blundell, Dr., iii. 14, note.

Body; comparative powers of different parts of, ii. 134; which are greater the nearer they are to the heart, *ib.* The structure of different parts produces a difference in the powers of action, *ib.*; and in their susceptibility of particular diseases, ii. 105. No one part of the body applied by Nature to two purposes with advantage, and instances of this in different animals, ii. 228.

——, influence on by the mind. (See *Imagination.*)

Bodies, foreign; of the extraction of, in gunshot wounds, iii. 550. Their approach to the surface accounted for, iii. 467, 479, notes.

Boerhaave, on the cause of inflammation, iii. 304.

Boils, i. 608.

Bones; Hunter's intended work on, i. 151. The earth of, not a part of the living body, i. 218. Their mode of growth illustrated, i. 253. Their diseases, i. 498. Inflammation of, i. 505, 514; iii. 277, 278, 530. Suppuration of, i. 513. Death of, i. 255, note. Exfoliation of, i. 514, 529. Absorption of, i. 255, note. Caries of, i. 499. Induration of, i. 500, 506, 514. Union of, i. 501. Of the extraction of dead pieces of, i. 530. Rickets, i. 531. Mollities ossium, i. 532. Exostosis, i. 533; iii. 533. Tumours of, i. 570. Venereal affections of, ii. 421, note. The union of may be destroyed by the poison of mercury, ii. 432, note. By scurvy, iii. 487.

Bordeu, calls the blood *la chair coulante*, i. 229.

Boughton, Sir T.; trial on the death of, i. 81. Hunter's evidence on the trial, i. 194.

Bougainville's Voyage, a passage from, ii. 144.

Bougies; their use in gonorrhœa, ii. 198, 213. In gleet, ii. 223, 224. Different kinds of, ii. 233, 252. Their use in stricture, ii. 233. Directions for passing them, ii. 235, 275. Frequently stop in the lacunæ of the urethra, ii. 237, note. Sometimes form a new passage on the side of the urethra, ii. 239, 253. Sometimes slip into the bladder, and occasion the patient to be cut for the stone, ii. 240. Mode of extracting them when a part remains still in the urethra, ii. 241. Description and use of the armed-bougie, ii. 246, note. Affect many parts by sympathy, ii. 251. Hollow, their use in stricture, ii. 266. How introduced, where the prostate gland is enlarged, ii. 280, 281.

Bowerbank, Mr. on the globules in the blood of insects, iii. 58, note.

Brain; preparations of, i. 170. Of the active and passive states of i. 259. Too much ascribed to it, i. 260. Whether formed before or after the nerves, i. 264, note. Injuries of, i. 487, 492, note. Inflammation of, i. 486, 489, note; iii. 531. Hydatids of, i. 574; identifiable with the *materia vitæ diffusa*, iii. 115. Is diffused through the whole body in many of the inferior animals, iii. 116 note. Peculiarity of its circulation, designed to protect it against pressure from sudden congestion, iii. 220, 224, note.

Brande, Mr., i. 28.

Breast, scrofulous, i. 594, 597. (See *Cancer.*)

Breath, rendered foul by rotten teeth, ii. 65. (See *Scurvy.*)

Brien, O', i. 106.

Brodie, Sir B., on the effects of cold, i. 287, note. On abscesses in bones, i. 514. On injuries of the head, i. 491. On hydrocele, i. 461.

Bromfield, Mr.; i. 25. His strictures on Mr. Hunter's operation for aneurism, i. 547.

Bubo; theory of its formation, ii. 354. Mistakes of authors relative to this subject, ii. 355. Situation and description of, ii. 357. May be formed in the lymphatics or lymphatic glands, ii. 358. How distinguished from other swellings, ii. 359. Of the time between the application of the venereal matter and the formation of, ii. 360. In the right groin, when occasioned by chancres, generally arises from sores situated on the right side of the penis, ii. 361. In women, its division, ii. 362. Of the inflammation of, ii. 363. Marks which distinguish it from other swellings of the glands, ii. 364. General reflections on its cure, ii. 368. Of the resolution of, *ib.* Is attended with different dispositions, which must be treated accordingly, ii. 370. Resolution of; the use of vomits in, *ib.* In the groin; the resolution of, ii. 371. In women; of the resolution of, ii. 372. In different parts of the body; treatment of, *ib.* Resolution of; the quantity of mercury necessary for, *ib.* Is more likely to suppurate if there is one in each groin than when single, ii. 373. Sometimes becomes scirrhous; its treatment, *ib.* Its treatment when it suppurates, ii. 374. The matter of is sometimes absorbed, iii. 512. Mercury is to be given during the suppuration of, ii. 374. Method of opening, *ib.* Consequences of, ii. 375. Degenerate sometimes into a sore of the scrofulous kind, ii. 375, 377. In some they spread to an amazing extent, ii. 379. Treatment of when it becomes stationary, *ib.*

Buchanan, Mr.; marries Agnes Hunter, i. 3. Fails in business, *ib.* His death, i. 13.

Buff of blood; consists of fibrin modified by disease, iii. 40, note. Of the relative proportions of solid and fluid parts in, in health and disease, *ib.* No guide for the repetition of venesection, *ib.* The quantity of, much influenced by the shape of the vessel and the quickness of its solidification, iii. 39, note. The cause of, iii. 38, note. In inflammation, iii. 354, 357.

Bugs; the bite of, poisonous, i. 615.

Buller, Judge; his strictures on Hunter's evidence, i. 54.

Bunion, i. 560.

Burke, Mr., his opinion of what is necessary to form a great man, i. 54.

Burns; mode of treating, iii. 265.

Burning the nerve of a tooth; method of performing, ii. 66. Reprobated, ii. 68, note. Of the ear, sometimes successful in the tooth-ache, ii. 66.

Burrows, Dr., on the power of coagulated blood to vascularize itself, iii. 269, note.

Bursæ, i. 449.

Butler, Bishop, his treatise on natural and revealed religion the fruit of twenty years' reflection, i. 276.

Byrne, C., i. 106.

C.

Cachexia; the worst forms of, induced by mercury, ii. 432, note.

Cæsarian operation, i. 448.

Calculi; i. 185. How formed, ii. 42, 54.

Calculous matter; frequently attaches itself to the ends of bougies when left in the bladder, ii. 251. Frequently fills up the cavity of the catheter when kept a long time in the bladder, ii. 298.

Callus; the nature of, i. 501, note, 502.

Calomel, its use in inflammation of the testicle, ii. 212, note.

Campbell, Lady, i. 41.

Camphor, its use in chordee, ii. 210.

Cancer; glands contaminated by, sometimes remain dormant for a long time, i. 309; and sometimes inflame without being contaminated, i. 329, 622. Diagnosis between cancer and scrofula of the testicle, i. 618; and of the breast, i. 598, 618. Symptoms and external appearances of, i. 618, 623. Progress of, i. 618, 624. Is strictly a local disease, i. 619. Predisposing causes of, i. 623. Parts most susceptible of, *ib.* Whether hereditary, *ib.* Morbid appearances of, i. 624. Treatment of, i. 625. By caustics, i. 626. By extirpation, *ib.*

Capacity for heat of the different bloods, employed to explain the functions of calorification, i. 281.

Capillaries; proofs of their muscularity, iii. 158. The peculiarity of their distribution constitutes them a distinct system, iii. 197, note. State of in inflammation, iii. 325, note.

Carbonic acid gas. (See *Acid.*)

Carbuncle, i. 602, 607; iii. 317. Treatment of, i. 609.

Caries, i. 499, 528. The excision of, stops the decay of teeth, ii. 65.

Carlisle, Sir A.; his introduction to Hunter, i. 115. His anatomical skill, i. 36. Anecdotes of, i. 14, 115.

Carswell, Dr., on the digestion of the stomach, i. 43.

Cartilage; not reproduced, i. 504, note; iii. 530. Inflammation of, iii. 530. Exfoliation of, i. 534. Absorption of, i. 535. Moveable, in the articulation of the jaws, described, ii. 5. Principal use of, ii. 6.

Cartilages, loose; how formed, i. 520; iii. 625.

Caruncles, in the urethra, ii. 277. Their cure, *ib.*

Case of inflammation and abscess of the abdomen, i. 422. Of aneurism of the aorta, *ib.* Of tumour of the dura mater, i. 423. Of ununited fracture of the thigh, i. 426. Of papular eruption, allowed to get well by scabbing, i. 429. Of Cæsarian operation, i. 448. Of chancre and eruptions, i. 478. Of sloughing from the application of a blister, i. 482. Of hæmatemesis, i. 483. Of fracture of the skull, which was trepanned two years after the accident, i. 488. Of hernia cerebri, i. 495. Of fractured patella, in which the extensor muscles were made to resume their action by a particular contrivance, i. 512. Of necrosis, i. 530. Of amputation at the shoulder joint, in which the cartilage was found unadherent two years afterwards, i. 535. Of secondary hæmorrhage after amputation, i. 543. Of secondary hæmorrhage after the operation for popliteal aneurism, i. 551. Of encysted tumour, in which the lining membrane afterwards formed a part of the external integument, i. 576. Of diseased joint, cured by mezereon, i. 599. Of carbuncle, i. 609. Of a tooth which was successfully transplanted, ii. 80, 101, 105. Of the enamel being worn away from the teeth in a peculiar manner, so as to give to them a peculiar truncated appearance, ii. 70, 71, note. Of a child under inoculation attacked with the measles, ii. 133; iii. 5. Of a gentleman, proving that a gonorrhœa may produce a lues venerea, ii. 145. Of a young woman from the Magdalen Hospital, showing that a gonorrhœa may continue two years, ii. 166. Of a gentleman, where a gonorrhœa continued a length of time without losing its virulence, *ib.* Of a gentleman, proving the same, ii. 167. Of a man where the cuticle of the glans came off, ii. 168. Of a young gentleman where the gonorrhœa was confined to the glans, ii. 169. Of a gentleman, showing how the venereal matter is communicated to the urethra, ii. 176. Of a woman having a fluor albus, and communicating a disease similar to gonorrhœa, ii. 186. Of a gentleman cured of a gonorrhœa almost immediately by taking ten grains of calomel, ii. 196. Of a gentleman under a course of mercury contracting a gonorrhœa, ii. 197. Of a gentleman, showing the use of blisters applied to the perinæum in removing disagreeable sensations which remain after the cure of a gonorrhœa, ii. 217. Of a gentleman's servant, showing the same, ii. 218. Of a chimney-sweeper cured of a stricture by the application of lunar caustic, ii. 244. Of a gentleman relieved in a stricture by a gonorrhœa, ii. 250. Of a gentleman, showing the same, *ib.* Of a soldier, where a new passage was made along the side of the urethra by a bougie, ii. 255. Its treatment and cure, *ib.* Of a gentleman where a mortification took place in the cellular membrane of the penis from urine diffused into it, ii. 261. Of a man in St. George's Hospital, showing that keeping extraneous bodies in the urethra prevents wounds made into that canal from healing, ii. 271. Of a man in St. George's Hospital, cured of a paralysis of the urethra, ii. 276. Of John Doby, a poor pensioner in the Charter-house, who died from a suppression of urine occasioned by a swelled prostate gland, ii. 279. Of a gentleman, showing the inconveniences arising from a swelling of the prostate gland, ii. 281. Of a gentleman, showing the use of blisters applied to the perinæum in spasmodic affections of the urethra accompanied with a paralysis of the bladder, ii. 290. Of a total suppression of urine relieved by a puncture in the bladder through the rectum, ii. 293. Two instances of the same, ii. 294. Of a sailor, where the urine passed from the bladder into the rectum, ii. 295. Of a gentleman, who was impotent with respect to one woman only, ii. 307. Of a young man cured of a seminal weakness by opium, ii. 309. Of a gentleman, where the semen passed into the bladder at the time of emission, ii. 310. Of a gentleman, where one of the testicles wasted entirely, ii. 312. Of a gentleman, showing the same, *ib.* Another instance of the same, ii. 313. Other cases, ii. 315. Of a gentleman, where seven weeks elapsed between the application of the venereal poison and the appearance of a chancre, ii. 319. Of a gentleman, where the penis was bent to one side at the time of erection, ii. 327. Of a gentleman, showing that mercurial frictions sometimes occasion ulcers on the tonsils which have the appearance of venereal ulcers, ii. 342. Another case, showing the same, *ib.* Of a gentleman, with a spreading ulcer of the prepuce cured by sea-bathing, ii. 350. Of a gentleman cured of ulcerations resembling chancres, by the lixivium saponarium, *ib.* Of a gentleman who had a swelling in the groin suspected to be venereal, ii. 366. Of an officer at Lisbon, where a bubo was resolved, though it contained matter, by sea-sickness, ii. 370. Of a gentleman, where a bubo degenerated into a sore of the scrofulous kind, ii. 376. Of a gentleman who had a gonorrhœa and two buboes, where a new disposition formed besides the venereal, ii. 377. Of a boy who swallowed some venereal matter without any ill consequences, ii. 384. Of a lady who met with the same accident, *ib.* Of a child who was supposed to infect its nurse with the lues venerea, ii. 388. Of a gentleman, proving that venereal complaints are often supposed to exist when they really do not, ii. 390. Of a man having the lues venerea, showing that the superficial parts, or those first in order, may come into action and be cured; while those parts which are second in order have only the disposition; but that they afterwards may come into action and be cured as those first in order were, ii. 400. Of a gentleman, showing the same, ii. 402. Of a lady who was salivated by a small quantity of red precipitate applied to sores. ii. 428. Of a gentleman, showing the effects of mercury on the constitution, ii. 431. Another instance of the same, *ib.* Of a gentleman, showing that the effects of mercury on the constitution are not sufficient for the cure of the lues venerea, it requiring its specific effects on the poison, as well as its sensible effects on the constitution, ii. 437. Of a gentleman, showing that the efficacy of electricity in the cure of diseases may be increased by mercury, ii. 455. Of a man in St. George's Hospital having the lues venerea, where a comparative trial was made of the effects of guaiacum and sarsaparilla, ii. 456. Of a woman in St. George's Hospital having the lues venerea, where the cure was attempted by opium, but without success, ii. 461. Of Luke Ward, in St. Bartholomew's Hospital, showing the inefficacy of opium in the lues venerea, and that it may sometimes act as a poison, *ib.* Of J. Morgan, in the same hospital, showing the use of opium in the cure of an ulcerated leg, ii. 462. Of a woman, where hemlock was of use in venereal sores which had put on a cancerous appearance, ii. 463. Of a gentleman infected with the yaws, ii. 472. Of a gentleman having a disease resembling the lues venerea, *ib.* Of a gentleman having a similar complaint, ii. 474. Of a lady infected with a disease similar to the lues venerea, by the transplanting of a tooth, ii. 483. Another instance in a young lady, ii. 484. Another in a gentleman, *ib.* Of milky blood, iii. 57. Of apoplexy, iii. 79. Of disease of the heart, with shrunken valves, iii. 80. Of disease of the heart, with communication between the ventricles, iii. 82. Of wounded crural artery, iii. 89. Of scarlet blood from the veins of the arm, iii. 91. Of fracture of the thigh in a person who was paralytic from lead, iii. 137. Of disease of the heart, attended with peculiar symptoms, iii. 193. Of ecchymosis of the leg and thigh, iii. 248. Of Lord Hertford's servant, who was tapped eight times, iii. 340. Of a gentleman, whose pulse became harder on bleeding, iii. 361. Of sizy blood, continuing after six bleedings, iii. 377. Of sizy blood attended with very weak powers, iii. 378. Of erysipelatous inflammation by the side of the anus, iii. 401. Of rigors, iii. 430, 431, 438. Of castration, attended with immediate death, iii. 431. Of suppuration of the cavity of the abdomen, which pointed in several places, iii. 477. Of fracture of the thigh-bone, which had not united, appearances three or four weeks after the accident, iii. 490. Of dissolution, attended by the absorption of anasarcous fluid before death, iii. 516. Of gun-shot wound in the cheek, iii. 555. Of gun-shot wound of the intestines, iii. 561. Of gun-shot wound through the body, which did well, iii. 564. Of wound of the lungs, by a small sword, iii. 568. Of inflammation of the veins of the arm, iii. 583. Of introsusception, iii.

589, 592. Of operation for popliteal aneurism by the author, iii. 598, 602, 603, 604, 605; by Mr. Lynn, iii. 605; by Mr. Birch, iii. 606; by Mr. Pott, iii. 608; by Mr. Cline, iii. 609; by Mr. Earle, iii. 611. Of horny excrescences from the head, iii. 632.

Cases of dentition attended with anomalous symptoms, ii. 110. Of gun-shot wounds which were left to themselves, iii. 549. Of operation for popliteal aneurism, iii. 598 et seq. and iii. 625. Of horny excrescences, iii. 631. Of a lady, two children, and a wet-nurse, infected with a disease resembling the lues venerea, ii. 475. Of three children and three wet-nurses having similar complaints, *ib.* Of diseases resembling the venereal disease, from transplanted teeth, ii. 483, 484.

Castle-street Museum; Hunter builds, i. 85. Opens to his friends, i. 107. Visited by eminent foreigners, i. 146.

Catalogue of Museum. (See *Museum.*)

Catheter in the urethra; mode of fixing it, ii. 270. Observations on the use of the, ii. 271. How introduced into the bladder when the prostate gland is enlarged, ii. 281. Of allowing it to remain in the urethra and bladder, ii. 297.

Cavendish, Lord; peculiarity of his case of stone in the bladder, i. 322.

Cavities circumscribed; inflammation of, i. 441.

Causation; often attributed to some accidental circumstance, iii. 25.

Cause and effect, the relation of, i. 208, note.

Caustics; how to apply them to the nerve of a tooth, ii. 66. Their use and application in stricture, ii. 242, 245, note, 267. Description of an instrument for conveying them to strictures in the urethra, ii. 244. And of the armed bougie, ii. 246, note; its chief effect is to relieve spasm, ii. 246, note; accidents attending its use in cases of stricture, ii. 247, note. Their use in opening abscesses, iii. 526. To be preferred to the knife in opening abscesses in irritable persons, i. 557. Their mode of action, i. 604, 605. Their use in cancer, i. 626.

Cautery actual; the use of, in diseases of the bones, i. 516, 528, 604. In cases of hæmorrhage, i. 541. In tetanus, i. 586, 588.

Cells, for the teeth; how formed, ii. 33. (See *Alveolar Processes.*)

Cellular tissue; preparations of the, i. 172. Inflammation of, iii. 518, note. Probably the regenerative tissue, iii. 271, note.

Chameleon; peculiarity in the structure of its tongue, i. 251; and vascular system, iii. 178, note.

Chancre; its poison the same as in gonorrhœa, ii. 143. Description of, ii. 316, 319, 321, note. Produced in three ways, ii. 317. May attack any part of the body, ii. 318. Not so frequent an effect of the venereal poison as the gonorrhœa, *ib.* Its seat, *ib.* Are to be distinguished more by their course and progress than by their present appearances, ii. 323, note. Of the distance of time between the application of the venereal poison and the appearance of, ii. 318. May produce a gonorrhœa by sympathy, ii. 320. An instance of its curing a gleet, *ib.* Its variation from constitution, ii. 321. Sometimes occasions a profuse bleeding, *ib.* Of, in women, ii. 327. Of the vagina, ii. 328, note. Observations on the treatment of, ii. 328. The constitution to be attended to in the cure of, ii. 329. Is a local complaint, but may infect the constitution by the absorption of its matter, ii. 330. May be destroyed in two ways, by excision or caustic, ii. 330. Neither of these methods to be relied on, ii. 331, note. Its cure, ii. 332. Local applications in, ii. 333. Is attended by particular dispositions, which must be considered in the cure, *ib.* Its cure by mercury given internally, ii. 340. Of the quantity of mercury necessary in the cure of, ii. 341. A kind of false one takes place sometimes after the cure of the true chancre, ii. 348. Consequences of; their treatment, ii. 344. Of dispositions to new diseases taking place during the cure of; their treatment, ii. 345.

Chara; flowers and fructifies in the hot-springs of Iceland, i. 293, note.

Chelsea Hospital, i. 7, 14.

Chemistry; applied to the investigation of the blood, i. 229, 355, notes. Has rendered important aids to physiology, iii. 12, note.

Cheselden, Mr.; anecdote of, i. 7.

Chilblains, i. 562.

Children, sympathies of; less determinate than in old persons, i. 324.

Chin, how projected forward in aged persons, ii. 33.

Cholera, how far occasioned by a vitiated state of the blood, iii. 46, note.

Chord, on the back of the penis; explanation of that appearance, ii. 358. Its treatment, ii. 370.

Chordee; its cause, ii. 170, 176. In some cases inflammatory, in others spasmodic, *ib.* Its treatment, ii. 210. The use of opium in, *ib.* The use of camphor in, ii. 210, 225. The use of electricity in, *ib.* The use of bark in, *ib.*

Christie, Mr., anecdote of, i, 138.

Christison, Dr., his work on poisons referred to, i. 353, note.

Chyle; the cause of the milkiness of the serum, iii. 56, note. Analogous to the blood, iii. 67, note. Is probably alive, iii. 117.

Chyme; the same from whatever substance it is elaborated, i. 230, 231.

Cicatrices, contraction of, i. 430.

Cicatrization, process of, i. 429, 554; iii. 500.

Cicuta. (See *Hemlock.*)

Cilia vibratory, of the mucous membranes; an important modern discovery, iii. 499.

Circulation of the blood; forces which assist in, iii. 229, note. Consequences of its interruption, ii. 55, note. Rapidity of, iii. 38, note, 210. Varies in different parts of the body, iii. 219. Dependence of, on the function of respiration, iii. 78, note. Manner in which it may be affected by obliteration of the valves of the heart, iii. 81. Gradual development of the organs of, in the zoological scale, iii. 100. Retarded in inflammation, iii. 326, note.

———, *capillary*; description of, iii. 196, note. State of in inflammation, iii. 325, note. Action of in the circulation of the blood, iii. 231, note.

———, *organs of*; i. 166; iii. 145.

Clarke, Dr. and Hunter, i. 75.

Clift, Mr., i. 131, 154.

——, *Mr. H.*, i. 154.

Climate; influence of in inducing a susceptibility to inflammation, iii. 275. Cause of, i. 294. The different means by which different animals are adapted to, i. 295, note. The effect of on disease, i. 354. In phthisis, i. 597. In scrofula, *ib.* On the lues venerea, ii. 399.

Cline, Mr., anecdotes of, i. 28, 53.

Clot; synonyms of, iii. 17, note. Composition and form of, varies according to many circumstances, iii. 25, 47. Contracts for several days, iii. 25; but in this respect does not differ from the curd of milk, iii. 30, note. Is said to be affected by various stimulants, iii. 128, note. In the heart and vessels during life, iii. 30. Reasons for doubting whether it is ever capable of becoming vascular, iii. 269, note. (See *Blood, Vascularity.*) Purulent deposits found in the centre of, iii. 457, note.

Clothing, warm; its advantages, in scrofula, i. 599.

Coagulation of the blood, i. 233; iii. 17. An inherent property of the fibrin, iii. 17, 20. Called an "act of contraction," iii. 23; which is compared to the action of life in the solids, iii. 33, 113. Necessary to the maintenance of life, iii. 20. Use of, in the œconomy, i. 234. Time required for, iii. 22, 23, note. Effect of cold on, iii. 26, 27. Of air on, *ib.* Of rest on, iii. 28. Retarded by contact of blood with blood, or with the living vessels, iii. 31. An act of life, iii. 34. Compared to union by the first intention, iii. 36, 267, note. Whether attended with a rise of temperature, iii. 35. Cause of, i. 238, 239; iii. 43, note. Accelerated by syncope, iii. 74, note. By heat, iii. 134. Power of, destroyed in many cases, i. 236, 238; iii. 42, note. Effect of various substances on, iii. 134, note.

Coagulum. (See *Clot.*)

Cocks, experiments on; in which their combs and wattles were frozen, iii. 109; and their testicles and spurs transplanted, ii. 56; iii. 256, 273.

Colchicum; the effect of, in inflammation, i. 401.

Cold; the negation of heat, i. 279, note; iii. 336. The generation of, in animals, i. 281, 292, 385; iii. 344. Its effects upon stricture, ii. 231. Upon the urethra, ii. 217. In disposing different parts of the body in receiving the venereal infection, ii. 400. Applied to the skin, affects the deeper-seated parts by sympathy, ii. 399. Effects of, when extreme, on the animal body, i. 284, note. Induces sleep, i. 285. In moderate degrees, acts as a stimulant, i. 286, 289, 345, 370, 481, 562. On its employment in mortification, iii. 8. In inflammation, iii. 265, 385. Effects of, on the coagulation of the blood, iii. 26, 27, notes. And on muscular fibre, *ib.*

Coleman, Professor, i. 48.

College of Surgeons. (See *Corporation.*)

Colour; advantage of a white, in animals, i. 295, note. Of inflamed parts, i. 383.

Committee; Hunter's revising, i. 101.

Compression of the brain, i. 487, 490, note.
Concretion, gouty; nature of, iii. 312, note.
Concussion of the brain, i. 487, 490, note; iii. 241, 243 notes. From gun-shot wounds, iii. 553, 570.
Consciousness; how used, in respect of the acts of an animal body, i. 232, 236, 255, 260, 264, 324, 361, 374, 398, 421, 430, 431, 524, 546, 553.
Constitution; an act of, what is to be understood by, i. 306, 339, 340, 483. Scorbutic, ii. 132. Treatment of, in the cure of gonorrhœa, ii. 204. Effects of inflammation in the perinæum and scrotum, on, ii. 267. To be attended to, in the cure of chancres, ii. 328. How infected by the matter of chancre, ii. 329. Irritable, consists in an increased disposition to act, without the power of acting, iii. 378, 381. Often affected in a degree disproportionate to the apparent cause, iii. 425. May be fatally depressed by simple violence, iii. 431.
Consumption; i. 596.
Contamination; the meaning of, ii. 396.
Contractility; a distinguishing mark of life, i. 242, note. Of the clot and muscular fibre, compared, iii. 43.
Cook's Voyage, quoted, ii. 143.
Copaiba; in gonorrhœa, ii. 208, note.
Copley Medal; Hunter receives, i. 107.
Copulation; of the requisites necessary for performing that act well, ii. 305.
Cornish, Mr., on the blood of torpid bats, iii. 33.
Corns, i. 560, 561.
Coronoid Process; in the upper jaw, described, ii. 2. The cells for the grinders formed in the root of, ii. 33.
Corporation of Surgeons; Hunter a member of, i. 34. Blamed by Sir J. Banks, i. 141. Accept the Hunterian Museum, i. 142. Obtain a royal charter, i. 143.
Correspondence. (See *Letters.*)
Corrosive sublimate; mode of giving it in the lues venerea, ii. 408, 442, note. A cure for itch, i. 618.
Cough; may be occasioned by the lues venerea, ii. 417.
Council of the College of Surgeons. (See *Museum Catalogue.*)
Counter-irritants, i. 406.
Coverings, external, i. 172.
Cowper's Glands; suppuration of, and fistula communicating with, i. 579; ii. 211. Affected in gonorrhœa, ii. 173, 178.
Cowpox and Smallpox form a hybridous disease, iii. 5, note.
Cranioscopy; the foundation on which it rests insecure, iii. 333.
Cranium; fractures of, i. 489. Peculiarities of, i. 493.
Crassamentum. (See *Clot.*)
Croonian Lectures, i. 50, 83.
Cruveilhier; his opinion respecting the reparative powers of the cellular tissue, iii. 271, note.
Crystals; Hunter's Collection of, i. 138.
Cubebs; in gonorrhœa, ii. 209, note.
Cuckoo; Hunter's letters on the, i. 37, 46, 91, 94, 104, 117. Stomach of, i. 46, 92. Jenner's paper on, i. 104.
Culley, Dr., i. 9.
Cuspidati, or canine teeth; particular description of, ii. 23. Their use, ii. 24. The frequent irregularity of, to what owing, ii. 88.
Cuticle; cracking of, a symptom of the lues venerea, ii. 408. Separation of from the cutis, how accounted for, i. 397, 554; iii. 349. New formed, nature of, i. 431; iii. 504.
Cutis; new-formed, nature of, iii. 502.

D.

Dancing, excited by sympathy, i. 321.
Davy, Dr., on buffy blood, i. 234.
——, *Sir H.*, on the effect of gases on the blood, iii. 28, note.
Dead Teeth; in what cases they are preferable to living ones, for transplantation, ii. 98. The objections they are liable to, ii. 101.

Death; the premonition of, i. 268. Difference between apparent nd absolute, i. 345. Convulsions of, i. 361.
Definitions; Mr. Hunter's objection to, i. 217.
Delirium; explanation of, i. 334, 364; iii. 436. In what respect it differs from insanity, i. 334, note.
Delusion; explanation of, i. 333, 354.
Denis and Emmerets, the first who performed transfusion on the human subject, iii. 13, note.
Dentes sapientiæ; particular description of those teeth, ii. 26. A frequent inconvenience in the cutting of, ii. 109. Violent pain from the cutting of, ii. 110.
Dentists; quackery of, ii. 58, note.
Dentition; cause of the pain in, explained, ii. 34, 105. Symptoms of, *ib.* Origin of these symptoms, ii. 106. Methods of relief and cure, ii. 108. Lancing the gums, *ib.* Contraction of the fingers and toes produced by, ii. 110.
Denudation; the decay of teeth by, described, ii. 70. (See *Scurvy.*)
Derivation, iii. 388, 394. (See *Revulsion.*)
Dessault's operation for aneurism, i. 98.
Development, laws of; in regard to the vascular system, iii. 184, note. In regard to the nervous system, iii. 329, note.
Diet, vegetable; in scrofula, of doubtful efficacy, i. 599.
Diet-Drinks; formulæ for, ii. 348. Their use in the lues venerea, ii. 460.
Digastricus; description and use of this muscle, ii. 11.
Digestion, i. 247, 248, note. Organs of, i. 161. Of the stomach, after death, i. 43, 165. Is suspended during hybernation, i. 286, note.
Digitalis; in inflammation, iii. 387.
Disease; the tendency of to destroy the body, i. 215. Curable and incurable, i. 300. Pathology of, ill understood, i. 301. Requires different occasional causes for its production, i. 309. Causes of, *ib.* Two cannot possibly exist in the same part at the same time, i. 313; ii. 132; iii. 2. Observations on, i. 314. Constitutional and local, reciprocally affect one another, i. 338, 485. Specific, i. 342, 554; iii. 306, 308, note, 367. Hereditary, i. 353. How affected by the mind, i. 359.
———, *Venereal*; Hunter's work on, i. 101. Its different forms, ii. 153. Varieties of, in different constitutions, ii. 154. Specific, observes a specific distance and extent, ii. 177, 395. A number of diseases said to be venereal which are not, ii. 423. Of the time necessary for the cure of its different forms, ii. 424. Of its prevention, ii. 464.
Diseases of the Teeth, specified, ii. 53.
——— *epidemic*; an observation on, ii. 152.
Dislocations, i. 518. Treatment of, *ib.*
Disposition to action; what is meant by, i. 269. May wear itself out, ii. 270. To be distinguished from action, i. 271, 300. And from susceptibility, i. 301, note. Is difficultly curable by medicine, i. 478; ii. 401.
Dispositions, diseased; meaning of, ii. 396; iii. 238. Division of, i. 308, 555. Always simple, i. 313. Of the irritable, i. 555. Of the indolent, i. 557. Of the cure of, i. 561. Are always more difficult of cure than the action, ii. 401. Actions which lead to restoration cannot be called diseased, iii. 239.
Dissolution, i. 341, 435; iii. 296, 506, 513.
Donellan, Capt., his trial, i. 81, 194.
Drawing of Teeth; the proper indication for, ii. 95. Consequence of deferring the operation too long, *ib.* Directions for its performance, *ib.* Remarks on the usual treatment of the gums, *ib.* How to stop the extraordinary bleeding of the gums, ii. 96. No bad consequences to be apprehended from breaking the alveolar processes, *ib.* Breaking of teeth, ii. 97. How to replace a tooth, drawn by mistake, ii. 100.
Drawings, Hunterian, i. 149.
Dreams; explanation of, i. 335. In what respect they differ from insanity, i. 337, note.
Dress; Hunter's style of, i. 133.
Dressings, may be advantageously dispensed with in many cases, i. 429.
Dropsy; the reparative powers often greatly reduced in, iii. 280.
——— *Ovarian*; proposal for extirpating the cysts in, i. 573, note.
Drowning; the question as to the probability of resuscitation from, iii. 32, note.
Dura mater; tumour of, i. 424; iii. 473. Wounds of, i. 451.

E.

Ear; burning of, useful in tooth-ache, ii. 66.

Earl's Court; Hunter's purchase of, i. 32. Description of, i. 120. Sale of, i. 137.

Ecchymosis, i. 388; iii. 244. The blood does not always coagulate in, iii. 33, 34. The effused blood in, is always dark-coloured, iii. 87.

Effect, ultimate; of an animal body, is the preservation and continuance of the species, i. 225, 273, 293.

Effusions, serous; in what respect they differ from the serum of the blood, iii. 21.

Egg; development of the chick in, i. 176. Drawings of, i. 177. Life of, i. 224; which is evinced by its resistance to cold and putrefaction, i. 228. Experiments on, iii. 106.

Elasticity; its properties and uses, in the animal body, i. 245; iii. 149, 155. Distinct from muscular action, i. 246, note.

Electricity; destroys the contractility of muscles, i. 228; promotes absorption, i. 431. Operates as a stimulant, i. 482. Its use in chordee, ii. 210. In the swelled testicle, ii. 214. In paralysis of the urethra, ii. 276. In paralysis of the bladder, ii. 290. In venereal warts, ii. 352. Its powers on diseases increased by mercury, ii. 455. Accelerates the coagulation of the blood, iii. 34. Is not identifiable with the vital principle, iii. 122, note.

Elephantiasis, i. 562.

Elliotson, Dr., i. 285, 294, notes.

Emaciation, iii. 11.

Emetics; their uses and effects, iii. 383. In abscesses, iii. 417. The second emetic does not need to be so powerful as the first, i. 276.

Eminent men; their small beginnings, i. 5.

Empyema; cases of, i. 442, 444; iii. 417.

Enamel of the teeth; description and use of, ii. 15. Experiments on, to ascertain the nature of its composition, ii. 15, note. Formation of, explained, ii. 41.

Endosmose and *Exosmose*, iii. 84, 85, note.

Epididymis; state of, in a swelled testicle, ii. 180, 213, 226.

Epistaxis; cure of, by oil of turpentine, i. 539.

Erection of the penis; how effected, i. 250. Painful, how prevented, ii. 210.

Erectile tissue; the structure of, i. 251.

Erethismus, mercurial; described, ii. 432, note.

Eruptions, venereal; variety of, baffles all description, ii. 409, note. Description of, ii. 410, note. Pustular, ii. 413, note. (See *Blotches*.)

Erysipelas; described, i. 398; iii. 314. The order of the effects of inflammation reversed in, iii. 284, 290, 315.

Escharotics; their use in destroying strictures in the urethra, ii. 243. In destroying warts, ii. 353.

Evacuations; seldom proper in specific diseases, i. 609.

Evaporation; one of the chief means by which the animal temperature is regulated, i. 289, note.

Exacerbations; the reason of, i. 381; iii. 431.

Examination, post mortem; of Hunter, i. 132. Of Sir J. Reynolds, i. 121.

Excrescences, horny; iii. 631.

Exercise; occasions the blood to become buffy, iii. 40, note.

Exfoliation of bone; i. 514, 525, 529.

Exostosis, i. 534. Sometimes arises from inflammation, iii. 533.

Experience; the only means by which we obtain a knowledge of the powers of medicines, iii. 366.

Experiments; made to prove that matter from sores in the lues venerea will not affect a person locally who has the lues venerea; but that matter from a gonorrhœa or chancre will, ii. 386. To ascertain the progress and effects of the venereal poison, ii. 417. Conclusion drawn from those experiments, ii. 419. To prove that mercury and its preparations are dissolved in the animal juices, ii. 453.

Extirpation, of tumours; often difficult, i. 567. Mode of, i. 569.

Extraction, of pieces of dead bone; i. 530. Of teeth, ii. 53, 54, note 95. The folly and mischief of, in many cases, ii. 47, 92, notes.

Eye; inflammation of, i. 449. Doubtful if ever venereal, ii. 417. Of the iris, undoubtedly venereal, *ib.* note.

F.

Face; how shortened in aged persons, ii. 32.
Facts; their use and value, i. 208.
Fainting. (See *Syncope*.)
Fangs of teeth; comparative observations on, ii. 26. How formed, ii. 40. Will continue sound when the tooth is destroyed, ii. 60. Swelling of, described, ii. 71.
Fat; unnatural accumulation of, i. 563. Uses of, iii. 12, note. The cause of the milky colour of the serum, iii. 56, note.
Fatness; the cause of, iii. 11, note.
Feelings; when powerful, prevent reasoning and voluntary motion, i. 260.
Feet, wet; effect of on the stomach, i. 325.
Fermentation, i. 217, note, 218. Not the cause of animal heat, i. 282. The venereal poison does not arise from, ii. 147.
Fever; two different kinds of, cannot exist at the same time, ii. 132. Its effects on gonorrhœa, ii. 205. Brings the lues venerea into action, ii. 400.
——, *hectic*, i. 324, 341, 431; ii. 131; iii. 433, 507. The effect of an incurable local disorder, i. 341; iii. 507. Hence it arises most readily from diseases of the bones and in scrofulous persons, i. 506. Sometimes an original constitutional disorder, i. 432; iii. 507. Does not depend on the absorption of pus, i. 433; iii. 509. Is not usually produced by large abscesses, until opened, iii. 511. Treatment of, i. 434; iii. 512.
——, *jail*. (See *Plague*.)
——, *suppurative*; iii. 424. Sometimes takes place in gonorrhœa, ii. 191.
——, *sympathetic inflammatory*, i. 324, 341; ii. 131; iii. 433. Does not necessarily attend union by the first intention, iii. 249. Is favourable when equal to and of the same nature as the existing inflammation, iii. 306. Violence of, depends on many circumstances, iii. 424.
Fibrin; solidity the natural state of, iii. 15. Described, iii. 23. Specific gravity of, iii. 22, 24, notes. The most important element of the blood, iii. 37. The relative proportion of, in the blood, varies, iii. 37, 46, notes. Is increased during inflammation and utero-gestation, iii. 37. Undergoes changes in the inflamed vessels, i. 367; iii. 353, note. Effused, becomes vascular, i. 367. And forms the medium of union of divided parts, iii. 267, note. And becomes of the same nature as the parts which afford it, i. 396.
Filing; the injurious effects of, on the teeth, ii. 81, note.
Fingers and toes; case of contraction of, produced by dentition, ii. 110.
Fistulæ, i. 426, 428, 577. Cure of, i. 581; iii. 572. Of the buccal glands, i. 578. Of Cowper's glands in the female, *ib.* Of the parotid gland, i. 579.
—— *lachrymales*, i. 578.
—— *in ano*, i. 579.
—— *in perinæo*; its cause, ii. 268. The occasion of aguish complaints, *ib.* Its cure, ii. 269. Description of the operation for, *ib.*
Fluor albus; sometimes communicates a disease similar to the gonorrhœa, ii. 186. Cure of, ii. 221, note; iii. 279.
Fluids, animal; the consequences of their stagnation pointed out, ii. 56.
Fœtal peculiarities, i. 178.
Fœtus; before birth has no sensation, i. 264. Acephalous, i. 265. Progress of the formation of the teeth in, ii. 33. May be infected *in utero* with the lues venerea by the matter which infected the mother, ii. 385. But not from the effects of that matter upon the mother, ii. 388. This opinion questioned, i. 354; ii. 476, notes. The blood of, does not contain fibrin, and therefore does not coagulate, iii. 37, note. Is more vascular than the adult, iii. 213.
Fomentations; their use in inflammation, iii. 386, 396, 413.
Fontana; his experiments referred to, ii. 164; iii. 30, note.
Food; on an artificial method of conveying into the stomach, in cases of paralysis of the muscles of deglutition, iii. 622.
Foot, Mr. Jesse; his calumnies of Hunter, i. 21. His Life of Hunter, i. xxi. 22. His work on the Venereal Disease, *ib.* His Life of Murphy, *ib.*
Fordyce, Dr., i. 44, 57, 85. His experiments quoted, ii. 291, 292.
Foreign bodies; their approach to the surface explained, iii. 300, 479, notes.
Formation, the order of, in the development of the fœtus, i. 264, note.

Fossils, Hunter's collection of, i. 148.
Fractures, simple, i. 439. Their mode of union, i. 501. Their treatment, i. 503. Period required for their union, i. 504.
——, *compound*, i. 440, 509. The question of amputation in such cases, i. 510; iii. 281, 575, notes. The danger of, *ib.*
—— *of the Cranium*, i. 489. From gun-shot wounds, iii. 553, 570.
—— *of the Thigh*, ununited, i. 426. Cause of, i. 504. Treatment of, i. 505.
Fragility; of the bones, i. 532, note. Of structure, one of the consequences of inflammation, iii. 532.
Frank, Dr., i. 146.
Freezing, Mr. Hunter's speculations on, as a method of prolonging life, i. 57, 284.
Fresne, M. Du, i. 146.
Friction; not the cause of animal heat, i. 281. A stimulus, i. 481.
Frost-bitten parts; the principle on which they should be restored, i. 603.
Frozen animals; may be recovered, i. 284; iii. 107, notes.
Functions; of sensation and voluntary motion, perfect in proportion to the proximity of the parts to the heart and brain, i. 274.

G.

Gaertner, Dr., i. 146.
Galvanism; accelerates coagulation, iii. 34, note. A delicate test of the presence of albumen, iii. 49, note.
Ganglions, i. 449.
Gangrene, iii. 318. (See *Mortification.*)
Garthshore, Dr., i. 28. And Hunter, i. 114. Kindness to Mrs. Hunter, i. 139.
Gases, effects of on the blood, iii. 28, note.
Gay Lussac and Thenard; their analysis of animal substances, iii. 20, note.
Gelatine; does not exist in the blood or animal secretions, iii. 20, 50, notes.
Gendrin, M., iii. 325, 457, notes.
Generation, organs of, multiplied in the lower animals, iii. 116, note. The ultimate object of life, i. 273, 293.
George's St., Hospital; Hunter a pupil at, i. 15. Disagreement amongst the surgeons of, i. 127. Appeal to the Governors of, i. 128. Death of Hunter at, i. 132.
Gillaroo Trout, i. 50.
Gland, prostate, swelling of, ii. 278. Its effects on the canal of the urethra, ii. 278, 280. Sometimes prevents a stone in the bladder being felt, ii. 279. Mode of detecting it, ii. 280. Its treatment, ii. 282. Should be perforated rather than puncture the bladder, in cases of retention of the urine, ii. 297, note. The use of hemlock in, ii. 283. The use of burnt sponge in, *ib.* Of the discharge of the secretion of, ii. 302. Mucus of; the distinction between it and the semen, ii. 203.
Glands, absorbent; swellings of, from sympathy, ii. 77, 182, 251, 256. Affected singly by the venereal poison, ii. 360. Those which are second in order are not affected by the venereal poison; the reason of this, *ib.* Swellings of, how distinguished from buboes, ii. 263.
—— *of the groin*; affected by sympathy in a gonorrhœa, ii. 177, 182. Of the urethra, their suppurations, how treated, ii. 172, 211. Of the groin, affected sympathetically by the use of bougies, ii. 251, 256.
——, *buccal*; obstruction of, i. 579. Fistula of, i. 578.
——, *conglomerate*; most susceptible of cancer, i. 618.
——, *Cowper's*; obstruction of, i. 578. Fistula of, *ib.*
——, *mesenteric*; do not form the red globules of the blood, iii. 68, note.
——, *parotid*; obstruction of, i. 579. Fistula of, *ib.*
Gleet; its cause, ii. 219. Its cure, ii. 221. Balsams, their use in, ii. 222. Injections to be used in, *ib.* The use of blisters in, ii. 224. The use of electricity in, ii. 225. Its treatment in women, *ib.* Attends upon stricture, ii. 229, 257. In consequence of a stricture, its cure, ii. 248. Cured by a chancre, an instance of, ii. 320.
Globules, blood, iii. 57. Teach nothing concerning the use of this fluid, i. 230. Their proportion to the serum, iii. 45, note. Uses of, *ib.* Size and shape of, iii. 62, note. Motion of, i. 242; iii. 63, 131, notes. Origin of, iii. 64, 67, notes. Probably the least important part of the blood, iii. 68. Whether the ultimate molecules of the solid textures, iii. 103, note. Become heavier in inflammation, iii. 356.

Globules, lymph, iii. 63, note.
——, *pus*, i. 317, note; iii. 449, 456, note. (See *Pus.*)
Gonorrhœa; may produce a lues venerea, ii. 146. Does not arise from ulcers in the urethra, ii. 159. Appears sometimes the day after receiving the infection, ii. 160. May be cured without mercury, ii. 159, 196. Virulent and simple; difficult to distinguish them, ii. 161. Frequently cures itself, ii. 163, 194, 199. Cannot be increased by the application of fresh matter, ii. 165. This opinion questioned, ii. 208, note. The first the severest; the succeeding ones generally milder; facts seeming to prove this, *ib.* Frequently continues a long time without losing its virulence, ii. 166, 215. Its seat in both sexes, ii. 168. Often confined to the glans, ii. 169. Its symptoms, ii. 171. Affects Cowper's glands, ii. 175. Of the discharge in, ii. 173. A variety of symptoms produced by sympathy in, ii. 177. Uncommon symptoms in, ii. 179. Its effects on the constitution in both sexes, ii. 191. Its cure, ii. 192. No specific medicine for, ii. 193. Different modes of practice in, ii. 195. As soon cured without mercury as with, ii. 196. May be contracted by a person under a course of mercury, ii. 197. How affected by fever, ii. 205. Treatment of occasional symptoms of, ii. 208. And gleet; the distinction between them not yet ascertained, ii. 215. Symptoms of, remaining after the disease is subdued, ii. 216. Supposed consequences of, ii. 227. Does not in general occasion stricture, ii. 232. Sometimes relieves a stricture, ii. 249. May be produced by a chancre sympathetically, ii. 320.
—— *in women*, ii. 186. Not easily distinguished from fluor albus, *ib.* The parts affected, ii. 187. Uncommon symptoms in, *ib.* Wears itself out in women as well as men, *ib.* Proofs of its existence in women, ii. 190. Its continuance, ii. 191. May exist without the patient knowing it, *ib.* Its cure, ii. 203.
Goods, Hunter's sale of, i. 138.
Gout, peculiar effect of, i. 244. Relieved by local action, i. 306. Ill formed, i. 307. Its connection with the secretion of uric acid, i. 353, note. Not hereditary, i. 358. Often produced by anxiety of mind, iii. 276.
Gouty Inflammation, iii. 311. More violent than common inflammation, *ib.* Has neither the adhesive or suppurative disposition, iii. 302. Cases where it should be repelled, iii. 371.
Grant, Dr., iii. 58, note.
Granulations, iii. 488. The second mode of union, i. 368. May take place independently of suppuration, iii. 490. Nature and properties of, i. 426; iii. 491. Formation and union of, i. 428; iii. 493. Longevity of, iii. 495. Contraction of, iii. 496. Of bones, i. 427, 504. Scrofulous, i. 594.
Gregorie, Abbé, i. 146.
Gregory, Dr., iii. 306, note.
Grinders; particularly described, ii. 25. Difference between those of the upper and lower jaw, ii. 26. The removal of the first, when decaying at an early age, recommended, ii. 92.
Growth of bones, illustrated, i. 253. Preternatural, of parts, i. 563.
Guaiacum; its uses in the lues venerea, ii. 460, 463.
Gum Guaiacum; its effects in the lues venerea, ii. 456.
Gums, the nature and use of, explained, ii. 29. How affected by dentition, ii. 34. Excrescences from, how to be treated, ii. 75, 76, notes. Effect of the scurvy on, ii. 80. Treatment of in this case, *ib.* Symptoms of the disorder vulgarly called the scurvy of, ii. 82. The cause of investigated, *ib.* Proper treatment of in this case, ii. 83 Callous thickenings of, *ib.* When of a cancerous nature require chirurgical treatment, ii. 84. Remarks on the common treatment of, in drawing teeth, ii. 95. Method of checking the extraordinary bleeding of, when a tooth is drawn, ii. 96. An attentive examination into the state of, necessary, when teeth are to be transplanted, ii. 97. When they ought to be cut, to facilitate dentition, ii. 108, 110, 111.
Gum-boils, the causes of, explained, ii. 72. Extraction of the affected tooth the only cure of, in the last resort, ii. 75, notes. How to open and dress them, *ib.* Treatment of, in the back part of the mouth, *ib.* (See *Abscess* and *Scurvy.*)
Gunning, Mr.; applies for an assistant, i. 107. His character, i. 127. Opposes Hunter, i. 128.
Guthrie, Mr., i. 549; iii. 576, notes.
Guy, Mr., i. 35.

H.

Habit; as applied to the body, i. 274, 276. The importance of, in respect of the mind, i. 277.

Hæmatemesis, case of, i. 483. Cured by oil of turpentine, i. 539.

Hæmatocele, i. 463, 631.

Hæmatosine, iii. 58, 66, notes.

Hæmoptysis; a precursor of phthisis, i. 597.

Hæmorrhage; capillary, i. 435. Cases of, i. 534, 543. Causes and kinds of, i. 536. Suppression of, i. 538, 541. Secondary, i. 542. From chancre; the use of oil of turpentine in, ii. 335. After gun-shot wounds not great in general, iii. 546.

Hereditary; how far diseases may be said to be so, i. 353. This property may be acquired, i. 357. Nature of gout and scrofula, i. 358. Of madness, i. 359. Of cancer, i. 623.

Hall, Dr. Marshall, i. 266, 293, 537; iii. 33. 87, notes.

Haller, Baron; his abstinence from wine, i. 10. He discovers the tubuli testis, i. 18. Describes the hernia congenita, *ib.*

Harmony, of the machine, i. 264; iii. 10, 125, note.

Harvey, Dr., on the life of the blood, iii. 104, note.

Hastings, Dr. C., on the state of the vessels in inflammation, iii. 326, note.

Hatchet, Mr., on the composition of shells, &c., i. 159.

Hawkins, Sir C., i. 25.

———, *Charles*, i. 127.

Head, pains of, relieved by amputation of the leg, i. 401. Injuries of, i. 486. (See *Cranium.*)

Health, the feeling of, often a precursor of disease, i. 311. Consists in the harmonious action of all the functions, i. 264; iii. 10, 125. Full, is not favourable for operations, iii. 281.

Heat; the antagonizing principle to attraction, i. 213, 278. The nature of, i. 279. Latent and absolute, the difference between, *ib.* Its effects on the body, i. 280, 315, 344, 482. Some effects of, similar to those of cold, i. 281, note. On its employment in mortification, iii. 8.

——, *vital*, Hunter's papers on, i. 57, 68. Experiments on, i. 59, 65; iii. 338. A certain standard of, necessary for the performance of the animal functions, i. 281, 285, 289. Which differs in different animals, i. 281, 288. And in different climates and seasons, i. 293; iii. 335, note. The causes of, i. 281, 288, 384; iii. 343. The author professes his ignorance on this subject, iii. 16, 335. Does not depend on respiration, i. 283. This opinion questioned, iii. 343, note. Is the effect of life, i. 283. Differs in different parts, i. 288, 289. How the standard of, is preserved, i. 291, 292. Of inflamed parts, i. 384, 397; iii. 335, 338. In fever, iii. 337. Referred to the stomach, i. 384; iii. 336. Of the vital parts, not affected by local inflammation, i. 385. How far dependent on the nervous system, iii. 343, note.

Heart; Hunter's affection of, i. 44, 94, 131, 244; iii. 193. Adhesions of to the pericardium, i. 444; iii. 348. Its action, cause of, iii. 188. How far dependent on respiration, iii. 78, note, 193. And on the nervous system, iii. 190, note. Immediate cause of, iii. 192, note. Diseases of the valves of; cases of, iii, 80, 193. Case of, in which the ventricles communicated, iii. 82. Case of, in which the coronary arteries were ossified, iii. 193. The influence of on the circulation, iii. 173. Varieties in the structure of in different animals, iii. 174, 183. Use of, iii. 176. Structure of, *ib.* Formation of, iii. 177. Size of, iii. 181. Contraction of, iii. 184. Cause of its impulse on the chest, iii. 185. Sounds of, iii. 186, note.

Hectic fever. (See *Fever.*)

Hellebore, a cure for scabies, i. 618.

Hemlock; successfully used in nervous pains of the jaws, ii. 85. In scrofula, i. 599; iii. 370. In swellings of the prostate gland, ii. 283. In what is called seminal weakness, ii. 304. In spreading ulcers of the prepuce, ii. 346. An instance of its having been taken in very large quantities, ii. 379. Its use in buboes, *ib.* In lues venerea, ii. 460, 463.

Hemiplegia; proceeds from the same cause as apoplexy, iii. 261.

Hérisson, M.; his sphygmometer, iii. 217, note.

Hernia, i. 448.

Hernia cerebri, arises from the support of the dura mater being removed, i. 495.
——— *congenita*; disputes respecting, i. 18.
——— *humoralis*; symptoms of, ii. 180.
Hewson, Mr.; succeeds Hunter, i. 23.
Hiccup, iii. 436.
Hip; diseases of, i. 595. The lengthening and shortening of the limb explained, *ib.*
Hoffman, Mr., on the arterialization of the blood, iii. 96, note.
Hollow Teeth; methods of stopping, ii. 68.
Home, Sir E., becomes Hunter's pupil, i. 44. Appointed to Plymouth Hospital, i. 72. Returns from Jamaica, i. 92. Becomes Hunter's assistant, i. 96. His paper on the Terebella, *ib.* Elected assistant surgeon to St. George's Hospital, i. 108. Publishes Hunter's work on inflammation, i. 123. Succeeds Hunter as lecturer on surgery, *ib.* Contests St. George's Hospital, i. 127. Present at Hunter's death, i. 131. Appointed Hunter's executor, i. 137. With Baillie, establishes the Hunterian oration, i. 146. Destroys the Hunterian MSS., i. 152. His numerous papers in the Phil. Trans., i. 153. On strictures, ii. 245, note. On the prostate gland, ii. 283, note. Experiments of, on suppuration, iii. 445. On introsusception, iii. 593. Two papers of, containing an account of Mr. Hunter's method of operating for popliteal aneurism, i. 117; iii. 594, 613. Paper of, on loose cartilages, i. 118; iii. 625. On horny excrescences, iii. 631.
——, *Miss*, i. 40.
Horny excrescences; observations on, iii. 631.
Humours; of the existence of, in the blood, i. 347, 352, note.
Hunter, James; account of, i. 2.
———, *John*; his birth and parentage, i. 1. Proceeds to London, i. 6. His first essay in anatomy, i. 7. A pupil of Cheselden, *ib.* His youthful freaks, i. 10. His advantageous position, *ib.* A pupil at St. Bartholomew's, i. 12. Revisits Scotland, i. 13. Enters at Oxford, i. 14. Resolves on his future course, *ib.* Enters at St. George's Hospital, i. 15. Becomes house surgeon, *ib.* His anatomical skill, *ib.* His dissection of the placenta, *ib.* Enters into partnership with his brother, i. 16. His part in anatomical disputes, i. 18. His paper on the descent of the testis, i. 19. Falls into ill health, i. 20. Becomes an army surgeon, *ib.* Goes abroad, *ib.* His private life and Foote's calumnies, i. 21. Returns to London, i. 23. Settles in practice, i. 24. His slow progress to fortune, i. 26. His ardour for the advance of his profession, i. 28. His carelessness of money, *ib.* Lectures on surgery, &c. *ib.* Recommences comparative anatomy, i. 30. His extensive plan of research, i. 31. His originality, i. 32. Purchases Earl's Court, *ib.* His amusements, *ib.* His dangerous encounters, i. 33. Elected an F.R.S., *ib.* Ruptures his tendo Achillis, i. 34. Elected surgeon to St. George's, *ib.* Elected member of the Corporation of Surgeons, *ib.* Receives house pupils, *ib.* Moves to Jermyn-street, i. 35. His friendship with Jenner, i. 37. His correspondence with Jenner (See *Letters*), i. 38. Publishes on the teeth, i. 40. Marries Miss Home, *ib.* His taste for society, i. 41. Routs and soirée, *ib.* His family, *ib.* His papers in the Phil. Trans. (See *Phil. Trans.*) Suffers from affection of the heart, i. 44, 244; iii. 193. Dissects torpedo, i. 46. Lectures on surgery, i. 47. His opinion of lecturing, i. 48. His character as a lecturer, *ib.* His disciples, i. 49. His papers on anatomical subjects, i. 50. Engages Mr. Bell, i. 51. Addicted to fits of passion and to swearing, i. 52. His punctuality, *ib.* Allotment of his time, i. 53. And Cline, anecdote of, *ib.* And Blizard, i. 54. Took but little repose, *ib.* His amusements few, i. 55. Projects a school of natural history, *ib.* Made surgeon extraordinary to the King, i. 57. Appointed Croonian lecturer, i. 58. Engaged in experiments on vital heat, i. 59, 66. Attacked with cerebral affection, i. 62. Visits Bath, i. 64. Returns to London, i. 65. Publishes second part of work on the teeth, i. 71. His professional gains, i. 72. His estimation of the cost of his museum, *ib.* His greediness for rarities, i. 75. Claims the discovery of the anatomy of the placenta, i. 76. His quarrel with Dr. Hunter, i. 77. His reconciliation, i. 80. Gives evidence on the trial of Donellan, i. 81. Elected F.S.B.L.G., i. 83. Completes his Croonian lectures, *ib.* Elected member of S.R.M.P. and A.R.C.P., i. 84. Purchases house in Leicester-fields, i. 85. Builds museum, *ib.* Assists to establish the Lyceum Medicum, *ib.* Assists to form Society for the Improvement of Medical and Chirurgical Knowledge, i. 86. His consultation with Taylor, i. 87. His paper on inflammation of the veins, i. 91. As an operator, i. 93. His opinion of operations, *ib.* His heart again affected, i. 94. Visits Tun-

bridge and Bath, i. 95. Returns to London, i. 96. Engages Home as his assistant, *ib.* Operates for aneurism, *ib.* Becomes deputy surgeon-general, i. 101. Publishes on syphilis, *ib.* Publishes on the animal œconomy, i. 102. Prints at home, *ib.* His expensive researches, i. 105. Obtains Byrne's body, i. 106. Receives the Copley medal, i. 107. Elected fellow of A.P.S., *ib.* Opens his museum, *ib.* Obtains assistant at St. George's, *ib.* Sits for his picture, i. 108. Patronizes Sharp, i. 109. And Mr. Thomas, anecdote of, i. 114. And Sir A. Carlisle, i. 115. And Mr. Lynn, i. 116. Loses his memory suddenly, i. 119. His love of life, *ib.* His residence at Earl's Court, i. 120. His toryism, &c., i. 121. Resigns his lectureship, i. 123. Preparing his work on inflammation, *ib.* Aids in establishing the Veterinary College, i. 125. Elected M.R.C.S.I. and M.C.P.S.E. *ib.* Disagrees with his colleagues, i. 127. Supports Home, versus Keate, *ib.* Resolves to appropriate pupils' fees, *ib.* His letter to his colleagues, i. 128. His letter to the governors of St. George's, *ib.* Undertakes the cause of two students, i. 131. Attends at St. George's, *ib.* His death, *ib.* Post mortem examination of, i. 132. His interment, i. 133. His personal appearance, *ib.* His character as a man, i. 134. As a surgeon, i. 135. As a naturalist, *ib.* His will, i. 137. His goods sold, i. 138. His library, *ib.* His crystallizations, *ib.* Epitaph on, Mrs. H.'s, i. 139. His anxiety about his museum, i. 149. His intended works, i. 150. His leaning to the Stahlian hypothesis, i. 255. His love of truth exemplified, ii. 19, note; iii. 121, notes.

Hunter, Dr. W.; a pupil of Cullen, i. 3. Settles in London, i. 4. Engages with Douglas, *ib.* Commences lecturing, *ib.* His narrow circumstances, i. 5. His anatomical disputes, i. 18. Offers to found a school of anatomy, i. 35. Builds a theatre in Windmill-street, *ib.* His quarrel with John, i. 76. His letter to the Royal Society, i. 77. His will, i. 80. His satisfaction in dying, i. 119.

———, *Mrs.*; her character and tastes, i. 40. Her parties, i. 41. Her letter to Jenner, i. 96. Desires to erect a monument to Hunter, i. 133. Her reduced circumstances, i. 137. Her pension, *ib.* Obtains a situation, i. 139. Her epitaph on Hunter, *ib.*

Hutchison, Mr. C., iii. 388.

Hybernation; the animal and organic functions suspended during, i. 244, note. Compared with ordinary sleep and torpor, i. 285, note.

Hydatids, i. 456, note, 572. Of the uterus, i. 573. Of the kidney, i. 574. Of the liver, *ib.* Of the lungs, *ib.* Of the brain, *ib.* Cancerous, i. 619.

Hydrargyri oxymurias; a delicate test of the presence of albumen, iii. 49, note. Use of in lues venerea, ii. 408, 442, note.

Hydrargyrum. (See *Mercury.*)

Hydrocele, i. 454. Causes of, i. 457. Spontaneous cure of, *ib.* Congenital, *ib.* Diagnosis of, i. 458. Varieties of, i. 461, note. Palliative cure of, i. 462. Different modes of radical cure of, i. 464. Causes of their failure, i. 470. Method by injection, i. 476, note.

————, *encysted*, i. 456.

Hydrocephalus, i. 488.

Hydrophobia; does not arise spontaneously, i. 615. Affects animals of different species, *ib.* Observations on, ii. 152, 383.

Hydrops pectoris; symptoms of, i. 442.

Hypertrophy; from chronic inflammation, i. 558, 563; iii. 533. Of the heart, cause of, iii. 82.

Hypopium, i. 450.

I.

Ice; of the application of in hæmorrhage of the urethra, ii. 210, note.

Identity, personal; the idea of, sometimes lost in dreams, i. 335, note. Curious case of, i. 336.

Idiosyncrasies, i. 611.

Imagination; the only active principle of the mind in sleep, i. 335, note. The influence of, i. 337, 359, 360; ii. 479; iii. 276.

Impotence; its causes, ii. 304. Depending on the mind, the cause of, ii. 305. From a want of proper correspondence between the actions of the different organs, ii. 308.

Impressions, i. 267. Insensibility to, acquired by custom, i. 274.

Incisores; the class of teeth so called, particularly described, ii. 22.

Incoagulability, of the blood, occurs under various circumstances, iii. 42, note.

Incrustations; on the teeth, the nature of explained, ii. 85. Mechanical, methods of removing, ii. 87. Chemical applications, *ib.* (See *Scaling.*)

Incubation; the yolk and albumen do not putrefy during, iii. 106.

Indians, East and West; their power of generating heat diminished, i. 293, note.

Induration; one of the effects of inflammation, i. 558, 563; iii. 532, note. Passing into ulceration, the constant and distinctive mark of the venereal irritation, ii. 321, note.

Infection; mode of preventing, i. 296, 314; ii. 140. May be received through the blood, i. 352, note. Venereal, the modes of, ii. 152. The opinion that it is received by matter only, and the practice founded on this dogma, questioned, ii. 141, note. May take place from simple chancrous induration, without breach of surface, ii. 142, note.

Inflammation; Mr. Hunter's treatise on, i. 123. Definition of, i. 393; iii. 297. Fundamental principles of, i. 365; iii. 268. The knowledge of a first principle in surgery, iii. 297. Division of, into adhesive, suppurative, and ulcerative, i. 366; ii. 135; iii. 282, 298. Into healthy and unhealthy, simple and specific, single and compound, iii. 298. Into such as affects the cellular membrane and body generally, and such as affects the outlets, iii. 298. The different degrees and kinds of, iii. 301. Consists in an increase of action and power, i. 365, 379, 381; iii. 7, 357, 372. Being a restorative action, is not to be considered as a disease, i. 365, 393; iii. 295, 305, 368, 406. Is allied to fever, iii. 275. Of the different causes which increase or diminish the susceptibility to, iii. 276. Of the parts most susceptible of, iii. 282. Of different organs and structures; produces very different effects on the constitution, iii. 277, 362. Causes of, i. 369, 371; iii. 304. How far the nervous system is concerned in the production of, iii. 328, note. Proximate cause of, i. 371; iii. 325, note. Is modified by the constitution, iii. 278, 307. By structure, i. 366, 373, 374; iii. 271, 274, 307, 310, note, 313, 370. By situation and position, iii. 272. By strength and weakness, i. 374; iii. 276, 278. Of the different degrees and kinds of inflammation, iii. 301. Spontaneous inflammation the most violent, *ib.* That from the death of a part the least so, iii. 302. Carbunculous, iii. 317. Chronic, i. 557. Critical, i. 370; iii. 303. Erysipelatous, i. 398, 556; iii. 290, 314, 401. Gouty, i. 369; iii. 302, 311. Irritable, i. 556; ii. 193; iii. 374, 378. Attended with mortification, iii. 318. Œdematous, iii. 314. Scrofulous, i. 590, 593; iii. 307, 419. Venereal, ii. 177. Inflammation of the bladder, i. 448. Of the bones, i. 505; iii. 277, 278, 530. Of the bursæ, i. 449. Of cartilages, iii. 530. Of the cellular membrane, iii. 316, 347, 528. Of the eye, i. 449. Of fibrous membranes, iii. 530. Of the joints, i. 449, 519. Of the lungs, i. 398; iii. 400. Of the lymphatics and veins, i. 451; iii. 519, 531, 581. Of mucous and serous membranes, i. 441; iii. 288, 529. Of muscles, iii. 531. Of the nerves and brain, i. 451; iii. 531. Of the pericardium, i. 444. Of the perinæum, and parts surrounding the urethra, ii. 262, 264, 266. Of the peritoneum, i. 445. Of the skin, iii. 528. Of the teeth, ii. 63, 67. Of the urethra, ii. 176. Effects of, on structure, 532, note. Primary, *ib.* Secondary, iii. 533, note. Effects of, on the constitution, i. 375; iii. 278. Where the part is equal to the act, the constitution does not sympathize, iii. 321, 330. Effects of, on the vascular system, i. 376.

——————, *Adhesive*; i. 393, 398; iii. 321. Action of the vessels in, iii. 321. Compared to a blush, iii. 322. From which, however, it is to be distinguished, iii. 324. The circulation in, accelerated, iii. 318, 323, 325. This opinion questioned, iii. 325, note. Colour of, i. 383; iii. 323, 326. Swelling of, i. 383; iii. 327. Pain of, i. 385; iii. 331. Heat of, i. 383, 397; iii. 335. Involves all the functions of a part, iii. 328, note. Effusions in, *ib.* Of the time that is required for its development, iii. 346. Of the uniting medium in, iii. 349. New vessels are formed in this medium, iii. 325, 351. (See *Blood, Fibrin, Vascularity.*) Of the state of the blood and pulse in, i. 381; iii. 354. Scabbing, iii. 362. General reflections on the resolution of inflammation, i. 386, 401; iii. 365. In what cases this should be attempted, iii. 369. Resolution, by constitutional means, i. 401; iii. 372. Evacuations less necessary now than formerly, iii. 276. By venesection, i. 402; iii. 373, 387, note. By purging, i. 405; iii. 383, 387, note. By emetics, iii. 383, 417. By local means, i. 402, 406; iii. 384, 396. By cold and lead, iii. 385. By warmth, as poultices and fomentations, i. 408; iii. 386, 396, 397, 413, 418. By mercury, digitalis, prussic acid, antimonial medicines and incisions, iii. 387, note. By colchicum, i. 401. By sympathy, derivation, and translation, i. 407; iii. 388. Uses of the adhesive inflammation, i. 398, note: iii. 399. Causes which limit the extension of, i. 394, 400; iii. 291, 268. In what cases and parts it is imperfect in its consequences, i. 399; iii. 346. Constitutional effects of, i. 400; iii. 362.

Inflammation, Suppurative, i. 409; iii. 403. Difficult to trace the chain of causes leading to, i. 410; iii. 404. Does not arise from the access of air, i. 409; iii. 405. Nor from the violence of action simply, iii. 406. Occurs most readily in canals, i. 411; iii. 408. Symptoms of, i. 411; iii. 408. Treatment of, where suppuration must take place, i. 412; iii. 411. Also where it has taken place, iii. 416. Of collections of matter without suppuration, i. 413; iii. 419. Of the effects of such collections of matter on the constitution, iii. 422. Of the effects of the suppurative inflammation on the constitution, iii. 424, 506. Divided into, first, the symptomatic fever; second, nervous affections; and third, hectic, iii. 433. Rigors, i. 411; iii. 427. Exacerbations, iii. 431. (See *Pus* and *Abscess*.)

———, *Ulcerative*, i. 423; iii. 459. Of the function of the absorbents, *ib.* Of the uses of this inflammation, iii. 463. Of the remote causes of absorption, iii. 564. Those of five kinds, iii. 565. Of the disposition of living parts to absorb, and be absorbed, iii. 565. Of interstitial absorption, iii. 469. Of progressive absorption, iii. 471. Of absorption attended with suppuration, called ulceration, i. 424; iii. 473. Is accompanied by a peculiar pain, i. 411; iii. 476. Of the relaxing process, which attends the approach of abscesses to the surface, i. 422; iii. 477. The approach of abscesses to the surface explained on another principle, iii. 479, note. Of the intention of the absorption of the body in disease, iii. 481. Modes of promoting absorption, iii. 482. Illustrations of ulceration, iii. 483. Granulations, i. 426; iii. 488. Nature and properties of, i. 427; iii. 491. Are disposed to unite with one another, i. 428; iii. 493. Longevity of granulations, iii. 495. Contraction of granulations, i. 429; iii. 497. Cicatrization, i. 430; iii. 500. The new cutis, i. 430; iii. 502. The new cuticle, i. 431; iii. 503. The new rete mucosum, *ib.*

Injections; different kinds of, used in gonorrhœa, ii. 198, 209, note. To be used frequently, ii. 199. Their effects, ii. 200. In what cases they are improper, *ib.* In gleet, ii. 223.

Injuries, which have no external communication, iii. 240. Those which have, iii. 251.

Inoculation; queries relative to that operation, ii. 133. Case of a child under inoculation attacked with measles, *ib.*

Inosculation, iii. 242.

Insanity; in what it differs from delirium and dreams, i. 335, note. Infrequent in India, i. 359. Hereditary, *ib.*

Insects; transformation of, i. 253, note. May be frozen and boiled, and yet recover, i. 284, 293, notes.

Instrument; description of one for conveying caustic to strictures, ii. 244.

Introsusception; paper on, iii. 587.

Iodine; in the blood, i. 355. In phagadenic ulcerations, ii. 349, note.

Iris; muscularity of, iii. 146, note.

Iritis; venereal, ii. 419, note.

Iron; in the blood, iii. 18, 54, notes. Sulpho-cyanate of, supposed by some to be the cause of the red colour of the blood, iii. 59, note.

Irritability; i. 315, 556. Restored by sleep, i. 266. Arises from weakness, i. 312. Consists in too great action compared with the powers, iii. 374, 378.

Irritants, i. 312, 314.

Irritation; specific, produced by the venereal poison, ii. 151. Venereal, can be kept up but a certain time in gonorrhœa, ii. 163, 193. Venereal, parts become so habituated to, as hardly to be affected by, ii. 166. Venereal, takes place more readily in those parts exposed to cold, ii. 398. Constitutional, often disproportionate to the apparent cause, iii. 425.

Itch, i. 617. Cure of, i. 618.

Itching; a peculiar mode of sensation, i. 262. The use of, i. 264.

J.

Jalap; its effects on the stomach when thrown into the veins, ii. 332.

James, Mr., iii. 321, note.

Jardin des Plantes, i. 147.

Jaundice; affects the teeth, ii. 19, note.

Jaw; the upper, its form, and the bones of which it is composed, ii. 1. Lower described, ii. 2. The articulation of the lower, explained, ii. 6. The several motions of which it is capable, *ib.* The muscles subservient to these motions, ii. 7. Critical remarks on these motions, ii. 12. The full usual number of teeth in each, ii. 21. Difference between the grinders in the upper and lower, ii. 26. The motion of in young and old persons, compared, ii. 31. The growth of, explained, ii. 44. Abscesses in, how to be treated, ii. 76. Caution relative to nervous pains in, ii. 84. Irregularities between, and the teeth, ii. 92. Method of rectifying the projection of the lower one, ii. 93. (See *Alveolar process.*)

Jelly. (See *Gelatine.*)

Jenner, Dr.; becomes Hunter's pupil, i. 36. His intimacy with Hunter, i. 37. His correspondence with Hunter (see *Letters.*) Settles at Berkeley, i. 38. Discovers vaccination, *ib.* Visits Hunter at Bath, i. 64. His disappointment, i. 69. His experiments on the tartar emetic, i. 86, 92. His observations on the migration of swallows, i. 91. His paper on the cuckoo, i. 104. Elected F.R.S., i. 117.

Johnson, Dr.; his Irish friend, i. 5. His fear of death, i. 119. His definition of genius, i. 134.

Joints; injuries of, i. 449, 510. False, i. 504, 519. Inflammation of, i. 519. Suppuration of, i. 522. Contracted, i. 516, 525, 582.

Juniors, Hunter's behaviour to his, i. 114.

Justamond, Mr., i. 28.

K.

Kay, Dr., his experiments adverted to in opposition to those of Bichat, iii. 78, 87, notes.

Keate, Mr.; his election to St. George's Hospital, i. 127.

Kidney; preparations of, i. 170. Hydatids of, i. 574.

Kingston, Mr., i. 35.

Knight, Mr.; his experiments on the direction of the germens and radicles of growing plants, iii. 287, note.

L.

Lacteals; discovery of, i. 250.

Lancet; the proper form of, for cutting the gums, ii. 109.

Lawrence, Mr.; his Hunterian oration, i. 146. On incisions in inflammation, iii. 388, note.

Lead; diminishes the powers of restoration, i. 557. Its use in gonorrhœa, ii. 202. In gleet, ii. 222. Pieces of, in the bladder, how removed, ii. 233. Its influence on the muscles, iii. 137, note. In inflammation, iii. 384, 385.

Le Canu, M.; his analysis of the blood, iii. 18, note. On the relative proportion of the different elements of the blood, iii. 43, note.

Lectures; early anatomical, i. 4. Dr. Hunter's, i. 6. Of W. and J. Hunter, i. 16. Of J. Hunter, i. 28, 47. Croonian, Hunter's, i. 58. Surgical, MS. of, lost, i. 123. On surgery, i. 207. Method and intention of, i. 219.

Lee, Dr. R., iii. 269, note.

Leeches; death of, from human blood, i. 354, note. An instance of, in which the blood remained fluid for ten weeks, iii. 33.

Leicester Fields; Hunter builds a house in, i. 85.

Leopards; Hunter's encounter with, i. 33.

Lepra; venereal, ii. 411, note.

Letters; of Lord Auckland to Sir J. Banks, i. 133. Of Sir J. Banks to Lord A., i. 141. Of J. Hunter to Sir J. Banks, i. 83, 84, 105, 122. Of J. H. to the Royal Society, i. 78. To his colleagues, i. 128. To Dr. Jenner, i. 37, 46, 55–76, 86–94, 103, 110, 116–118. Of Mrs. Hunter to Dr. Jenner, i. 96. Of Wm. Hunter to the Royal Society, i. 77.

Leuchorrhœa. (See *Fluor albus.*)

Leverian Museum, i. 147.

Library; Hunter's, i. 138.

Lice; body, live after being boiled, i. 294, note.

Lichen; venereal, description of, ii. 411, note.

Life; a power superadded to common matter, i. 214, 221; iii. 120, note. Definition of, i. 223; iii. 2, 120, 126, notes. The cause of all actions, i. 217, 219. A simple property, i. 221, 223; iii. 120, note. Is not the result of organization, i. 221, 242; iii.

121, note. Or of action, i. 224; iii. 124, note. Possibly may arise from the arrangement of the ultimate molecules, i. 221; iii. 121, note. This idea illustrated by magnetism, i. 221; iii. 122, note. Is also ascribed to the *materia vitæ diffusa*, iii. 122, note. Is modified in its phænomena by organization, i. 223; iii. 124, note. Has been identified, but improperly, with galvanism, iii. 123, note. The propagation and preservation of the species, the end of, i. 225, 273, 293.

Life; of the blood, i. 231; iii. 103, 127, note. The argument for, a cumulative one, iii. 133, note.

—— of the teeth, ii. 19, note.

Ligatures; caution respecting their use, iii. 302, note.

Lightning; destroys the coagulability of the blood and the contractility of muscles, iii. 114.

Lint; use of, in dressing wounds, iii. 414.

Lip; cancer of, i. 629.

Liquor sanguinis; iii. 21, 24, notes.

Liver; the reason why diseases of are more frequent in hot climates, i. 295, note. Hydatids of, i. 574.

Living; above par, the pernicious effect of, iii. 276; mode of, under a course of mercury, ii. 440, 445.

Lixivium Saponarium; its use in ulcerations resembling chancres, ii. 350.

Lizards; Hunter's experiments on, i. 21.

Locked jaw; iii. 379. (See *Tetanus*.)

Locomotion; organs of, i. 158.

Lotions; of the use of, in inflammation, iii. 396.

Lower and King; the first who practised transfusion on the human subject, in this country, iii. 13, note.

Lues Venerea; never combined with the itch or scurvy, ii. 132. And smallpox may appear at the same time, but not in the same parts, *ib.* Produced by a gonorrhœa, ii. 145. The cause of other diseases, ii. 155. The different ways in which it is communicated, ii. 381. Of the nature of the sores or ulcers proceeding from the, ii. 382. Does not contaminate the different secretions, ii. 383. This opinion questioned, ii. 477, note. Sores in the; the matter from, compared with that from chancres and buboes, ii. 385. Sores in the; the matter of, not venereal, *ib.* A person having the, may be affected locally by the application of matter from a gonorrhœa or chancre, ii. 386. Of the local effects arising from the, considered as critical, ii. 391. Of the symptomatic fever in the, ii. 393. Of the local and constitutional forms of the disease never interfering with each other, ii. 393. Of its supposed termination in other diseases, ii. 394. Of the specific distance of the venereal inflammation in the, ii. 395. Of the parts most susceptible of the, ii. 396. Of the time and manner in which the parts are affected in the, *ib.* Summary of the doctrine on the, *ib.* Parts affected in the, are divided into two orders, namely, first in order of parts, and second in order of parts, ii. 398, 425. Takes place more readily in those parts which are exposed to cold, ii. 398. Is brought into action by fever, ii. 400. Symptoms of the, ii. 405. Of the time necessary for its appearance, *ib.* Of the symptoms of the first stage of, ii. 407. Of the symptoms of the second stage of, ii. 420. Of the effects of the poison, on the constitution in the, ii. 422. General observations on the cure of the, ii. 423. The poison in the, circulates with the blood; but its effects are local and may be cured locally, ii. 425. The parts first in order are easier of cure than those second in order, ii. 426. Of continuing mercury while the swelling of the parts second in order still continues, *ib.* Of the use of mercury in the cure of, ii. 426, 468, note. Preparation of mercury and mode of applying it in the, ii. 427. Of the quantity of mercury necessary to be given in the cure of the, ii. 433. Of the length of time mercury should be continued for the cure of the, ii. 343. Of the cure of the, in the second or third stage, ii. 344. Of the local treatment in the, ii. 346. Of the effects remaining after its cure, and of the diseases sometimes produced by the cure, ii. 457. General observations on the medicines usually given for the cure of, ii. 460. Of the continuance of the spitting in, 464. Of diseases resembling the, which have been mistaken for it, ii. 466. Error on this subject, ii. 467, note, particularly as to the grounds of distinction between syphilitic and pseudo-syphilitic diseases, *ib.* Supposed to be communicated by transplanting of a tooth, *ib.*

Lumbar abscess. (See *Abscess.*)

Lungs; inflammation of, i. 398; iii. 400.

Lyceum Medicum, i. 85.
Lymph, coagulable, of a scirrhous tumour will contaminate the glands, i. 620. Objection to the term, iii. 17. (See *Fibrin.*)
Lymphatics; their functions discovered, i. 18, 251. Hunter's intended work on, i. 20. Preparations of, i. 160. Diseases of in gonorrhœa, ii. 184. Inflammation of, iii. 319, 531, notes. (See *Absorption.*)

M.

Macaire and Marcet; their ultimate analysis of the blood, iii. 20, note.
Machine; the animal body contrasted with a, i. 242.
Madder; the effects of, on the teeth of a young pig, ii. 17. (See *Ossification.*)
Majendie, M. and his dogs, i. 76. His experiments of injecting air into the veins, iii. 28, note. On the formation of the red globules, iii. 64, note.
Magnetism, Animal, i. 337
Man; distinguished by his reason, i. 260. Standard heat of, i. 289. Whether to be ranked in the class of carnivorous animals, from his teeth, ii. 52, note.
Marcet, Dr.; his analysis of the serum, iii. 18, note.
Marriage; Hunter's, i. 40.
Martin's, St., in the Fields; Hunter interred there, i. 133.
Masseter muscle; its description and uses, ii. 7.
Mastication; the several motions of the under-jaw in, ii. 6. Action of the teeth in, ii. 30.
Materia vitæ diffusa; what meant by, iii. 115, note, 333, 334, 335, 429, 436.
Matter; the existence of, known only by our senses, i. 210. An abstract idea of, i. 212. Difference between common and organic, i. 214. How one passes into the other, unknown, i. 219.
Matter; of a sore, not pernicious to that sore, ii. 164. This opinion questioned, ii. 208, note. Venereal, may be taken into the stomach without producing any bad consequences, ii. 384.
Mayo, Mr.; iii. 42, 62, note.
Measles; case of, in which it took the lead of smallpox, i. 513; iii. 5.
Mechanics; in what respect the power in, differs from that in an animal body, i. 242, 267.
Medical and Chirurgical Society, i. 86. Hunter's contributions to, on inflammation of the veins, i. 91. On paralysis of the œsophagus, i. 110. On introsusception, i. 117. On aneurism, *ib.* Jenner's paper to, on emetic tartar, i. 92.
Medicines; the action of, i. 476. Our ignorance on this subject, iii. 366. Is only learnt from experience, iii. 278, note.
Membranes, mucous; inflammation of, i. 411; iii. 475, 529, note. Do not bear or require much depletion, ii. 208; iii. 529, note.
———, *serous*; inflammation of, i. 441, 529, note. Rarely affected primarily with ulceration, iii. 466.
———, *inorganized*; produced by the coagulation and organization of fibrin, iii. 36.
———, *cellular*; very susceptible of the adhesive and suppurative inflammations, iii. 282. And also of the ulcerative, iii. 466. Further observations on inflammation of this tissue, iii. 528, note.
———, *fibrous*; inflammation of, iii. 530, note.
Memory; Hunter's loss of, i. 119. As applied to the body, compared with the same faculty of the mind, i. 274.
Menses; the blood in, is not globular, and does not coagulate, iii. 35, 85, 115.
Mercury; assists the absorbents in removing callous parts, i. 430. In diseases of the bones, i. 507. The taking of, destructive to the transplantation of teeth, ii. 98. Unnecessary in the cure of a gonorrhœa, ii. 196. In inflammation of the testicle, ii. 212. Combined with mucilage, preferable to oily substances when used externally, ii. 333. Sometimes produces ulcers on the tonsils, which are taken for venereal, ii. 342. When rubbed into the thigh for the cure of a chancre, sometimes occasions swelling of the glands of the groin, ii. 343. Cautions respecting its use in phagadenic ulcerations, ii. 349, note. And pseudo-syphilitic disorders, ii. 468, note. How to be used in the resolution of buboes, ii. 368, 371. Of the quantity necessary for the resolution of buboes, ii. 373. To be used during the suppuration of buboes, ii. 374. Appears sometimes to lose its power on the body, ii. 376. Of the use of, in the cure of lues venerea, ii. 426. Preparation of, and mode of applying it in the

lues venerea, ii. 427. The most convenient way of introducing it into the constitution, ii. 429. Its action, ii. 430, 436. Its effects on the constitution, and parts capable of secretion, ii. 430, 455. Its effects as a poison, ii. 432, note. Never gets into the bones in the form of a metal, ii. 432. Of the quantity necessary to be given for the cure of the lues venerea, ii. 433, 438, 444. Its effects on the mouth, ii. 434. Of its sensible effects upon parts, *ib.* Does not act by evacuation, ii. 435, 454. Of the different methods of giving mercury externally and internally, ii. 438, 440. When mixed with the saliva may act as a gargle upon ulcers in the throat, ii. 439. Mode of living under a course of, ii. 440, 445. Of the different preparations of, and their combination with other medicines, ii. 440, 443. Of the length of time it should be continued for the cure of the lues venerea, ii. 443. Of correcting some of the effects of, ii. 448. Of the form of the different preparations of, when in the circulation, ii. 452. Is dissolved in the animal juices, ii. 453. Of the operation of, on the venereal poison, ii. 454. Increases the efficacy of electricity in the cure of diseases, ii. 455. The effect of on inflammation, i. 401; iii. 387, notes.

Mercury, perchloride of. (See *Corrosive sublimate.*)

———, protochloride of. (See *Calomel.*)

Mercurius calcinatus; its use in preventing a lues venerea from a gonorrhœa, ii. 207. In the lues venerea, ii. 441.

Metastasis; the laws which govern, iii. 389, note.

Mezereon; the uses of, in diseases of the bones, i. 509. In scrofula, i. 599. In lues venerea, ii. 460.

Miasmata; infectious, effects of, i. 296. How destroyed, *ib.*

Microscope; the indications of, to be received with much caution, iii. 60, note.

Middleton, Mr., i. 101.

Migratory animals, i. 91, 294.

Milk teeth; progress of the formation of, in the fœtus, ii. 33. (See *Dentition.*)

Mimosa; actions of the, i. 328.

Mind; influence of, on the body, iii. 276.

Molares; origin of the formation of, in the fœtus, ii. 34.

Mollities ossium, differs from rickets principally in regard to age, i. 532.

Moon; the influence of, on diseases, i. 346.

Morgan, Dr., iii. 410, note.

———, *Mr.*, on inflammation, iii. 427, note.

Mortification, i. 602; iii. 7, 318. Arises from the action being greater than the power, i. 603; iii. 8. Of the teeth, symptoms of, ii. 59. And Death, not the same, ii. 60, note. Inquiry into the cause of, ii. 62. Prevention and cure of, ii. 65. Takes place in the extremities of tall people, and why, ii. 134. Of two kinds, ii. 136. Its cause, *ib.* Its treatment hitherto in part improper, ii. 137. Its cure, i. 604; ii. 137; iii. 8. The use of bark in, *ib.* The use of opium in, *ib.* In consequence of diffusion of urine into the cellular membrane of the scrotum; its treatment, ii. 260. Occasions the blood to coagulate in the vessels, iii. 31, 42, note. From deficient innervation, iii. 329, note.

Munro, Dr.; his disputes with the Hunters, i. 18.

Muscles; loss of power of, consequent on injuries, i. 264, 439, 513, 517, 524. Contraction of, in diseases of the joints, i. 516. Wasting of, i. 524. Colour of, iii. 69, 199. Experiments on, iii. 109. General observations on their action, iii. 145. The involuntary, the strongest, iii. 148. Of the elongation of, iii. 150. Inflammation of, iii. 531, note.

Museum; Hunter's, cost of, i. 72. His wishes respecting, i. 137. Pitt refuses to purchase, *ib.* Letter from Lord Auckland to Sir J. Banks respecting, *ib.* Reply of Sir J. Banks to Lord Auckland, i. 139. Parliamentary committee, i. 141. Purchased by Parliament, *ib.* Offered to the College of Physicians, i. 142. Accepted by the Corporation of Surgeons, *ib.* Curators of, appointed, i. 145. New building planned, *ib.* Parliamentary grants for, *ib.* Visited by eminent foreigners, i. 146. New building completed, *ib.* Lectures established at, *ib.* Hunterian orations, *ib.* Contents of, i. 148. MS. catalogue of, i. 151. Physiological department, i. 156. Dry preparations, i. 179. Osteology, *ib.* Monsters, i. 181. Natural history, i. 183. Pathology, i. 184.

———, *Catalogue of*; Hunter's anxiety to complete, i. 149. Sir E. Home engages to form, i. 152. Supineness of Council respecting, i. 153. In course of publication, i. 154.

N.

Nails; the separation of, a symptom of the lues venerea, ii. 409.
Napoleon; his retreat from Moscow, disastrous consequences of, i. 287, note.
Nash, Mr.; his claims to the discovery of vaccination, i. 39.
Natural History; a project for a school of, by Mr. Hunter, i. 55. Department, in the Museum, i. 183.
Naturalist; Hunter, as a, i. 135.
Necrosis; i. 515, 529. Of the mode of operating for, i. 530.
Nerves; i. 259. Olfactory, i. 19. Preparations of, i. 170. Do not cause or support life, i. 232, 264. Of the modes of impression which they are capable of, i. 261, 353. May exist without the brain, i. 264, note. Are sometimes included in ligatures without bad consequences, i. 541. Of the teeth, if exposed, the seat of tooth-ache, ii. 50, 53. Method of protecting them, ii. 54. Method of burning them, ii. 66. Reproduction of, iii. 120.
Nervous system; probably exists in all animals, i. 260, note. Influence of, on the blood, i. 354. Influence of, on inflammation, i. 378; iii. 328, 531, notes.
Nitric acid; its use in ptyalism, ii. 451, note.
Nodes, Venereal; description of, ii. 420. Treatment of, ii. 446. Use of blisters in, ii. 447. Of abscesses in, consequence of, *ib.* Of exfoliation in, consequence of, ii. 448. On tendons, ligaments, and fasciæ, their treatment, *ib.*
Nurses; who suckle children, supposed to have the lues venerea, how affected, ii. 387.
Nutrition; the function of, i. 247. Impaired when the nerves are destroyed, iii. 329, note. Is perverted or modified by inflammation, iii. 522, note.

O.

Œconomy, animal; Hunter publishes his work on, i. 102. The final purposes of accomplished by a succession of actions, arising out of one another, i. 273.
Œdema; consequent on cancer, i. 629.
Ointment; mercurial, a cure for the itch, i. 618.
Olecranon; fracture of, i. 511. Treatment of, i. 513.
Onanism; how far pernicious to the constitution, ii. 304, 305, note.
Operations; Hunter's opinion of, i. 93. Difficult to judge of their expediency, i. 210. The cause of their failure often obscure, *ib.* Should not be rashly undertaken, i. 465. The circumstances which should determine the propriety of in cancer, i. 627. Do not succeed in persons of full health, iii. 281.
Operator; Hunter as a, i. 93.
Ophthalmia, i. 449.
Opium; in irritable persons, i. 556. In mortification, i. 604; ii. 237. In priapism, ii. 173. In gonorrhœa, ii. 201. In chordee, ii. 210. In stricture, ii. 235. In spasmodic affections of the urethra, ii. 301. In seminal weakness, ii. 309. In phimosis, ii. 338. In the lues venerea, ii. 441, 460. In soreness of the mouth from mercury, ii. 451. An instance where it was given in very large quantities, ii. 462. In inflammation, iii. 412.
Organization; the proper notion of, i. 222, 241. Not the cause of life, i. 242. Of effused blood. (See *Blood, Vascularity.*) Gradual development of in the animal scale, i. 264; iii. 184, notes.
Organs; vital, unmanageable in inflammation, i. 374.
O'Shaughnessy, Dr.; his analysis of the blood, iii. 20, note.
Ossification; the general progress of, different from the formation of the teeth, ii. 18. Of a tooth upon the pulp explained, ii. 39.
Osteological department of the Museum, i. 179.
Ovum; development of, i. 176, 178.
Owen, Mr. R.; on the placenta, i. 16. Appointed assistant curator, i. 154. Forms the catalogue of the physiological series, i. 155.
Oxford; Hunter enters at, i. 14.
Oxygen; its effects on respiration, iii. 20, note.

P.

Pain; the nature of, i. 262, 361, 385, note. Why it is not felt by a part when it is struck by a musket-ball, i. 263. Dark people less susceptible of, than fair, i. 308,

Inflammation of different parts and in different stages of its progress is characterized by peculiarities of, i. 397 ; iii. 331, 476, 562.

Paracentesis Thoracis, i. 443.

——— *abdominis*; cases of, in which the wound did not close, iii. 280.

Parotid gland; fistula of, i. 579.

Partnership; of W. and J. Hunter, i. 15. Of W. Hunter and Hewson, i. 23.

Paralysis; of the urethra, ii. 276. Its cure, *ib*. Of the bladder from obstruction to the passage of the urine, ii. 287. Of the bladder, its cure when it arises from obstruction owing to pressure or spasm, ii. 289. Of the acceleratores muscles; its cure, ii. 301.

Paraphimosis; its cause, ii. 322. Natural, description of, ii. 325. From disease, description of, *ib*. From chancres, the treatment of, ii. 339. Operation for, ii. 340.

Parasitical animals; an enumeration of several species, iii. 256, note.

Patella; fracture of, i. 511.

Pathology; humoral, considered, i. 347, 352. The foundation of, is laid in experience, iii. 277, note.

Pearls; Hunter's, i. 105.

Pearson, John, ii. 457, note.

Peculiarities of animals, i. 173.

Penis; the structure of, i. 251. Sensation of, i. 262. Cancer of, i. 330.

Pericardium; inflammation of, i. 444; iii. 348. Use of, iii. 180.

Perinæum; fistula of, i. 580. Operations on, in cases of retention of urine, from strictures, ii. 296, note.

Period, latent; of diseases, what meant by, i. 309, 312.

Periosteum; of the teeth, described, ii. 2.

Peritoneum; inflammation of, i. 445. In puerperal women, i. 446. After tapping, i. 447.

Personal appearance; Hunter's, i. 133.

Philosophical Transactions; Hunter's contributions to, on the Proteus of Ellis, i. 33. On the digestion of the stomach after death, i. 43. On the torpedo, i. 47. On the gizzard trout, i. 50. On the air-receptacles of birds, *ib*. On the recovery of drowned persons, i. 57. On vital heat, i. 57, 68. On the free-martin, i. 73. On smallpox during pregnancy, i. 80. On the change of plumage in birds, *ib*. On the ear in fishes, i. 84. On the wolf, jackal, and dog, i. 105, 117. On whales, i. 105. On bees, i. 122. Home's papers in, i. 153. Dr. Jenner's, on the cuckoo, i. 104.

Phimosis; its cause, ii. 322. Natural, description of, ii. 325. From disease, description of, *ib*. Its treatment when produced by or attended with chancre, ii. 334, 339, note. Produced by chancres, the common operation for, ii. 336. Of the constitutional treatment of, ii. 338, 339, note.

Phlebitis; i. 451 ; iii. 319, 581. Causes and treatment of, i. 452; iii. 582, 585. Frequency of, in the horse, i. 452; iii. 583.

Phthisis Pulmonalis, i. 596. The blood often buffy in the latter stages of, iii. 40, note.

Physician-Anatomists, i. 5.

Physiology; study of, much aided by comparative anatomy, disease, and monstrosities, i. 220. A complex science, embracing many different branches of knowledge, iii. 125, note.

Picture; Hunter's, by Sir J. Reynolds, i. 108.

Pictures; Hunter's love of, i. 38.

Pins and *needles*; traverse the body without exciting pain or inflammation, iii. 287. The stomachs of animals which feed in bleaching-fields often stuck full of, without inconvenience, *ib*.

Piracy; literary, complained of by Hunter, i. 84; iii. 2.

Pitcairn, Dr. D.; in consultation with Hunter, i. 610.

Placenta; anatomy of, i. 15, 76.

Plague; the poison of, affects the constitution in a specific manner, iii. 307.

Plant Sensitive; motions of the, i. 328.

Plaster; stimulant, to promote suppuration, iii. 418.

Pleura; very susceptible of inflammation, i. 442.

Plunkett; the cancer-curer, anecdote of, i. 625.

Poison; venereal, its origin doubtful, ii. 138. Began in the human race, and in the parts of generation, ii. 139. Its nature, *ib*. Its effects, ii. 140. Propagated by matter, ii. 140, 192. Its action, ii. 142. Its greater or less acrimony, *ib*. It affects very differently different people, *ib.* The same in gonorrhœa as in chancre, ii. 143. This opinion questioned, ii. 146, note. How communicated to the inhabitants of the South Sea Islands, ii. 145. Produces different forms of the disease; how this happens, ii. 145. The cause of its poisonous quality, ii. 147. Does not arise from fermentation, ii. 149. Its effects arise from a specific irritation, ii. 151. Affects the body in two different ways, locally and constitutionally, ii. 153. Of the time between the application and effect, ii. 160. Applied to a sore will often produce the venereal irritation, ii. 165. May be absorbed in three different ways, ii. 356. When absorbed may affect the lymphatics themselves, or the lymphatic glands, forming buboes in each, ii. 357, 358. Of the time between its application and the formation of a bubo, ii. 360. Affects but one gland at a time, *ib.* Never affects the glands which are second in order; the reason of this, ii. 361. Sometimes only irritates the glands to disease, producing in them scrofula, ii. 366. Experiments made to ascertain the progress and effects of the, ii. 417. Of its effects on the constitution in the lues venerea, ii. 422. Circulates with the blood in the lues venerea; but its effects are local, and may be cured locally, ii. 425. Of the operation of mercury on the, ii. 454.

Poisons; the effects of, i. 355, note. General considerations on, i. 611. Of the different ways in which they affect the body, i. 612, 616; iii. 427, note. Mineral, i. 613. Vegetable, i. 614. Animal, *ib.* Morbid, i. 615; ii. 138. Modes of receiving, i. 616. New, are rising up every day, ii. 477. Particular, affect particular structures, iii. 6. Do not essentially alter the inflammatory action, iii. 300.

Polypi, i. 568. Of the uterus, *ib.*

Position; the effect of, on the progress and cure of disease, iii. 272.

Potash; hydriodate of, its use in phagadenic ulcerations, ii. 349, note.

———; ferro-cyanate of, a delicate test of the presence of albumen, iii. 49, note.

Potassa Fusa; when and how it should be used, i. 603.

Pott, Mr.; his improvements in surgery, i. 13. His disputes with Hunter, i. 18. His life and character, i. 111. His strictures on Mr. Hunter's operation for aneurism, i. 547.

Poultices; in inflammation, i. 412; iii. 397, 413. Of sea-water, in scrofula, i. 600. Stimulant, so as to promote suppuration, iii. 418.

Practice; Hunter's dislike of, i. 28. Amount of, i. 40, 72. Slow progress in, i. 26.

Predispositions; require an exciting cause for their development, i. 306.

Pregnancy; state of the blood in, iii. 357.

Pressure; a cause of absorption and thickening, i. 256, 421, 464; iii. 466. A stimulus, i. 481.

Prevost and *Dumas*; on the blood-globules, iii. 64, note.

Principle, aromatic; of the blood, iii. 54, note.

————, of conservation and repair; inherent in an animal body, iii. 269.

————, vital; unlike any power or property in physics, i. 223. Used synonymously with simple animal life, i. 217, 318. Reasons for retaining the term, iii. 125, note. The presence of, prevents substances from acting as foreign bodies, iii. 256.

Principles; the value of in surgery, i. 208, 365; iii. 297. Secondary, i. 275. Connexion between, in the higher animals, i. 264, 318. Mechanical and chemical, often introduced into the animal œconomy, i. 217; iii. 125, note.

———— proximate; of organized bodies, i. 215, 216, 218, notes. Easily convertible into one another, iii. 37, 41, 45, 55, notes.

Printing; carried on in Hunter's house, i. 102.

Processions; Hunter's dislike of, i. 121.

Professional men; their slow progress, i. 25.

Projection; of the under jaw, method of rectifying, ii. 94.

Propagation and *Preservation* of the species, the ultimate end of life, i. 225, 273, 293.

Prostate Gland. (See *Gland.*)

Prout, Dr.; on the salts of the blood, iii. 47, note. On animal chemistry, iii. 67, note.

Prussic acid; in inflammation, iii. 387, note.

Psoriasis venereal; description of, ii. 412, note.

Pterygoidœi muscles; their description and use, ii. 10.

Ptyalism, ii. 434, 464. Of the use of nitric acid in, ii. 451, note.

Pulse; the state of, in disease, i. 362. In inflammation, i. 376, 382; iii. 354, 358. In inflammation of different textures and organs, iii. 362. How far an indication for bleeding can be derived from, i. 404; iii. 360, 379. In different animals, iii. 194.

Cause of, iii. 216. Is the result of the combined action of the heart and arteries and the part affected, iii. 359, 362. Rises after bleeding, iii. 362. Sometimes even becomes harder, iii. 361.

Punctuality; Hunter's, i. 52. Baillie's, i. 53.

Pupils; Hunter's, i. 28, 34, 49. Fees of, disputes respecting, i. 127.

Purging; in inflammation, i. 406; iii. 382.

Pus, i. 414; iii. 438. General opinion of the formation of, iii. 440, 457, note. Experiments to ascertain the progress of suppuration, iii. 444. To be regarded as the result of secretion, iii. 410, 422, 440, 457, note. Production of, independently of inflammation, i. 413; iii. 419. This opinion questioned, iii. 421, note. Properties of, i. 414; iii. 449. Of the distinction between pus and mucus, i. 417. Has all the specific qualities of the part which produces it, iii. 452. And is not injurious to the parts which secrete it, ii. 165, 453; iii. 452. This opinion questioned, ii. 228, note, Corrosive, i. 418; iii. 452. Uses of, i. 419; iii. 455. From diseased bones, i. 516; iii. 455. Scrofulous, i. 594; iii. 417. Composition of, iii. 456, note. Progress of, towards the surface, iii. 479, note, 520. Is found in unorganized coagula, iii. 457, note.

Putrefaction; peculiar kind of, attended with emphysema, i. 226. Is slower in taking place in young and inflammatory than in old and healthy blood, iii. 124, 128, 132, notes.

Q.

Queensbury, case of the Duke of, who broke his tendo Achillis, i. 264, 439.

R.

Rabbit-mouth; means of rectifying, ii. 91.

Rabbits; experiments on, of freezing their ears, iii. 108, 323.

Ramollissement, iii. 532, note.

Raspail, M.; on the formation of the red globules, iii. 64, note.

Reading and *Reflection*; their advantages compared, i. 210.

Reason; the result of sensation, i. 259. The distinguishing attribu'e of man, i. 260. Sometimes active during sleep, i. 335.

Redness; in inflammation, accounted for, i. 383. Sometimes deficient, i. 397, note.

Relaxation; of the skin, precedes the approach of an abscess to the surface, iii. 477.

Replacing of a tooth drawn by mistake, instruction for, ii. 100.

Reproduction; organs of, i. 174.

Repulsion, i. 210; iii. 388, 391.

Resistance; of heat and cold, in animals, i. 289.

Respiration; organs of, i. 169. Artificial, mode of producing, iii. 76. Connection of, with the circulation, iii. 78, note. Importance of, iii. 86. Changes effected by, on the blood, iii. 90, 92, notes.

Resolution; of inflammation, i. 387, 400.

Rest; effect of, on coagulation, iii. 28, 30, 33, notes.

Restoration; the powers of, in inflammation, i. 309, 501, 555. Greater in youth than in age, i. 484. Of joints, extremely limited, i. 519. Different from resistance to disease, iii. 3, note.

Resurrection-men; Hunter a favourite with, i. 10.

Rete-mucosum, i. 431; iii. 505.

Revulsion, i. 321, 407; iii. 388, 395.

Reynolds, Sir J.; his picture of Hunter, i. 108. His death and funeral, i. 121.

Rickets, i. 531; ii. 18.

Rigors; depend on the novelty of an unaccustomed action or impression, i. 379; iii. 358. How far the stomach is concerned in their production, iii. 346, 429. To be regarded as a proof of debility, iii. 358, 430.

Roche, M. de la, i. 289, 290.

Roget, Dr., iii. 79, note.

Roof, of the mouth; osteological description of, ii. 1.

Rot, the; in sheep, i. 572.

Rotting, of the teeth; symptoms and consequences of, ii. 59. Inquiry into the cause

of, ii. 62. Whether a rotten tooth has any contaminating power, *ib.* Symptoms of inflammation, ii. 63. Is cured only by extraction, ii. 65. The breath rendered foul by, *ib.* Prevention a cure of, ii. 66.
Royal Society; Hunter elected a fellow of, i. 33. (See *Phil. Trans.*)
Running hard; destroys the coagulability of the blood and the contractility of muscles, iii. 114.
Rupia venereal; description of, ii. 412, note.
Russian savans; their opinion of Hunter's museum, i. 147.

S.

Sacculi mucosi, inflammation of and cure, i. 449.
Sacs; adventitious, formed for the lodgement of bullets, glass, &c., iii. 289.
Salivation; occasioned by a sore being dressed with red precipitate, ii. 428.
Salts, of the blood; their relative quantity in health and disease, iii. 46, note. Their supposed uses, *ib.*
Sarsaparilla; its use in spreading ulcers of the prepuce, ii. 346. In buboes, ii. 380. In the lues venerea, ii. 456, 460, 463.
Scabbing, i. 429; iii. 262, 264.
Scabies, i. 617.
Scalds, iii. 265.
Scaling of teeth; the utility of this operation, ii. 54. Caution in, ii. 87.
Scarifications; the danger of, in anasarca, i. 603. In mortification, i. 604. In carbuncle, i. 610.
Schultz, M., iii. 63, 197, notes.
Schwilgue; on the composition of pus, iii. 457, note.
Scion tooth; instructions for the choice of, ii. 99.
Scorpions; may poison and destroy one another, i. 614.
Scrofula; observations on, i. 590; ii. 155, 156, 216, 219, 432, note; iii. 307, 417, 419. Brutes subject to, i. 590. Predisposing causes of, i. 308, 592. Not hereditary, i. 358, 591. Parts most subject to, i. 591. Of climates and seasons, in reference to this disease, i. 592. Susceptibility to, may be acquired, *ib.* Progress of, i. 593. Appearances of, i. 594. Of the testicle, i. 597. Of the breast, *ib.* Medical treatment of, i. 598. Surgical treatment of, i. 600.
Scrotum; relaxation of the, the cause of, ii. 305.
Scurvy; effects of that disorder on the gums and alveolar processes, ii. 80. Is the first object of cure, ii. 81. Of the gums, ii. 82.
Seasons; influence of, on disease, i. 345, 592.
Secretion, i. 250. Rapidity of, iii. 38, note. Influence of the nervous system on, iii. 329, note.
Secretions; uses of, i. 250. Of the skin, acid in rheumatism, i. 353, note.
Sedatives; effects of, i. 314.
Seeing; the sense of, compared with that of feeling, i. 212.
Sensation; cannot exist without the brain and nerves, i. 259. Delusive, from sympathy and when the nerves are injured, explained, i. 261, 326. Is only to be perceived within certain limits of time and space, i. 263. In healthy persons is in proportion to the nerves and vascularity of the part, i. 263; iii. 200. But not in disease, iii. 334. Does not exist in the unborn fœtus, i. 264. May be produced in any part by fixing the attention to that part, i. 337. Continued, exhausts life, i. 266. Some actions, independenr of, i. 264, 318. Suspended during sleep, i. 335. Of inflamed parts, i. 378.
Senses; organs of, preparations of, i. 171. How to be considered, i. 261.
Sensibility and *Contractility*; the distinguishing properties of an animal body, i. 242, note.
——— of the teeth; accounted for, ii. 50, note. Of diseased parts, not in proportion to the quantity of nerves, iii. 334.
Serosity; account of, iii. 50.
Serum, iii. 39. Analysis of, iii. 18, note. Proportion of, to crassamentum, iii. 25, 47, notes. Specific gravity of, iii. 47, note. Becomes lighter in inflammation, iii. 356. Proportion of albumen in, in health and disease, iii. 45, note. Sometimes separates before coagulation, iii. 46. Colour of, iii. 47. Coagulation of, iii. 49. Milky, iii. 55.

Sharp, Samuel, i. 25.
——, *William*, i. 4.
——, the engraver, i. 109.
Shedding of teeth; the process of, explained, ii. 43. The necessity of a new set, pointed out, ii. 46.
Sickness; produced by a bougie, i. 311, 320. By an enema, i. 311.
Silica; its solution compared to that of the albumen in the serum, iii. 49, note.
Simpson, Dr., iii. 410, note.
Skin; sympathy of, with the stomach, i. 325. Seems to be the cause of the susceptibility of the absorbents to receive venereal irritation, ii. 361. Inflammation of, iii. 528, note.
Skinning. (See *Cicatrization.*)
Sleep; small portion of, required by Hunter, i. 54. The nature of, i. 265.
Sloughing; the causes of, i. 602. Mode in which the dead parts are detached, i. 606. Sores, from contusion, treatment of, iii. 266. (See *Mortification.*)
Smallpox; case of, which was checked by the occurrence of measles, i. 313; iii. 5. The pits left by, caused by a sloughing of the cutis, i. 426. May be received in utero, i. 354, note. Effects its own cure, i. 616. Matter, immaterial from what subject taken, ii. 143. The reason why a person cannot be infected twice with, ii. 392. And cow-pox, are sometimes combined, iii. 5, note.
Snakes; instances of, where they have remained fat for several months, without taking food, iii. 12, note.
Society; Hunter's early position in, i. 10. His taste for, i. 41.
Soda; the use of, in carbuncle, i. 610.
Soemmerring, A. Von; his letter, on being elected F.R.S., i. 73.
Softening, of the tissues, in inflammation, iii. 532, note.
Soirée; Hunter's conduct at, i. 41.
Solander, Dr., how affected by cold, i. 286.
Somnambulism, i. 335.
Sores, fungated, i. 629. (See *Ulcer, Chancre.*)
South Sea Islands; inhabitants of, how affected with lues venerea, ii. 143.
Species; the meaning of this term, as applied to disease, iii. 1.
Sphacelus, i. 226. (See *Mortification.*)
Sponge, burnt; its efficacy in scrofula, i. 599.
Specific gravity; of the blood, iii. 22, note. Of milky serum, iii. 46, note. Of serum and serous effusions, iii. 47, note.
Speech, depends on the respiration being partially under the will, iii. 194.
Spleen; the red globules not formed in, iii. 68, note.
Spots of blood; tests for distinguishing them from other stains, iii. 54, note.
Sprains, i. 517.
Stevens, Dr.; on the salts of the blood, iii. 46, note. His theory of arterialization examined, iii. 94, note.
Stimuli; the nature of, explained, i. 269. Carried to their utmost extent, act as sedatives, i. 269, 477, 479. This exemplified by cold, i. [illegible] Effects of, i. 314, 479. In mortification, iii. 8.
Stimulus; of necessity, the sense in which this term is employed, i. 236, 308, 316, 361, 509, 560; iii. 32, 34. Called also a sympathetic stimulus, iii. 146, note. Of death, i. 227, 239, 269, 446; iii. 114, note. Of imperfection, called also the irritation or consciousness of imperfection, i. 232, 255, 387, 398; iii. 239. Of nature, i. 238. Of want, or hunger, i. 270, 311. Of weakness, i. 529.
Stoker, Dr., iii. 39.
Stoll, Dr., i. 146.
Stomach; sympathy of, with other parts, i. 245, 248, 325, 378; iii. 346, 429. With the mind, i. 249. With the skin, i. 325. The principal part in the lower animals, i. 247. The powers of, *ib.* The effects of inflammation on, i. 278; iii. 362. The seat of simple animal life, i. 378, 379; iii. 429. The source of heat and cold, i. 384; iii. 336, 345. Is often multiplied in the lower animals, iii. 116.
Stone in the bladder; indicated by pain in the left arm, i. 322.
Stopping of hollow teeth; method of performing, ii. 68, 69, note.
Strangury; the use of blisters in, ii. 218. Its cause, ii. 273.
Strawberries; sometimes act as a poison, i. 611.
Strength; in what sense this term is used, iii. 277.

Strength and weakness; how they modify the phenomena of inflammation, i. 374; iii. 276, 278.

——— *and action*. (See *Action*.)

Stricture; different kinds of, ii. 229. Permanent, description of, ii. 230. Affected by cold, ii. 231. Its cause, *ib.* Common to most passages in the body, *ib.* In general not the effect of the venereal complaint, ii. 232. May arise in consequence of any long-continued irritation of the urinary organs, ii. 233, note. Its cure by dilatation, ii. 234. Use of bougies in, ii. 235. Frequently attended with spasms, *ib.* Its cure by ulceration, ii. 238. Occasions an increase in the strength of the bladder, ii. 241. Use and application of caustic to, ii. 242, 245, note, 267. In women, observations on, ii. 246. In women, its cure, ii. 248. Attended with spasmodic affection, ii. 249. Sometimes relieved by a gonorrhœa, *ib.* Spasmodic, its treatment, ii. 250. Permanent, diseases in consequence of, ii. 257. Bad effects of travelling in, ii. 274.

Striking the teeth; a mode of detecting those that are unsound, ii. 71, note.

Structure; the influence of, in disease, i. 343, 366, 373, 374, 484; iii. 271, 282, 527. Experiments to prove that there is considerable inequality in this respect, iii. 273. Is altered by inflammation, iii. 527, note. New formed, generally assumes the nature of the surrounding parts, iii. 115.

Stumps of teeth; the state in which they usually remain, ii. 60.

Styptics, i. 538.

Substances, foreign; their approach to the surface described and explained, i. 373, 423; iii. 479, note. In the blood, i. 352, note.

Sugar; one of the best restoratives of the kind we are acquainted with, ii. 445.

Sulphur; a cure for the itch, i. 618. Its use in correcting some of the effects of mercury, ii. 450.

Supernumerary teeth; the origin of, accounted for, ii. 51. Ought to be removed, ii. 93.

Suppression of urine; how relieved, ii. 287. Operations for the cure of, ii. 290.

Suppuration; i. 409; iii. 403. Symptoms of, i. 379, 411; iii. 408. What are the conditions of structure most favourable to, iii. 283, note. Principally occurs in the external parts, iii. 287; and mucous canals, i. 411; iii. 289. Sometimes takes the lead of the adhesive, constituting the diffuse suppurative inflammation, iii. 347. Causes of, i. 410; iii. 404. May take place without breach of surface, iii. 410, 422, 441; and without inflammation, iii. 419. This opinion questioned, iii. 421, note. Analogous to secretion, iii. 444. Treatment of, i. 412; iii. 408. Treatment of, when suppuration must take place, iii. 411; and also when it has taken place, iii. 416. Constitutional effects of, iii. 424. Of its not answering the common final intention in a gonorrhœa, ii. 159. (See *Pus, Abscess, Suppurative Inflammation*.)

Surfaces, sécreting and nonsecreting; what they are, ii. 145. Of the best for absorption, ii. 427.

Surgeons; eminent, and their pupils, i. 35. College of. (See *Corporation*.)

———; French military, superior to the English, before the time of Hunter, iii. 541, note.

Surgery; state of, before Pott, i. 13. Pott's improvements in, *ib.* State of, before Hunter, i. 30.

Susceptibility; of impressions, i. 267; of disease, i. 301. Greater in some persons than in others, i. 304. Kinds of, i. 305. May often be known by concomitant circumstances, i. 308.

Sutures; remarks on, iii. 265.

Swallows; migration of, i. 91.

Swearing; Hunter addicted to, i. 28, 52.

Swelling; in inflammation, i. 383, 397; iii. 327. White, i. 596.

Sympathy; i. 371; iii. 6. May be regarded as a secondary principle, introduced into the œconomy of the higher order of animals, i. 371. Of the stomach, as universal as that of the brain, i. 248. Of the stomach with other organs, i. 245, 248, 325; iii. 346, 429. With the mind, i. 249. Of the vital principle, i. 226, 264. Connection of principles of action, in the living body, i. 318. Between different individuals, i. 320. Of natural and diseased, and their classification, i. 320; ii. 131. Constitutional, i. 322; iii. 6, 433. Certain parts sympathize more strongly than others, i. 324. Of similar and dissimilar, i. 325. Between the body and mind, i. 329. Of the mind with the living principle, *ib.* Uses of sympathy in the animal œconomy, i. 330. Of delusion, i. 331. The cause of the disorders incident to dentition, ii. 106. The symptoms of, in children, often more violent than the parts immediately affected, ii. 107. How adults are affected by it, *ib.* To be cured by local applications, ii. 108. Partial, divided into remote, contiguous, and continuous, ii. 132; iii. 7. Between the urethra and the cutting of a tooth, an instance of, ii. 33, 161. Occasions a variety of symptoms in gonorrhœa, ii. 51, 177. In gonorrhœa, occasions swellings in the testicles, ii. 177, 213. And in the absorbent glands, ii. 182. Sometimes cures a gleet, ii. 224. Occasions affections of many parts during the use of bougies, ii. 251, 256. Between the skin and deeper-seated parts, when cold is applied to the former, ii. 399. In inflammation, i. 376; iii. 291, 388, 393, 427, 433. Of repulsion, revulsion, translation, and derivation, iii. 393.

Symptoms; what so called, i. 310, 311, 361. Premonitory, i. 268, 311. The knowledge of, important, i. 320. Delusive, i. 353.

Syncope, i. 266.

Syphilis. (See *Lues Venerea.*)

Syphilitic and pseudo-syphilitic diseases; the distinction between, ii. 467, note.

System, absorbent; affected in two ways, by irritation and the absorption of matter, ii. 182. (See *Absorbent.*)

——, *vascular*; general considerations on, iii. 145. (See *Heart, Arteries, Veins.*)

T.

Tænia; found alive in carp that have been boiled, i. 293, note. Each joint of, the seat of a separate ovary, iii. 116, note.

Taliacotian operation; cases in which the principle of, is applicable, iii. 256, note.

Taylor, a quack, and Hunter, i. 87.

Teething, i. 324.

Teeth; Hunter's work on, i. 40, 71. The sockets for, how formed, ii. 3. The alveolar processes belong rather to them than to the jaws, ii. 4. Description and use of the enamel of, ii. 15. The interior substance of, ii. 16. Whether vascular or not, ii. 17, 18, note. The growth of, different from that of bones, ii. 18. The growth of not affected by rickets, *ib.* The cavity in, ii. 19. The periosteum of, ii. 20. The natural situation of, *ib.* The full number of, ii. 21. The several classes of, *ib.* The incisores, ii. 22. The cuspidati, ii. 23. The bicuspides, ii. 24. The grinders, ii. 25. Their fangs, ii. 27. Articulation of, ii. 28. Action of, from the motion of the lower jaw, ii. 29. The cells for, how formed, ii. 32. Formation of, in the fœtus, ii. 33. Cause of the pain in dentition explained, ii. 34. Adult, progress of their formation, ii. 82. A third set sometimes formed in old age, ii. 35. Manner of formation, ii. 37, note. Process of shedding described, ii. 43. First and second sets connected by a communicating chord, ii. 44, note. Reason of the shedding of, ii. 46. How the cavity fills up with new matter as they wear down, ii. 47. Whether they continued to grow after being completely formed, ii. 48. The sensibility of, accounted for, ii. 50. Supernumerary, how they originate, ii. 51. How they affect the voice, *ib.* Whether man is proved to be a carnivorous animal by his teeth, ii. 52. The diseases they are subject to, ii. 53. On the extraction of, ii. 54, note. Of cleaning them, ii. 54. Transplantation of, ii. 55. The practice of, reprobated, ii. 56, note. Of venereal diseases supposed to be produced by transplantation, ii. 466, 483. Transplantation produces a disease which is sometimes more difficult of cure than the venereal, ii. 488. Decay of, by rotting, ii. 59. Inquiry into the cause of their rotting, ii. 62. Whether a rotten tooth has any contaminating power, *ib.* Symptoms of inflammation, ii. 63. The pain of, brought on by circumstances unconnected with the disease, ii. 65. Prevention and cure of rottenness in, *ib.* Methods of burning the nerve, ii. 66. Methods of stopping them where hollow, ii. 68. Decay of, by denudation, ii. 70. Swelling of the fangs described, ii. 71. The nature and causes of gum-boils, ii. 72. Treatment of, ii. 75, and note. Incrustation of extraneous matter upon, ii. 85. Mechanical methods of removing, ii. 87. Chemical applications to, *ib.* Irregularity in the position of, to what owing, ii. 88. The operation of moving them described, ii. 90. Cautions as to the extraction of those that are irregular, ii. 91. Method of rectifying what is called the rabbit-mouth, *ib.* The proper indications for drawing them, ii. 95. Consequence of deferring the operation too long, *ib.* Directions for the performance, *ib.* Instructions for the transplantation of, ii. 97.

Temperament, i. 307. (See *Susceptibility.*)

Temperature. (See *Animal Heat. Climate.*)

Temporal muscle; description and use of, ii. 9.
Tendo Achillis; rupture of, i. 34, 264, 436, 438.
Tendons; injuries of, i. 439.
Testis; descent of, i. 18. Anatomy of, *ib.* Pulpy; the diagnosis between and hydrocele, i. 459, 468. Scrofulous, i. 469, 594, 597. Cancerous, i. 629. Seldom associated with hydrocele, i. 469. Swelling of, arises from sympathy in gonorrhœa, ii. 179, 213, 320. Swelled, symptoms of, ii. 179. Its treatment, ii. 212. Swelling of, is not venereal, ii. 179, 212. This opinion questioned, ii. 182, note. Sometimes produced by the gout, ii. 182. Affected sympathetically from the use of bougies, ii. 251, 256. Of the decay of, ii. 311, 315; iii. 533.
Tetanus, i. 324, 583; iii. 437. In animals, i. 584. Causes of, i. 585; iii. 431. Treatment of, i. 587.
Thackrah, Mr.; his explanation of the milky appearance of the blood, iii. 55, note.
Thomas, Mr.; his anecdotes of Hunter, i. 114.
Thomson, Dr. J., iii. 410.
Thought; the importance of established habits of, i. 277.
Throats; venereal sore, described, ii. 415, note.
Tic Douloureux; the periodic character of, distinguishes those cases which arise from constitutional causes from those which arise from the teeth, ii. 85, note.
Tickling; a peculiar mode of sensation, i. 262.
Tiedemann and *Gmelin*, i. 295.
Tiger; Mr. Hunter's purchase of, i. 29.
Time; Hunter's distribution of, i. 53. His great economy of, *ib.*
Tissue erectile; structure of, i. 251.
Tissues elementary; endowed with life and the powers of reproduction and reparation in very different degrees, iii. 271, 527, notes. (See *Structure.*)
Tommasini, Sig., iii. 388, note.
Tongue; state of, in disease, i. 363. Ulcers of, are seldom venereal, ii. 398.
Tonsils; venereal ulcers of, description of, ii. 413, 415, note. Tumefaction of, *ib.* Excoriation of, ii. 414, 458.
Toothache; is caused by the exposure of the nerve of the tooth to the air, ii. 50, 53. How to stop a hollow tooth, ii. 54. Method of burning the nerve, ii. 66. Other modes of treatment, *ib.* Cautions in relation to nervous pains in the jaws, ii. 84. Instructions for the drawing of teeth, ii. 95.
Torpedo; anatomy of the, i. 40.
Torpor and *Sleep*; the difference between, i. 286. Digestion suspended during the former, *ib.*
Torsion; of arteries, is an unsafe substitute for the ligature, i. 540, note.
Toryism; Hunter's, i. 121.
Touch; the sense of, common to all the organs of the senses, i. 261.
Trail, Dr., iii. 55, note.
Trances, iii. 32, note. (See *Swoons.*)
Transformations; of structure, are supposed by some to be referrible to inflammation, iii. 533, note.
Transfusion, i. 541. History of, iii. 13, note.
Translation; of disease, iii. 388, 395.
Transplantation of teeth; facility of this operation, ii. 55. Successful performance of, ii. 80. General remarks on, ii. 97. Necessary attentions to the state of the gums and sockets, *ib.* In what cases dead teeth are preferable to living ones, ii. 98. In what cases it ought not to be attempted, *ib.* Ought not to be attempted on persons while taking of mercury, *ib.* The proper age for the performance of, ii. 99. Directions for the choice of scion teeth, *ib.* Of replacing a sound tooth when drawn by mistake, ii. 100. Successful instance of replaced teeth, ii. 101. Of dead teeth, *ib.* How teeth are to be fixed and tied, ii. 102. How the patient is to conduct himself, ii. 103. Accidents to which transplanted teeth are liable, ii. 103, 466, 483, 488. Evidences of a living union between transplanted teeth and their sockets, *ib.* The practice of, reprobated, ii. 56, 104, notes.
Trephine; the operation of, when required, i. 492, 494, 496, notes. Dangers of, i. 495, note.
Trout Gillaroo, i. 50.
Truncated teeth; a peculiar appearance of, ii. 71, note.
Tubercles; i. 567. Venereal, description of, ii. 410, note. Ulcerating, resemble rupia, ii. 415, note.

Tumours; general observations on, i 314, 566. Origin of, i. 367, 559, 567, notes. Removal of, i. 567, 569. Encysted, i. 567, note, 571, 574. Bony, i. 570. Cuticular, i. 575. Of the gums, require the extraction of stumps or diseased teeth, ii. 76, note. Horny, iii. 632.

Turner, Dr.; on the coagulation of albumen, iii. 49, note. On the arterialization of the blood, iii. 96, note.

Turpentine; the styptic powers of, i. 483, 539; ii. 335.

U.

Ulceration, i. 380, 428; iii. 459, 473, 483. (See *Ulcerative Inflammation, Absorption.*)

Ulcers; fungated, i. 630. Irritable, i. 553. Indolent, i. 557. The causes which retard their cure, i. 552. Venereal, of the nature of, ii. 382. Phagadenic, ii. 324, note. Phagadenic, description of, ii. 347, note. The secondary symptoms from this kind peculiarly severe and intractable, ii. 348, note. Of the tonsils, description of, ii. 413.

Union by the first intention, i. 367; iii. 34, 118, 238. The uses of, i. 368. Is not attended with sympathetic fever, iii. 249. Of the period after which it would be improper to attempt this union, iii. 253. Of the coagulating lymph or bond of union, iii. 254, note; 349. Of the time required for this process, iii. 255, 346. Practical observations respecting, iii. 257. Is probably not effected, as Mr. Hunter supposed, through the medium of the blood, but by coagulable lymph, iii. 43, 132, 267, notes. Of strength and weakness, in facilitating or retarding this process, iii. 280. Does not take place sometimes in dropsical people, *ib.* Is sometimes destroyed in consequence of constitutional diseases, as scurvy and mercury, ii. 432, note; iii. 487.

Ure, Dr.; on the red colour of the blood, iii. 59, note.

Urea; in the blood, i. 352, note.

Uredo Nivalis; grows and flowers under the snow, i. 293, note.

Ureter and *Kidney*; affected in a gonorrhœa, ii. 179. Of the distension of the ureters, ii. 299.

Urethra; case where a disorder of, was produced by dentition, ii. 110. Ulcers in the, not produced in a gonorrhœa, ii. 158, 232. A short history relative to that subject, ii. 158. An instance of its sympathising with the cutting of a tooth, ii. 161. Is sometimes the seat of the gout and rheumatism, ii. 162. Its action, ii. 173. What parts of the, furnish the matter in a gonorrhœa, ii. 174. Bleeding of, ii. 145. How affected by inflammation, ii. 176. Bleedings from, their treatment, ii. 209. Suppuration of its glands, how treated, ii. 211. Observations on its uses, ii. 228. Obstructions of, the different kinds of, *ib.* Parts of the, most subject to stricture, ii. 230. Lacunæ of, a bougie frequently stops in them, ii. 237. Different kinds of obstructions which take place in that canal, ii. 242. Sometimes a new passage is made along the side of the urethra by bougies; the treatment and cure of that accident, ii. 258. Enlargement of, ii. 257. Inflammation of the parts surrounding the, treatment of, ii. 264, 266. Abscesses near the, their treatment, ii. 264, 265. Spasmodic affections of the, ii. 273. Their cause, *ib.* Their cure, ii. 274. Paralysis of, ii. 276; its cure, *ib.*; the use of cantharides in, *ib.* And bladder contract and relax alternately, ii. 284. Inconveniences which arise when these actions do not take place regularly, ii. 285. Their treatment, ii. 286. Mucus of, the discharge of, ii. 302.

Urine; state of, in disease, i. 362. Albuminous, i. 552, note. Affords an indication for bleeding, i. 405. Coagulation of, by Goulard's extract, iii. 52, note. Rendered alkaline by mercury, ii. 207, note; or reduction of the general strength, ii. 208, note. Of a new passage formed for the, ii. 258. The mischief it occasions by being diffused into the cellular membrane of the scrotum and neighbouring parts, ii. 259. Description of an operation to prevent it, ii. 260. To be drawn off frequently in suppressions of, ii. 260, 290. Suppression of, how relieved, ii. 287. Retention of, operations for the cure of, ii. 290, 296, note. Suppression of, the use of calomel and opium in, ii. 294. Should never be retained a length of time in the bladder, ii. 301.

Uterus; tubercles of, i. 568. Hydatids of, i. 573.

V.

Valves; of arteries, iii. 202. Of the heart, construction of, iii. 179. (See *Heart.*)

Variola. (See *Smallpox.*)

Vascular system. (See *System.*)
Vascularity; of coagulated blood, i. 236, 238, 368, 439; iii. 34, 115, 119, 243, 268, note, 350. Of granulations, i. 427; iii. 492. Of parts, is in proportion to the duty they have to perform, i. 383; iii. 99, 199. Of the teeth, ii. 18, note. Is greater in proportion in the fœtus than in the adult, iii. 213.
Vegetable food; its tendency to keep the teeth clean, ii. 51.
Vegetables; nutrition of, i. 215. Composition of, i. 216. Exist under great ranges of temperature, i. 293. Compared with animals, i. 329. The reason why the sap of, does not freeze at low temperatures, iii. 107. Their tendency to the surface explained, iii. 285.
Vegetations, fibrinous, iii. 30, note.
Veins; described, i. 250; iii. 221. Inflammation of, Hunter's paper on, i. 91; iii. 319, 581, notes. Varicose, i. 560. Valves of, iii. 223. Anastomosis of, iii. 225. Cause of the unintermittent current in, iii. 227. Pulsation of, iii. 228. How far they assist the general circulation, iii. 229, note.
Vena portæ; instances in which it did not terminate in the liver, iii. 86, note.
Venereal disease; Hunter's work on, i. 101. Contains many theoretical doctrines, ii. 125; and hasty generalizations, ii. 129. Is full, however, of practical observations of the highest value, *ib.* (See *Disease.*)
——— *matter*, is changed by absorption, i. 257.
Venesection; the use of, i. 402. Effects of, i. 537. In phthisis, *ib.* In gonorrhœa, ii. 205. In chordee, ii. 210. Seldom proper in specific inflammations, i. 609. The first blood which flows is the darkest, iii. 91. Rules for its employment, i. 404; iii. 374, 376. Sometimes followed by increased quickness and hardness of the pulse, iii. 362.
Ventricles; case of communication between the, iii. 83. Contract together, iii. 194.
Vesiculæ seminales; their use, ii. 175. Are seldom diseased, ii. 283. Of the discharge of the secretion of, ii. 302. Mucus of, the distinction between it and the semen, ii. 164.
Vessels, blood; general observations on, iii. 195. Actively dilate in inflammation, iii. 321. This opinion questioned, iii. 327, note. Of the formation of new, in coagulable lymph, iii. 350. State of in inflammation, iii. 268, note. (See *Vascular system, Vascularity, Arteries, Veins*, &c.)
Veterinary College, established, i. 125.
Vipers; the bite of, i. 615. An observation on its poison, ii. 164.
Vines, Mr., iii. 40, note.
Vita propria, of Blumenbach, iii, 123, note.
Vivification, i. 215, 230, 231.
Voice, how affected by the teeth, ii. 51.
Volition, i. 260. Is lost during sleep, i. 334.
Vomits; their use in swelled testicle, ii. 164. In resolving buboes, ii. 370; iii. 417.
Voyages; recommended in phthisis, i. 597. In scrofula, i. 598.

W.

Wadd, Mr. W., i. 29.
Wardrop, Mr.; case by, in which a very extensive surface was healed by scabbing, iii. 263, note.
Warner, Mr., i. 25.
Warts, i. 568. Venereal, their treatment, ii. 351.
Watson, Mr. H., anecdote of William Hunter, i. 5. Discovers the tubuli testis, i. 18. On the Gillaroo trout, i. 50.
Weakness. (See *Strength.*)
——— *seminal*; its cause, ii. 309. The use of opium in, ii. 310. Its cure, ii. 311.
Weather; the state of, affects the spirits, i. 611.
Wens, i. 567.
Westminster Abbey; Mrs. Hunter's wish to erect a monument in, to Hunter, i. 133.
White swelling, i. 596.
White's New South Wales, i. 118.
Whitloes, i. 425; iii. 486. Much more painful than other inflammations, *ib.*
Will, Hunter's; i. 137.
Willan, Dr., iii. 5, note.
Williams, Dr. C. J. B., on the arterialization of the blood, iii. 96, note.

Willis; circle of, use of, iii. 208.
Wind; the Sirocco, i. 291, note. The Harmettan, i. 297.
Wine; of its use in mortification, iii. 8.
Women more affected by the imagination than men, i. 360.
Woodville, Dr., iii. 5, note.
Wounds; division of, i. 388; iii. 240. Which communicate externally, i. 390; iii. 251. Which do not communicate externally, i. 388; iii. 240. Of the different modes of treating, iii. 251, 257. Of the brain, i. 487, 492, note. State of, affected by the atmosphere, i. 297. And by the constitution, iii. 239.
———, *gunshot*, iii. 541. Difference between and common wounds, iii. 542. Kinds of, iii. 547. Treatment of, iii. 548, 576. The impropriety of enlarging, iii. 548. Penetrating, of the abdomen, iii. 559. Penetrating, of the chest, iii. 566.

Y.

Yawning, an effect of sympathy, i. 321.
Yaws; case of a gentleman infected with, ii. 382. Description of, ii. 472.

END OF THE THIRD VOLUME.

PRINTED BY RICHARD AND JOHN E. TAYLOR,
RED LION COURT, FLEET STREET.

www.ingramcontent.com/pod-product-compliance
Ingram Content Group UK Ltd.
Pitfield, Milton Keynes, MK11 3LW, UK
UKHW040701180125
453697UK00010B/324